Biomarkers of Neurological Diseases

Biomarkers of Neurological Diseases

Editor: Noah Benge

STATES
ACADEMIC PRESS
www.statesacademicpress.com

www.statesacademicpress.com

STATES
ACADEMIC PRESS

Cataloging-in-Publication Data

Biomarkers of neurological diseases / edited by Noah Benge.
p. cm.
Includes bibliographical references and index.
ISBN 978-1-63989-789-6
1. Nervous system--Diseases. 2. Biochemical markers. 3. Neurology. I. Benge, Noah.
RC346 .B56 2023
616.8--dc23

States Academic Press,
109 South 5th Street,
Brooklyn, NY 11249, USA

ISBN 978-1-63989-789-6 (Hardback)

Contents

Preface

It is often said that books are a boon to mankind. They document every progress and pass on the knowledge from one generation to the other. They play a crucial role in our lives. Thus I was both excited and nervous while editing this book. I was pleased by the thought of being able to make a mark but I was also nervous to do it right because the future of students depends upon it. Hence, I took a few months to research further into the discipline, revise my knowledge and also explore some more aspects. Post this process, I begun with the editing of this book.

Neurological diseases are disorders of the nervous system that affect the functioning of the brain and the nerves found throughout the human body and the spinal cord. The most common neurological disorders are epilepsy, Alzheimer's disease, migraine, stroke, Parkinson's disease, multiple sclerosis and cerebral palsy. The term biomarker or biological marker refers to a biological molecule found in blood, tissues or other body fluids, which indicates a normal or abnormal process, a condition, or a disease. Biomarkers help to diagnose a disease or condition, or to detect the disease progression, and record the effect of new drugs and therapeutic strategies as they are generated. Neurological biomarkers are used to diagnose a variety of neurological disorders and to monitor the advancement of these diseases or effect of the treatment. This process aids in predicting outcomes, determining interventions, and evaluating the therapeutic responses. This book is compiled in such a manner, that it will provide an in-depth knowledge about neurological biomarkers. It is a vital tool for all researching or studying the biomarkers of neurological diseases.

I thank my publisher with all my heart for considering me worthy of this unparalleled opportunity and for showing unwavering faith in my skills. I would also like to thank the editorial team who worked closely with me at every step and contributed immensely towards the successful completion of this book. Last but not the least, I wish to thank my friends and colleagues for their support.

Editor

1

Pretreatment with Risperidone Ameliorates Systemic LPS-Induced Oxidative Stress in the Cortex and Hippocampus

Md. Mamun Al-Amin[1], Md. Faiyad Rahman Choudhury[1], Al Saad Chowdhury[1], Tahsinur Rahman Chowdhury[1], Preeti Jain[1], Mohsin Kazi[2], Musaed Alkholief[2], Sultan M. Alshehri[2] and Hasan Mahmud Reza[1]**

[1] *Department of Pharmaceutical Sciences, North South University, Dhaka, Bangladesh,*

[2] *Department of Pharmaceutics, College of Pharmacy, King Saud University, Riyadh, Saudi Arabia*

Correspondence:
Mohsin Kazi
mkazi@ksu.edu.sa
Hasan Mahmud Reza
hasan.reza@northsouth.edu

Risperidone (RIS), an atypical antipsychotic has been found to show anti-inflammatory effect against lipopolysaccharide (LPS)-induced inflammation. *In vitro* study has revealed that RIS inhibits the LPS-induced reactive oxygen species (ROS) formation. We investigated the antioxidant effects of RIS on LPS-induced oxidative stress markers in *Swiss albino* mice. Ten weeks old male *Swiss albino* mice (30 ± 2 g) were pretreated with either distilled water (control) or RIS (3 mg/kg) for 7 days. On day 8, animals were challenged with a single dose of LPS (0.8 mg/kg) while control animals received distilled water only. The animals were sacrificed after 24 h of LPS administration and tissue samples were collected. RIS administration significantly ($p < 0.05$) reduced the LPS-induced elevated levels of lipid peroxidation product malondialdehyde (MDA), advanced protein oxidation products, and nitric oxide (NO) in the cortex. Catalase (CAT) and superoxide dismutase (SOD) levels were also diminished while the level of glutathione (GSH) was enhanced. Hippocampus data showed that RIS significantly ($p < 0.05$) reduced the LPS-induced increased levels of MDA and NO, and SOD activity. Our results suggest that LPS-induced neuronal oxidative damage can be alleviated by the pretreatment with RIS and the effect is shown presumably by scavenging of the ROS by risperidone as an antioxidant.

Keywords: brain, psychiatric disease, oxidative stress, risperidone, LPS

INTRODUCTION

The brain is a specialized restricted region separated by blood–brain barrier (BBB). Endothelial cells, astrocytes, and microglial cells are the vital elements that conserve the features of BBB. Endothelial cells create a tight junction and electrical resistance of BBB, thus selectively permitting external substances to penetrate through. On the other hand, astrocytes and microglial cells provide a distinct immune mechanism to the brain. However, under inflammatory state, BBB becomes leaky and allows the access of undesirable components, such as immune cells, inflammatory molecules, and albumin to the brain. Entrance of pro-inflammatory cytokines; tumor necrosis factor-alpha (TNF-α), interleukin-6 (IL-6) has been shown to be associated with the progression of Parkinson's disease (Smith et al., 2012), Alzheimer's disease (Minagar et al., 2002), and schizophrenia (O'Brien et al., 2008; Al-Amin and Reza, 2014). Inflammatory cytokines (IL-1 or IL-6, TNF-α); nitric oxide (NO); and reactive oxygen species (ROS) may also mediate neurodegeneration (Gebicke-Haerter, 2001; Vallieres et al., 2002). Under inflammatory condition, microglia becomes activated resulting in the release of cytotoxic mediators; such as NO, TNF-α, IL-1β, and ROS. Overproduction of these mediators has been found to be toxic to the neurons which leads to neuronal death (Cui et al., 2012).

Inflammatory agents such as LPS (lipopolysaccharide) has been used to simulate a range of brain diseases; depression (Medeiros et al., 2015), schizophrenia (Zhu et al., 2014a), autism (Kirsten et al., 2015), Parkinson's disease (Sharma and Nehru, 2015), Alzheimer's disease (El-Sayed and Bayan, 2015) in rodents. LPS is a major component of the cell wall of gram negative bacteria and a potent activator of the inflammatory response, particularly of microglia. LPS at a dose of 1 g/ml (intraperitoneal injection) enhances the permeability of the BBB and increases the production of ROS in the brain (Zhao et al., 2014; Yu et al., 2015). While, most of the studies have discussed the inflammatory mechanism of LPS, several studies have explained LPS-induced oxidative damage in the brain (Noworyta-Sokolowska et al., 2013). For example, ROS formation is accelerated by LPS, which causes a significant alteration in NO, malondialdehyde (MDA), GSH, superoxide dismutase (SOD), and CAT levels in brain disease (Sharma and Nehru, 2015). Previous studies have shown that an increased level of pro-inflammatory cytokines (e.g., TNF-α, INF-γ, and IL-6) can be the basis of formation of ROS, MDA, AOPP, CAT, SOD, and GSH (Zhang et al., 2003; Rukmini et al., 2004; Yao et al., 2006; Dean et al., 2009).

Peripheral systemic administration of LPS has shown to produce neuro-inflammation and oxidative stress in the brain (Ho et al., 2015). Single-dose of LPS is adequate to stimulate the production of inflammatory cytokines; IL-1β, IL-6, and TNF-α in the prefrontal cortex and hippocampus (Sulakhiya et al., 2014; Ho et al., 2015; Li et al., 2015). Previous research has indicated that a single dose of systemic LPS could enhance the production of MDA – a lipid peroxidation marker, nitrite- a reactive nitrogen species marker, while reduce GSH level in the rat (Shukla et al., 2008). On the other hand, RIS, a second generation atypical antipsychotic, which is prescribed for the treatment of schizophrenia, schizoaffective disorders, bipolar disorders, and behavioral irritability in autistic patients, was used to improve the situation given that the anti-inflammatory activity of RIS is mediated through the reduction of TNF-α, INF-γ, and IL-6 (Al-Amin et al., 2013; MacDowell et al., 2013; Ajami et al., 2014), and prevention of microglial activation (Zhu et al., 2014b). The antioxidant effect of RIS has been reported previously. *In vitro* human U937 cell culture study by Chen et al. (2013) revealed that RIS inhibits LPS-induced ROS formation. A recent study on first episode drug naïve schizophrenic patient demonstrates that 11 weeks-long treatment with RIS lowers lipid peroxidation (Noto et al., 2015). Moreover, RIS treatment reduces elevated SOD level in schizophrenic patient (Zhang et al., 2012). In animal model of schizophrenia, RIS has been found to enhance the level of GSH, while reduce SOD and MDA (Stojković et al., 2012) levels. Neuroprotective properties exhibited by RIS could be attributed to microglial activation or antioxidant maintenance mechanisms in the cerebral cortex and hippocampus (Yan et al., 2014). The aim of this study was to investigate the effect of risperidone (RIS) on the LPS-induced oxidative stress in the prefrontal cortex and hippocampus.

MATERIALS AND METHODS

Animals

Male *Swiss albino* (10 weeks old weighing 30–32 g) mice (n = 24) were obtained and 6 mice per cage (Tecniplast, Italy) were housed in humidity controlled environment at a temperature of 25 ± 1°C on a 12 h light/day cycle, with liberal access to food and water. Prior to the testing, the mice were allowed to get habituated to the testing rooms for 1 week. The mice were divided into four groups; Ctrl (control) (n = 6), LPS (lipopolysaccharide, I.P.) (n = 6), RIS (risperidone) (n = 6), and RIS+LPS (risperidone + LPS) (n = 6). RIS was administered at a dose of 3 mg/kg once daily, for 7 days. LPS (*Escherichia coli*, Sigma Aldrich), was administered only once on day 8 at a concentration of 0.8 mg/kg with the water for injection (WFI). All experimental procedures were approved by the institutional ethical committee, North South University (NSU/PHA/2014/133-046), Dhaka, Bangladesh. Animals were handled in accordance with the international principles guiding the usage and handling of experimental animals (United States National Institute for Health Publication, 1985).

Preparation of RIS and LPS

Risperidone powder (99.8%) was obtained as a gift from General Pharmaceuticals, Ltd., Dhaka, Bangladesh. RIS was dissolved in distilled water and administered orally at a dose of 3 mg/kg (O'Sullivan et al., 2014). LPS (10 μg/μl) (Zhu et al., 2014b) was dissolved in WFI and a single dose was administered via IP route. The concentration of the administered risperidone dose was 900 μg/ml. The control animals received 100 μl of distilled water orally. LPS group received LPS at a dose of 0.8 mg/kg body weight. The working concentration of LPS was 240 μg/mL. LPS + Risperidone group received LPS (0.8 mg/kg) and Risperidone (3 mg/kg). Risperidone group received risperidone at a dose of 3 mg/kg.

Tissue Collection

Mice were euthanized using 200 μl of ketamine (50 mg/ml, ACI Pharmaceuticals, Ltd., Bangladesh). The animals were sacrificed by decapitation. The entire brain was rapidly removed cautiously and kept in a Petri dish on ice. Then cortex, hippocampus regions were dissected from the brain. Liver tissue was also collected. Homogenate of various brain regions, 10% (w/v) were prepared in phosphate buffer saline (PBS) (10 mM, pH 7.0) using Ultra-Turrax T25 (United States) homogenizer. Homogenized tissue samples were sonicated at 5 s cycle for 30 s using an ultrasonic processor and centrifuged at 10,000 rpm (RCF 11200) for 10 min. The supernatant was diluted with 0.1x PBS buffer and preserved in −20°C. The clear supernatants were collected for the biochemical analysis.

Biochemical Test

The following biochemical tests were conducted in triplicate.

Determination of the Level of MDA

Lipid peroxidation was evaluated colorimetrically as described previously (Niehaus and Samuelsson, 1968). Briefly, 0.1 ml of tissue homogenate (Tris-HCl buffer, pH 7.5) was treated with 2 ml of (1:1:1 ratio) TBA-TCA-HCl reagent (2-thiobarbituric acid 0.37%, 0.25 N HCl and 15% TCA) and placed in water bath (70°C) for 15 min and cooled. The absorbance of clear supernatant was measured against reference blank at a wavelength of 535 nm. The level of MDA was measured by using standard curve and expressed as nmol/mg of tissue.

Determination of the Level of APOP

Determination of advanced protein oxidation products (APOPs) was carried out spectrophotometrically as described by Witko-Sarsat et al., 1996). Concisely, 50 μl of plasma, which was diluted 1:2 with PBS and chloramine T (0–100 μmol/l) were used for the preparation of calibration curve. PBS was used as blank. One hundred μl of 1.16 M potassium iodide and 50 μl of acetic acid were added to each well and absorbance was measured immediately at a wavelength of 340 nm. Concentration of APOP was expressed as μmol/mg of tissue.

Determination of the Level of NO

Nitric oxide was assayed according to the method described by Tracey et al. (1995). In this assay, Griess-Illosvoy reagent was modified by using naphthyl ethylene diaminedihydrochloride (0.1% w/v) instead of 1-napthylamine (5%). The reaction mixture (3 ml) containing brain homogenates (1.5 ml) and PBS (1.5 ml) was incubated at 25°C for 15 min. Rest of the process was followed as described previously (Al-Amin et al., 2015). A pink colored chromophore was formed in diffused light. The absorbance was measured at a wavelength of 540 nm against the corresponding blank. NO level was determined by using standard curve and expressed as nmol/mg of tissue.

Determination of the Activity of CAT

The activity of catalase enzyme was assayed spectrometrically at a wavelength of 240 nm (Sinha, 1972). The reaction mixture (1.5 ml) contained 1.0 ml of 0.01 M phosphate buffer (pH 7.0), 0.1 ml of tissue homogenate (supernatant) and 0.4 ml of 2 M H_2O_2. The reaction was stopped by the addition of 2.0 ml of dichromate-acetic acid reagent (5% potassium dichromate and glacial acetic acid were mixed in 1:3 ratio). The activity of catalase was expressed as the percent change in absorption between initial and subsequent at 1 min interval.

Determination of the Activity of SOD

The activity of SOD was assayed by a modified procedure by Ma et al. (2010). Briefly, 300 μL of reaction mixture contained 50 mM sodium phosphate (pH 7.8), 13 mM methionine, 75 mM nitrobluetetrazolium (NBT), 2 mM riboflavin, 100 mM EDTA, and 20 μl of plasma. The change in absorbance of the sample was then recorded at a wavelength of 560 nm after the production of blue formazan. The activity of SOD was determined as changes of absorption between initial and subsequent at 30 s interval divided by initial absorption. Results were expressed as percentage activity of SOD enzyme.

Determination of the Level of GSH

Glutathione in the brain was evaluated based on the method described by Ellman (1959). Briefly, 1 ml of plasma was added with 2.7 ml of phosphate buffer (0.1 M, pH 8) and 0.2 ml of 5, 5-dithio-bis (2-nitrobenzoic acid). The color developed was determined immediately at 412 nm. Results of glutathione assay was expressed as μmol/mg of protein.

Data Analysis

All the biochemical tests were carried out in triplicate and data were represented as mean ± SEM (standard error of mean). One-way ANOVA was conducted followed by suitable *post hoc* test to analyze the main effect of treatment on the dependent variables among four treatment groups. Oxidative stress markers (MDA, APOP, NO, GSH, CAT, and SOD) were considered as dependent variables. All analyses were carried out in SPSS 16, and graphs were prepared using GraphPad prism (version 6.0, GraphPad Software, Inc.). The difference was considered significant when *p*-value was at least less than 0.05.

RESULTS

Effect of Risperidone on Lipid Peroxidation (MDA)

There was a significant main effect of risperidone treatment on MDA level [$F_{(3,20)} = 10.04$, $p < 0.001$] in the prefrontal cortex (**Figure 1A**). *Post hoc* multiple comparison test indicated an increased level of MDA in the LPS group ($M = 62.67$, $SD = 13.15$) than the control ($M = 35.11$, $SD = 5.72$), LPS+RIS ($M = 59.17$, $SD = 1.64$) and RIS ($M = 47.67$, $SD = 12.78$) groups.

There was a noticeable main effect of treatment on MDA level [$F_{(3,20)} = 6.70$, $p = 0.002$] in the hippocampus (**Figure 1B**) also. *Post hoc* analysis exhibited an increased level of MDA in the LPS ($M = 60.67$, $SD = 0.73$) than the control ($M = 47.00$, $SD = 9.83$) group. Interestingly, LPS+RIS ($M = 52.33$, $SD = 3.28$) group had a lower level of MDA than LPS ($M = 60.67$, $SD = 0.73$) group. However, there was no significant effect of treatment on MDA [$F_{(3,18)} = 2.75$, $p = 0.07$] level in the liver (**Figure 1C**).

Effect of Risperidone on Advanced Protein Oxidation Product (APOP)

There was a significant main effect of treatment on APOP [$F_{(3,20)} = 7.66$, $p < 0.001$] in the prefrontal cortex (**Figure 2A**). *Post hoc* analysis showed an enhanced level of AOPP in the LPS ($M = 144.7$, $SD = 12.86$) than the control ($M = 100.2$, $SD = 23.71$) group. LPS+RIS ($M = 113.8$, $SD = 18.56$), group showed a lower level of MDA than LPS ($M = 144.7$, $SD = 12.84$) group indicating effectiveness of risperidone treatment.

The noticeable main effect of treatment on AOPP [$F_{(3,20)} = 4.63$, $p < 0.01$] in the hippocampus is shown in **Figure 2B**. *Post hoc* test displayed an elevated level of AOPP

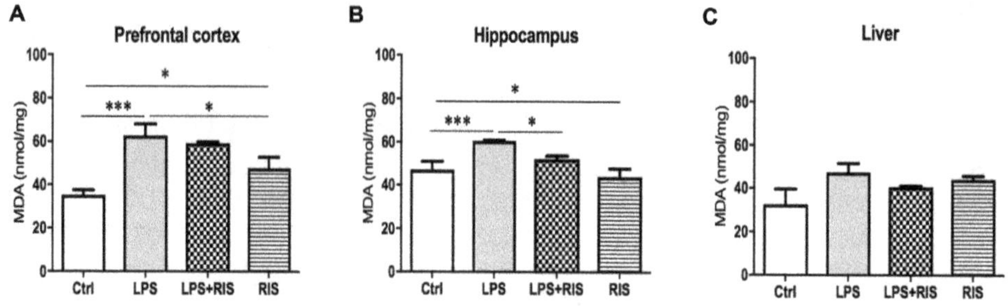

FIGURE 1 | Effect of various treatments on the level of lipid peroxidation (MDA). Groups are Ctrl (control), LPS (lipopolysaccharide), LPS+RIS (lipopolysaccharide + risperidone), and RIS (risperidone). The level of MDA was assayed from the prefrontal cortex **(A)**, hippocampus **(B)**, and liver **(C)** tissues. Values are represented as mean ± SEM. *Post hoc* multiple comparison test namely, "Newman–Keuls" test was used to compare between groups. $n = 6$ per group. $^{*}p < 0.05$, $^{**}p < 0.01$, $^{***}p < 0.001$.

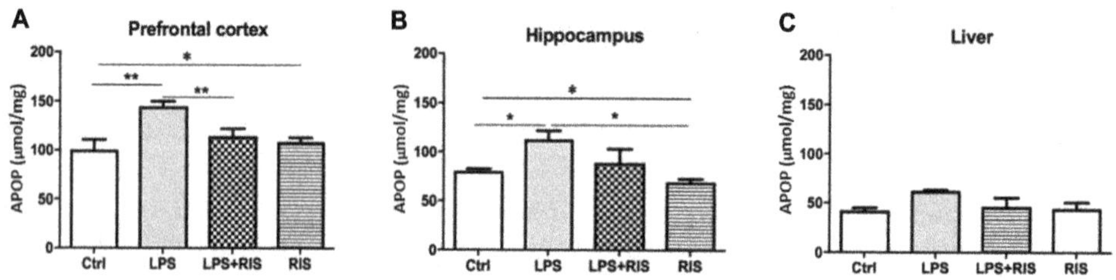

FIGURE 2 | Effect of various treatments on the level of advanced protein oxidation products (APOPs). Groups are Ctrl (control), LPS (lipopolysaccharide), LPS+RIS (lipopolysaccharide + risperidone), and RIS (risperidone). The level of AOPP was determined from the prefrontal cortex **(A)**, hippocampus **(B)**, and liver **(C)** tissues. Values are represented as mean ± SEM. *Post hoc* multiple comparison test namely, "Newman–Keuls" test was used to compare between groups. $n = 6$ per group. $^{*}p < 0.05$, $^{**}p < 0.01$, $^{***}p < 0.001$.

in the LPS (M = 112.3, SD = 21.44) than control (M = 80.33, SD = 4.92), LPS+RIS (M = 89.17, SD = 34.25), and RIS (M = 69.50, SD = 7.66) groups. No significant main effect of treatment on AOPP in the liver [$F_{(3,18)} = 2.67$, $p = 0.07$] was observed (**Figure 2C**).

Effect of Risperidone on Nitric Oxide (NO)

A significant main effect of RIS treatment on NO [$F_{(3,20)} = 15.28$, $p < 0.001$] level was observed in the prefrontal cortex (**Figure 3A**). *Post hoc* analysis showed an enhanced level of NO in the LPS (M = 7.72, SD = 3.07) than the control (M = 1.84, SD = 0.19) group. LPS+RIS (M = 4.23, SD = 0.88) group showed a decreased level of NO than LPS (M = 7.72, SD = 3.07) group.

There was a noticeable main effect of treatment on NO [$F_{(3,20)} = 259.2$, $p < 0.001$] level in the hippocampus (**Figure 3B**). *Post hoc* test disclosed an increased level of NO in the LPS group (M = 7.60, SD = 0.61) as compared to control (M = 1.83, SD = 0.38). LPS+ RIS (M = 3.02, SD = 0.34) group mice showed a diminished level of NO than LPS (M = 7.60, SD = 0.61) only group. As shown in **Figure 3C**, a significant main effect of treatment on NO [$F_{(3,19)} = 32.74$, $p < 0.001$] was observed in the liver also. *Post hoc* study showed a higher level of NO in the LPS (M = 6.80, SD = 0.32) than the control (M = 3.55, SD = 1.19) group. However, no significant difference was found between LPS+RIS (M = 6.48, SD = 0.23) and LPS mice groups.

Effect of Risperidone on Catalase (CAT) Level

The main effect of treatment on CAT was noteworthy [$F_{(3,17)} = 53.59$, $p < 0.001$] in the prefrontal cortex (**Figure 4A**). *Post hoc* analysis indicated an increased level of CAT in the LPS (M = 85.50, SD = 3.83) than the control (M = 11.69, SD = 2.36) group. Importantly, LPS+ RIS (M = 29.73, SD = 11.16) mice had a reduced level of CAT than LPS (M = 85.50, SD = 3.83) only group.

There was no significant main effect of treatment on CAT [$F_{(3,20)} = 2.58$, $p = 0.08$] in the hippocampus (**Figure 4B**). However, there was an obvious main effect of treatment on CAT [$F_{(3,19)} = 9.68$, $p < 0.001$] in the liver (**Figure 4C**). *Post hoc* multiple comparison analysis exhibited a higher activity of CAT in the LPS (M = 65.34, SD = 2.55) than control (M = 17.48, SD = 3.85), LPS+RIS (M = 51.78, SD = 19.26) and RIS (M = 55.67, SD = 22.59) groups.

Effect of Risperidone on Superoxide Dismutase (SOD) Level

Risperidone treatment showed a significantly strong main effect on SOD level [$F_{(3,20)} = 36.32$, $p < 0.001$] in the prefrontal cortex (**Figure 5A**). *Post hoc* analysis exhibited an increased SOD level in the LPS (M = 21.43, SD = 0.61) than the control (M = 11.69, SD = 2.37) group. LPS+RIS (M = 14.86, SD = 2.91) mice showed a significantly lower level of SOD than LPS

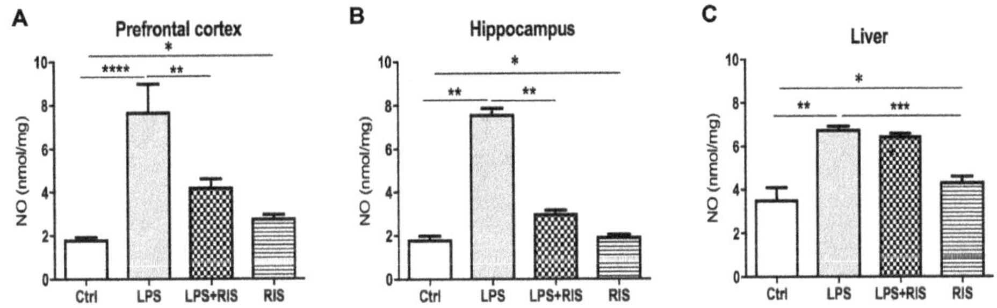

FIGURE 3 | Effect of various treatments on the level of nitric oxide (NO). Groups are Ctrl (control), LPS (lipopolysaccharide), LPS+RIS (lipopolysaccharide + risperidone), and RIS (risperidone). NO was measured from the prefrontal cortex **(A)**, hippocampus **(B)**, and liver **(C)** tissues. Values are represented as mean ± SEM. *Post hoc* multiple comparison test namely, "Newman–Keuls" test was used to compare between groups. $n = 6$ per group. *$p < 0.05$, **$p < 0.01$, ***$p < 0.001$, ****$p < 0.0001$.

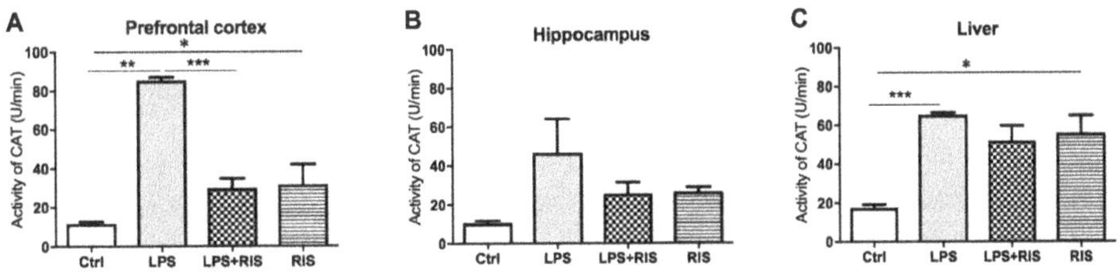

FIGURE 4 | Effect of various treatments on the activity of catalase (CAT). Groups are Ctrl (control), LPS (lipopolysaccharide), LPS+RIS (lipopolysaccharide + risperidone), and RIS (risperidone). CAT activity was measured from the prefrontal cortex **(A)**, hippocampus **(B)**, and liver **(C)** tissues. Values are represented as mean ± SEM. *Post hoc* multiple comparison test namely, "Newman–Keuls" test was used to compare between groups. $n = 6$ per group. *$p < 0.05$, **$p < 0.01$, ***$p < 0.001$.

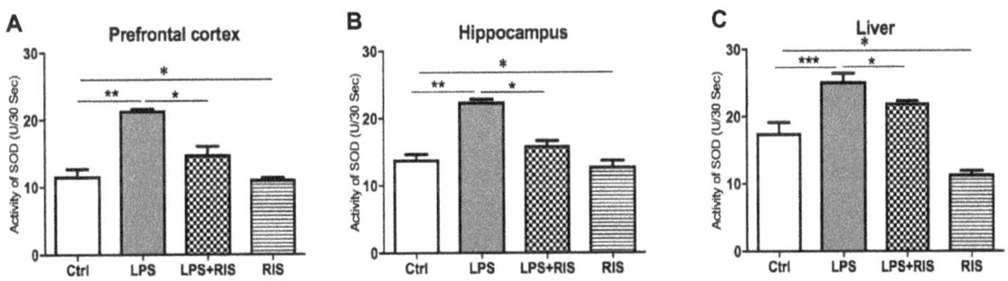

FIGURE 5 | Effect of various treatments on the activity of superoxide dismutase (SOD). Groups are Ctrl (control), LPS (lipopolysaccharide), LPS+RIS (lipopolysaccharide + risperidone), and RIS (risperidone). SOD activity was measured from the prefrontal cortex **(A)**, hippocampus **(B)**, and liver **(C)** tissues. Values are represented as mean ± SEM. *Post hoc* multiple comparison test namely, "Newman–Keuls" test was used to compare between groups. $n = 6$ per group. *$p < 0.05$, **$p < 0.01$, ***$p < 0.001$.

($M = 21.43$, $SD = 0.61$) which demonstrates the effectiveness of the treatment.

The main effect of treatment on SOD [$F_{(3,20)} = 40.94$, $p < 0.001$] level in the hippocampus is shown in **Figure 5B**. *Post hoc* analysis exhibited a significantly higher SOD level in the LPS ($M = 22.54$, $SD = 0.78$) than control ($M = 13.92$, $SD = 1.75$). Interestingly, LPS+RIS ($M = 15.94$, $SD = 0.24$) mice showed a lower SOD activity than LPS ($M = 22.54$, $SD = 0.78$) mice. There was a noticeable main effect of treatment on SOD [$F_{(3,20)} = 34.81$, $p < 0.001$] in the liver (**Figure 5C**). *Post hoc* test revealed a significant elevation of SOD in LPS group ($M = 25.30$, $SD = 2.79$) than the control ($M = 17.54$, $SD = 3.91$). By contrasts, LPS+RIS ($M = 22.08$, $SD = 0.70$) group showed a reduced SOD level than LPS group.

Effect of Risperidone on the Level of Glutathione (GSH)

There was a significant main effect of treatment on GSH [$F_{(3,20)} = 4.19$, $p = 0.018$] level in the prefrontal cortex (**Figure 6A**). *Post hoc* multiple comparison analysis displayed a reduced level of GSH in the LPS ($M = 131.5$, $SD = 2.74$) group than the control ($M = 158.2$, $SD = 5.49$). By contrasts, LPS+RIS ($M = 151.8$, $SD = 17.72$) mice showed a higher glutathione level than LPS mice.

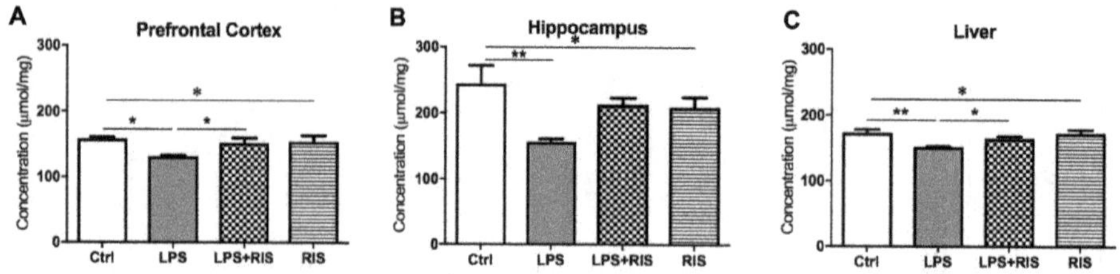

FIGURE 6 | Effect of various treatments on the level of glutathione (GSH). Groups are Ctrl (control), LPS (lipopolysaccharide), LPS+RIS (lipopolysaccharide + risperidone), and RIS (risperidone). GSH was measured from the prefrontal cortex **(A)**, hippocampus **(B)**, and liver **(C)** tissues. Values are represented as mean ± SEM. *Post hoc* multiple comparison test namely, "Newman–Keuls" test was used to compare between groups. $n = 6$ per group. $^{*}p < 0.05$, $^{**}p < 0.01$, $^{***}p < 0.001$.

There was a noticeable main effect of treatment on GSH [$F_{(3,20)} = 4.75$, $p = 0.011$] level in the hippocampus (**Figure 6B**). *Post hoc* test revealed a significantly reduced level of GSH in the LPS ($M = 156.3$, $SD = 10.60$) than the control ($M = 244.3$, $SD = 67.65$) group. Moreover, LPS+RIS ($M = 213.0$, $SD = 24.55$) mice showed no significant difference than LPS treated mice.

There was a significant main effect of treatment on GSH [$F_{(3,20)} = 5.86$, $p = 0.004$] level in the liver (**Figure 6C**). *Post hoc* test displayed a significant reduction of GSH in LPS ($M = 152.3$, $SD = 1.37$) than control ($M = 173.0$, $SD = 12.68$). In addition, LPS+RIS ($M = 165.0$, $SD = 7.64$) mice showed a significantly higher level of GSH than LPS mice.

DISCUSSION

The present study was designed to evaluate the neuroprotective effect of risperidone pre-treatment on the acute peripheral LPS-induced oxidative damage in different regions of the brain in *Swiss albino* mice. We found that the level of oxidative damage in the prefrontal cortex and hippocampus were markedly enhanced following intraperitoneal LPS administration. However, pretreatment with risperidone improved most of the oxidative stress parameters in the hippocampus and cortex.

Our results showed that LPS causes a significant detrimental effect on the prefrontal cortex and hippocampus by increasing the breakdown of lipids and proteins. Moreover, LPS enhanced the level of NO and diminished the level of glutathione. In response to this damage, the level of antioxidant enzymes, catalase and SOD were elevated It is possible that the administration of LPS increased the activity of antioxidant enzymes in the brain regions. Our results are consistent with the previous findings (Al-Amin et al., 2013; MacDowell et al., 2013; Cauwels et al., 2014; Jia et al., 2014; Su et al., 2014; Zhang et al., 2015). We also found that RIS treatment reduces LPS-induced increased MDA level in the hippocampus but not in the liver. Also, LPS+RIS group showed reduction in LPS-induced increase in NO levels in the hippocampus and cortex. These results are consistent with the studies performed on RIS (Shioda et al., 2012). Furthermore, LPS+RIS improved the level of AOPP in the cortex and hippocampus. Our results indicate that RIS treatment increased the level of glutathione in the cortex and liver, which is in agreement with a previous study (Stojković et al., 2012).

The effect of RIS treatment on the level of glutathione in LPS-induced neuroinflammatory model has not been studied in the past. However, a previous study reported that LPS reduces the level of glutathione (Yamada et al., 2006). In addition, RIS could reverse phencyclidine-induced reduced glutathione levels in the rat brain (Stojković et al., 2012). Consistent with this finding, we also report that RIS may reverse LPS-induced reduced glutathione levels.

Upon analyzing the levels of the antioxidant enzymes catalase and SOD, we found that RIS pretreatment improves the activity of catalase in the cortex and hippocampus.

Our observation that the level of SOD was improved in the brain is consistent with several previous studies (Zhang et al., 2012; Yan et al., 2014). All these findings taken together, asserts that pretreatment with RIS can rescue the LPS-induced oxidative stress in the brain.

The damaging effect of LPS due to oxidative stress in the brain has been demonstrated in the previous studies as well (Shukla et al., 2008; Del Angel-Meza et al., 2011; Tomaz et al., 2014; Ho et al., 2015). The organelle that encounters the oxidative stress most is the mitochondria. Mitochondria produce energy by the breakdown of glucose with the help of oxygen. It is noted that the brain requires almost 20% of the total oxygen intake to produce energy. Mitochondria in the neural cells are constantly producing highly reactive free radicals as by product during the metabolic processes. The excess amount of free radicals may cause the damage to proteins, lipids and even the neural function (Lohr, 1991; Lohr and Browning, 1995). Unfortunately, neural cells are poorly equipped to defend against oxidative damage (Mahadik and Mukherjee, 1996). The underlying reason of this poor defensive system is due to the sensitivity of lipids to the free radicals, failure of adult neurons to reproduce and compensate destroyed DNA and poor activity of antioxidant enzymes namely glutathione, catalase, and SOD (Cohen, 1984). Impaired antioxidant defense system has been reported to be associated with neuropsychiatric diseases (Lohr, 1991; Lohr and Browning, 1995; Salim, 2014), such as, schizophrenia (Li et al., 2006), autism (McGinnis, 2004), depression (Michel et al., 2012), bipolar mood disorder (Erdem et al., 2014). In this study, treatment with risperidone showed decrease in the LPS-induced high levels of oxidative markers in the distinct brain regions. We report that the administration of RIS in LPS-induced stress model might be promising in improving the deficits due to oxidative stress.

Accumulating evidences suggest the neuroprotective potential of RIS (Lauterbach et al., 2010) via antioxidant immunomodulatory activity. A study with 22 schizophrenic patients demonstrated that RIS possesses significant antioxidant activity (Gilca et al., 2014). Moreover, RIS treatment lowers lipid peroxidation on 51 first episode schizophrenic patients treated with risperidone for 11 weeks. Noto et al. (2015), suggested that RIS enhances antioxidant defense against lipid peroxidation possibly through PON1 (paraoxonase 1) antioxidant enzyme. Immunomodulatory potential of RIS was observed when given with celecoxib as an add-on therapy in schizophrenia (Müller et al., 2002). Animal model of gerbil stroke revealed that post-treatment with RIS provides neuroprotection presumably via attenuation of microglial activation as well as maintenance of the antioxidants (Yan et al., 2014). RIS also shows the antioxidant activity by lowering the glutathione level in phencyclidine-treated rat brain (Stojković et al., 2012). RIS has also been found effective in preventing microglia activation and improves behavioral deficits when LPS was administered directly to the hippocampus in neonatal rats (Zhu et al., 2014b).

In this study, LPS was administered only once on day 8. We have observed that acute LPS administration increased immobility time in the behavioral test. We have not incorporated behavioral data in this study since acute LPS administration causes immediate effect on behavioral level. We have conducted open field test and tail suspension test; both tests have shown a significant increase in immobile phase following LPS administration (data not shown) as consistent with the previous studies (Frenois et al., 2007; O'Connor et al., 2008). LPS at a dose of 25, 50, 100, or 1000 μg/kg caused suppressed behavior in the open field test (Yirmiya et al., 1994), while LPS at 0.63 or 1.25 μg/kg exhibited diminished locomotor activity at 2 h (Dunn and Swiergiel, 2005), reduced distance traveled at 6 h and poor exploration behavior in 24 h (Biesmans et al., 2013). It is noted that we used 0.8 mg/kg (800 μg/kg) (El-Sayed and Bayan, 2015) single dose to induce behavioral impairment. LPS at a dose of 1 and 5 μg/kg once dose has been shown to produce long immobility time in the TST (Dunn and Swiergiel, 2005).

Lipopolysaccharide directly enhances the production of inflammatory cytokines. Therefore, the determination of the cytokines in this study could have provided insights into the effect of RIS in the LPS-induced impairment at the molecular level. Despite this limitation, our study is novel in some respects. To the best of our knowledge, this study is the first to report the role of RIS in the LPS-induced six oxidative stress markers in the two important brain regions that are involved in cognitive function, learning and memory formation. Moreover, liver data provided additional evidence on overall condition besides the brain. Our findings further support the hypothesis that RIS possesses a significant antioxidant property that could be studied further in details. There are several possible explanations in favor of the current outcomes (i) RIS may regulate the production of GSH, CAT, and SOD to combat against ROS, (ii) RIS might diminish the formation of ROS, (iii) RIS, itself is involved in neutralizing the already formed ROS, (iv) RIS is possibly associated with the regulation of GSH, SOD, and CAT forming genes. Future work can be undertaken to gain insight into the mechanisms underlying the antioxidant activity of RIS in improving the stress condition induced by LPS.

CONCLUSION

The present study was designed to determine the effect of risperidone on systemic LPS-induced oxidative damage in the specific brain regions and liver. The study has demonstrated that risperidone is effective in reversing LPS-mediated behavioral impairment and subsequent oxidative stress. In conclusion, our findings suggest that risperidone may possess some neuro-protective effects through reduction of oxidative stress parameters. The results of this research support the notion that RIS diminishes the production of ROS possibly through the regulation of antioxidant enzymes in the brain. We further propose that RIS may contribute to the improvement in brain diseases due to its protective effects against the endotoxin-linked oxidative damage in the brain.

AUTHOR CONTRIBUTIONS

MAA-A and HMR participated in the design of the experimental work. MAA-A, MFRC performed experiments and analyzed the data. ASC and TRC provided technical support. PJ and HMR contributed to preparation, editing and critically revising the manuscript for important intellectual content. MK, MA and HMR corrected drafts and obtained the funding. SMA contributed in the manuscript during the revision period and shared his experience in editing the manuscript. All authors read and approved the final manuscript.

ACKNOWLEDGMENTS

The authors are very grateful to the Deanship of Scientific Research and Research Centre, College of Pharmacy, King Saud University, Riyadh, Saudi Arabia for their funding and support.

REFERENCES

1. Ajami, A., Abedian, F., Hamzeh Hosseini, S., Akbarian, E., Alizadeh-Navaei, R., and Taghipour, M. (2014). Serum TNF-alpha, IL-10 and IL-2 in schizophrenic patients before and after treatment with risperidone and clozapine. *Iran. J. Immunol.* 11, 200–209.
2. Al-Amin, M. M., Rahman, M. M., Khan, F. R., Zaman, F., and Mahmud Reza, H. (2015). Astaxanthin improves behavioral disorder and oxidative stress in prenatal valproic acid-induced mice model of autism. *Behav. Brain Res.* 286, 112–121. doi: 10.1016/j.bbr.2015.02.041
3. Al-Amin, M. M., and Reza, H. M. (2014). Neuroinflammation: contemporary anti-inflammatory approaches. *Neurosciences* 19, 87–92.
4. Al-Amin, M. M., Uddin, M. M. N., and Mahmud Reza, H. (2013). Effects of antipsychotics on the inflammatory response system of patients with schizophrenia in peripheral blood mononuclear cell cultures. *Clin. Psychopharmacol. Neurosci.* 11, 144–151. doi: 10.9758/cpn.2013.11.3.144
5. Biesmans, S., Meert, T. F., Bouwknecht, J. A., Acton, P. D., Davoodi, N., De Haes, P., et al. (2013). Systemic immune activation leads to neuroinflammation and sickness behavior in mice. *Mediators Inflamm.* 2013:271359. doi: 10.1155/2013/271359

6. Cauwels, A., Bultinck, J., De Zwaef, R., Vandendriessche, B., Magez, S., and Brouckaert, P. (2014). Nitric oxide production by endotoxin preparations in TLR4-deficient mice. *Nitric Oxide* 36, 36–43. doi: 10.1016/j.niox.2013.11.001
7. Chen, M. L., Wu, S., Tsai, T. C., Wang, L. K., and Tsai, F. M. (2013). Regulation of macrophage immune responses by antipsychotic drugs. *Immunopharmacol. Immunotoxicol.* 35, 573–580. doi: 10.3109/08923973.2013.828744
8. Cohen, G. (1984). Oxy-radical toxicity in catecholamine neurons. *Neurotoxicology* 5, 77–82.
9. Cui, Y. Q., Jia, Y. J., Zhang, T., Zhang, Q. B., and Wang, X. M. (2012). Fucoidan protects against lipopolysaccharide-induced rat neuronal damage and inhibits the production of proinflammatory mediators in primary microglia. *CNS Neurosci. Ther.* 18, 827–833. doi: 10.1111/j.1755-5949.2012.00372.x
10. Dean, O. M., van den Buuse, M., Bush, A. I., Copolov, D. L., Ng, F., Dodd, S., et al. (2009). A role for glutathione in the pathophysiology of bipolar disorder and schizophrenia? Animal models and relevance to clinical practice. *Curr. Med. Chem.* 16, 2965–2976. doi: 10.2174/092986709788803060Del Angel-Meza, A. R., Dávalos-Marín, A. J., Ontiveros-Martinez, L. L., Ortiz, G. G., Beas-Zarate, C., Chaparro-Huerta, V., et al. (2011). Protective effects of tryptophan on neuro-inflammation in rats after administering lipopolysaccharide. *Biomed. Pharmacother.* 65, 215–219. doi: 10.1016/j.biopha. 2011.02.008
11. Dunn, A. J., and Swiergiel, A. H. (2005). Effects of interleukin-1 and endotoxin in the forced swim and tail suspension tests in mice. *Pharmacol. Biochem. Behav.* 81, 688–693. doi: 10.1016/j.pbb.2005.04.019
12. Ellman, G. L. (1959). Tissue sulfhydryl groups. *Arch. Biochem. Biophys.* 82, 70–77. doi: 10.1016/0003-9861(59)90090-6
13. El-Sayed, N. S., and Bayan, Y. (2015). Possible role of resveratrol targeting estradiol and neprilysin pathways in lipopolysaccharide model of Alzheimer disease. *Adv. Exp. Med. Biol.* 822, 107–118. doi: 10.1007/978-3-319-08927-0_12
14. Erdem, M., Akarsu, S., Pan, E., and Kurt, G. Y. (2014). Bipolar disorder and oxidative stress. *J. Mood Disord.* 4, 70–79. doi: 10.5455/jmood.20131205 063815
15. Frenois, F., Moreau, M., O'Connor, J., Lawson, M., Micon, C., Lestage, J., et al. (2007). Lipopolysaccharide induces delayed FosB/DeltaFosB immunostaining within the mouse extended amygdala, hippocampus and hypothalamus, that parallel the expression of depressive-like behavior. *Psychoneuroendocrinology* 32, 516–531. doi: 10.1016/j.psyneuen.2007.03.005
16. Gebicke-Haerter, P. J. (2001). Microglia in neurodegeneration: molecular aspects. *Microsc. Res. Tech.* 54, 47–58. doi: 10.1002/jemt.1120
17. Gilca, M., Piriu, G., Gaman, L., Delia, C., Iosif, L., Atanasiu, V., et al. (2014). A study of antioxidant activity in patients with schizophrenia taking atypical antipsychotics. *Psychopharmacology* 231, 4703–4710. doi: 10.1007/s00213-014-3624-0
18. Ho, Y. H., Lin, Y. T., Wu, C. W., Chao, Y. M., Chang, A. Y., and Chan, J. Y. (2015). Peripheral inflammation increases seizure susceptibility via the induction of neuroinflammation and oxidative stress in the hippocampus. *J. Biomed. Sci.* 22:46. doi: 10.1186/s12929-015-0157-8
19. Jia, M., Jing, Y., Ai, Q., Jiang, R., Wan, J., Lin, L., et al. (2014). Potential role of catalase in mice with lipopolysaccharide/D-galactosamine-induced fulminant liver injury. *Hepatol. Res.* 44, 1151–1158. doi: 10.1111/hepr.12220
20. Kirsten, T. B., Queiroz-Hazarbassanov, N., Bernardi, M. M., and Felicio, L. F. (2015). Prenatal zinc prevents communication impairments and BDNF disturbance in a rat model of autism induced by prenatal lipopolysaccharide exposure. *Life Sci.* 130, 12–17. doi: 10.1016/j.lfs.2015.02.027
21. Lauterbach, E. C., Victoroff, J., Coburn, K. L., Shillcutt, S. D., Doonan, S. M., and Mendez, M. F. (2010). Psychopharmacological neuroprotection in neurodegenerative disease: assessing the preclinical data. *J. Neuropsychiatry Clin. Neurosci.* 22, 8–18. doi: 10.1176/appi.neuropsych.22.1.8
22. Li, H.-C., Chen, Q.-Z., Ma, Y., and Zhou, J.-F. (2006). Imbalanced free radicals and antioxidant defense systems in schizophrenia: a comparative study. *J. Zhejiang Univ. Sci. B* 7, 981–986. doi: 10.1631/jzus.2006.B0981
23. Li, R., Zhao, D., Qu, R., Fu, Q., and Ma, S. (2015). The effects of apigenin on lipopolysaccharide-induced depressive-like behavior in mice. *Neurosci. Lett.* 594, 17–22. doi: 10.1016/j.neulet.2015.03.040
24. Lohr, J. B. (1991). Oxygen radicals and neuropsychiatric illness. Some speculations. *Arch. Gen. Psychiatry* 48, 1097–1106. doi: 10.1001/archpsyc.1991. 01810360061009
25. Lohr, J. B., and Browning, J. A. (1995). Free radical involvement in neuropsychiatric illnesses. *Psychopharmacol. Bull.* 31, 159–165.
26. Ma, L., Liu, J., Li, N., Wang, J., Duan, Y., Yan, J., et al. (2010). Oxidative stress in the brain of mice caused by translocated nanoparticulate TiO2 delivered to the abdominal cavity. *Biomaterials* 31, 99–105. doi: 10.1016/j.biomaterials.2009.0 9.028
27. MacDowell, K. S., García-Bueno, B., Madrigal, J. L., Parellada, M., Arango, C., Micó, J. A., et al. (2013). Risperidone normalizes increased inflammatory parameters and restores anti-inflammatory pathways in a model of neuroinflammation. *Int. J. Neuropsychopharmacol.* 16, 121–135. doi: 10.1017/S1461145711001775
28. Mahadik, S. P., and Mukherjee, S. (1996). Free radical pathology and antioxidant defense in schizophrenia: a review. *Schizophr. Res.* 19, 1–17. doi: 10.1016/0920- 9964(95)00049-6
29. McGinnis, W. R. (2004). Oxidative stress in autism. *Altern. Ther. Health Med.* 10, 22–36.
30. Medeiros, I. U., Ruzza, C., Astha, L., Guerrini, R., Romão, P. R. T., Gavioli, E. C., et al. (2015). Blockade of nociceptin/orphanin FQ receptor signaling reverses LPS-induced depressive-like behavior in mice. *Peptides* 72, 95–103. doi: 10.1016/j.peptides.2015.05.006
31. Michel, T. M., Pulschen, D., and Thome, J. (2012). The role of oxidative stress in depressive disorders. *Curr. Pharm. Des.* 18, 5890–5899. doi: 10.2174/ 138161212803523554
32. Minagar, A., Shapshak, P., Fujimura, R., Ownby, R., Heyes, M., and Eisdorfer, C. (2002). The role of macrophage/microglia and astrocytes in the pathogenesis of three neurologic disorders: HIV-associated dementia, Alzheimer disease, and multiple sclerosis. *J. Neurol. Sci.* 202, 13–23. doi: 10.1016/S0022-510X(02) 00207-1
33. Müller, N., Riedel, M., Scheppach, C., Brandstätter, B., Sokullu, S., Krampe, K., et al. (2002). Beneficial antipsychotic effects of celecoxib add-on therapy compared to risperidone alone in schizophrenia. *Am. J. Psychiatry* 159, 1029–1034. doi: 10.1176/appi.ajp.159.6.1029
34. Niehaus, W. G., and Samuelsson, B. (1968). Formation of malonaldehyde from phospholipid arachidonate during microsomal lipid peroxidation. *Eur. J. Biochem.* 6, 126–130. doi: 10.1111/j.1432-1033.1968.tb00428.x
35. Noto, C., Ota, V. K., Gadelha, A., Noto, M. N., Barbosa, D. S., Bonifácio, K. L., et al. (2015). Oxidative stress in drug naive first episode psychosis and antioxidant effects of risperidone. *J. Psychiatr. Res.* 68, 210–216. doi: 10.1016/j.jpsychires. 2015.07.003
36. Noworyta-Sokolowska, K., Gorska, A., and Golembiowska, K. (2013). LPS-induced oxidative stress and inflammatory reaction in the rat striatum. *Pharmacol. Rep.* 65, 863–869. doi: 10.1016/S1734-1140(13)71067-3
37. O'Brien, S. M., Scully, P., and Dinan, T. G. (2008). Increased tumor necrosis factor-alpha concentrations with interleukin-4 concentrations in exacerbations of schizophrenia. *Psychiatry Res.* 160, 256–262. doi: 10.1016/j.psychres.2007.1 1.014
38. O'Connor, J. C., Lawson, M. A., André, C., Moreau, M., Lestage, J., Castanon, N., et al. (2008). Lipopolysaccharide-induced depressive-like behavior is mediated by indoleamine 2,3-dioxygenase activation in mice. *Mol. Psychiatry* 14, 511– 522. doi: 10.1038/sj.mp.4002148
39. O'Sullivan, D., Green, L., Stone, S., Zareie, P., Kharkrang, M., Fong, D., et al. (2014). Treatment with the antipsychotic agent, risperidone, reduces disease severity in experimental autoimmune encephalomyelitis. *PLoS One* 9:e104430. doi: 10.1371/journal.pone.0104430
40. Rukmini, M. S., D'Souza, B., and D'Souza, V. (2004). Superoxide dismutase and catalase activities and their correlation with malondialdehyde in schizophrenic patients. *Indian J. Clin. Biochem.* 19, 114–118. doi: 10.1007/BF02894268
41. Salim, S. (2014). Oxidative stress and psychological disorders. *Curr. Neuropharmacol.* 12, 140–147. doi: 10.2174/1570159X11666131120230309
42. Sharma, N., and Nehru, B. (2015). Characterization of the lipopolysaccharide induced model of Parkinson's disease: role of oxidative stress and neuroinflammation. *Neurochem. Int.* 87, 92–105. doi: 10.1016/j.neuint. 2015.06.004
43. Shioda, K., Nisijima, K., Kasai, M., Yoshino, T., and Kato, S. (2012). Risperidone attenuates the increase of extracellular nitric oxide and glutamate levels in serotonin syndrome animal models. *Neurosci. Lett.* 528, 22–26. doi: 10.1016/ j.neulet.2012.08.083
44. Shukla, R., Tyagi, E., and Kumar, R. (2008). Protective effect of COX and NOS inhibitors on LPS induced oxidative stress in rat. *Ann. Neurosci.* 15, 6–10. doi: 10.5214/ans.0972.7531.2008.150102
45. Sinha, A. K. (1972). Colorimetric assay of catalase. *Anal. Biochem.* 47, 389–394. doi: 10.1016/0003-2697(72)90132-7
46. Smith, A. J., Das, A., Ray, K. S., and Banik, N. L. (2012). Role of pro-inflammatory cytokines released from microglia in neurodegenerative diseases. *Brain Res. Bull.* 87, 10–20. doi: 10.1016/j.brainresbull.2011.10.004
47. Stojkovic', T., Radonjic', N. V., Velimirovic', M., Jevtic', G., Popovic', V., Doknic', M., et al. (2012). Risperidone reverses phencyclidine induced decrease in glutathione levels and alterations of antioxidant defense in rat brain. *Prog. Neuropsychopharmacol. Biol. Psychiatry* 39, 192–199. doi: 10.1016/j.pnpbp. 2012.06.013
48. Su, Z., Mo, Z., Liao, J.-B., Feng, X.-X., Liang, Y.-Z., Zhang, X., et al. (2014).

Usnic acid protects LPS-induced acute lung injury in mice through attenuating inflammatory responses and oxidative stress. *Int. Immunopharmacol.* 22, 371–378. doi: 10.1016/j.intimp.2014.06.043
49. Sulakhiya, K., Kumar, P., Jangra, A., Dwivedi, S., Hazarika, N. K., Baruah, C. C., et al. (2014). Honokiol abrogates lipopolysaccharide-induced depressive like behavior by impeding neuroinflammation and oxido-nitrosative stress in mice. *Eur. J. Pharmacol.* 744, 124–131. doi: 10.1016/j.ejphar.2014.09.049
50. Tomaz, V. S., Cordeiro, R. C., Costa, A. M., de Lucena, D. F., Nobre Júnior, H. V., de Sousa, F. C., et al. (2014). Antidepressant-like effect of nitric oxide synthase inhibitors and sildenafil against lipopolysaccharide-induced depressive-like behavior in mice. *Neuroscience* 268, 236–246. doi: 10.1016/j.neuroscience.2014.03.025
51. Tracey, W. R., Tse, J., and Carter, G. (1995). Lipopolysaccharide-induced changes in plasma nitrite and nitrate concentrations in rats and mice: pharmacological evaluation of nitric oxide synthase inhibitors. *J. Pharmacol. Exp. Ther.* 272, 1011–1015.
52. Vallieres, L., Campbell, I. L., Gage, F. H., and Sawchenko, P. E. (2002). Reduced hippocampal neurogenesis in adult transgenic mice with chronic astrocytic production of interleukin-6. *J. Neurosci.* 22, 486–492. doi: 10.1523/JNEUROSCI.22-02-00486.2002
53. Witko-Sarsat, V., Friedlander, M., Capeillere-Blandin, C., Nguyen-Khoa, T., Nguyen, A. T., Zingraff, J., et al. (1996). Advanced oxidation protein products as a novel marker of oxidative stress in uremia. *Kidney Int.* 49, 1304–1313. doi: 10.1038/ki.1996.186
54. Yamada, H., Arai, T., Endo, N., Yamashita, K., Fukuda, K., Sasada, M., et al. (2006). LPS-induced ROS generation and changes in glutathione level and their relation to the maturation of human monocyte-derived dendritic cells. *Life Sci.* 25, 926–933. doi: 10.1016/j.lfs.2005.05.106
55. Yan, B. C., Park, J. H., Ahn, J. H., Kim, I. H., Park, O. K., Lee, J.-C., et al. (2014). Neuroprotection of posttreatment with risperidone, an atypical antipsychotic drug, in rat and gerbil models of ischemic stroke and the maintenance of antioxidants in a gerbil model of ischemic stroke. *J. Neurosci. Res.* 92, 795–807. doi: 10.1002/jnr.23360
56. Yao, J. K., Leonard, S., and Reddy, R. (2006). Altered glutathione redox state in schizophrenia. *Dis. Markers* 22, 83–93. doi: 10.1155/2006/248387
57. Yirmiya, R., Rosen, H., Donchin, O., and Ovadia, H. (1994). Behavioral effects of lipopolysaccharide in rats: involvement of endogenous opioids. *Brain Res.* 648, 80–86. doi: 10.1016/0006-8993(94)91908-9
58. Yu, H. Y., Cai, Y. B., and Liu, Z. (2015). Activation of AMPK improves lipopolysaccharide-induced dysfunction of the blood-brain barrier in mice. *Brain Inj.* 29, 777–784. doi: 10.3109/02699052.2015.1004746
59. Zhang, X. Y., Cao, J. B., Zhang, L. M., Li, Y. F., and Mi, W. D. (2015). Deferoxamine attenuates lipopolysaccharide-induced neuroinflammation and memory impairment in mice. *J. Neuroinflammation* 12:20. doi: 10.1186/s12974-015-0238-3
60. Zhang, X. Y., Zhou, D. F., Cao, L. Y., Chen, D. C., Zhu, F. Y., and Wu, G. Y. (2003). Blood superoxide dismutase level in schizophrenic patients with tardive dyskinesia: association with dyskinetic movements. *Schizophr. Res.* 62, 245–250. doi: 10.1016/S0920-9964(02)00352-3
61. Zhang, X. Y., Zhou, D. F., Shen, Y. C., Zhang, P. Y., Zhang, W. F., Liang, J., et al. (2012). Effects of risperidone and haloperidol on superoxide dismutase and nitric oxide in schizophrenia. *Neuropharmacology* 62, 1928–1934. doi: 10.1016/j.neuropharm.2011.12.014
62. Zhao, Z., Hu, J., Gao, X., Liang, H., and Liu, Z. (2014). Activation of AMPK attenuates lipopolysaccharide-impaired integrity and function of blood-brain barrier in human brain microvascular endothelial cells. *Exp. Mol. Pathol.* 97, 386–392. doi: 10.1016/j.yexmp.2014.09.006
63. Zhu, F., Zhang, L., Ding, Y. Q., Zhao, J., and Zheng, Y. (2014a). Neonatal intrahippocampal injection of lipopolysaccharide induces deficits in social behavior and prepulse inhibition and microglial activation in rats: implication for a new schizophrenia animal model. *Brain Behav. Immun.* 38, 166–174. doi: 10.1016/j.bbi.2014.01.017
64. Zhu, F., Zheng, Y., Ding, Y., Liu, Y., Zhang, X., Wu, R., et al. (2014b). Minocycline and risperidone prevent microglia activation and rescue behavioral deficits induced by neonatal intrahippocampal injection of lipopolysaccharide in rats. *PLoS One* 9:e93966. doi: 10.1371/journal.pone.0093966

2

MRI-Based Mapping of Cerebral Propagation in Amyotrophic Lateral Sclerosis

Hans-Peter Müller and Jan Kassubek*

Department of Neurology, University of Ulm, Ulm, Germany

***Correspondence:**
Jan Kassubek
jan.kassubek@uni-ulm.de

Neuropathological studies revealed the propagation of amyotrophic lateral sclerosis (ALS) in a sequence of four separate disease-related regional patterns. Diffusion tensor imaging (DTI)-based analysis was established for the individual mapping of sequential disease spreading in ALS as the *in vivo* transfer to neuroimaging. The aim of this review is to summarize cross-sectional and longitudinal results of these technical approaches in ALS as an *in vivo* tool to image ALS propagation stages. This concept was also applied to restricted phenotypes of ALS, e.g., lower motor neuron disease (LMND) or primary lateral sclerosis (PLS). In summary, the regional disease patterns in the course of ALS have been successfully mapped by DTI *in vivo* both cross-sectionally and longitudinally so that this technique might have the potential as a read-out in clinical trials.

Keywords: amyotrophic lateral sclerosis, motor neuron disease, diffusion tensor imaging, fractional anisotropy, magnetic resonance imaging

INTRODUCTION

The potential of neuroimaging as a technical biological marker for cerebral microstructural alterations in neurodegenerative diseases like motor neuron disorders (MND) is under investigation (Turner et al., 2011, 2012). This review was designed to summarize diffusion tensor imaging (DTI)-based approaches for mapping the established propagation patterns in the brain in amyotrophic lateral sclerosis (ALS) and its variants (restricted phenotypes Ludolph et al., 2015). Classification of MND is a challenge of growing importance given that the therapeutic portfolio for ALS might expand in the future, as reflected in the efforts to revise the diagnostic criteria (Ludolph et al., 2015). With respect to the clinical presentation of ALS, the current revision of the El Escorial criteria addressed a validated staging system, and it was held that the development of non-invasive investigations including MRI will assist (Ludolph et al., 2015). For the staging concept, post-mortem studies of the brain pathology of ALS based on phosphorylated 43 kDa TAR DNA-binding protein (pTDP-43) revealed a possible dissemination in a regional sequence of four disease-related patterns (Braak et al., 2013; Brettschneider et al., 2013; Jucker and Walker, 2013), with the sequential protein pathology spreading initially from the motor neocortex toward the spinal cord and brainstem, followed by spreading to frontal, parietal and, ultimately, anteromedial temporal lobes (Ludolph and Brettschneider, 2015). This corticoefferent spreading model has been transferred *in vivo* to MRI-based concepts by *in silico* models (Schmidt et al., 2016), microstructural data (Kassubek et al., 2014, 2018b), and functional connectivity analysis (Schulthess et al., 2016). Specifically, DTI can be used to detect pathology within the corresponding neuronal white matter (WM) tracts and to obtain *in vivo* staging at an individual patient level by fiber-tract of interest (TOI)-based DTI mapping, i.e., a hypothesis-driven approach that revealed sequential involvement of the corresponding WM tracts in cross-sectional data (Kassubek et al., 2014) and longitudinal data (Kassubek et al., 2018b). To assess the axonal damage and myelin degradation, the statistical analysis of DTI metrics can be performed by various approaches: (1) unbiased voxelwise comparison by whole brain-based spatial statistics (WBSS) (Müller et al., 2012) or tractwise comparison by tract-based spatial statistics (TBSS) (Smith et al., 2006), or (2) hypothesis-guided tract-based quantification by analyzing DTI metrics in tract systems by probabilistic tools (Sarica et al., 2017), or TOI-based tractwise fractional anisotropy statistics (TFAS) (Müller et al., 2007b). In this review, results of DTI-based cross sectional and longitudinal analyses in ALS were summarized including applications to clinical variants, i.e., lower motor neuron disease (LMND) and primary lateral sclerosis (PLS).

DTI DATA ANALYSIS TECHNIQUES

The post-processing and statistical analysis of WBSS and TFAS was performed by use of the analysis software tensor imaging and fiber tracking (TIFT) (Müller et al., 2007a). In order to assess the axonal damage and myelin degradation, DTI metrics effects at the group level are reported by voxelwise WBSS comparison (Müller et al., 2012) and tract-based quantification by TOI-based TFAS (Müller et al., 2007b). Standard pre-processing procedures contain quality control of the DTI data including elimination of corrupted DTI volumes (Müller et al., 2011), motion correction of individual DTI data sets, in case of longitudinal data an alignment of baseline data and follow-up data by a halfway rigid-brain co-registration (Menke et al., 2014), normalization to the Montreal Neurological Institute (MNI) stereotaxic standard space (i.e., non-linear and iterative normalization to a study specific template - Müller et al., 2012), and, in case of DTI data from different scanners, a 3-D inter-protocol correction which can be applied ex post facto (Rosskopf et al., 2015). The covariate age should be regressed out due to an age dependency of FA values (Lim et al., 2015). In case of longitudinal analyses, the FA differences between the baseline and follow-ups were normalized to an identical time interval representing comparable disease durations for all patients before group level comparison as previously described in detail (Kassubek et al., 2018b), in order to control for variable follow-up intervals. Post-processing and statistical analysis was performed by a differentiated analysis, i.e., unbiased WBSS (Müller et al., 2012) that statistically compares voxelwise FA values of two subject groups and hypothesis-based tractwise quantification by analyzing FA values along tract systems (TFAS - Müller et al., 2007b).

Fiber tracts were reconstructed from an averaged DTI data set of MNI transformed controls' data (Müller et al., 2007b) by a seed-to-target approach (Kassubek et al., 2014, 2018b); here, for a given pathway, the corresponding TOI is defined by all tracts that originate in a defined seed ROI and end in a target ROI. For quantification of the directionality of the underlying tract structures, the TFAS technique (Müller et al., 2007b) was applied. The four-stage corticoefferent sequential axonal spread of pTDP-43 has been transferred *in vivo* by a hypothesis-driven TOI-based analysis that revealed sequential involvement of the corresponding WM tracts in cross-sectional data (Kassubek et al., 2014) and longitudinal data (Kassubek et al., 2018b). Staging categorization for a given patient at the individual level is possible using an FA-based categorization scheme with sequential involvement of the specific tract structures (Kassubek et al., 2014, 2018b).

IN VIVO TRANSFER OF THE STAGING CONCEPT

The TOI-Based Staging Approach

The hypothesis-guided TOI-based staging approach was suggested to image the neuropathologically proposed sequential progression of ALS in the respective cerebral tract systems, i.e., the CST (as a correlate of ALS-stage 1), the corticorubral and corticopontine tracts (ALS stage 2), the corticostriatal pathway (ALS stage 3), and the proximal portion of the perforant path (ALS stage 4) (Kassubek et al., 2014). The statistical analyses of TOIs showed differences between ALS patients and healthy controls for all tract systems; the significance level of the cross-sectional comparison at the group level in the corresponding fiber tracts was lower, the higher ALS-stage was (Kassubek et al., 2014). After a cross-sectional study with 111 ALS patients and 74 healthy controls with MRI data from 1.5T as well as at 3.0T scanners, a follow-up (mono-centre) study confirmed the results in 382 ALS patients and 149 healthy controls (Kassubek et al., 2018b). In a subsample of 67 ALS patients and 31 healthy controls who obtained at least one follow-up scan after a median of 6 months, longitudinal FA changes showed significant alterations in ALS patients compared with healthy controls in all ALS-related tracts as well as for the grand average of all tract systems (Kassubek et al., 2018b).

By applying the *in vivo* categorization cascade at the individual level (Kassubek et al., 2014), staging categorization for the baseline scans of 387 ALS patients revealed that 72% of the ALS patients were categorized into ALS stages with a homogeneous distribution over the stages. The longitudinal follow-up study with 67 patients with ALS demonstrated that 27% of the longitudinally scanned ALS patients showed an increase in ALS stage after about 4 months, while the other ALS patients remained stable or had already been classified as ALS stage 4 (Kassubek et al., 2018b).

The Unbiased Approach Confirms Results at the Cross-Sectional and Longitudinal Group Level

A multicentre study of eight contributing centers with 253 ALS patients and 189 healthy controls (Müller et al., 2016) confirmed the most significant alterations to be localized in the CST (corresponding to stage 1) and found additional significant WM tract changes in the frontal lobe, the brainstem, and hippocampal regions (corresponding to stages 2–4). The localization of these DTI-based *in vivo* results were in accordance with the definition of the post-mortem neuropathological stages (Brettschneider et al., 2013; Braak et al., 2017).

In a longitudinal study with 67 ALS patients and 31 healthy controls and an average inter-scan interval of 6 months (Kassubek et al., 2018b), longitudinal significant FA alterations were also observed in the CST, the frontal lobe, the brainstem, and in hippocampal regions, that way imaging longitudinal alterations of FA during disease progression.

Hypothetical Longitudinal FA Dependence in ALS Patients

The cross-sectional and longitudinal FA alterations in ALS patients for unbiased WBSS and hypothesis-guided TFAS suggested a hypothetical FA alteration model for the mean FA values in ALS staging-related tract systems (**Figure 1**). After a certain time interval after disease onset in the ALS patients, FA alterations at the group level appear first in the CST; these FA alterations increase during the disease course, and FA alterations in the corticopontine and corticorubral tract as well as in the corticostriatal pathway can be observed. Finally, FA alterations in the proximal portion of the perforant path contribute to the FA alteration pattern. This hypothetical course is based upon the assumption of almost linear FA alterations. However, there is no proof yet which mathematical model (linear or polynomial) could be assumed for the FA decrease. A solution to this challenge could be the analysis of high-frequency DTI scanning (monthly or even bi-weekly) in a group of about 10 ALS patients during the course of the disease.

A study with 65 DTI scans from ALS patients and healthy controls with several follow-up measurements (Baldaranov et al., 2017) showed an FA decrease in the CST that correlated with the revised ALS functional rating scale (ALS-FRS-R – Cedarbaum et al., 1999). In other studies, both the clinical severity as assessed by the slope of the ALS-FRS-R and the disease duration significantly correlated with the resulting staging scheme (Kassubek et al., 2014, 2018b). Furthermore, the results were recently supplemented by neuropsychological data: 139 patients with ALS were tested with the Edinburgh Cognitive and Behavioral ALS screen (ECAS), in addition to DTI brain measures of pathological spread. Executive function, memory and disinhibited behavior were selected for cognitive staging criteria, since these cognitive functions are attributed to cerebral areas analogous to the pattern of MRI markers of TDP-43 pathology, showing that cognitive impairment follows specific patterns in ALS and, in analogy to DTI-based staging, these patterns are useful to set up a cognitive staging (Lulé et al., 2018).

APPLICATION OF THE *IN VIVO* STAGING APPROACH TO PHENOTYPIC VARIANTS OF ALS

Lower Motor Neuron Disease and Primary Lateral Sclerosis

The current revision of the El Escorial criteria for ALS addressed restricted phenotypes in the sense of clinical variants (Ludolph et al., 2015). Adult LMND without clinically overt upper motor neuron (UMN) pathology accounts for about 10% of all cases of MND types and is also traditionally named progressive muscular atrophy (PMA) (Norris et al., 1993; Traynor et al., 2000). On the other hand, PLS is considered a MND which almost exclusively affects UMN (Wais et al., 2017).

In a monocentric study of 37 LMND patients vs. 53 healthy controls, WM microstructure showed characteristic alteration patterns in patients with LMND (clinically differentiated in fast and slow progressors according to van den Berg-Vos et al., 2003), especially along the CST with regional FA reductions in the motor system; the TOI-based tract-specific analysis in fast progressing LMND showed significant FA reductions in ALS-related tracts beyond the CST when compared to slow progressors or healthy controls (Rosenbohm et al., 2016). These results were confirmed by a bicentric study of 65 LMND patients compared to 92 matched healthy controls and 101 matched ALS patients with a "classical" phenotype: the tract-specific analysis demonstrated significant alterations in ALS-related tract systems for fast progressing LMND patients vs. slow progressors and healthy controls (Müller et al., 2018a).

There is also a longstanding debate if PLS could be classified as a disease entity separate from ALS or as a slowly progressing ALS variant with UMN predominance (Singer et al., 2007). In the revision of the El Escorial criteria, PLS is described as a restricted phenotype that evolves into ALS in the majority of patients (Ludolph et al., 2015). *In vivo*, the analysis of WM integrity by regional FA reductions in 50 PLS patients vs. 50 controls showed the alterations along the CST and additionally in frontal and prefrontal brain areas in PLS and ALS patients (Müller et al., 2018b). The ALS-staging-related tract-specific analysis demonstrated identical alterations of ALS-related tract systems for PLS and ALS when compared with controls and showed no differences for the comparison between ALS and PLS (Müller et al., 2018b).

APPLICATION OF THE *IN VIVO* STAGING APPROACH TO BEHAVIORAL VARIANT OF FRONTOTEMPORAL DEMENTIA

The characteristic longitudinal distribution pattern of the underlying pTDP-43 pathology in the behavioral variant of frontotemporal dementia (bvFTD) across specific brain regions was demonstrated (Brettschneider et al., 2014). The *in vivo* staging approach was transferred to bvFTD (without MND) and showed an alteration pattern in the involved major WM tracts (Kassubek et al., 2018a): the TOIs of bvFTD-pattern 1 (uncinate fascicle), 2 (corticostriatal pathway) and 4 (optic radiation) demonstrated significant differences for bvFTD patients vs. controls, whereas the TOI representing the CST (bvFTD-pattern 3) showed no differences for bvFTD vs. controls. Aspects of the heterogeneous neuropathology of bvFTD which is based upon pTDP-43 only in about 50% of the cases are an issue of discussion (Kassubek et al., 2018a).

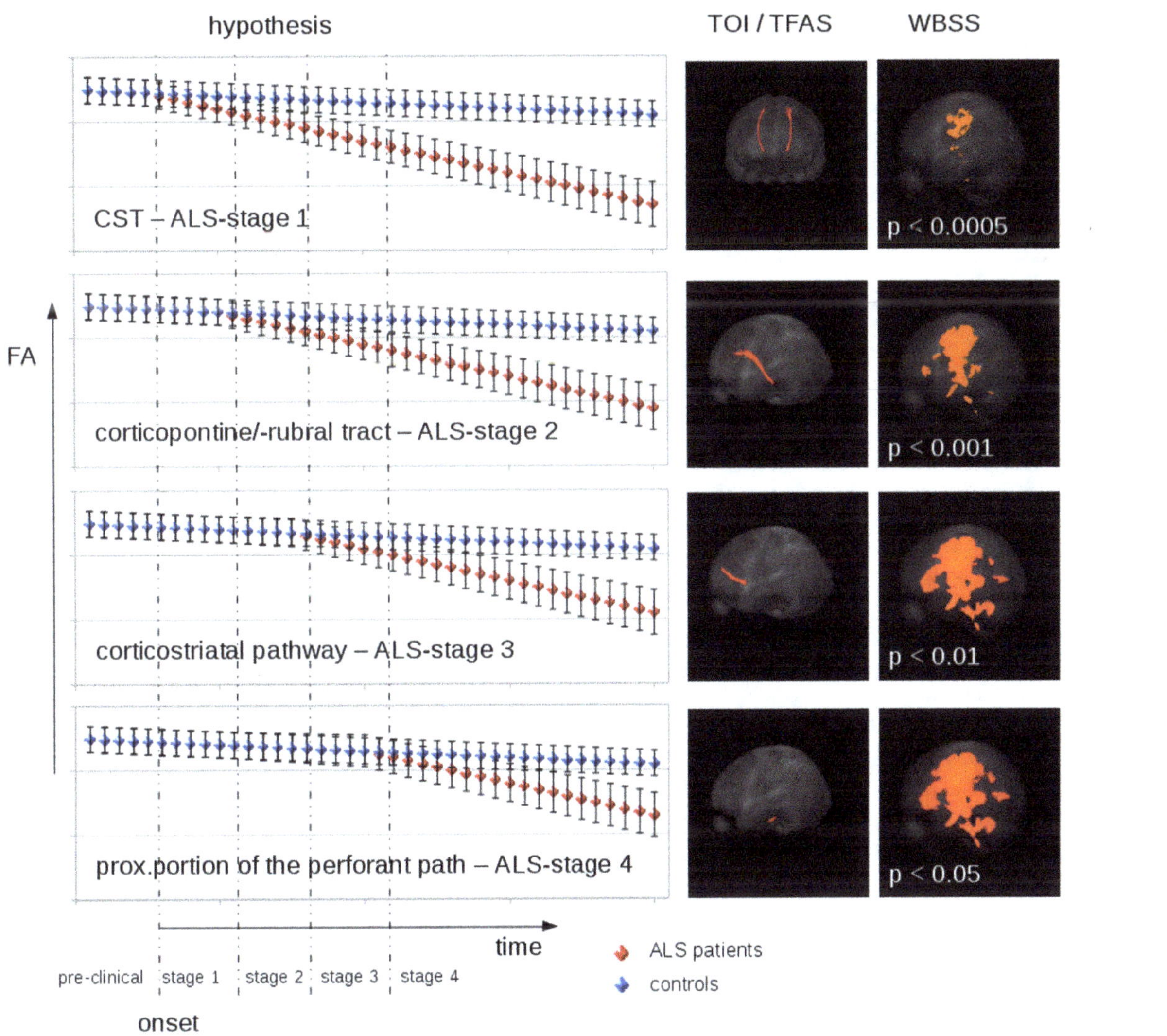

FIGURE 1 | Hypothetical FA development/decrease model for the mean FA values in ALS staging related tract systems. Left panel: At baseline, mean FA was supposed to be identical in patients and controls (with individual error bars). After a certain time interval after disease onset, FA alterations appear first in the CST (related to ALS stage 1). During the disease course, these FA alterations manifest, and FA alterations in frontal and prefrontal areas as well as in the brain stem are observed (corticopontine and corticorubral tract as well as corticostriatal pathway, related to ALS stages 2 and 3, respectively). With higher disease duration, FA alterations in the CST further decrease and alterations in hippocampal areas (proximal portion of the perforant path, related to ALS stage 4) contributed to the FA alteration pattern. Central panel: Projectional views of fiber tracts used for tractwise fractional anisotropy statistics (TFAS) for each of the four stages. Right panel: Projectional views of the corresponding whole brain-based spatial statistics (WBSS).

DISCUSSION

In this review, the approach to use DTI metrics in the assessment of axonal damage and myelin degradation in ALS is specifically addressed. An unbiased voxelwise comparison by WBSS (Müller et al., 2012) is an approach to assess microstructural alterations with an imaging resolution in the order of millimeters. WBSS directly compares DTI metrics of subjects at the group level after stereotaxic normalization for the whole brain without any prior restriction to specific brain areas. On the other hand, a tractwise comparison by TOI-based TFAS (Müller et al., 2007b) addresses DTI-based alterations along specific tract structures both at the group level and at the individual level; the hypothesis-guided TOI approach provides a higher statistical accuracy compared to voxelwise analysis since the whole tract structure is taken into account. An alternative approach to assess ALS-related microstructural alterations is TBSS (Smith et al., 2006; Agosta et al., 2010) that aims at analyzing changes in WM across individuals, that way relying on the precise changes in WM across individuals. TBSS is a probabilistic method that generates multiple solutions to reflect the variability or uncertainty of the estimated fiber orientation restricting the statistical comparisons to the centers of WM tracts after non-linear registration (using FA measurements to realign subjects and extract the centers of WM tracts).

In vivo Imaging of TDP-43 Pathology in ALS and Its Variants

Post-mortem studies demonstrated a concept for patterns of TDP-43 pathology in ALS with a sequential progression of pTDP-43 aggregates (Braak et al., 2013), the task remained to investigate if *in vivo* neuroimaging measures might be identified that were consistent with these patterns of pTDP-43 progression (Kassubek et al., 2018a). The TOI-based staging approach (Kassubek et al., 2014) was able to map *in vivo* the proposed neuropathological progression of ALS cross-sectionally as well as longitudinally, that way supporting DTI as a candidate technical marker to image ALS stages *in vivo* (Kassubek et al., 2018b). The microstructural alterations were supplemented by alterations in functional brain organization: specific intrinsic functional connectivity networks revealed significantly increased functional connectivity for the motor network (as the correlate of the neuropathological stage 1), the brainstem network (neuropathological stage 2), the ventral attention network (neuropathological stage 3), and the default mode/hippocampal network (neuropathological stage 4) in a cross-sectional as well as in a longitudinal study design (Schulthess et al., 2016). Increased functional connectivity is strongly indicative for abnormal brain functioning. First, patterns of increased functional connectivity in ALS that result from abnormally strong functional coupling within a specific functional brain network have been attributed to a gradual loss of the inhibitory influence (Douaud et al., 2011). Second, the patterns of increased functional connectivity also present as a network expansion (Schulthess et al., 2016) which is a commonly observed phenomenon in neurodegenerative diseases (Gorges et al., 2015). A straightforward interpretation of adaptive changes is that additional brain areas become functionally integrated, i.e., additional functionally segregated resources are recruited for compensating the ongoing cell loss in within-network modules in order to maintain "normal" performance (Hillary and Grafman, 2017). The application of the *in vivo* techniques to specific MND phenotypes (ALS variants) demonstrates central nervous system involvement of the corticofugal tracts in fast progressive LMND, in support of the hypothesis that LMND is an ALS variant (Müller et al., 2018a). Furthermore, the clinical approach to the phenotype of PLS as an ALS variant was confirmed, in accordance with the latest revision of the El Escorial criteria (Agosta et al., 2015a; Ludolph et al., 2015), in favor of the conclusion that these patients can be treated like ALS and also may be included into clinical trials of ALS (Müller et al., 2018a).

Hypothesis Guided Tract-Based Analysis

The DTI-based TOI approach is a microstructural correlate of the progressive pathological process; this analysis technique identifies defined anatomical tract systems that represent the proposed progression patterns based upon histopathology (Braak et al., 2013) and are not *per se* determined by a data-driven analysis (Kassubek et al., 2018a). The approach of analyzing a "propagation pattern" is longitudinal in nature. Thus, the analysis according to the progression concept – which has been developed on the basis of cross-sectional post-mortem data – targets the identification of patterns that can be consistently found in a diverse group of neurodegenerative disorders, each of which entails the aggregation of abnormal protein inclusions in characteristic locations (Jucker and Walker, 2013). The longitudinal access of categorizing patients with ALS could be by longitudinal DTI scans followed by confirmation by post-mortem pathology analyses, i.e., the combination of the *in vivo* staging with post-mortem classification in the same subjects. However, the availability of such data is limited. The role of other neuroimaging modalities including molecular imaging has to be evaluated in future studies.

Limitations

A limitation of the staging categorization is that only about 80% of the MND patients could be categorized. This is a technique-immanent limitation as thresholds for the differentiation between patients and controls were defined in a data-driven approach. Due to an incomplete separation between ALS patients and controls (the sensitivity is about 80%), not all patients would be classifiable (Kassubek et al., 2014). The definition of optimized thresholds by repeated control scans or an increased number of control scans might increase the sensitivity and thus the percentage of categorized MND patients. A further limitation of present neuroimaging approaches is the lack of autopsy-confirmed data (Kassubek et al., 2018a); thus, the TOI-based analysis only provides a plausible surrogate pattern for *in vivo* "staging" for the pathology in the ALS cohorts. Finally, since DTI is a quantitative imaging technique, suboptimal acquisition, data processing and analysis approaches can affect the quality and reliability of DTI-derived metrices (Jones, 2010).

Summary

Many neurodegenerative diseases feature characteristic patterns of early neuronal and regional vulnerability, with increasing evidence that misfolded protein aggregates can spread by a self-perpetuating process, and novel neuroimaging techniques can help elucidating how these disorders spread across brain networks (Agosta et al., 2015b). Measurement of WM tract involvement seems to be a valid surrogate to assess the *in vivo* spreading of pathological proteins and seems to be a valid approach to provide insights into the trajectory of processes of neurodegeneration (Agosta et al., 2015b) in order to move neuroimaging "from snapshots to motion picture" according to Schuster and co-workers (Schuster et al., 2015).

In ALS as one of the neurodegenerative diseases with such a propagation pattern, the analysis of the neuropathologically defined structures demonstrated a characteristic alteration pattern of the involved WM pathways cross-sectionally as well as longitudinally (Kassubek et al., 2018a); at present, no direct neuroimaging marker for pTDP-43 exists, but previous neuropathological studies have shown the correlation between the degree of pTDP-43 aggregation and axonal loss (Geser et al., 2009). The DTI-based analysis of microstructural integrity is a different approach compared to analysis techniques like regional volumetric studies that directly measure regional atrophy or intrinsic functional connectivity analysis (Filippi et al., 2015). Thus, the investigation of microstructural integrity by the DTI/TOI-based approach has potential to serve as a non-invasive *in vivo* neuroimaging marker.

The DTI-based techniques have the potential for future use in the work-up of individual patients, they potentially enlarge the spectrum of non-invasive biological markers as a neuroimaging-based read-out for clinical studies (Kassubek et al., 2018a). These studies also could be used for the identification of patients that could be elected for trials targeting at treating the specific histopathologic abnormalities causing MND (Kassubek et al., 2018a). DTI-based scores may provide a different target information to currently available scores for longitudinal screening, as a candidate read-out for future disease-modifying strategies on the transmission of TDP-43 in ALS (Kassubek et al., 2018b).

AUTHOR CONTRIBUTIONS

H-PM and JK conceived and designed the study, collected and interpreted the data, and wrote the manuscript.

FUNDING

This underlying studies were supported by the German Research Foundation (Deutsche Forschungsgemeinschaft, DFG Grant No. LU 336/15-1) and the German Network for Motor Neuron Diseases (BMBF 01GM1103A).

REFERENCES

1. Agosta, F., Al-Chalabi, A., Filippi, M., Hardiman, O., Kaji, R., Meininger, V., et al. (2015a). The El Escorial criteria: strengths and weaknesses. *Amyotroph. Lateral Scler. Frontotemporal. Degener.* 16, 1–7. doi: 10.3109/21678421.2014.964258
2. Agosta, F., Pagani, E., Petrolini, M., Caputo, D., Perini, M., Prelle, A., et al. (2010). Assessment of white matter tract damage in patients with amyotrophic lateral sclerosis: a diffusion tensor MR imaging tractography study. *AJNR Am. J. Neuroradiol.* 31, 1457–1461. doi: 10.3174/ajnr.A2105
3. Agosta, F., Weiler, M., and Filippi, M. (2015b). Propagation of pathology through brain networks in neurodegenerative diseases: from molecules to clinical phenotypes. *CNS Neurosci. Ther.* 21, 754–767. doi: 10.1111/cns.12410
4. Baldaranov, D., Khomenko, A., Kobor, I., Bogdahn, U., Gorges, M., Kassubek, J., et al. (2017). Longitudinal Diffusion Tensor Imaging-based assessment of tract alterations: an application to amyotrophic lateral sclerosis. *Front. Hum. Neurosci.* 11:567. doi: 10.3389/fnhum.2017.00567
5. Braak, H., Brettschneider, J., Ludolph, A. C., Lee, V. M., Trojanowski, J. Q., and Del Tredici, K. (2013). Amyotrophic lateral sclerosis–a model of corticofugal axonal spread. *Nat. Rev. Neurol.* 9, 708–714. doi: 10.1038/nrneurol.2013.221
6. Braak, H., Neumann, M., Ludolph, A. C., and Del Tredici, K. (2017). Does sporadic amyotrophic lateral sclerosis spread via axonal connectivities? *Neurol. Int. Open* 1, E136–E141. doi: 10.1055/s-0043-111375
7. Brettschneider, J., Del Tredici, K., Irwin, D. J., Grossman, M., Robinson, J. L., Toledo, J. B., et al. (2014). Sequential distribution of pTDP-43 pathology in behavioral variant frontotemporal dementia (bvFTD). *Acta Neuropathol.* 127, 423–439. doi: 10.1007/s00401-013-1238-y
8. Brettschneider, J., Del Tredici, K., Toledo, J. B., Robinson, J. L., Irwin, D. J., Grossman, M., et al. (2013). Stages of pTDP-43 pathology in amyotrophic lateral sclerosis. *Ann. Neurol.* 74, 20–38. doi: 10.1002/ana.23937
9. Cedarbaum, J. M., Stambler, N., Malta, E., Fuller, C., Hilt, D., Thurmond, B., et al. (1999). The ALSFRS-R: a revised ALS functional rating scale that incorporates assessments of respiratory function. BDNF ALS Study Group (Phase III). *J. Neurol. Sci.* 169, 13–21. doi: 10.1016/S0022-510X(99)00210-5
10. Douaud, G., Filippini, N., Knight, S., Talbot, K., and Turner, M. R. (2011). Integration of structural and functional magnetic resonance imaging in amyotrophic lateral sclerosis. *Brain* 134, 3470–3479. doi: 10.1093/brain/awr279
11. Filippi, M., Agosta, F., Grosskreutz, J., Benatar, M., Kassubek, J., Verstraete, E., et al. (2015). Progress towards a neuroimaging biomarker for amyotrophic lateral sclerosis. *Lancet Neurol.* 14, 786–788. doi: 10.1016/S1474-4422(15)00134-9
12. Geser, F., Martinez-Lage, M., Robinson, J., Uryu, K., Neumann, M., Brandmeir, N. J., et al. (2009). Clinical and pathological continuum of multisystem TDP-43 proteinopathies. *Arch. Neurol.* 66, 180–189. doi: 10.1001/archneurol.2008.558
13. Hillary, F. G., and Grafman, J. H. (2017). Injured brains and adaptive networks: the benefits and costs of hyperconnectivity. *Trends Cogn. Sci.* 21, 385–401. doi: 10.1016/j.tics.2017.03.003
14. Jones, D. K. (2010). Precision and accuracy in diffusion tensor magnetic resonance imaging. *Top. Magn. Reson. Imaging* 21, 87–99. doi: 10.1097/RMR.0b013e31821e56ac
15. Jucker, M., and Walker, L. C. (2013). Self-propagation of pathogenic protein aggregates in neurodegenerative diseases. *Nature* 501, 45–51. doi: 10.1038/nature12481
16. Kassubek, J., Müller, H.-P., Del Tredici, K., Brettschneider, J., Pinkhardt, E. H., Lulé, D., et al. (2014). Diffusion tensor imaging analysis of sequential spreading of disease in amyotrophic lateral sclerosis confirms patterns of TDP-43 pathology. *Brain* 137, 1733–1740. doi: 10.1093/brain/awu090
17. Kassubek, J., Müller, H.-P., Del Tredici, K., Hornberger, M., Schroeter, M. L., Müller, K., et al. (2018a). Longitudinal diffusion tensor imaging resembles patterns of pathology progression in behavioral variant frontotemporal dementia (bvFTD). *Front. Aging Neurosci.* 10:47. doi: 10.3389/fnagi.2018.00047
18. Kassubek, J., Müller, H.-P., Del Tredici, K., Lulé, D., Gorges, M., Braak, H., et al. (2018b). Imaging the pathoanatomy of amyotrophic lateral sclerosis in vivo: targeting a propagation-based biological marker. *J. Neurol. Neurosurg. Psychiatry* 89, 374–381. doi: 10.1136/jnnp-2017-316365
19. Lim, S., Han, C. E., Uhlhaas, P. J., and Kaiser, M. (2015). Preferential detachment during human brain development: age- and sex-specific structural connectivity in diffusion tensor imaging (DTI) data. *Cereb. Cortex* 25, 1477–1489. doi: 10.1093/cercor/bht333
20. Ludolph, A., Drory, V., Hardiman, O., Nakano, I., Ravits, J., Robberecht, W., et al. (2015). A revision of the El Escorial criteria - 2015. *Amyotroph. Lateral Scler. Frontotemporal. Degener.* 16, 291–292. doi: 10.3109/21678421.2015.1049183
21. Ludolph, A. C., and Brettschneider, J. (2015). TDP-43 in amyotrophic lateral sclerosis - is it a prion disease? *Eur. J. Neurol.* 22, 753–761. doi: 10.1111/ene.12706
22. Lulé, D., Böhm, S., Müller, H.-P., Aho-Özhan, H., Keller, J., Gorges, M., et al. (2018). Cognitive phenotypes of sequential staging in amyotrophic lateral sclerosis. *Cortex* 101, 163–171. doi: 10.1016/j.cortex.2018.01.004
23. Menke, R. A., Körner, S., Filippini, N., Douaud, G., Knight, S., Talbot, K., et al. (2014). Widespread grey matter pathology dominates the longitudinal cerebral MRI and clinical landscape of amyotrophic lateral sclerosis. *Brain* 137, 2546–2555. doi: 10.1093/brain/awu162
24. Müller, H.-P., Agosta, F., Riva, N., Spinelli, E. G., Comi, G., Ludolph, A. C., et al. (2018a). Fast progressive lower motor neuron disease is an ALS variant: a two-centre tract of interest-based MRI data analysis. *Neuroimage Clin.* 17, 145–152. doi: 10.1016/j.nicl.2017.10.008
25. Müller, H.-P., Gorges, M., Kassubek, R., Dorst, J., Ludolph, A. C., and Kassubek, J. (2018b). Identical patterns of cortico-efferent tract involvement in primary lateral sclerosis and amyotrophic lateral sclerosis: a tract of interest-based MRI study. *Neuroimage Clin.* 18, 762–769. doi: 10.1016/j.nicl.2018.03.018
26. Müller, H.-P., Süßmuth, S. D., Landwehrmeyer, G. B., Ludolph, A., Tabrizi, S. J., Klöppel, S., et al. (2011). Stability effects on results of diffusion tensor imaging analysis by reduction of the number of gradient directions due to motion artifacts: an application to presymptomatic Huntington's disease. *PLoS Curr.* 3:RRN1292. doi: 10.1371/currents.RRN1292
27. Müller, H.-P., Turner, M. R., Grosskreutz, J., Abrahams, S., Bede, P., Govind, V., et al. (2016). A large-scale multicentre cerebral diffusion tensor imaging study in amyotrophic lateral sclerosis. *J. Neurol. Neurosurg. Psychiatry* 87, 570–579. doi: 10.1136/jnnp-2015-311952
28. Müller, H.-P., Unrath, A., Huppertz, H.-J., Ludolph, A. C., and Kassubek, J. (2012). Neuroanatomical patterns of cerebral white matter involvement in

different motor neuron diseases as studied by diffusion tensor imaging analysis. *Amyotroph. Lateral Scler.* 13, 254–264. doi: 10.3109/17482968.2011.653571

29. Müller, H. P., Unrath, A., Ludolph, A. C., and Kassubek, J. (2007a). Preservation of diffusion tensor properties during spatial normalization by use of tensor imaging and fibre tracking on a normal brain database. *Phys. Med. Biol.* 52, N99–N109.
30. Müller, H.-P., Unrath, A., Sperfeld, A. D., Ludolph, A. C., Riecker, A., and Kassubek, J. (2007b). Diffusion tensor imaging and tractwise fractional anisotropy statistics: quantitative analysis in white matter pathology. *Biomed. Eng. Online* 6:42. doi: 10.1186/1475-925X-6-42
31. Norris, F., Shepherd, R., and Denys, E. (1993). Onset, natural history and outcome in idiopathic adult motor neuron disease. *J. Neurol. Sci.* 118, 48–55. doi: 10.1016/0022-510X(93)90245-T Rosenbohm, A., Müller, H.-P., Hübers, A., Ludolph, A. C., and Kassubek, J. (2016). Corticoefferent pathways in pure lower motor neuron disease: a diffusion tensor imaging study. *J. Neurol.* 263, 2430–2437. doi: 10.1007/s00415-016-8281-2
32. Rosskopf, J., Müller, H.-P., Dreyhaupt, J., Gorges, M., Ludolph, A. C., and Kassubek, J. (2015). Ex post facto assessment of diffusion tensor imaging metrics from different MRI protocols: preparing for multicentre studies in ALS. *Amyotroph. Lateral Scler. Frontotemporal. Degener.* 9, 1–10. doi: 10.3109/21678421.2014.977297
33. Sarica, A., Cerasa, A., Valentino, P., Yeatman, J., Trotta, M., Barone, S., et al. (2017). The corticospinal tract profile in amyotrophic lateral sclerosis. *Hum. Brain Mapp.* 38, 727–739. doi: 10.1002/hbm.23412
34. Schmidt, R., de Reus, M. A., Scholtens, L. H., van den Berg, L. H., and van den Heuvel, M. P. (2016). Simulating disease propagation across white matter connectome reveals anatomical substrate for neuropathology staging in amyotrophic lateral sclerosis. *Neuroimage* 124, 762–769. doi: 10.1016/j.neuroimage.2015.04.005
35. Schulthess, I., Gorges, M., Müller, H.-P., Lulé, D., Del Tredici, K., Ludolph, A. C., et al. (2016). Functional connectivity changes resemble patterns of pTDP-43 pathology in amyotrophic lateral sclerosis. *Sci. Rep.* 6:38391. doi: 10.1038/srep38391
36. Schuster, C., Elamin, M., Hardiman, O., and Bede, P. (2015). Presymptomatic and longitudinal neuroimaging in neurodegeneration - from snapshots to motion picture: a systematic review. *J. Neurol. Neurosurg. Psychiatry* 86, 1089–1096. doi: 10.1136/jnnp-2014-309888
37. Singer, M. A., Statland, J. M., Wolfe, G. I., and Barohn, R. J. (2007). Primary lateral sclerosis. *Muscle Nerve* 35, 291–302. doi: 10.1002/mus.20728
38. Smith, S. M., Jenkinson, M., Johansen-Berg, H., Rueckert, D., Nichols, T. E., Mackay, C. E., et al. (2006). Tract-based spatial statistics: voxelwise analysis of multi-subject diffusion data. *Neuroimage* 31, 1487–1505. doi: 10.1016/j.neuroimage.2006.02.024
39. Traynor, B. J., Codd, M. B., Corr, B., Forde, C., Frost, E., and Hardiman, O. M. (2000). Clinical features of amyotrophic lateral sclerosis according to the El Escorial and Airlie house diagnostic criteria. *Arch. Neurol.* 57, 1171–1176. doi: 10.1001/archneur.57.8.1171
40. Turner, M. R., Agosta, F., Bede, P., Govind, V., Lulé, D., and Verstraete, E. (2012). Neuroimaging in amyotrophic lateral sclerosis. *Biomark. Med.* 6, 319–337. doi: 10.2217/bmm.12.26
41. Turner, M. R., Grosskreutz, J., Kassubek, J., Abrahams, S., Agosta, F., Benatar, M., et al. (2011). Towards a neuroimaging biomarker for amyotrophic lateral sclerosis. *Lancet Neurol.* 10, 400–403. doi: 10.1016/S1474-4422(11)70049-7
42. van den Berg-Vos, R. M., Visser, J., Franssen, H., de Visser, M., de Jong, J. M., Kalmijn, S., et al. (2003). Sporadic lower motor neuron disease with adult onset: classification of subtypes. *Brain* 126, 1036–1047. doi: 10.1093/brain/awg117
43. Wais, V., Rosenbohm, A., Petri, S., Kollewe, K., Hermann, A., Storch, A., et al. (2017). The concept and diagnostic criteria of primary lateral sclerosis. *Acta Neurol. Scand.* 136, 204–211. doi: 10.1111/ane.12713

3

Machine Learning in Amyotrophic Lateral Sclerosis: Achievements, Pitfalls and Future Directions

Vincent Grollemund[1,2], Pierre-François Pradat[3,4,5], Giorgia Querin[3,4], François Delbot[1,6], Gaétan Le Chat[2], Jean-François Pradat-Peyre[1,6,7] and Peter Bede[3,4,8]*

[1] Laboratoire d'Informatique de Paris 6, Sorbonne University, Paris, France, [2] FRS Consulting, Paris, France, [3] Laboratoire d'Imagerie Biomédicale, INSERM, CNRS, Sorbonne Université, Paris, France, [4] APHP, Département de Neurologie, Hôpital Pitié-Salpêtrière, Centre Référent SLA, Paris, France, [5] Northern Ireland Center for Stratified Medecine, Biomedical Sciences Research Institute Ulster University, C-TRIC, Altnagelvin Hospital, Londonderry, United Kingdom, [6] Département de Mathématiques et Informatique, Paris Nanterre University, Nanterre, France, [7] Modal'X, Paris Nanterre University, Nanterre, France, [8] Computational Neuroimaging Group, Trinity College, Dublin, Ireland

***Correspondence:**
Vincent Grollemund
vincent.grollemund@lip6.fr

Background: Amyotrophic Lateral Sclerosis (ALS) is a relentlessly progressive neurodegenerative condition with limited therapeutic options at present. Survival from symptom onset ranges from 3 to 5 years depending on genetic, demographic, and phenotypic factors. Despite tireless research efforts, the core etiology of the disease remains elusive and drug development efforts are confounded by the lack of accurate monitoring markers. Disease heterogeneity, late-stage recruitment into pharmaceutical trials, and inclusion of phenotypically admixed patient cohorts are some of the key barriers to successful clinical trials. Machine Learning (ML) models and large international data sets offer unprecedented opportunities to appraise candidate diagnostic, monitoring, and prognostic markers. Accurate patient stratification into well-defined prognostic categories is another aspiration of emerging classification and staging systems.

Methods: The objective of this paper is the comprehensive, systematic, and critical review of ML initiatives in ALS to date and their potential in research, clinical, and pharmacological applications. The focus of this review is to provide a dual, clinical-mathematical perspective on recent advances and future directions of the field. Another objective of the paper is the frank discussion of the pitfalls and drawbacks of specific models, highlighting the shortcomings of existing studies and to provide methodological recommendations for future study designs.

Results: Despite considerable sample size limitations, ML techniques have already been successfully applied to ALS data sets and a number of promising diagnosis models have been proposed. Prognostic models have been tested using core clinical variables, biological, and neuroimaging data. These models also offer patient stratification opportunities for future clinical trials. Despite the enormous potential of ML in ALS research, statistical assumptions are often violated, the choice of specific statistical models is seldom justified, and the constraints of ML models are rarely enunciated.

Conclusions: From a mathematical perspective, the main barrier to the development of validated diagnostic, prognostic, and monitoring indicators stem from limited sample sizes. The combination of multiple clinical, biofluid, and imaging biomarkers is likely to increase the accuracy of mathematical modeling and contribute to optimized clinical trial designs.

Keywords: amyotrophic lateral sclerosis, machine learning, diagnosis, prognosis, risk stratification, clustering, motor neuron disease

1. INTRODUCTION

Amyotrophic Lateral Sclerosis (ALS) is an adult-onset multi-system neurodegenerative condition with predominant motor system involvement. In Europe, its incidence varies between 2 or 3 cases per 100 000 individuals (Hardiman et al., 2017) and its prevalence is between 5 and 8 cases per 100 000 (Chiò et al., 2013b). An estimated 450 000 people are affected by ALS worldwide according to the ALS Therapy Development Institute. While no unifying pathogenesis has been described across the entire spectrum of ALS phenotypes, the incidence of the condition is projected to rise in the next couple of decades (Arthur et al., 2016) highlighting the urgency of drug development and translational research. Given the striking clinical and genetic heterogeneity of ALS, the considerable differences in disability profiles and progression rates, flexible individualized care strategies are required in multidisciplinary clinics (den Berg et al., 2005), and it is also possible that precision individualized pharmaceutical therapies will be required.

Depending on geographical locations, the terms "ALS" and "Motor Neuron Disease" (MND) are sometimes used interchangeably, but MND is the broader label, encompassing a spectrum of conditions, as illustrated by **Figure 1**. The diagnosis of ALS requires the demonstration of Upper (UMN) and Lower Motor Neuron (LMN) dysfunction. The diagnostic process is often protracted. The careful consideration of potential mimics and ruling out alternative neoplastic, structural, and infective etiologies, is an important priority (Hardiman et al., 2017). ALS often manifests with subtle limb or bulbar symptoms and misdiagnoses and unnecessary interventions in the early stage of the disease are not uncommon (Zoccolella et al., 2006; Cellura et al., 2012). Given the limited disability in early-stage ALS, many patients face a long diagnostic journey from symptom onset to definite diagnosis which may otherwise represent a valuable therapeutic window for neuroprotective intervention. Irrespective of specific healthcare systems the average time interval from symptoms onset to definite diagnosis is approximately 1 year (Traynor et al., 2000). ALS is now recognized as a multi-dimensional spectrum disorder. From a cognitive, neuropsychological perspective, an ALS-Frontotemporal Dementia (FTD) spectrum exists due to shared genetic and pathological underpinnings. Another important dimension of the clinical heterogeneity of ALS is the proportion of UMN / LMN involvement which contributes to the spectrum of Primary Lateral Sclerosis (PLS), UMN-predominant ALS, classical ALS, LMN-predominant ALS, and Progressive Muscular Atrophy (PMA), as presented in **Figure 1**.

The genetic profile of MND patients provides another layer of heterogeneity. Specific genotypes such as those carrying the *C9orf72* hexanucleotide expansions or those with Super Oxide Dismutase 1 (*SOD1*) mutations have been associated with genotype-specific clinical profiles. These components of disease heterogeneity highlight the need for individualized management strategies and explain the considerable differences in prognostic profiles. Differences in survival due to demographic, phenotypic, and genotypic factors are particularly important in pharmaceutical trials so that the "treated" and "placebo-control" groups are matched in this regard.

With the ever increasing interest in Machine Learning (ML) models, a large number of research papers have been recently published using ML, classifiers, and predictive modeling in ALS (Bede, 2017). However, as these models are usually applied to small data sets by clinical teams, power calculations, statistical assumptions, and mathematical limitations are seldom discussed in sufficient detail. Accordingly our objective is the synthesis of recent advances, discussion of common shortcomings and outlining future directions. The overarching intention of this paper is to outline best practice recommendations for ML applications in ALS.

2. METHODS

Machine learning is a rapidly evolving field of applied mathematics focusing on the development and implementation of computer software that can learn autonomously. Learning is typically based on training data sets and a set of specific instructions. In medicine, it has promising diagnostic, prognostic, and risk stratification applications and it has been particularly successful in medical oncology (Kourou et al., 2015).

2.1. Main Approaches

Machine learning encompasses two main approaches; "supervised" and "unsupervised" learning. The specific method should be carefully chosen based on the characteristics of the available data and the overall study objective.

"Unsupervised learning" aims to learn the structure of the data in the absence of either a well-defined output or feedback (Sammut and Webb, 2017). Unsupervised learning models can help uncover novel arrangements in the data which

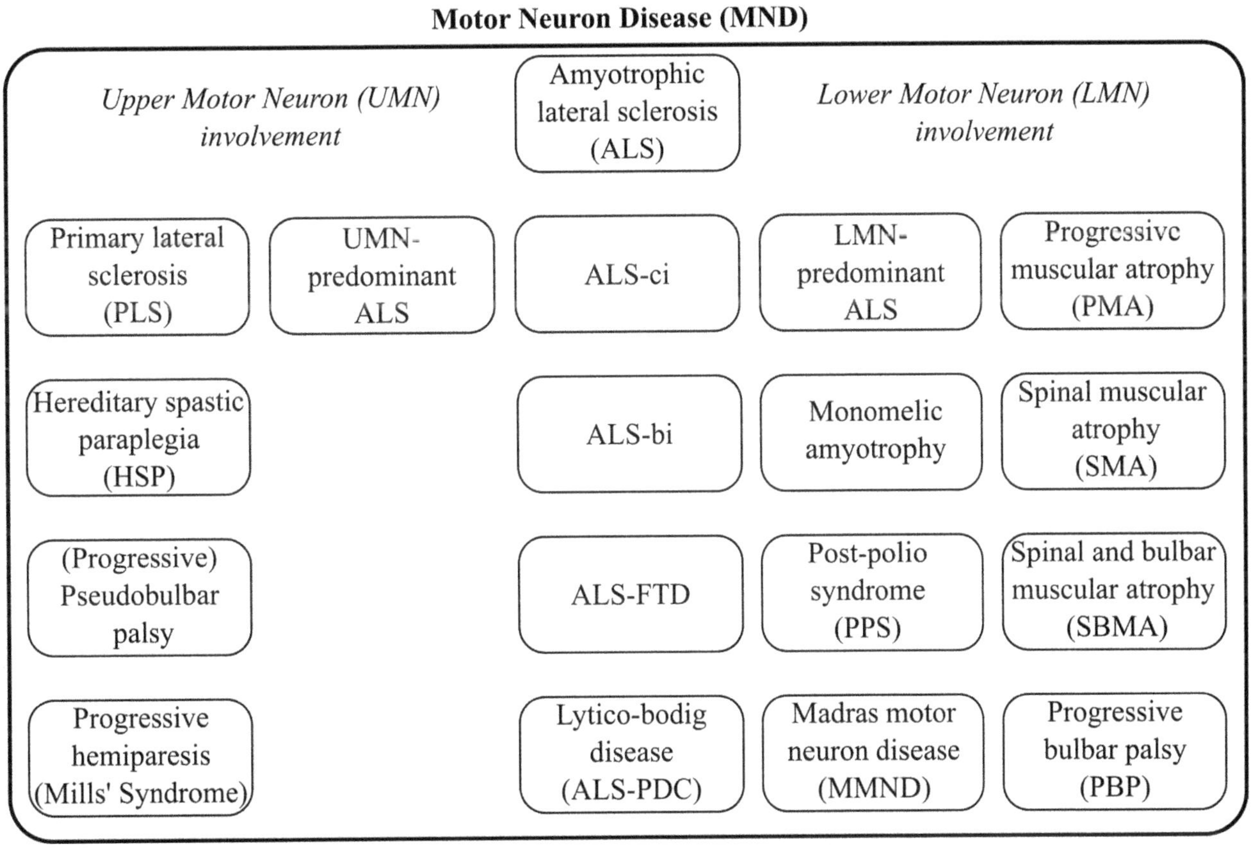

FIGURE 1 | The clinical heterogeneity of Motor Neuron Disease common phenotypes and distinct syndromes.

in turn can offer researchers new insights into the problem itself. Unsupervised learning can be particularly helpful in addressing patient stratification problems. Clustering methods can be superior to current clinical criteria, which are often based on a limited set of clinical observations, rigid thresholds, and conservative inclusion/exclusion criteria for class membership. The K-means algorithm is one of the most popular methods. It recursively repeats two steps until a stopping criterion is met. First, samples are assigned to the closest cluster, which are randomly initialized, then cluster centers are computed based on the centroid of samples belonging to each cluster. Unsupervised learning methods have been successfully used in other fields of medicine (Gomeni and Fava, 2013; Marin et al., 2015; Beaulieu Jones and Greene, 2016; Ong et al., 2017; Westeneng et al., 2018). **Figure 2** represents an example of a patient stratification scheme using an unsupervised learning algorithm.

Supervised learning focuses on mapping inputs with outputs using training data sets (Sammut and Webb, 2017). Supervised learning problems can be divided into either classification or regression problems. Classification approaches allocate test samples into specific categories or sort them in a meaningful way (Sammut and Webb, 2017). The possible outcomes of the modeled function are limited to a set of predefined categories. For example, in the context of ALS, a possible classification task is to link demographic variables, clinical observations, radiological measures, etc. to diagnostic labels such as "ALS," "FTD," or "healthy." Schuster et al. (2016b), Bede et al. (2017), Ferraro et al. (2017), and Querin et al. (2018) have implemented diagnostic models to discriminate between patients with ALS and healthy subjects. Regression problems on the other hand, deal with inferring a real-valued function dependent on input variables, which can be dependent or independent of one another (Sammut and Webb, 2017). For instance, in the context of prognosis, a possible regression task could consist of designing a model which accurately predicts motor decline based on clinical observations (Hothorn and Jung, 2014; Taylor A. A. et al., 2016). When a regression task deals with time-related data sequences, often called "longitudinal data" in a medical context, it is referred to as "time series forecasting." The core characteristics of the data, which are most likely to define group-membership are referred to as "features."

2.2. Common Machine Learning Models

While a plethora of ML models have been developed and successfully implemented for economic, industrial, and biological applications (Hastie et al., 2009; Bishop, 2016; Goodfellow et al., 2017), this paper primarily focuses on ML

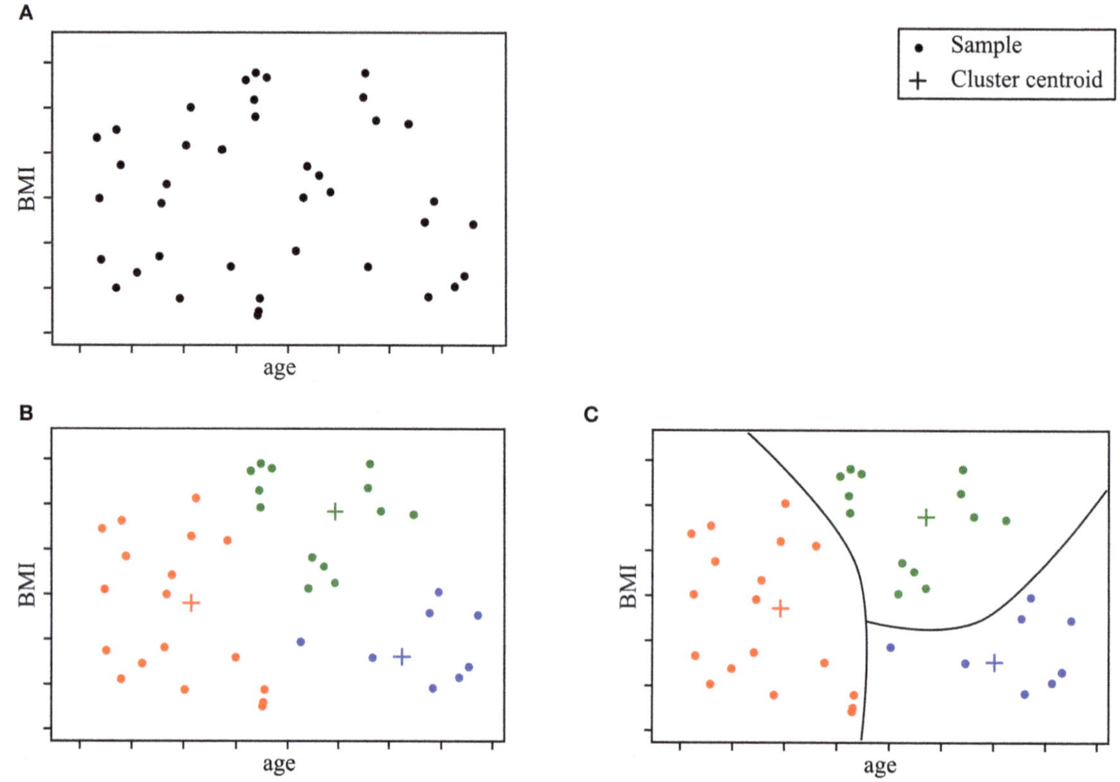

FIGURE 2 | Clustering model for patient stratification. The available data consist of basic clinical features; age and BMI. Given this specific ALS patient population, the objective is to explore if patients segregate into specific subgroups. After running a clustering algorithm, we obtain clusters and cluster memberships for each patient. Further analysis of shared traits within the same cluster can help identify novel disease phenotypes. **(A)** Initial data samples without output. **(B)** Identify cluster and cluster membership. **(C)** Stratify samples based on shared feature traits.

methods utilized in ALS research. These include Random Forests (RF) (Hothorn and Jung, 2014; Ko et al., 2014; Beaulieu-Jones and Greene, 2016; Sarica et al., 2016; Taylor A. A. et al., 2016; Ferraro et al., 2017; Fratello et al., 2017; Huang et al., 2017; Jahandideh et al., 2017; Seibold et al., 2017; Pfohl et al., 2018; Querin et al., 2018), Support Vector Machines (SVM) (Srivastava et al., 2012; Welsh et al., 2013; Beaulieu-Jones and Greene, 2016; Bandini et al., 2018; D'hulst et al., 2018), Neural Networks (NN) (Beaulieu-Jones and Greene, 2016; van der Burgh et al., 2017), Gaussian Mixture Models (GMM) (Huang et al., 2017), Boosting methods (Jahandideh et al., 2017; Ong et al., 2017), k-Nearest Neighbors (k-NN) (Beaulieu-Jones and Greene, 2016; Bandini et al., 2018). Generalized linear regression models are also commonly used (Gordon et al., 2009; Taylor A. A. et al., 2016; Huang et al., 2017; Li et al., 2018; Pfohl et al., 2018), but will not be presented here. Please refer to Bishop (2016) for additional information on linear modeling. Our review of ML model families does not intend to be comprehensive with regards to ML models utilized in other medical subspecialties. Additional models with successful implementation in neurological conditions include Latent Factor models (Geifman et al., 2018) and Hidden Markov Models (HMM) (Martinez-Murcia et al., 2016) which have been successfully implemented in Alzheimer disease cohorts.

2.2.1. Random Forests

Tree-based methods partition the input space into sets that minimize an error function, impurity, or entropy (Hastie et al., 2009). A decision tree is a tree-based method that can be described as a series of bifurcations with yes/no questions. To compute the output of a data sample, one needs to start at the top of the tree, and iteratively decide where to go next based on the answer. **Figure 3** illustrates an example of a decision tree for diagnosis modeling in ALS.

"Random Forest" (RF) is a ensemble method based on decision trees. By relying on multiple learning algorithms to combine their results, ensemble methods obtain a more efficient prediction model. Each tree in the RF is built on a random subset of the training data and available features. This increases robustness to outliers and generalizability. The final estimation is the average or majority of the trees' estimation depending on whether the target is a regression or classification task (Louppe, 2014). Most RFs contain more than a hundred decision trees and decision tree length and width can also be sizable depending on the number of input features. In ML, the term "interpretability" refers to the degree to which the machine's decision is comprehensible to a human observer (Miller, 2017). While global model interpretability is de facto rather low, RFs evaluate feature importance with regards to its discriminatory power.

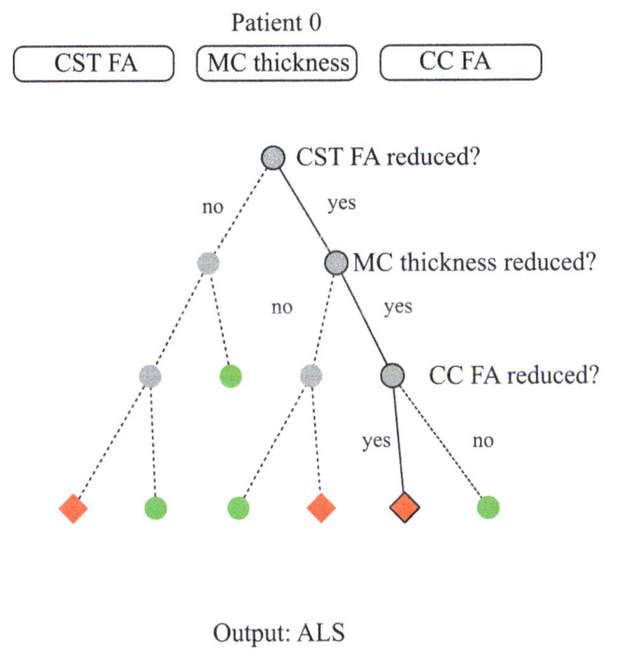

FIGURE 3 | Decision tree model for diagnosis. The available data consist of three basic neuroimaging features: average Corticospinal Tract (CST) Fractional Anisotropy (FA), Motor Cortex (MC) thickness, and average Corpus Callosum (CC) FA. For patient 0, these features are reduced CST FA, reduced MC thickness, reduced CC FA. The target is to classify subjects between healthy and ALS subjects. Establishing a diagnosis requires to run through the decision tree till there are no more questions to answer. At step 1, the closed question directs to the right node due to patient 0's CST pathology. At step 2, the closed question directs to the right node due to patient 0's MC pathology. At step 3, the closed question directs to the left node due to patient 0 CC involvement. Step 3 is the last step as there is no more steps below. The diagnosis for patient 0 is the arrival cell value which is ALS.

Feature relevance is appraised based on the error function upon which the decision trees were built. Extremely Randomized Trees (Extra Trees) have shown promising results for discriminating patients suffering from Progressive Supranuclear Palsy (PSP) and Multiple System Atrophy (MSA) using speech analysis (Baudi et al., 2016). Please refer to Breiman (2001) for a more thorough description of decision trees and RFs and to Rokach (2016) and Shaik and Srinivasan (2018) for a general overview of forest models and their evolution. **Figure 4** illustrates a possible diagnostic application of RF in ALS.

2.2.2. Support Vector Machines

Support Vector Machines (SVM) map input data into high dimensional spaces, called feature spaces, using a non-linear mapping function (Vapnik, 2000). They define a hyperplane that best separates the data. While traditional linear modeling is performed in the input space, SVMs perform linear modeling after projecting the data into another space. The features which discriminate in the projected space, also known as "feature space," derive from input features but these are not readily interpretable. The feature space hyperplane is defined by a limited set of training points called support vectors, hence the name of the method. The chosen hyperplane maximizes the margins between the closest data samples on each side of the hyperplane, which is why SVMs are also referred to as "large margins classifier." These vectors are identified during the "learning phase" after solving a constrained optimization problem. SVMs work as a "black box" as the logic followed by the model cannot be directly interpreted. SVM were state-of-the-art models before being outperformed by NN architecture. That being said, SVM models can adjust well to imaging specific tasks such as anomaly detection using one class SVM. Medical applications of one class SVMs have addressed the issues of tumor detection (Zhang et al., 2004) or breast cancer detection (Zhang et al., 2014). Please refer to Bishop (2016) for more information on SVMs. **Figure 5** illustrates an example of a SVM used to predict prognosis in ALS.

2.2.3. Neural Networks

A "perceptron," also called "artificial neuron," is a simplified representation of a human neuron. It is defined by its afferents (inputs), the inputs' respective weights and a non-linear function. The perceptron's output is the linear combination of its inputs onto which the non-linear function is applied. The linear combination consists of the sum of the multiplications of each input and their respective weight. Perceptrons can be compiled, the output of one perceptron providing the input of the next perceptron. The resulting structure is called a "multi-layer perceptron" which is the most common Neural Network (NN) framework. The contribution of each input to the neuron is modulated by its respective weight which is commonly regarded as a "synapse." NN structures are chosen based on manual tuning and model weights are selected using iterative optimization methods. The stochastic gradient descent method is one of the most popular approaches. Specific model architectures are optimally-suited for specific data types such as "Recurrent NNs" (RNN) for time series or "Convolutional NNs" (CNN) for images. Deep learning models are NN models with significant depth or number of layers (hence the name deep learning) and extensive height or number of nodes per layer, which strongly limits their direct interpretability, similarly to SVMs. Deep learning models are currently state-of-the-art in multiple domains, specifically those which deal with imaging data. Substantial achievements were reached in the field of oncology with regards to melanoma (Esteva et al., 2017), breast cancer and prostate cancer detection (Litjens et al., 2016). Advanced neural network architecture such as the Generative Adversarial Networks (GAN) (Goodfellow et al., 2014) have been tested in a medical imaging synthesis (Nie et al., 2017) or patient record generation (Choi et al., 2017) contexts. Please refer to Goodfellow et al. (2017) for additional material on NNs, Amato et al. (2013) for NN applications in medical diagnosis, Lisboa and Taktak (2006) for NN models in decision support in cancer and Suzuki (2017). **Figure 6** provides a schematic example of NNs to aid prognostic modeling in ALS using a two layer multi-layer perceptron.

2.2.4. Gaussian Mixture Models

Gaussian Mixture Models (GMM) are probabilistic models which can be used in supervised or unsupervised learning. The model hypothesis is that the data can be modeled as

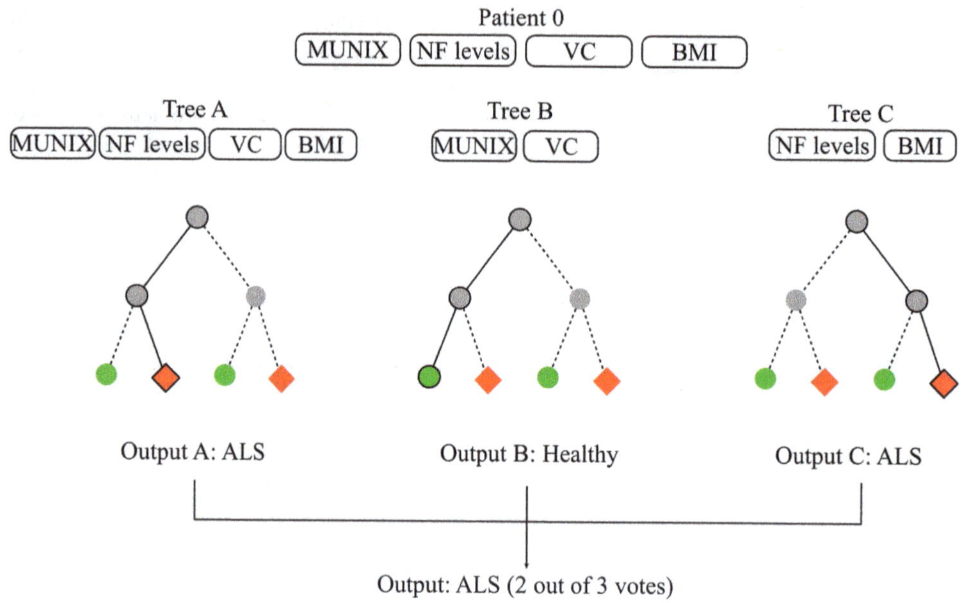

FIGURE 4 | Random forest for diagnosis. The available data consist of basic biomarkers features which are MUNIX, CSF Neurofilament (NF) levels, Vital Capacity (VC), and BMI. The objective is to classify subjects between healthy and ALS patients. The RF contains 3 decisions trees which use different feature subsets to learn a diagnosis model. Tree A learns on all available features, Tree B learns on MUNIX and VC, Tree C learns on NF levels and BMI. Each tree proposes a diagnosis. RF diagnosis is computed based on the majority vote of each of the trees contained in the forest. Given that two out of three trees concluded that patient 0 had ALS, the final diagnosis suggested by the model is ALS.

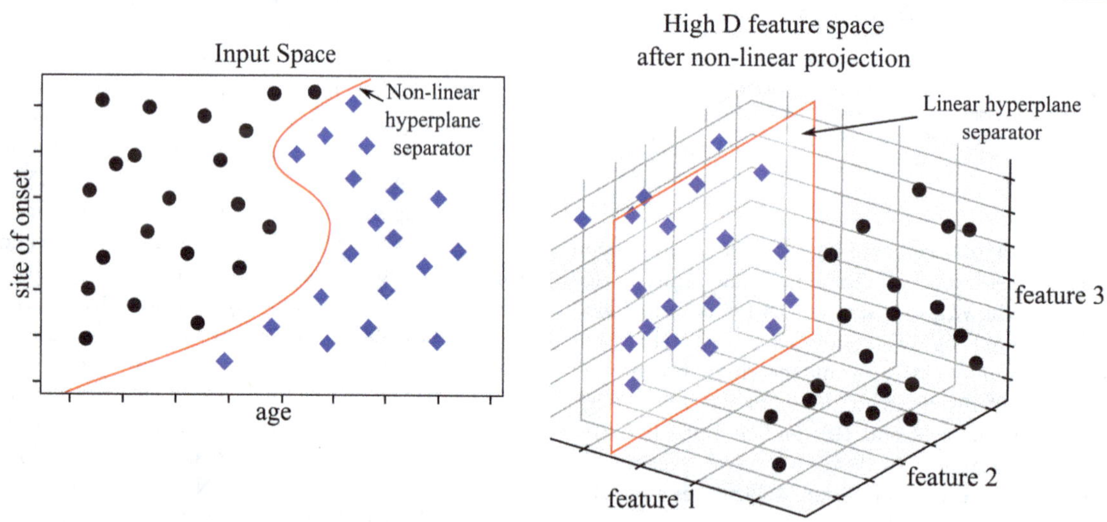

FIGURE 5 | SVM model for prognosis. The available data consist of basic clinical and demographic features; age and site of onset. The objective is to classify patients according to 3-year survival. In the input space (where features are interpretable), no linear hyperplane can divide the two patient populations. The SVM model projects the data into a higher dimensional space—in our example a three dimensional space. The set of two features is mapped to a set of three features. In the feature space, a linear hyperplane can be computed which discriminates the two populations accurately. The three features used for discrimination are unavailable for analysis and interpretability is lost in the process.

a weighted-sum of finite Gaussian-component densities. Each density component is characterized by two parameters: a mean vector and a covariance matrix. Component parameters are estimated using the "Expectation Maximization" (EM) algorithm based on maximizing the log likelihood of the component densities. Inference is performed by drawing from the estimated mixture of Gaussian densities. GMM has achieved good results in medical applications, including medical imaging (de Luis-García et al., 2011) and diagnosing of PD (Khoury et al., 2019). Please refer to Rasmussen (2005) for additional material on GMMs,

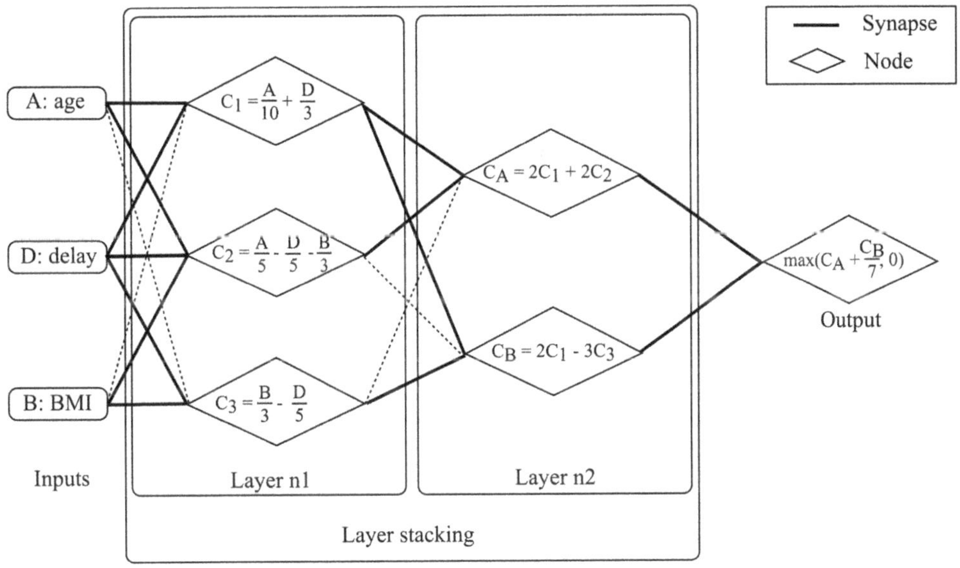

FIGURE 6 | Neural Network model for prognosis. The available data consist of basic demographic and clinical features: age, BMI and diagnostic delay. For patient 0, these features are 50, $15 kg/m^2$, and 15 months, respectively. The objective is to predict ALSFRS-r in 1 year. The multi-layer perceptron consists of two layers. Nodes are fed by input with un-shaded arrows. At layer 1, the three features are combined linearly to compute three node values, C_1, C_2, and C_3. C_1 is a linear combination of age and delay, C_2 is a linear combination of age, delay and BMI, and C_3 is a linear combination of BMI and delay. For patient 0, computing the three values returns 10, 2, and 2 for C1, C2, and C3, respectively. At layer 2, outputs from layer 1 (i.e., C_1, C_2, and C_3) are combined linearly to compute two values, C_A and C_B. C_A is a linear combination of C_1 and C_2 while C_B is a linear combination of C_1 and C_3. For patient 0, computing the two values gives 24 and 14 for C_A and C_B, respectively. Model output is computed after computing linear combination of C_A and C_B and applying a non-linear function (in this case a maximum function which can be seen as a thresholding function which accepts only positive values). The output is the predicted motor functions decline rate. For patient 0, the returned score is 26.

Moon (1996) for more information on the EM algorithm and Roweis and Ghahramani (1999) for a global overview of Gaussian mixture modeling.

2.2.5. k-nearest Neighbors

k-Nearest Neighbors (k-NN) is an instance-based model. Inference is performed according to the values of its nearest neighbors. The advantage of the model is that limited training is required: all of the training data is kept in memory and is used during the prediction phase. Based on a selected distance function, the K most similar neighbors to the new sample are identified. The new sample's label is the average of its nearest neighbors' label. An advanced version of the method is called Fuzzy k-NN (Fk-NN) which has been used to diagnose PD based on computational voice analyses (Chen et al., 2013). Please refer to Bishop (2016) for more information on k-NN models and Aha et al. (1991) for a review on instance-based ML models.

2.2.6. Boosting Methods

Boosting algorithms are ensemble methods: they rely on a combination of simple classifiers. In contrast to RF models, which are made up of decision trees and output a result based on the average or majority vote of the decision belonging to the RF mode, boosting algorithms are based on simple classifiers. The concept behind boosting is combining multiple "weak" (performance wise) learning models. This combination provides a more robust model than working with a simple base model. Model learning is based on finding the right weighting of the weak learners which make up the model to learn an efficient global model. Recent applications of boosting models include analysis of genetic information to inform on breast cancer prognosis (Lu et al., 2019) and cardiac autonomic neuropathy (Jelinek et al., 2014). Please refer to Bishop (2016) for more information on boosting methods and (Schapire, 2003) for a general overview of boosting methods.

As opposed to relying on a single ML model, models have been increasingly used in combination. For example, NN has been combined with a RF in Beaulieu-Jones and Greene (2016) where the NN output is fed into the RF model. Learning sub-models on specific feature sets have been used to feed sub-model outputs to another ML model as in Fratello et al. (2017) which trained two RF models on different imaging data sets (functional and structural MRI features) and combined intermediate outputs as the final model output. Model combination and model integration can significantly enhance overall performance, but the complexity of both approaches is often underestimated. ML model constraints are even more stringent when used as part of combined or integrated models.

2.3. The Limitations of Machine Learning Approaches

ML models have considerable advantages over traditional statistical approaches for modeling complex datasets. Most ML models, including the six approaches presented above, do not require stringent assumptions on data characteristics.

They offer novel insights by identifying statistically relevant correlations between features and, in the case of supervised learning, of a specific outcome. Despite the pragmatic advantages, the application of ML models requires a clear understanding of what determines model performance and the potential pitfalls of specific models. The most common shortcomings will be discussed in the following section. Concerns regarding data analyses will be examined first, which include data sparsity, data bias, and causality assumptions. Good practice recommendations for model design will then be presented, including the management of missing data, model overfitting, model validation, and performance reporting.

2.3.1. Data Sparsity

"Data sparsity" refers to working and interpreting limited data sets which is particularly common in medical applications. Medical data is often costly, difficult to acquire, frequently require invasive (biopsies, spinal fluid), uncomfortable (blood tests), or time consuming procedures (Magnetic Resonance Imaging). Other factors contributing to the sparsity of medical data include strict anonymization procedures, requirements for informed consent, institutional, and cross-border data management regulations, ethics approvals, and other governance issues. The processing, storage, and labeling of medical data is also costly and often requires specific funding to upkeep registries, DNA banks, brain banks, biofluid facilities, or magnetic resonance repositories (Turner et al., 2011; Bede et al., 2018b; NEALS Consortium, 2018; Neuroimaging Society in ALS, 2018). Multicenter protocols are particularly challenging and require additional logistics, harmonization of data acquisition, standardized operating procedures, and bio-sample processing, such as cooling, freezing, spinning, staining, etc.

Most ML models have originally been intended, developed, and optimized for huge quantities of data. Accordingly, the generalizability of most ML models depends heavily on the number of samples upon which it can effectively learn. Additionally, there is the "curse of dimensionality." The number of samples required for a specific level of accuracy grows exponentially with the number of features (i.e., dimensions) (Samet, 2006). If the number of samples is restrictively low, then the features lose their discriminating power, as all samples in the dataset seem very distinct from one another (Pestov, 2007). ML models learn the underlying relationship between data samples through feature correlations. This requires the ability to discriminate between similar and dissimilar samples in the dataset. Calculating the Sample to Feature Ratio (SFR), i.e., the number of samples available per feature, is a simple way to assess whether the sample size is satisfactory for a given model. An "SFR" of around 10–15 is often considered the bare minimum (Raudys, 2001), but this is based on historical statistical models and may be insufficient for working with complex ML models. Working with a low SFR can lead to both model "underfitting" or "overfitting." These concepts will be introduced below.

2.3.2. Data Bias

Discussing data bias is particularly pertinent when dealing with medical data. Most ML models assume that the training data used is truly representative of the entire population. The entire spectrum of data distribution should be represented in the training data, just as observed in the overall population, otherwise the model will not generalize properly. For example, if a model is presented with a phenotype which was not adequately represented in the training data set, the model will at best label it as an "outlier" or at worst associate it to the wrong category label. Medical data are particularly prone to suffer from a variety of data biases which affect recorded data at different analysis levels (Pannucci and Wilkins, 2010). The four most common types of bias include: study participation bias, study attrition bias , prognostic factor measurement bias, and outcome measurement bias (Hayden et al., 2013). In ALS, study participation bias, - a.k.a. "clinical trial bias," is by far the most significant. It affects prognostic modeling in particular, as patients in clinical trials do not reflect the general ALS population: they are usually younger, tend to suffer from the spinal form of ALS and have longer survival (Chio et al., 2011). Unfortunately, very little can be done to correct for participation bias *post-hoc*, therefore its potential impact needs to be carefully considered when interpreting the results. Study attrition bias also influences ALS studies as data censoring is not always systematically recorded. "Censoring" is a common problem in medical research; it refers to partially missing data, typically to attrition in longitudinal studies. Prognostic factor measurements can be influenced by subjective and qualitative medical assessments and by "machine bias" in imaging data interpretation. The single most important principle to manage these factors, especially if limited data are available, is overtly discussing the type of bias affecting a particular study, and openly reporting them.

2.3.3. Causality Assumption

ML models identify strong (i.e., statistically significant) correlations between input features and the output in the case of supervised learning. Models can only capture observed correlations which are fully contained within the training data. Causality between features and the output cannot be solely established based on significant correlations in the dataset, especially when working with small and potentially unrepresentative population samples. Causality is sometimes inferred based on ML results which can be misleading.

2.4. Good Practice Recommendations

2.4.1. Feature Selection

Identifying the most appropriate features is a crucial step in model design. In "sparse data" situations, the number of features should be limited to achieve an acceptable SFR and to limit model complexity. Various feature selection and engineering approaches exist, which can be chosen and combined depending on primary study objectives. It can be performed manually based on a priori knowledge or using a RF model which ranks data features based on feature importance. This method is commonly used in medical contexts as it easily gives a broad overview of the feature set. Dimension reduction is another option, with linear methods such as Principal Component Analysis (PCA) or Independent Component Analysis (ICA) and non-linear methods such as manifold learning methods. Automated feature selection methods, such as the "wrapper" or "filtering," undergo an iterative, sometimes time-consuming process where features are selected based on their impact on overall model performance. Finally, provided that sufficient data are available, NN Auto Encoders (AE) models can also reliably extract relevant features. To this day, feature selection and engineering cannot be fully automated and human insight is typically required for manual tuning of either the features or the algorithms performing feature selection. Please refer to Guyon et al. (2006) for further information on feature selection strategies, Fodor (2002) for an overview of dimension reduction techniques and (Lee and Verleysen, 2007) for additional material on non-linear dimension reduction.

2.4.2. Missing Data Management

While most ML models require complete data sets for adequate learning, medical data are seldom complete and missing features are also common. Missing data may originate from data censoring in longitudinal studies or differences in data acquisition. One common approach to missing data management is the discarding of incomplete samples. This has no effect on model design provided there is sufficient data left and that sample distribution is unaltered after discarding. This strategy usually requires large volumes of data with only a small and random subset of missing records. This condition however is rarely met in a clinical setting, where data is sparse, and missing data patterns are typically not random. Missing data can often be explained by censoring or specific testing procedures. Discarding data in these situations may increase data bias as it alters the sample distribution. The first step to missing data management is therefore to explore the mechanisms behind missing data features. Features can be "missing completely at random," without modifying the overall data distribution, "missing at random," when missing feature patterns are based on other features available in the dataset or "non-missing at random" for the remaining cases. Depending on the type of missing data, an appropriate imputation method should be selected. Basic data imputation methods, such as mean imputation, work well on "missing completely at random" cases but induce significant bias for "missing at random" scenarios. In this case, advanced imputation methods such as "Multiple Imputation using Chained Equations" (MICE) (van Buuren, 2007) or "Expectation Maximization" (EM) (Nelwamondo et al., 2007) algorithms operate well. Recently, missing data imputation has been managed using Denoising Auto-Encoders (DAE) models (Nelwamondo et al., 2007; Costa et al., 2018), which have a specific NN architecture. MICE and EM algorithms are statistical methods which substitute missing feature values with feature values from the most similar records in the training set. DAE models build a predictive model using the data available with no missing features to assess substitution values."Non-missing at random" patterns are usually dealt with missing at random imputation methods, but this induces bias in data which needs to be specifically acknowledged. Please refer to Little (2002) for general principles on missing data management and (Rubin, 1987) for missing data imputation for "non-random missing" patterns.

2.4.3. Model Overfitting

Each model design is invariably associated with a certain type of error. "Bias" refers to erroneous assumptions associated with a model, i.e., certain interactions between the input and the output may be overlooked by the model. 'Variance' refers to errors due to the model being too sensitive to training data variability. The learnt model may be excessively adjusted to the training data and poorly generalizable to the overall population if it has only captured the behavior of the training dataset. "Irreducible error" is inherent to model design and cannot be dealt with *post-hoc*. "Bias" and "variance" are interlinked, which is commonly referred to as the "bias-variance trade-off." A high level of bias will lead to model "underfitting," i.e., the model does not represent adequately the training data. A high level of variance will lead to model "overfitting," i.e., the model is too specific to the training data. Overfitting is critical, as it is easily overlooked when evaluating model performance and with the addition of supplementary data, the model will not be able to accurately categorize the new data. This severely limits the use of "overfitted" models. Complex models tend to "overfit" more than simpler models and they require finer tuning. Carefully balancing variance and bias is therefore a key requirement for ML model design. Please refer to Bishop (2016) for more information on overfitting.

2.4.4. Validation Schemes

Working with an optimal validation scheme is crucial in ML. Validation schemes usually split available data into "training" and "testing" datasets, so that performance can be assessed on novel data. Training and testing data should share the same distribution profile, which in turn should be representative of the entire population. Overfitting is a common shortcoming of model designs and carefully chosen validation schemes can help to avoid it. Several validation frameworks exist, "hold out validation" and "cross validation" being the two most popular. The former splits the initial dataset into two sets, one for training the other for testing. The latter performs the same splitting but multiple times. The model is learned and tested each time and the overall performance is averaged. Nevertheless, caution should be exercised in a sparse data context as validation schemes do not compensate well for poorly representative data. Please refer to Bishop (2016) for additional considerations regarding validation schemes.

2.4.5. Harmonization of Performance Evaluation and Reporting

Formal and transparent performance assessments are indispensable to compare and evaluate in ML frameworks. To achieve that, standardized model performance metrics are required. In classification methods, model evaluation should include sensitivity and specificity, especially in a diagnostic context. Sensitivity (or "recall") is the true positive rate, and specificity is the true negative rate. "Accuracy" and Area Under the "Receiver Operating Curve" (ROC) metrics can be added but should never be used alone to characterize model performance. Accuracy is the average of sensitivity and specificity. ROC is used to represent sensitivity and specificity trade-offs in a classifier model (Fawcett, 2004). The ROC space represents the relationship between the true positive rate (i.e., sensitivity) and the false positive rate (which is 1 - specificity). Given a threshold sensitivity rate, the prediction model will return a specificity rate, adding a data point to the ROC. Multiple thresholding enables the generation of the ROC curve. Perfect predictions lead to 100% sensitivity and 100% specificity (i.e., 0% false positives) which leads to an Area Under the ROC (AUC) of 1. Random predictions will return a 50% accuracy rate which is represented by a continuous straight line connecting the plot of 0% sensitivity with 100% specificity and the plot of 100% sensitivity with 0% specificity, which leads to an AUC of 0.5. Accuracy can hide a low specificity rate if there is a class imbalance and AUC can be misleading as it ignores the goodness of fit of the model and predicted probability values (Lobo et al., 2008). In regression approaches, Root Mean Squared Error (RMSE) (also referred to as Root Mean Square Deviation) and R^2, the coefficient of determination, are good metrics. R^2 represents the ratio of explained variation over the total variation of the data (Draper and Smith, 1998). The closer this index is to one, the more the model explains all the variability of the response data around its mean. Hence the model fits the data well. It is advisable to report multiple performance index for model evaluation as each metric reflects on a different aspect of the model. Using confidence intervals when possible is another good practice, as it conveys the uncertainty relative to the achieved error rate. General reporting guidelines for model design and model evaluation are summarized in the Transparent Reporting of a multivariate prediction model for Individual Prognosis or Diagnosis, or TRIPOD, statement (Moons et al., 2015).

Both "supervised" and "unsupervised" learning approaches have a role in clinical applications, the former for diagnosis and prognosis, the latter for patient stratification. There are a large number of ML models available, but recent work in medicine has primarily centered on three models: RF, SVM, and NN models. The advantages and drawbacks of the specific models are summarized in **Table 1** (Hastie, 2003). The following factors should be considered when implementing ML models for a specific medical project:

Data limitation considerations:

- SFR assessment
- Data bias assessment
- Causality assumptions

Model design considerations:

- Feature selection with regards to SFR
- Missing data management
- Overfitting risk assessment
- Validation framework selection
- Performance metric selection
- Comprehensive model performance reporting.

3. RESULTS

Diagnostic, prognostic, and risk stratification papers were systematically reviewed to outline the current state of the art in ML research efforts in ALS. Consensus diagnostic criteria, established monitoring methods, and validated prognostic indicators provide the gold standard to which emerging ML applications need to be compared to.

3.1. Current Practices in ALS

3.1.1. Current Practices in ALS for Diagnosis

The diagnosis of ALS is clinical, and the current role of neuroimaging, electrophysiology, and cerebrospinal fluid (CSF) analyses is to rule out alternative neurological conditions which may mimic the constellation of symptoms typically associated with ALS. Patients are formally diagnosed based on the revised El Escorial criteria (Brooks, 1994; Brooks et al., 2000; de Carvalho et al., 2008) which achieve low false negative rates (0.5%), but suffer from relatively high false positive rates (57%) (Goutman, 2017). As most clinical trials rely on the El Escorial criteria for patient recruitment, erroneous inclusions cannot be reassuringly ruled out (Agosta et al., 2014). Additionally, misdiagnoses are not uncommon in ALS (Traynor et al., 2000) and these, typically early-stage, ALS patients may be left out from pharmaceutical trials.

3.1.2. Established Prognostic Indicators

Providing accurate prognosis and survival estimates in the early-stage ALS is challenging, as these are influenced by a myriad of demographic, genetic and clinical factors. There is a growing consensus among ALS experts that the most important determinants of poor prognosis in ALS include, bulbar-onset, cognitive impairment, poor nutritional status, respiratory compromise, older age at symptom onset, and carrying the hexanucleotide repeat on *C9orf72* (Chiò et al., 2009). Functional disability is monitored by the revised ALS Functional Rating Scale (ALSFRS-r) worldwide (Cedarbaum et al., 1999), which replaced the AALS scale (Appel ALS) (Appel et al., 1987). The ALSFRS-r is somewhat subjective as it is based on reported abilities in key domains of daily living, such as mobility, dexterity, respiratory and bulbar function. Despite its limitations, such as being disproportionately influenced by lower motor neuron dysfunction, the ALSFRS-r remains the gold standard instrument to monitor clinical trials outcomes. Prognostic modeling in ALS is typically approached in two ways; either focusing on survival or forecasting functional decline.

3.1.3. Current Practices in ALS for Patient Stratification

Current patient stratification goes little beyond key clinical features and core phenotypes. These typically include sporadic vs. familial, bulbar vs. spinal, ALS-FTD vs. ALS with no cognitive impairment (ALSnci) (Turner et al., 2013). A number of detailed patient classification schemes have been proposed based on the motor phenotype alone, as in Mora and Chiò (2015) and (Goutman, 2017): "classic," "bulbar," "flail arm," "flail

TABLE 1 | Overview of model pros & cons, updated from Hastie (2003).

Characteristics	Neural network	SVM	Decision tree	RF	Generelized linear model	Gaussian mixture model	k-NN	Boosting
Model complexity	High	High	Low	Fair	Low	High	Low	Fair
Sensitivity to data sparsity	High	High	Low	Fair	Low	High	High	Fair
Sensitivity to data bias	High	High	High	High	High	High	High	High
Interpretability	Poor	Poor	Fair	Poor	Good	Poor	Good	Poor
Predictive power	Good	Good	Poor	Good	Poor	Good	Poor	Good
Ability to extract linear combinations of features	Good	Good	Poor	Poor	Poor	Poor	Poor	Poor
Natural handling of missing values	Poor	Poor	Good	Good	Poor	Good	Good	Good
Robustness to outliers in input space	Poor	Poor	Good	Good	Fair	Good	Good	Good
Computational scalability	Poor	Poor	Good	Good	Good	Poor	Poor	Good

SVM, Support Vector Machine; RF, Random Forest; k-NN, k-Nearest Neighbors.

leg," "UMN-predominant," "LMN-predominant," "respiratory-onset," "PMA,""PLS," "Mills' syndrome," etc. Patients may also be classified into cognitive phenotypes such as ALS with cognitive impairment (ALSci), ALS with behavioral impairment (ALSbi), ALS-FTD, ALS with executive dysfunction (ALSexec) (Phukan et al., 2011), as presented in **Figure 1**. Diagnostic criteria for these phenotypes tend evolve, change and are often revisited once novel observations are made (Strong et al., 2017). Irrespective of the specific categorization criteria, these classification systems invariably rely on clinical evaluation, subjective observations, choice of screening tests, and are subsequently susceptible to classification error (Goutman, 2017). Adhering to phenotype definitions can be challenging, as performance cut-offs for some categories, such as cognitive subgroups (i.e., ALSbi/ ALSci) may be difficult to implement (Strong et al., 2009; Al-Chalabi et al., 2016). Al-Chalabi et al. (2016) used muscle bulk, tone, reflexes, age at onset, survival, diagnostic delay, ALSFRS-r decline, extra-motor involvement, symptom distribution, and family history as key features for patient stratification. ALS and FTD share common aetiological, clinical, genetic, radiological and pathological features and the existence of an ALS-FTD spectrum is now widely accepted. Up to 15% of patients develop frank dementia (Kiernan, 2018) and 60% show some form of cognitive or behavioral impairment (Phukan et al., 2011; Elamin et al., 2013; Kiernan, 2018). The presence of cognitive impairment is hugely relevant for machine-learning applications because neuropsychological deficits have been repeatedly linked to poorer survival outcomes (Elamin et al., 2011), increased caregiver burden (Burke et al., 2015), specific management challenges (Olney et al., 2005), and require different management strategies (Neary et al., 2000; Hu et al., 2009).

Clinical staging systems

One aspect of patient stratification is to place individual patients along the natural history of the disease by allocating them to specific disease phases or "stages." The utility of staging in ALS is 2-fold; it guides the timing of medical interventions (non-invasive ventilation, gastrostomy, advance directives) and also allows the separation of patients early in their disease trajectory from "late-phase" patients in clinical trials. Three staging systems have been recently developed; Kings' (Roche et al., 2012), MiToS (Chiò et al., 2013a), and Fine Till 9 (FT9) (Thakore et al., 2018). While the MiToS stage can be directly calculated based on ALSFRS-r scores, the Kings' stage is a derived measure. It is noteworthy, that the stages and the ALSFRS-r score are highly correlated (Balendra et al., 2014a). Both staging systems have been cross-validated, compared and they are thought to reflect on different aspects of the disease (Hardiman et al., 2017). The MiToS system is more sensitive to the later phases of the disease, while Kings' system reflects more on the earlier phases of ALS. The FT9 system is not partial to earlier or later stages. The FT9 framework defines stages based on ALSFRS-r subscores, using 9 as a threshold after testing different values on the PRO-ACT dataset. One of the criticism of MiToS, is that stage reversion is possible and that it does not directly capture disease progression (Balendra et al., 2014b). Ferraro et al. (2016) compared MiToS and King clinical staging systems and Thakore et al. (2018) compared all three systems on PRO-ACT data.

Current diagnostic approaches in ALS are suboptimal and often lead to considerable diagnostic delay. Prognostic protocols are not widely validated and current patient stratification frameworks don't represent the inherent heterogeneity of ALS. Accordingly, machine-learning approaches have been explored to specifically address these three issues.

3.2. Results in Diagnosis

3.2.1. Advances in Biomarker Research

The majority of ML research projects focus on the development, optimization, and validation of diagnostic biomarkers. These typically include clinical, biofluid, and neuroimaging indicators. Diagnostic model performance depends on the feature's ability to describe how the disease affects the subjects. Optimal diagnostic biomarkers should not only discriminate between ALS patients and healthy controls but also between ALS patients and patients with mimic or alternative neurological conditions (Bede, 2017). Ideally, an optimal diagnostic model should have outstanding early-stage sensitivity and specificity so that patients can be recruited into clinical trials early in their disease.

Clinical biomarker research

MUNIX (Fathi et al., 2016) is a non-invasive neurophysiological method which is extensively used in both clinical and research settings. It may also have the ability to capture pre-symptomatic motor neuron loss (Escorcio-Bezerra et al., 2018), therefore it has the potential to confirm early-stage disease in suspected cases. An earlier diagnosis would in turn enable the earlier initiation of neuroprotective therapy with established drugs and more importantly, earlier entry into clinical trials.

Biological biomarker research

Cerebrospinal Fluid (CSF) Neurofilaments (NF) are regarded as one of the most promising group of "wet" biomarkers in ALS (Rossi et al., 2018; Turner, 2018). Typically, research studies assess both Neurofilament Light (NF-L) chain and phosphorylated Heavy (pNF-H) chain levels that are released due to axonal degeneration and can be detected in the CSF and serum. Studies have consistently shown increased CSF pNF-H levels in ALS and up to ten times higher levels than in patients with Alzheimer disease (Brettschneider et al., 2006) or other neurological conditions (Gresle et al., 2014; Steinacker et al., 2015). Even though ALS studies have consistently detected raised pNF-H concentrations, these values vary considerably in the different reports. CSF NF-L levels were linked to reduced pyramidal tract Fractional Anisotropy (FA) and increased Radial Diffusivity (RD) (Menke et al., 2015) and NF-L levels are also thought to correlate with progression rates (Tortelli et al., 2014). Other biological biomarkers include proxies of oxidative stress, such as CSF 4-hydroxy-2,3-nonenal (4-HNE) (Simpson et al., 2004) or 3-nitrotyrosine (3-NT) (Tohgi et al., 1999). Neuroinflammation is another important feature of ALS, and several studies have detected an increase in inflammation-associated molecules, such as interleukin-6 (IL-6) and TNF alpha ($TNF - \alpha$) (Moreau et al., 2005) and galectin-3 (GAL-3) (Zhou et al., 2010). Increased levels of CSF Chitotriosidase-1 (CHIT1) is thought to indicate increased microglial activity (Varghese et al., 2013). Raised levels of CSF hydrogen sulfide (H_2S) was also reported in ALS, which is released by astrocytes and migrolia and is known to be toxic for motor neurons (Davoli et al., 2015). These are all promising wet biomarkers, indicative of disease-specific pathological processes and it is likely that a panel of several biomarkers may be best suited for diagnostic purposes.

Genetic biomarker research

A shared pathological hallmark of neurodegenerative conditions is protein aggregation. The accumulation of the Transactive Response DNA Binding Protein 43 (*TDP-43*) is the most consistent pathological finding in approximately 95% of ALS cases (Neumann et al., 2006). Given the widespread aggregation and accumulation of *TDP-43* in FTD-ALS spectrum, *TDP-43* detection, measurement or imaging is one of the most promising biomarkers strategies. A recent meta-analysis evaluated the diagnostic utility of CSF *TDP-43* levels in ALS (Majumder et al., 2018) and found that increased levels may be specific to ALS, as *TDP-43* levels are significantly raised compared to FTD as well. Reports on *SOD1* levels in the CSF of ALS patients have been inconsistent; some studies detected increased levels (Kokić et al., 2005) whereas others have identified decreased levels (Ihara et al., 2005) or levels comparable to controls (Zetterström et al., 2011).

Proteomics biomarker research

Beyond the interpretation of clinical and imaging data, ML models have an increasing role in genetics, RNA processing and proteomics (Bakkar et al., 2017). Using IBM Watson 5 new RNA-Binding Proteins (RBPs) were identified which were previously not linked to ALS; Heterogeneous nuclear ribonucleoprotein U (*hnRNPU*), Heterogeneous nuclear ribonucleoprotein Q (*SYNCRIP*), Putative RNA-binding protein 3 (*RBMS3*), ell Cycle Associated Protein 1 (*Caprin-1*) and Nucleoporin-like 2 (*NUPL2*). ML models play an important role in modern genetic analyses (Libbrecht and Noble, 2015) but considerable variations exist in their application between various medical subspecialties. One of the roles of ML in genomics is to identify the location of specific protein-encoding genes within a given DNA sequence (Mathé et al., 2002). In the field of proteomics, ML has been extensively utilized to predict 3-dimensional folding patterns of proteins. Approaches such as Deep Convolutional Neural Fields (DeepCNF) have been successful in predicting secondary structure configurations (Wang et al., 2016). In proteomics, ML models are also utilized for loop modeling, and protein side-chain prediction (Larranaga et al., 2006).

Imaging biomarker research

Neuroimaging offers unique, non-invasive opportunities to characterize disease-associated structural and functional changes and imaging derived metrics have been repeatedly proposed as candidate biomarkers (Turner et al., 2011; Agosta et al., 2018a; Bede et al., 2018b). The primary role of MRI in current clinical practice is the exclusion of alternative structural, neoplastic and inflammatory pathology in the brain or spinal cord which could manifest in UMN or LMN dysfunction similar to ALS. Diffusion tensor imaging (DTI) has gained a lot of attention as DTI-derived metrics, such as FA, Mean Diffusivity (MD), RD, or Axial Diffusivity (AD) have already been successfully used to identify ALS patients in ML models (RF) (Bede et al., 2017; Querin et al., 2018). The DTI signature of ALS is firmly established thanks to a myriad of imaging studies, and it includes the commissural fibers of the corpus callosum and the bilateral Corticospinal Tract (CST) (Turner et al., 2009; Bede et al., 2014). The latter has been associated to clinical UMN dysfunction, as well as rate of progression in specific sub-regions (Schuster et al., 2016a). White matter degeneration in frontal and temporal regions have been linked to cognitive and behavioral measures (Agosta et al., 2010; Christidi et al., 2017) and specific genotypes (Bede et al., 2013a). While callosal (Filippini et al., 2010; Bede et al., 2013a) and CST (Agosta et al., 2018b) degeneration seems to be a common ALS-associated signature, frontotemporal and cerebellar white matter degeneration seems to be more specific to certain phenotypes (Prell and Grosskreutz, 2013; Bede et al., 2014). From a gray matter perspective, motor cortex atrophy is a hallmark finding irrespective of specific genotypes and phenotypes (Bede et al., 2012) which is readily captured by cortical thickness or volumetric measures. Other gray matter regions, such as frontal (Lulé et al., 2007), basal ganglia (Bede et al., 2013c, 2018a; Machts et al., 2015), or cerebellar regions (Prell and Grosskreutz, 2013; Batyrbekova et al., 2018) may be more specific to certain patient cohorts. What is important to note, is that considerable white matter degeneration can already be detected around the time of diagnosis which progress relatively little, as opposed to the incremental gray matter findings in the post-symptomatic phase of the disease (Bede and Hardiman, 2017; Menke et al., 2018). The relevance of these observations is that white matter metrics may be particularly suitable for diagnostic models, whereas gray matter metrics in monitoring applications.

3.2.2. Overview of Research in Diagnosis

ML methods have already been extensively tested to aid the diagnosis of ALS (Gordon et al., 2009; Welsh et al., 2013; Sarica et al., 2016; Schuster et al., 2016b; Bede et al., 2017; Ferraro et al., 2017; Fratello et al., 2017; D'hulst et al., 2018; Li et al., 2018; Querin et al., 2018). Diagnostic models are typically developed within a classification framework with limited category labels, such as "healthy" vs. "ALS." Srivastava et al. (2012) implemented a model to discriminate patients within the Spinal Muscular Atrophy (SMA) spectrum. A similar attempt has not been made in ALS yet but could prove very valuable. A number of imaging features have been explored in recent years (Sarica et al., 2016; Schuster et al., 2016b; Bede et al., 2017; Ferraro et al., 2017; Fratello et al., 2017; D'hulst et al., 2018; Querin et al., 2018).

Performance was highest using combined imaging metrics (Bede et al., 2017) outperforming diagnostic models relying solely on clinical features (Li et al., 2018) which typically achieve up to 68% sensitivity and 87% specificity. Current models however are severely limited by small sample sizes and achieve lower true positive rates than the El Escorial's criteria but dramatically improve false negative rates. In general, diagnostic models based on imaging data achieve a sensitivity above 80% which is very encouraging especially given the emergence of larger data sets (Müller et al., 2016). It is crucial to evaluate model performance in comparison to the current gold standard criteria and report both sensitivity (true positive rate) and specificity (true negative rate). Additional metrics seem also necessary such as accuracy and AUC which provides a global indication of the model's performance.

Performance analysis

Welsh et al. (2013),Schuster et al. (2016b),Bede et al. (2017),Ferraro et al. (2017),Fratello et al. (2017),D'hulst et al. (2018), and Querin et al. (2018) only used single-centre imaging data for their model design. Bede et al. (2017) used a canonical discriminant function and achieved an accuracy of 90% (for 90% sensitivity and 90% specificity). Sarica et al. (2016),Ferraro et al. (2017),Fratello et al. (2017), and Querin et al. (2018) used RFs achieving accuracy rates between 77.5 and 86.5%. Schuster et al. (2016b) used a binary logistic regression model and reached 78.4% (90.5% sensitivity and 62.5% specificity). Welsh et al. (2013) and D'hulst et al. (2018) used SVMs reaching an accuracy of 71 and 80%, respectively. A relatively low accuracy of 71% (Welsh et al., 2013) and low specificity of 12.5% (D'hulst et al., 2018) may stem from model overfitting. The complexity of SVM models, class imbalance (D'hulst et al., 2018), data sparsity (Welsh et al., 2013) are some of the factors which may contribute to their relatively poorer performance. Li et al. (2018) used a linear regression model based on clinical data and reached 77.5% accuracy, 68% sensitivity and 87% specificity. Half of the studies (Welsh et al., 2013; Sarica et al., 2016; Bede et al., 2017; D'hulst et al., 2018; Querin et al., 2018) focused on discriminating ALS patients from healthy controls. Four studies (Gordon et al., 2009; Ferraro et al., 2017; Fratello et al., 2017; Li et al., 2018) went further and attempted to identify ALS within a range of neurological diseases including patients with Parkinson's Disease (PD), Kennedy's Disease (KD), PLS, etc. Srivastava et al. (2012) focused on identifying specific SMA phenotypes. Please refer to **Table 2** for an overview of ML papers focusing on the diagnosis of ALS.

Technical analysis

From a methods point of view, all of the above papers overtly present their pre-processing pipeline (Sarica et al., 2016; Schuster et al., 2016b; Bede et al., 2017; Ferraro et al., 2017; Fratello et al., 2017; D'hulst et al., 2018; Querin et al., 2018) and feature selection strategy (Gordon et al., 2009; Srivastava et al., 2012; Welsh et al., 2013; Sarica et al., 2016; Schuster et al., 2016b; Bede et al., 2017; Fratello et al., 2017; Querin et al., 2018). Imaging analyses need to take the effect of age, gender, and education on MRI data into account, as these have a major impact on white and gray matter metrics. Studies control for these demographic factors differently; while age is generally adjusted for (Zhang et al., 2018), the effect of gender (Bede et al., 2013b) and education (Cox et al., 2016) are often overlooked which can affect model development. Judicious feature selection is paramount as model complexity is directly related to the number of features fed into the model. Limiting model complexity, especially in the context of sparse data is crucial to avoid model overfitting. Feature selection is often based, either on group comparisons or a priori imaging or pathological information. Features often include imaging measures of key, disease-associated anatomical regions, such as measures of the motor cortex or pyramidal tracts (Bede et al., 2016). Existing studies use very different validation schemes to test model performance. Cross-validation is the most commonly used (Srivastava et al., 2012; Sarica et al., 2016; Schuster et al., 2016b; Fratello et al., 2017; Querin et al., 2018), followed by holdout validation (Bede et al., 2017; Ferraro et al., 2017) and leave-one-out validation (Welsh et al., 2013; D'hulst et al., 2018). While robust validation schemes are essential, they don't circumvent overfitting especially when limited data are available. "Cross validation" and "leave-one-out" approaches are generally more robust than holdout validation. Special caution should be exercised with regards to validation reports in sparse data situations, where validation schemes have a limited ability to assess model performance. Querin et al. (2018) and Li et al. (2018) both show SFR higher than ten (15 and 12 ,respectively) which comply with minimum SFR recommendations (Raudys, 2001).

TABLE 2 | Research overview: diagnosis.

Key	Dataset(s) origin	Dataset(s) type	Dataset(s) length	Scope	Biomarker(s) type	Pre-processing (if any)	Validation (if any)	Model(s) tested	Performance
Gordon et al., 2009	Eleanor and Lou Gehrig MDA/ALS Research Center	Real-life	34	ALS, UMN, PLS	Clinical	FS	None described	Linear regression	-
Srivastava et al., 2012	Boston Children Hospital	Real-life	46	SMA phenotypes	Clinical, genetic	FS	CV	SVM	AUC (0.928)
Welsh et al., 2013	Michigan MND Clinic	Real-life	63	ALS, healthy	Imaging	FS	LOOV	SVM	AUC:0.7, Acc:71%, Spec:74%, Sens:68.8%
Sarica et al., 2016	Catanzaro Magna Graecia University	Real-life	48	ALS, healthy	Clinical, imaging	SP, FS	CV	RF	Acc:80%
Schuster et al., 2016b	Trinity College Dublin	Real-life	147	ALS, healthy	Imaging	SP, FS	CV	Logistic regression	Acc:78.4%, Sens:90.5%, Spec:62.5%
Bede et al., 2017	Trinity College Dublin	Real-life	150	ALS, healthy	Imaging	SP, FS	HOV	Discriminant function	Acc:90%, Sens:90%, Spec:90%
Ferraro et al., 2017	MND Clinics in Northern Italy	Real-life	265	ALS, UMN, ALS mimics	Imaging	SP	HOV	RF	Acc:87%, Spec:75%, Sens:92%
Fratello et al., 2017	UK PD Brain Bank	Real-life	120	ALS, PD, healthy	Imaging	SP, FS	CV	RF	Acc:80%
D'hulst et al., 2018	University Hospital Leuven and Turino ALS Center	Real-life	370	ALS, healthy	Imaging	SP	LOOV	SVM	Acc:80%, Sens:85%, Spec:12.5%
Li et al., 2018	Australia	Clinical trial	81	ALS, KD, ALS mimics	Clinical	FS	None described	Linear regression	Acc:77.5%, Sens:68%, Spec:87%
Querin et al., 2018	Pitiè Salpêtrière Hospital	Real-life	105	ALS, healthy	Imaging	SP	CV	RF	AUC:0.96, Acc:86.5%, Sens:88%, Spec:85%

CV, Cross Validation; LOOV, Leave One Out Validation; HOV, Hold Out Validation; AUC, Area under the ROC Curve; Acc, Accuracy; Sens, Sensitivity; Spec, Specificity; PD, Parkinson's Disease; FS, Feature Selection; SP, Signal Processing.

3.3. Results in Prognosis

3.3.1. Advances in Biomarker Research

As the precise mechanisms of disease propagation in ALS are largely unknown (Ravits, 2014; Ayers et al., 2015), research has focused on the identification of candidate prognostic biomarkers including potential clinical, biological, imaging, and genetic indicators. Prognostic model performance depends on the feature's ability to capture the disease spread. Optimal prognostic biomarkers should not only discriminate between different ALS phenotypes but categorize individual patients to common disease progression rates (slow vs. fast progressors) (Schuster et al., 2015).

Clinical biomarker research

Several recent studies examined the specific impact of psychosocial factors, cognitive impairment, nutritional status and respiratory compromise, on prognosis. Psychosocial adjustments in ALS may have an under-recognized impact on prognosis (Matuz et al., 2015). The potential effect of mood on disease progression has only been investigated on a relatively small number of samples to date (Johnston et al., 1999).

Biological biomarker research

Recent research suggests that prognostic modeling that does not rely on a priori hypotheses could lead to more accurate prognostic models than does driven by pre-existing hypotheses. For instance, elevations in Creatine Kinase (CK) were linked to LMN involvement and faster disease progression (Rafiq et al., 2016; Goutman, 2017) using the PRO-ACT data (Ong et al., 2017).

Genetic biomarker research

In a clinical setting, genetic testing is often only performed in familial forms of ALS. *C9orf72* repeat expansions account for

40% of hereditary ALS cases and 10% of sporadic ALS cases (Goutman, 2017) and hexanucleotide repeats are associated with specific clinical traits (Byrne et al., 2012). More than 30 genes have been implicated in the pathogenesis of ALS to date and samples are often screened for Angiogenin (*ANG*), Dynactin subunit 1 (*DCTN1*), Fused in sarcoma (*FUS*), Optineurin (*OPTN*), *SOD1*, Transactive Response DNA Binding Protein (*TARDBP*), Ubiquilin (*UBQLN2*), Valosin-Containing Protein (*VCP*) (Chen et al., 2013; Renton et al., 2013; Taylor J. P. et al., 2016), Alsin Rho Guanine Nucleotide Exchange Factor (*ALS2*), Polyphosphoinositide phosphatase (*FIG4*), Probable Helicase Senataxin (*SETX*), Spatacsin (*SPG11*), Vesicle-Associated membrane protein-associated Protein B/C (*VAPB*) (Chen et al., 2013; Renton et al., 2013), Heterogeneous nuclear ribonucleoprotein A1 (*HNRNPA1*), Profilin 1 (*PFN1*), Sequestosome 1 (*SQSTM1*) (Renton et al., 2013; Taylor J. P. et al., 2016), Coiled-coil-helix-coiled-coil-helix domain-containing protein 10 (*CHCHD10*), Matrin 3 (*MATR3*), Serine/Threonine-protein Kinase (*TBK1*) (Taylor J. P. et al., 2016), sigma-1 receptor (*SIGMAR1*), Diamine oxidase (*DAO*) (Chen et al., 2013), Charged multivesicular body protein 2b (*CHMP2B*), Ataxin-2 (*ATXN2*), Neurofilament Heavy (NEFH), Elongator complex protein 3 (*ELP3*) (Renton et al., 2013) as well as Receptor tyrosine-protein kinase (*ERBB4*), Unc-13 homolog A (*UNC13A*), Peripherin (*PRPH*), TATA-binding protein-associated factor 2N (*TAF15*), Spastin (*SPAST*), Lamin-B1 (*LMNB1*), Sterile alpha and TIR motif-containing protein 1 (*SARM1*), *C21orf2*, (never in mitosis gene a)-related kinase 1 (*NEK1*), Granulin Precursor (*GRN*), Microtubule Associated Protein Tau (*MAPT*) and Presenilin 2 (*PSEN2*). IBM Watson software has been successfully utilized to identify other candidate genes; such as *hnRNPU*, *SYNCRIP*, *RBMS3*, *Caprin-1* and *NUPL2* (Bakkar et al., 2017). Genomic research teams have increasingly capitalized on ML methods worldwide, as they can handle copious amounts of data for systematic processing, genomic sequence annotation, DNA pattern recognition, gene expression prediction, and the identification of genomic element combinations (Libbrecht and Noble, 2015).

The benefit of multiparametric datasets

Early machine learning efforts have been hampered by the lack of large data sets in ALS, which is increasingly addressed by the availability of large international repositories, such as those maintained by NISALS (Müller et al., 2016; Neuroimaging Society in ALS, 2018), NEALS (NEALS Consortium, 2018), and PRO-ACT which includes more than 10 000 patient records from 23 clinical trials in total. Similar initiatives had been carried out in other neurological conditions, as part of the Alzheimer's Disease Neuroimaging Initiative (ADNI) (Mueller et al., 2005), the Parkinson's Progression Marker's Initiative (PPMI) (Marek et al., 2011) and Tract HD (Tabrizi et al., 2012). Emerging large data sets, like PRO-ACCT, also serve as validation platforms for previously identified biomarkers. For example, vital capacity was identified as early as 1993 (Schiffman and Belsh, 1993) as a predictor of disease progression and proved relevant in the Prize4Life challenge (Küffner et al., 2014). Other validated biomarkers include creatinine (Atassi et al., 2014; Küffner et al., 2014; Ong et al., 2017), BMI (Atassi et al., 2014; Küffner et al., 2014; Ong et al., 2017), CK (Ong et al., 2017), Alkaline Phosphatase (ALP)(Küffner et al., 2014; Ong et al., 2017), albumin (Ong et al., 2017), total birilubin (Ong et al., 2017), and uric acid (Atassi et al., 2014). Other predictive clinical features such as onset at age, region of onset, and respiratory compromise have long been firmly established (Chio et al., 2009; Creemers et al., 2014).

3.3.2. Overview of Research in Prognosis

While prognostic forecasting has historically been undertaken using traditional statistical approaches in ALS (Ince et al., 2003; Forbes, 2004; Visser et al., 2007; Coon et al., 2011; Atassi et al., 2014; Elamin et al., 2015; Marin et al., 2015; Rong et al., 2015; Tortelli et al., 2015; Wolf et al., 2015; Knibb et al., 2016; Reniers et al., 2017), ML models have an unprecedented potential to identify novel prognostic indicators (Gomeni and Fava, 2013; Hothorn and Jung, 2014; Ko et al., 2014; Beaulieu-Jones and Greene, 2016; Taylor A. A. et al., 2016; Huang et al., 2017; Jahandideh et al., 2017; Ong et al., 2017; Schuster et al., 2017; Seibold et al., 2017; van der Burgh et al., 2017; Bandini et al., 2018; Pfohl et al., 2018; Westeneng et al., 2018). Most prognostic models use clinical features to determine prognosis in ALS but two recent papers enriched their clinical data with imaging measures (Schuster et al., 2017; van der Burgh et al., 2017). Seven studies designed their prediction model around both clinical and biological data, (Hothorn and Jung, 2014; Ko et al., 2014; Beaulieu-Jones and Greene, 2016; Huang et al., 2017; Jahandideh et al., 2017; Ong et al., 2017; Seibold et al., 2017) and nine studies developed their prognostic model based on PRO-ACT data, (Gomeni and Fava, 2013; Hothorn and Jung, 2014; Ko et al., 2014; Beaulieu-Jones and Greene, 2016; Taylor A. A. et al., 2016; Huang et al., 2017; Jahandideh et al., 2017; Ong et al., 2017; Seibold et al., 2017). Prognosis is typically defined either as functional decline or survival and is either approached as a classification problem with predefined categories or as a regression problem with a specific survival or functional thresholds. The most accurate regression approach had a RMSE of 0.52 (with regards to the ALSFRS rate) (Hothorn and Jung, 2014) and one of the most accurate classification method (Ko et al., 2014) reached 66% accuracy, 66% sensitivity, and 65% specificity using a RF. Bandini et al. (2018) achieved 87% accuracy with a SVM model a fairly complex model built on only 64 samples - which puts the model at a high risk of overfitting. For outcome prediction as a regression problem, best results were reached by Pfohl et al. (2018) using a RF. For outcome prediction as a classification problem, best performance was achieved by Westeneng et al. (2018) with 78% accuracy using a multivariate Royston-Parmar model.

Statistical methods

Previous prognostic studies in ALS primarily used traditional statistical approaches, mostly Cox regressions, mixed effect models and Kaplan-Meier estimators. These models have relatively stringent data assumptions which limit model validity and limit data exploration. Nevertheless, they were instrumental in identifying key prognosis indicators in ALS, such as diagnostic delay (Forbes, 2004; Elamin et al., 2015; Marin et al., 2015; Wolf et al., 2015; Knibb et al., 2016; Reniers et al., 2017), age at symptom onset (Forbes, 2004; Marin et al., 2015; Wolf et al., 2015; Knibb et al., 2016; Reniers et al., 2017), functional disability (Visser et al., 2007; Elamin et al., 2015; Marin et al., 2015; Wolf et al., 2015; Reniers et al., 2017), El Escorial categorization (Forbes, 2004; Marin et al., 2015; Wolf et al., 2015), comorbid FTD or executive dysfunction (Elamin et al., 2015; Wolf et al., 2015; Knibb et al., 2016), site of onset (Forbes, 2004; Elamin et al., 2015), Riluzole therapy (Forbes, 2004; Knibb et al., 2016), vital capacity (Visser et al., 2007), muscle weakness (Visser et al., 2007), involvement of body regions (Visser et al., 2007), gender (Wolf et al., 2015), BMI (Atassi et al., 2014), presence of *C9orf72* mutations (Reniers et al., 2017). Other prognostic studies focused on the macrophage marker Cluster of Differentiation 68 (*CD68*) (Ince et al., 2003), neuropsychological deficits (Coon et al., 2011), creatinine and uric acid levels (Atassi et al., 2014), tongue kinematics (Rong et al., 2015), anatomical spread (Tortelli et al., 2015), and LMN involvement (Reniers et al., 2017). A number of studies have specifically focused on survival (Forbes, 2004; Visser et al., 2007; Coon et al., 2011; Atassi et al., 2014; Elamin et al., 2015; Marin et al., 2015; Tortelli et al., 2015; Wolf et al., 2015; Reniers et al., 2017). Ince et al. (2003) performed an a posteriori analysis of disease progression based on MRI data. Coon et al. (2011) analyzed the impact of language deficits and behavioral impairment on survival. Rong et al. (2015) assessed the implications of early bulbar involvement. To this date, most reliable predictive features are clinical factors, but similar approaches can be extended to biofluid, genetic, and imaging data. Both ML and traditional statistical approaches perform better with multi-modal data. Existing ML studies in ALS show considerable differences in their methodology and validation approaches. Please refer to **Table 3** for an overview of ALS papers focusing on prognostic modeling.

Performance analyses

RF is the most commonly used model in ALS, implemented in eight of the fourteen reviewed studies (Hothorn and Jung, 2014; Ko et al., 2014; Beaulieu-Jones and Greene, 2016; Taylor A. A. et al., 2016; Huang et al., 2017; Jahandideh et al., 2017; Seibold et al., 2017; Pfohl et al., 2018) and it is also one of the best performing methods (Beaulieu-Jones and Greene, 2016; Taylor A. A. et al., 2016; Huang et al., 2017; Pfohl et al., 2018). Boosting, another ensemble method, was tested by Jahandideh et al. (2017) and Ong et al. (2017). The boosting algorithm outperformed the RF model in Jahandideh et al. (2017). NN models were used successfully in two studies: Beaulieu-Jones and Greene (2016) and van der Burgh et al. (2017). Regression models have also been extensively used in ALS, including generalized linear models (Taylor A. A. et al., 2016; Huang et al., 2017; Pfohl et al., 2018), Royston-Parmar models for Westeneng et al. (2018), and non-linear Weibull models (Gomeni and Fava, 2013). Regression models, despite their stringent assumptions, have great potential in clinical applications (Westeneng et al., 2018). Seibold et al. (2017) used an innovative RF approach to establish the impact of Riluzole therapy on functional decline and survival. Out of the ten models built on clinical data, nine were based on PRO-ACT data (Gomeni and Fava, 2013; Hothorn and Jung, 2014; Ko et al., 2014; Beaulieu-Jones and Greene, 2016; Taylor A. A. et al., 2016; Huang et al., 2017; Jahandideh et al., 2017; Ong et al., 2017; Seibold et al., 2017).

Prognosis in ALS is typically either addressed as a classification or a regression problem. In studies using the classification approach, categories are defined based on functional decline (Gomeni and Fava, 2013; Ko et al., 2014; Ong et al., 2017; Westeneng et al., 2018), survival (Schuster et al., 2017; Pfohl et al., 2018), or disease phase (Bandini et al., 2018). Studies using the regression approach predicted survival (Beaulieu-Jones and Greene, 2016; Huang et al., 2017; van der Burgh et al., 2017; Pfohl et al., 2018), Riluzole effect (Seibold et al., 2017), functional decline (Hothorn and Jung, 2014; Taylor A. A. et al., 2016), or respiratory function (Jahandideh et al., 2017). ALSFRS-r is invariably used in these studies, highlighting that it remains the gold standard instrument to monitor disease progression. Most prognostic models rely solely on clinical features,sometimes enriched with biological data. Radiological data are seldom used in these models, and often rely on relatively small datasets; Schuster et al. (2017) included 69 and van der Burgh et al. (2017) 135 subjects. Despite their considerable sample size limitations, these models achieved relatively promising results with accuracy rates above 79%. Unfortunately, as in the case of diagnostic modeling, large datasets of imaging data, especially longitudinal, are still relatively difficult to acquire in single-centre settings.

A variety of metrics have been utilized for model performance evaluation. For classification tasks, these typically include AUC, specificity and sensitivity, accuracy and concordance (C-index), and for regression methods, RMSE, R^2, mean absolute error, and Pearson correlations between real and predicted estimates are usually reported. Approximately half of the reviewed papers used RF to assess variable importance (Hothorn and Jung, 2014; Huang et al., 2017; Jahandideh et al., 2017; Ong et al., 2017; Seibold et al., 2017; Pfohl et al., 2018; Westeneng et al., 2018). Pfohl et al. (2018) carried out correlation analysis and PCA component projection analysis which proved very instructive. Gamma glutamyl-transferase, was identified as a potential prognostic indicator by Ong et al. (2017). Despite the obvious advantages, model testing is only rarely carried out on external data sets (Jahandideh et al., 2017) for which population data should ideally be used (Taylor A. A. et al., 2016). Many referral centres develop models based on local datasets (Schuster et al., 2017; van der Burgh et al., 2017; Pfohl et al., 2018), which are more accessible than population-based data. Population-based data are increasingly available thanks to national (Donaghy et al., 2009; Talman et al., 2016) and regional (Rosenbohm et al., 2017) registries and increasingly thanks to international consortia (Turner et al., 2011; Müller et al., 2016; Westeneng et al., 2018).

The direct comparison of model performances in ALS ML studies is challenging as performance metrics, prediction targets, sample sizes and study designs are hugely divergent. There is little evidence that a specific type of input data, clinical features alone or clinical data enriched with other data types, enhances model performance. This is due to the lack of large

TABLE 3 | Research overview: prognosis with statistical models.

Key	Dataset(s) origin	Dataset(s) type	Dataset(s) length	Scope	Biomarker(s) type	Pre-processing (if any)	Validation (if any)	Model(s) tested
Ince et al., 2003	Newcastle upon Tyne MND clinic	Real-life	81	Progression	Imaging	None described	Not required	Univariate analysis
Forbes, 2004	Scottish ALS-MND Register	Population	1226	Outcome	Clinical	None described	Not required	Cox time dependent regression modeling
Visser et al., 2007	Dutch university hospitals	Real-life	37	Outcome	Clinical, genetic, biological	None described	Not required	Univariate analysis
Coon et al., 2011	Mayo Clinic	Real-life	56	Outcome	Clinical, imaging	None described	Not required	KM analysis
Atassi et al., 2014	PRO-ACT	Clinical trial	8635	Outcome, progression	Clinical, biological	Data cleaning	Not required	Multivariate analysis
Elamin et al., 2015	Irish and Italian (Piemonte) ALS registry	Population	326	Outcome	Clinical, genetic	FS	HOV	Proportional hazards Cox
Marin et al., 2015	FRALim register	Population	322	Outcome	Clinical	None described	Not required	Cox regression (KM)
Rong et al., 2015	-	Clinical trial	66	Progression	Clinical	FS	Not required	Linear Mixed Effect, KM analysis
Tortelli et al., 2015	University of Bari MND Center	Clinical trial	145	Outcome	Clinical	None described	Not required	Bivariate model for correlation
Wolf et al., 2015	Rhineland-Palatinate Register	Population	193	Outcome	Clinical	FS	Not required	Cox proportional hazards
Knibb et al., 2016	South-East England Register	Population	575	Outcome, progression	Clinical	MVR	CV	Cox proportional hazards, ACT
Reniers et al., 2017	University Hospitals Leuven	Real-life	396	Outcome	Clinical	None described	Not required	Univariate and multivariate Cox regression

HOV, Hold Out Validation; CV, Cross Validation; ACT, Accelerated Failure Time; KM, Kaplan Meier; MVR, Missing Value Removal; FS, Feature Selection.

scale databases which routinely store biological samples and imaging data along with clinical observations. It is likely that the incorporation of genetic, biological, and imaging features, will improve prognostic modeling. Some studies candidly discuss their methodological limitations, and model overfitting is the most often cited shortcoming. Data censoring is often mentioned when using PRO-ACT data and selection bias when relying on clinical trial data. Most studies discuss the issues around feature selection and the importance of limiting feature dimension. Model interpretability concerns are sometimes raised when using NN models (van der Burgh et al., 2017). Westeneng et al. (2018) published their findings according to the methodology introduced by Moons et al. (2015) setting an example of performance reporting. Please refer to **Tables 4, 5** for an overview of ML studies in ALS focusing on prognostic projections.

Data management approaches

Most studies perform some kind of data pre-processing, such as feature selection (Gomeni and Fava, 2013; Ko et al., 2014; Taylor A. A. et al., 2016; Huang et al., 2017; Jahandideh et al., 2017; Schuster et al., 2017; Bandini et al., 2018; Pfohl et al., 2018; Westeneng et al., 2018), signal processing (Schuster et al., 2017; van der Burgh et al., 2017; Bandini et al., 2018), and address missing data (Hothorn and Jung, 2014; Beaulieu-Jones and Greene, 2016; Taylor A. A. et al., 2016; Huang et al., 2017; Jahandideh et al., 2017; Ong et al., 2017; Seibold et al., 2017; Pfohl et al., 2018; Westeneng et al., 2018). Feature importance analysis prior to model design provides important insights before feature selection (Hothorn and Jung, 2014; Taylor A. A. et al., 2016; Huang et al., 2017; Jahandideh et al., 2017; Ong et al., 2017; Seibold et al., 2017; Pfohl et al., 2018). Feature selection

TABLE 4 | Research overview: Prognosis with ML models (1/2).

Key	Dataset(s) origin	Dataset(s) type	Dataset(s) length	Scope	Biomarker(s) type	Pre-processing (if any)	Validation (if any)	Model(s) tested	Performance	Framework
Gomeni and Fava, 2013	PRO-ACT	Clinical trial	338	Progression	Clinical	FS	HOV	non-linear Weibull	AUC:0.96	Classification
Hothorn and Jung, 2014	PRO-ACT	Clinical trial	1822	Progression	Clinical, biological	MVI, VIA	HOV	RF	RMSE:0.52 (ALSFRS rate), PC:40%	Regression
Ko et al., 2014	PRO-ACT	Clinical trial	1822	Progression	Clinical, biological	FS	HOV	RF	Spec:66%, Sens:65%, Acc:66%	Classification
Beaulieu-Jones and Greene, 2016	PRO-ACT	Clinical trial	3398	Outcome	Clinical, biological	MVI	CV	NN, RF, SVM, k-NN, DT, NN with RF (best)	AUC:0.692	Classification
Taylor A. A. et al., 2016	PRO-ACT, Emery ALS Clinic	Clinical trial, real-life	4372	Progression	Clinical	FS, MVR, VIA	HOV	GLM, RF (best)	R^2:58.2%, MC:0.942, ME:-0.627 (ALSFRS score)	Regression
van der Burgh et al., 2017	University Medical Center Utrecht	Real-life	135	Outcome	Clinical, imaging	SP	HOV	NN	Acc:84.4%	Classification
Huang et al., 2017	PRO-ACT	Clinical trial	6565	Outcome	Clinical, biological	FS, MVR, VIA	CV	GP, Lasso, RF (best)	C-ind:0.717	Regression
Jahandideh et al., 2017	PRO-ACT, NEALS	Clinical trial, population	4406	Progression	Clinical, biological	FS, MVI, VIA	CV	RF, XGBoost, GBM (best)	RMSE:0.635 (FVC), R^2:66.9%	Regression
Ong et al., 2017	PRO-ACT	Clinical trial	1568-6355	Progression, outcome	Clinical, biological	MVR, VIA	CV	Boosting	For P: AUC:0.82, Acc:56.5%, Spec:74%, Sens:39%, For O: AUC:0.83, Acc:76.7%, Spec:76.1%, Sens:77.3%	Classification

CV, Cross Validation; HOV, Hold Out Validation; AUC, Area under the ROC Curve; Acc, Accuracy; Sens, Sensitivity; Spec, Specificity; MC,Model Calibration; ME, Mean Error; PC, Pearson's Correlation; DT, Decision Tree; GLM, Generalized Linear Model; k-NN, k-Nearest Neighbors; FS, Feature Selection; MVI, Missing Value Imputation; VIA, Variable Importance Analysis; MVR, Missing Value Removal; P, Progression; O, Outcome; C-ind, Concordance; GP, Gaussian Process; GBM, Gradient Boosting Model; SP, Signal Processing; FVC, Forced Vital Capacity.

is automated when using RF, NN, or boosting models. Missing data management is crucial when dealing with medical data sets as it has a strong impact on data bias and overall model performance. Huang et al. (2017),Seibold et al. (2017),Taylor A. A. et al. (2016), and Ong et al. (2017) discarded data samples with missing features which can introduce further bias in sparse data situations. Mean imputation, which is a simple imputation method, was performed by Jahandideh et al. (2017) and Hothorn and Jung (2014). Simple imputation methods can increase bias in data as these methods assume missing 'completely at random' characteristics which rarely reflect real-life scenarios. Consequently, multiple imputation approaches such as NN approaches (Beaulieu-Jones and Greene, 2016) or MICE (Westeneng et al., 2018) are favored. With few exceptions, Seibold et al. (2017), most studies report their validation framework in detail. Cross-validation schemes are used by some (Beaulieu-Jones and Greene, 2016; Huang et al., 2017; Jahandideh et al., 2017; Ong et al., 2017; Bandini et al., 2018; Pfohl et al., 2018; Westeneng et al., 2018) and hold out validation schemes are implemented by others (Gomeni and Fava, 2013; Hothorn and Jung, 2014; Ko et al., 2014; Taylor A. A. et al., 2016; van der Burgh et al., 2017). Dataset population ranges between 64 and 11 475 samples which explains the considerable methodological differences in pre-processing, data analysis and overall model design. SFR ranges between < 1 (with 135 samples for 2 376 features (van der Burgh et al., 2017)) to close to 1100 (with 6 565 samples for 6 features (Huang et al., 2017)). Small SFRs are mostly due to either data type scarcity (Schuster et al., 2017; van der Burgh et al., 2017; Bandini et al., 2018) or the use of complex models such as NN (Beaulieu-Jones and Greene, 2016).

TABLE 5 | Research overview: Prognosis with ML models (2/2).

Key	Dataset(s) origin	Dataset(s) type	Dataset(s) length	Scope	Biomarker(s) type	Pre-processing (if any)	Validation (if any)	Model(s) tested	Performance	Framework
Schuster et al., 2017	Trinity College Dublin	Real-life	69	Outcome	Clinical, imaging	SP, FS	CV	Logistic regression	Spec:83.34%, Sens:75%, Acc:79.19%	Classification
Seibold et al., 2017	PRO-ACT	Clinical trial	2534-3306	Progression, outcome	Clinical, biological	MVR, VIA	None	RF	Treatment effect on outcome and progression	Regression
Bandini et al., 2018	-	Clinical trial	64	Progression	Clinical	SP, FS	CV	k-NN, SVM (best)	Spec:86.1%, Sens:88.8%, Acc:87%	Classification
Pfohl et al., 2018	Emery ALS Clinic	Real-life	801	Outcome	Clinical	MVI, FS, VIA	CV	GLM, RF (best)	RMSE:547 +/-46 days, R^2:52%, AUC:0.85	Regression, Classification
Westeneng et al., 2018	14 European ALS centers	Real-life	11475	Outcome	Clinical	FS, MVI	CV	MRP	Acc:78%, MC:1.01, AUC:0.86	Classification

CV, Cross Validation; AUC, Area under the ROC Curve; Acc, Accuracy; Sens, Sensitivity; Spec, Specificity; MC, Model Calibration; GLM, Generalized Linear Model; k-NN, k-Nearest Neighbors; MRP, Multivariate Royston-Parmar; FS, Feature Selection; MVI, Missing Value Imputation; VIA, Variable Importance Analysis; MVR, Missing Value Removal;SP, Signal Processing.

Six studies have used less than nine features for model design (Gomeni and Fava, 2013; Hothorn and Jung, 2014; Ko et al., 2014; Huang et al., 2017; Ong et al., 2017; Westeneng et al., 2018) reaching SFRs over 100 samples per feature.

3.4. Advances in Risk Stratification

Accurate patient stratification is not only essential for clinical trial designs but also for individualized patient care (Kiernan, 2018). Current stratification strategies are surprisingly limited and do not utilize patient clustering for pharmaceutical research and medical interventions. Only two drugs have been approved by the FDA to treat ALS to date: Riluzole (Rilutek) and Edavarone (Radicava). While there is some debate if the maximal therapeutic benefit of Riluzole may be in late-stage disease (Dharmadasa et al., 2018; Fang et al., 2018), recent research suggest that Edavarone effect may be superior in the earlier phases of ALS (Goutman, 2017; Kiernan, 2018). It is also noteworthy, that past clinical trials were primarily based on heterogeneous ALS populations. The inconclusive findings of admixed cohorts may not apply to specific patient subgroups (Bozik et al., 2014) or presymptomatic cohorts. Rigorous patient stratification would have an important role in addressing these shortcomings. Unsupervised learning methods, such as the one carried out by Beaulieu-Jones and Greene (2016) using denoised autoencoder and t-distributed Stochastic Neighbor Embedding (t-SNE), provide novel means of monitoring patients. However, as for most unsupervised learning methods, selecting the appropriate number of patient clusters requires extensive empirical testing.

3.4.1. Overview of Stratification Initiatives

Patient stratification in ALS is often explored from a prognostic perspective (Visser et al., 2007; Gomeni and Fava, 2013; Ko et al., 2014; Elamin et al., 2015; Marin et al., 2015; Beaulieu-Jones and Greene, 2016; Ong et al., 2017; van der Burgh et al., 2017; Pfohl et al., 2018; Westeneng et al., 2018) approaching it as a classification problem and patient categories are defined to build the model. Balendra et al. (2014a) analyzed progression patterns using the King's staging system. Clinical stages are potential input variables for stratification, and therapeutic intervention can be tested based on disease subgroups or disease stage.

Patient stratification was performed based on clinical observations alone in seven recent studies (Visser et al., 2007; Balendra et al., 2014a; Ko et al., 2014; Elamin et al., 2015; Burke et al., 2017; van der Burgh et al., 2017; Pfohl et al., 2018). Variables, such as limb involvement (Visser et al., 2007), disease-stage (Balendra et al., 2014a), ALSFRS-r decline (Ko et al., 2014), executive dysfunction (Elamin et al., 2015), behavioral impairment (Burke et al., 2017), and survival (van der Burgh et al., 2017; Pfohl et al., 2018) have been used for patient stratification. Other studies relied on unsupervised techniques to identify patient subgroups. These methods either used model estimation (Gomeni and Fava, 2013; Westeneng et al., 2018), K-means (Ong et al., 2017), a tree-growing algorithm called Recursive Partitioning and Amalgation (Marin et al., 2015) or NNs with a denoising autoencoder (Beaulieu-Jones and Greene, 2016). Clustering was performed either based on clinical features alone (Gomeni and Fava, 2013; Marin et al., 2015; Westeneng et al., 2018) or based on clinical features and biological data (Beaulieu-Jones and Greene, 2016; Ong et al., 2017).

Contrary to supervised learning problems, unsupervised learning methods do not have clear and easily presentable performance metrics. Possible options include the description of inter- and intra-patient subgroup distances and outlier distribution. The optimal number of models (equivalent to cluster number) can be identified using an iterative procedure for studies based on model estimation (Gomeni and Fava, 2013; Westeneng et al., 2018).

Clustering methods

Patient clustering was performed on various datasets in ALS; clinical trial data (Gomeni and Fava, 2013; Balendra et al., 2014a; Ko et al., 2014; Ong et al., 2017), "real-life data" (Visser et al., 2007; van der Burgh et al., 2017; Pfohl et al., 2018; Westeneng et al., 2018) and population data (Elamin et al., 2015; Marin et al., 2015; Burke et al., 2017). The term "real-life" data is used to samples which derive from local recruitment, typically single-center non-pharmacological studies, where data are acquired prospectively but do not represent entire populations. Access to large patient databases with limited missing data is fundamental to the development of accurate stratification schemes. Recent initiatives such as the Prize4Life challenge (Küffner et al., 2014), the PRO-ACT database and Euro-MOTOR consortium (Rooney et al., 2017; Visser et al., 2018) have proven invaluable resources for research and should be continued and expanded. PRO-ACT's main limitation with regards to patient stratification is its inclusion bias. Working with population data leads to more representative results as clinical trial datasets tend to be associated with considerable bias. The identification of specific patient subgroups is most accurate when the data truly represents an entire patient population.

The maximum number of clusters does not typically exceed five in ALS research; Gomeni and Fava (2013), Ko et al. (2014), Beaulieu-Jones and Greene (2016), Ong et al. (2017), and Pfohl et al. (2018) work with only two patient subgroups, Visser et al. (2007), Elamin et al. (2015), van der Burgh et al. (2017), and Burke et al. (2017) with three patient subgroups, Marin et al. (2015) with four patient subgroups and Balendra et al. (2014a); Westeneng et al. (2018) with five patient subgroups. Depending on the available data, feature type, and data source working with a limited number of clusters may be desirable. This can be particularly challenging in ALS, where a number of phenotypes contribute to clinical heterogeneity. Identifying the correct number of clusters is a common problem in unsupervised learning which can only be solved with *ad-hoc* analyses. Please refer to **Tables 6, 7** for an overview of studies focusing on risk stratification in ALS.

ALS studies approach patient stratification in strikingly different ways. Visser et al. (2007) proposed an innovative PMA strategy which is based on limb involvement and focuses on symmetrical vs. asymmetrical limb weaknesses. Current ALS phenotyping already considers aspects of limb involvement, but this could be extended to adopt more detailed characterization. Gomeni and Fava (2013) divided patients into slow- and fast-progressing groups based on non-linear Weibull model estimation, which can account for linear, sigmoid or exponential evolutions. Two clusters were retained based on model fitting, as three-cluster attempts proved less conclusive. Balendra et al. (2014a) explored King's stages (Roche et al., 2012) on LiCALS and Mito Target data and demonstrated a viable alternative to ALSFRS-r and traditional patient stratification strategies. Clinical staging is thought to represent pathological stages better than ALSFRS-r. Alternative clinical staging systems, such as MiToS (Chiò et al., 2013a) or Fine'Till 9 (Thakore et al., 2018) could be tested further to assess if they are more sensitive in the earlier or later stages of the disease. Ko et al. (2014) performed an interesting patient classification study based on ALSFRS-r decline but choice of threshold, 0.6 ALSFRS-r point / month was not expounded. Elamin et al. (2015) divided patients into three risk groups based on a scoring system, which was based on site of onset, ALSFRS-r, and executive dysfunction. Marin et al. (2015) identified four groups using an unsupervised ML technique: Recursive partitioning and amalgamation. Membership rules were derived from analyzing ALSFRS-r decline and El Escorial criteria. Beaulieu-Jones and Greene (2016) investigated PRO-ACT survival data using denoising autoencoders, a deep learning model, and used the visualization algorithm t-SNE to visualize how the NN model had divided the subjects according to short vs. long survival. These results are particularly promising as NN models can work well without extensive feature selection. van der Burgh et al. (2017) segregated patients into three classes based on survival times defined by Elamin et al. (2015). Burke et al. (2017) proposed three subgroups for clustering based on executive dysfunction ("non-significant," "mild," and "severe symptoms") using the Beaumont Behavioral Inventory (Elamin et al., 2016), a questionnaire on patient behavior completed by the patient and caregivers. Ong et al. (2017) used unsupervised ML techniques Partitioning Around Medoids and K-Means to identify patient clusters for disease progression and survival. Partitioning Around Medoids and K-Means differ on cluster computing as the former computes the medoid (data point whose average dissimilarity with the other data points is minimal) while the latter computes the average value. Two clusters were optimally suited for both algorithms. Pfohl et al. (2018) used empirically defined survival times based on clinician experience. Westeneng et al. (2018) identified five patient groups after Royston-Parmar model analysis and estimation. Differing patient stratification strategies can be successfully combined as demonstrated by Burke et al. (2017) who analyzed cognitive impairment stratification with regards to King's clinical staging system.

4. DISCUSSION

4.1. Summary of Main Findings

4.1.1. Diagnosis

ML models have been increasingly explored in diagnostic applications in ALS. These models have the potential to supersede the current gold standard diagnostic approach which is based on clinical evaluation and uses the El Escorial criteria. The El Escorial criteria is thought to suffer from low specificity (Goutman, 2017). Recent ML models in ALS have reached comparable sensitivity and specificity values to the El Escorial criteria. The main barriers to model performance stem from limited data availability for training and poor sample to feature ratios. Future strategies should centre on models using multimodal data, and models which discriminate phenotypes

TABLE 6 | Research overview: Patient stratification (1/2).

Key	Dataset(s) origin	Dataset(s) type	Dataset(s) length	Scope	Approach	Clustering feature(s)	Number of clusters found
Visser et al., 2007	Dutch university hospitals	Real-life	37	Progression	Clinical observations	Limb involvement	3
Gomeni and Fava, 2013	ProACT	Clinical trial	338	Progression	Unsupervised (non-linear Weibull model estimation)	Clinical features	2
Balendra et al., 2014a	LiCALS, Mito Target	Clinical trial	725	Progression	Clinical observations	Clinical stages	5
Ko et al., 2014	ProAct	Clinical trial	1822	Progression	Clinical observations	ALSFRS decline rate	2
Elamin et al., 2015	Irish ALS registry, Italy (Piemonte Region)	Population	326	Outcome	Clinical observations	Score based on onset type, ALSFRS rate an executive disfunction	3
Marin et al., 2015	FRALim register	Population	322	Outcome	Unsupervised (RECPAM)	Clinical features	4

RECPAM, Recursive Partitioning and Amalgation.

TABLE 7 | Research overview: Patient stratification (2/2).

Key	Dataset(s) origin	Dataset(s) type	Dataset(s) length	Scope	Approach	Clustering feature(s)	Number of clusters found
Beaulieu-Jones and Greene, 2016	ProAct	Clinical trial	3398	Outcome	Unsupervised learning (DA)	Clinical and biological features	2
van der Burgh et al., 2017	University Medical Center Utrecht	Real-life	135	Outcome	Clinical observations	Survival time based on Elamin2015 categories	3
Burke et al., 2017	Irish ALS Register	Population	383	Progression	Clinical observations	Behavioral impairment based on BBI score	3
Ong et al., 2017	ProAct	Clinical trial	1568-6355	Progression, outcome	Unsupervised (PAM and K-Means)	Clinical and biological features	2x2
Pfohl et al., 2018	Emery ALS Clinic	Real-life	801	Outcome	Clinical observations	Survival time (empirical)	2
Westeneng et al., 2018	14 European ALS centers	Real-life	11475	Outcome	Unsupervised (RP model estimation)	Clinical features	5

DA, Denoising Autoencoders; PAM, Partitioning Around Medoids; RP, Royston-Parmar; BBI, Beaumont Behavioral Inventory.

within the ALS spectrum and distinguish ALS from disease-controls. Optimally, these models should be developed to enable an early, definite, and observer independent diagnosis of ALS.

4.1.2. Prognosis

The development of accurate prognostic models attracts considerable interest, and is fuelled by initiatives like the challenge launched by Prize4Life (Küffner et al., 2014). Prognostic model performance depends heavily on each feature's relevance to disease propagation. Current models rely primarily on clinical findings and laboratory tests which might not be sufficient to predict disease evolution. Despite these challenges, recent models have provided a reasonable gross estimate of death risk (Ong et al., 2017), survival (Schuster et al., 2017; van der Burgh et al., 2017; Westeneng et al., 2018) and progression rates (Ong et al., 2017). The most important constraints of prognostic modeling stem from significant data bias, limited data availability, poor missing data management, and limited sample to feature ratios. Performance reporting should be standardized for model comparisons, reproducibility, and benchmark development. Future studies should include multimodal data, multiple timepoints, include ALS patients with comorbid FTD and appraise disease progression in terms of clinical stages instead of solely relying on ALSFRS-r. Effective prognostic modeling should also account for disease heterogeneity to provide patients and clinicians with accurate prognostic insights across multiple phenotypes.

4.1.3. Risk Stratification

Novel computerized risk stratification initiatives are urgently required in ALS, as this aspect of ALS research has been relatively ignored to date. Existing studies tend to stratify patients according to rather basic categorization rules, limiting their analyses to a restricted number of clusters and focusing mostly on clinical features. Future research should focus on working with multimodal and longitudinal datasets and analyzing model-derived clustering with commonly used ALS phenotypes. Optimized patient stratification schemes will undoubtedly improve clinical trial design and has the potential to identify clinically relevant ALS subtypes.

5. CONCLUSIONS

ML models have enormous academic and clinical potential in ALS. With the increasing availability of large datasets, multicentre initiatives, high-performance computer platforms, open-source analysis suites, the insights provided by flexible ML models are likely to supersede those gained from conventional statistical approaches. The choice of the ML model need to be carefully tailored to a proposed application based on the characteristics of the available data and the flexibility, assumption and limitation profile of the candidate model. While ALS research to date has overwhelmingly relied on conventional ML approaches, emerging models and neural network architectures have considerable potential to advance the field. Novel models such as "black box" methods however may suffer from similar pitfalls than established algorithms. The meticulous evaluation of data characteristics, appraisal of data bias, missing data, sample to feature ratio is indispensable irrespective of the choice of ML model. Novel models may have outperformed traditional approaches, but data constraints and limitations are often overlooked. Model overfitting is the most commonly encountered shortcoming of recent studies which limits the generalizability of a proposed model. Transparent performance assessment using standardized metrics, robust missing data management and adherence to reporting guidelines are key requirements for future machine learning studies in ALS. Despite the drawbacks of current models and the methodological limitations of recent studies, the momentous advances in the field suggest that ML models will play a pivotal role in ALS research, drug discovery, and individualized patient care.

AUTHOR CONTRIBUTIONS

VG contributed to the design of the study, analyzed the data, and wrote the first draft of the manuscript. VG, GL, PB, FD, J-FP-P, and P-FP contributed to the revision of the manuscript. VG, GL, PB, FD, J-FP-P, P-FP, and GQ read and approved the final version.

FUNDING

VG, GL, J-FP-P, and FD contributions were made within a SORBONNE UNIVERSITE/CNRS and FRS Consulting partnership which received funding from MESRI grant CIFRE 2017/1051. PB and the Computational Neuroimaging Group in Trinity College Dublin is supported by the Health Research Board (HRB - Ireland; HRB EIA-2017-019), the Andrew Lydon scholarship, the Irish Institute of Clinical Neuroscience IICN - Novartis Ireland Research Grant, the Iris O'Brien Foundation, and the Research Motor Neuron (RMN-Ireland) Foundation.

REFERENCES

1. Agosta, F., Al-Chalabi, A., Filippi, M., Hardiman, O., Kaji, R., Meininger, V., et al. (2014). The el escorial criteria: strengths and weaknesses. *Amyotroph. Lateral Scler. Frontotemporal Degener.* 16, 1–7. doi: 10.3109/21678421.2014. 964258
2. Agosta, F., Pagani, E., Petrolini, M., Caputo, D., Perini, M., Prelle, A., et al. (2010). Assessment of white matter tract damage in patients with amyotrophic lateral sclerosis: a diffusion tensor MR imaging tractography study: Fig 1. *Am. J. Neuroradiol.* 31, 1457–1461. doi: 10.3174/ajnr.a2105
3. Agosta, F., Spinelli, E. G., and Filippi, M. (2018a). Neuroimaging in amyotrophic lateral sclerosis: current and emerging uses. *Expert Rev. Neurother.* 18, 395–406. doi: 10.1080/14737175.2018.1463160
4. Agosta, F., Spinelli, E. G., Marjanovic, I. V., Stevic, Z., Pagani, E., Valsasina, P.,et al. (2018b). Unraveling ALS due toSOD1mutation through the combination of brain and cervical cord MRI. *Neurology* 90, e707–e716. doi: 10.1212/wnl.0000000000005002
5. Aha, D. W., Kibler, D., and Albert, M. K. (1991). Instance-based learning algorithms. *Mach. Learn.* 6, 37–66. doi: 10.1007/bf00153759
6. Al-Chalabi, A., Hardiman, O., Kiernan, M. C., Chiò, A., Rix-Brooks, B., and van den Berg, L. H. (2016). Amyotrophic lateral sclerosis: moving towards a new classification system. *Lancet Neurol.* 15, 1182–1194. doi: 10.1016/s1474-4422(16)30199-5
7. Amato, F., López, A., Peña-Méndez, E. M., Van˘hara, P., Hampl, A., and Havel, J. (2013). Artificial neural networks in medical diagnosis. *J. Appl. Biomed.* 11, 47–58. doi: 10.2478/v10136-012-0031-x
8. Appel, V., Stewart, S. S., Smith, G., and Appel, S. H. (1987). A rating scale for amyotrophic lateral sclerosis: description and preliminary experience. *Ann. Neurol.* 22, 328–333. doi: 10.1002/ana.410220308
9. Arthur, K. C., Calvo, A., Price, T. R., Geiger, J. T., Chiò, A., and Traynor, B. J. (2016). Projected increase in amyotrophic lateral sclerosis from 2015 to 2040. *Nat. Commun.* 7:12408. doi: 10.1038/ncomms12408
10. Atassi, N., Berry, J., Shui, A., Zach, N., Sherman, A., Sinani, E., et al. (2014). The PRO-ACT database: design, initial analyses, and predictive features. *Neurology* 83, 1719–1725. doi: 10.1212/wnl.0000000000000951
11. Ayers, J. I., Fromholt, S. E., O'Neal, V. M., Diamond, J. H., and Borchelt, D. R. (2015). Prion-like propagation of mutant SOD1 misfolding and motor neuron disease spread along neuroanatomical pathways. *Acta Neuropathol.* 131, 103–114. doi: 10.1007/s00401-015-1514-0
12. Bakkar, N., Kovalik, T., Lorenzini, I., Spangler, S., Lacoste, A., Sponaugle, K., et al. (2017). Artificial intelligence in neurodegenerative disease research: use of IBM watson to identify additional RNA-binding proteins altered in amyotrophic lateral sclerosis. *Acta Neuropathol.* 135, 227–247. doi: 10.1007/s00401-017- 1785-8
13. Balendra, R., Jones, A., Jivraj, N., Knights, C., Ellis, C. M., Burman, R., et al. (2014a). Estimating clinical stage of amyotrophic lateral sclerosis from the ALS functional rating scale. *Amyotroph. Lateral Scler. Frontotemporal Degener.* 15, 279–284. doi: 10.3109/21678421.2014.897357
14. Balendra, R., Jones, A., Jivraj, N., Steen, I. N., Young, C. A., Shaw, P. J., et al. (2014b). Use of clinical staging in amyotrophic lateral sclerosis for phase 3 clinical trials. *J. Neurol. Neurosurg. Psychiatry* 86, 45–49. doi: 10.1136/jnnp-2013-306865
15. Bandini, A., Green, J. R., Wang, J., Campbell, T. F., Zinman, L., and Yunusova,

Y. (2018). Kinematic features of jaw and lips distinguish symptomatic from presymptomatic stages of bulbar decline in amyotrophic lateral sclerosis. *J. Speech Lang. Hear. Res.* 61:1118. doi: 10.1044/2018 jslhr-s-17-0262

16. Batyrbekova, M., Prell, T., Stubendorff, B., Steinbach, R., Bokemeyer, M., et al. (2018). P48. progression of cerebellar involvement in amyotrophic lateral sclerosis as seen by SUIT/ CAT12 voxel-based morphometry and d50 disease modelling. *Clin. Neurophysiol.* 129, e86–e87. doi: 10.1016/j.clinph.2018.04.686 Baudi, K., Brodu, N., Rusz, J., and Klempir, J. (2016). "Objective discrimination between progressive supranuclear palsy and multiple system atrophy using speech analysis," in *38th Annual International Conference of the IEEE Engineering in Medicine and Biology Society* (Orlando, FL).
17. Beaulieu-Jones, B. K., and Greene, C. S. (2016). Semi-supervised learning of the electronic health record for phenotype stratification. *J. Biomed. Informatics* 64, 168–178. doi: 10.1016/j.jbi.2016.10.007
18. Bede, P. (2017). From qualitative radiological cues to machine learning: MRI-based diagnosis in neurodegeneration. *Future Neurol.* 12, 5–8. doi: 10.2217/fnl-2016-0029
19. Bede, P., Bokde, A., Elamin, M., Byrne, S., McLaughlin, R. L., Jordan, N., et al. (2012). Grey matter correlates of clinical variables in amyotrophic lateral sclerosis (ALS): a neuroimaging study of ALS motor phenotype heterogeneity and cortical focality. *J. Neurol. Neurosurg. Psychiatry* 84, 766–773. doi: 10.1136/jnnp-2012-302674
20. Bede, P., Bokde, A. L. W., Byrne, S., Elamin, M., McLaughlin, R. L., Kenna, K., et al. (2013a). Multiparametric MRI study of ALS stratified for the c9orf72 genotype. *Neurology* 81, 361–369. doi: 10.1212/wnl.0b013e31829c5eee Bede, P., Elamin, M., Byrne, S., and Hardiman, O. (2013b). Sexual dimorphism in ALS: exploring gender-specific neuroimaging signatures. *Amyotroph. Lateral Scler. Frontotemporal Degener.* 15, 235–243. doi: 10.3109/21678421.2013.865749
21. Bede, P., Elamin, M., Byrne, S., McLaughlin, R. L., Kenna, K., Vajda, A., et al. (2013c). Basal ganglia involvement in amyotrophic lateral sclerosis. *Neurology* 81, 2107–2115. doi: 10.1212/01.wnl.0000437313.80913.2c
22. Bede, P., Elamin, M., Byrne, S., McLaughlin, R. L., Kenna, K., Vajda, A., et al. (2014). Patterns of cerebral and cerebellar white matter degeneration in ALS: Figure 1. *J. Neurol. Neurosurg. Psychiatry* 86, 468–470. doi: 10.1136/jnnp-2014-308172
23. Bede, P., and Hardiman, O. (2017). Longitudinal structural changes in ALS: a three time-point imaging study of white and gray matter degeneration. *Amyotroph. Lateral Scler. Frontotemporal Degener.* 19, 232–241. doi: 10.1080/21678421.2017.1407795
24. Bede, P., Iyer, P. M., Finegan, E., Omer, T., and Hardiman, O. (2017). Virtual brain biopsies in amyotrophic lateral sclerosis: diagnostic classification based on *in vivo* pathological patterns. *Neuroimage Clin.* 15, 653–658. doi: 10.1016/j.nicl.2017.06.010
25. Bede, P., Iyer, P. M., Schuster, C., Elamin, M., Mclaughlin, R. L., Kenna, K., et al. (2016). The selective anatomical vulnerability of ALS: 'disease-defining' and 'disease-defying' brain regions. *Amyotroph. Lateral Scler. Frontotemporal Degener.* 17, 561–570. doi: 10.3109/21678421.2016.1173702
26. Bede, P., Omer, T., Finegan, E., Chipika, R. H., Iyer, P. M., Doherty, M. A., et al. (2018a). Connectivity-based characterisation of subcortical grey matter pathology in frontotemporal dementia and ALS: a multimodal neuroimaging study. *Brain Imaging Behav.* 12, 1696–1707. doi: 10.1007/s11682-018-9837-9
27. Bede, P., Querin, G., and Pradat, P.-F. (2018b). The changing landscape of motor neuron disease imaging. *Curr. Opin. Neurol.* 31, 431–438. doi: 10.1097/wco.0000000000000569
28. Bishop, C. M. (2016). *Pattern Recognition and Machine Learning*. New York, NY: Springer.
29. Bozik, M. E., Mitsumoto, H., Brooks, B. R., Rudnicki, S. A., Moore, D. H., Zhang, B., et al. (2014). A *post-hoc* analysis of subgroup outcomes and creatinine in the phase III clinical trial (EMPOWER) of dexpramipexole in ALS. *Amyotroph. Lateral Scler. Frontotemporal Degener.* 15, 406–413. doi: 10.3109/21678421.2014.943672
30. Breiman, L. (2001). Random forests. *Mach. Learn.* 45, 5–32. doi: 10.1023/a:1010933404324
31. Brettschneider, J., Petzold, A., Sussmuth, S. D., Ludolph, A. C., and Tumani, H. (2006). Axonal damage markers in cerebrospinal fluid are increased in ALS. *Neurology* 66, 852–856. doi: 10.1212/01.wnl.0000203120.85850.54
32. Brooks, B. R. (1994). El escorial world federation of neurology criteria for the diagnosis of amyotrophic lateral sclerosis. *J. Neurol. Sci.* 124, 96–107. doi: 10.1016/0022-510x(94)90191-0
33. Brooks, B. R., Miller, R. G., Swash, M., and Munsat, T. L. (2000). El escorial revisited: revised criteria for the diagnosis of amyotrophic lateral sclerosis. *Amyotroph. Lateral Scler. Other Motor Neuron Disord.* 1, 293–299. doi: 10.1080/146608200300079536
34. Burke, T., Elamin, M., Galvin, M., Hardiman, O., and Pender, N. (2015). Caregiver burden in amyotrophic lateral sclerosis: a cross-sectional investigation of predictors. *J. Neurol.* 262, 1526–1532. doi: 10.1007/s00415-015-7746-z
35. Burke, T., Pinto-Grau, M., Lonergan, K., Bede, P., O'/Sullivan, M., Heverin, M., et al. (2017). A cross-sectional population-based investigation into behavioral change in amyotrophic lateral sclerosis: subphenotypes, staging, cognitive predictors, and survival. *Ann. Clin. Transl. Neurol.* 4, 305–317. doi: 10.1002/acn3.407
36. Byrne, S., Elamin, M., Bede, P., Shatunov, A., Walsh, C., Corr, B., et al. (2012). Cognitive and clinical characteristics of patients with amyotrophic lateral sclerosis carrying a c9orf72 repeat expansion: a population-based cohort study. *Lancet Neurol.* 11, 232–240. doi: 10.1016/s1474-4422(12) 70014-5
37. Cedarbaum, J. M., Stambler, N., Malta, E., Fuller, C., Hilt, D., Thurmond, B., et al. (1999). The ALSFRS-r: a revised ALS functional rating scale that incorporates assessments of respiratory function. *J. Neurol. Sci.* 169, 13–21. doi: 10.1016/s0022-510x(99)00210-5
38. Cellura, E., Spataro, R., Taiello, A. C., and Bella, V. L. (2012). Factors affecting the diagnostic delay in amyotrophic lateral sclerosis. *Clin. Neurol. Neurosurg.* 114, 550–554. doi: 10.1016/j.clineuro.2011.11.026
39. Chen, H.-L., Huang, C.-C., Yu, X.-G., Xu, X., Sun, X., Wang, G., et al. (2013). An efficient diagnosis system for detection of parkinson's disease using fuzzy k-nearest neighbor approach. *Expert Syst. Appl.* 40, 263–271. doi: 10.1016/j.eswa.2012.07.014
40. Chio, A., Canosa, A., Gallo, S., Cammarosano, S., Moglia, C., Fuda, G., et al. (2011). ALS clinical trials: do enrolled patients accurately represent the ALS population? *Neurology* 77, 1432–1437. doi: 10.1212/wnl.0b013e318232ab9b
41. Chiò, A., Hammond, E. R., Mora, G., Bonito, V., and Filippini, G. (2013a). Development and evaluation of a clinical staging system for amyotrophic lateral sclerosis. *J. Neurol. Neurosurg. Psychiatry* 86, 38–44. doi: 10.1136/jnnp-2013-306589
42. Chiò, A., Logroscino, G., Hardiman, O., Swingler, R., Mitchell, D., Beghi, E., et al. (2009). Prognostic factors in ALS: a critical review. *Amyotroph. Lateral Scler.* 10, 310–323. doi: 10.3109/17482960802566824
43. Chiò, A., Logroscino, G., Traynor, B., Collins, J., Simeone, J., Goldstein, L., et al. (2013b). Global epidemiology of amyotrophic lateral sclerosis: a systematic review of the published literature. *Neuroepidemiology* 41, 118–130. doi: 10.1159/000351153
44. Chio, A., Mora, G., Calvo, A., Mazzini, L., Bottacchi, E., Mutani R et al. (2009). Epidemiology of ALS in italy: a 10-year prospective population-based study. *Neurology* 72, 725–731. doi: 10.1212/01.wnl.0000343008.26874.d1
45. Choi, E., Biswal, S., Malin, B., Duke, J., Stewart, W. F., and Sun, J. (2017). "Generating multi-label discrete patient records using generative adversarial networks," in *Proceedings of Machine Learning Research, PMLR Volume 68, Machine learning for Healthcare Conference* (Boston, MA).
46. Christidi, F., Karavasilis, E., Zalonis, I., Ferentinos, P., Giavri, Z., Wilde, E. A., et al. (2017). Memory-related white matter tract integrity in amyotrophic lateral sclerosis: an advanced neuroimaging and neuropsychological study. *Neurobiol. Aging* 49, 69–78. doi: 10.1016/j.neurobiolaging.2016.09.014
47. Coon, E. A., Sorenson, E. J., Whitwell, J. L., Knopman, D. S., and Josephs, K. A. (2011). Predicting survival in frontotemporal dementia with motor neuron disease. *Neurology* 76, 1886–1892. doi: 10.1212/wnl.0b013e31821d767b
48. Costa, A. F., Santos, M. S., Soares, J. P., and Abreu, P. H. (2018). "Missing data imputation via denoising autoencoders: the untold story," in *Advances in Intelligent Data Analysis XVII* (Hertogenbosch, NL: Springer International Publishing), 87–98.
49. Cox, S. R., Dickie, D. A., Ritchie, S. J., Karama, S., Pattie, A., Royle, N. A., et al. (2016). Associations between education and brain structure at age 73 years, adjusted for age 11 IQ. *Neurology* 87, 1820–1826. doi: 10.1212/wnl.0000000000003247
50. Creemers, H., Grupstra, H., Nollet, F., van den Berg, L. H., and Beelen, A. (2014). Prognostic factors for the course of functional status of patients with ALS: a systematic review. *J. Neurol.* 262, 1407–1423. doi: 10.1007/s00415-014-7564-8
51. Davoli, A., Greco, V., Spalloni, A., Guatteo, E., Neri, C., Rizzo, G. R., et al. (2015). Evidence of hydrogen sulfide involvement in amyotrophic lateral sclerosis. *Ann. Neurol.* 77, 697–709. doi: 10.1002/ana.24372
52. de Carvalho, M., Dengler, R., Eisen, A., England, J. D., Kaji, R., Kimura, J., et al. (2008). Electrodiagnostic criteria for diagnosis of ALS. *Clin. Neurophysiol.* 119, 497–503. doi: 10.1016/j.clinph.2007.09.143
53. de Luis-García, R., Westin, C.-F., and Alberola-López, C. (2011). Gaussian

mixtures on tensor fields for segmentation: applications to medical imaging. *Comput. Med. Imaging Graph.* 35, 16–30. doi: 10.1016/j.compmedimag.2010.09.001

54. den Berg, J. P. V., Kalmijn, S., Lindeman, E., Veldink, J. H., de Visser, M., der Graaff, M. M. V., et al. (2005). Multidisciplinary ALS care improves quality of life in patients with ALS. *Neurology* 65, 1264–1267. doi: 10.1212/01.wnl.0000180717.29273.12
55. Dharmadasa, T., Matamala, J. M., Howells, J., Vucic, S., and Kiernan, M. C. (2018). 10. phenotypic variability in motor neuron disease: site of onset and patterns of disease spread. *Clin. Neurophysiol.* 129, e4–e5. doi: 10.1016/j.clinph.2017.12.023
56. D'hulst, L., Weehaeghe, D. V., Chiò, A., Calvo, A., Moglia, C., Canosa, A., et al. (2018). Multicenter validation of [18f]-FDG PET and support-vector machine discriminant analysis in automatically classifying patients with amyotrophic lateral sclerosis versus controls. *Amyotroph. Lateral Scler. Frontotemporal Degener.* doi: 10.1080/21678421.2018.1476548. [Epub ahead of print].
57. Donaghy, C., O'Toole, O., Sheehan, C., Kee, F., Hardiman, O., and Patterson, V. (2009). An all-ireland epidemiological study of MND, 2004-2005. *Eur. J. Neurol.* 16, 148–153. doi: 10.1111/j.1468-1331.2008.02361.x
58. Draper, N. R., and Smith, H. (1998). *Applied Regression Analysis.* John Wiley & Sons, Inc.
59. Elamin, M., Bede, P., Byrne, S., Jordan, N., Gallagher, L., Wynne, B., et al. (2013). Cognitive changes predict functional decline in ALS: a population-based longitudinal study. *Neurology* 80, 1590–1597. doi: 10.1212/wnl.0b013e31828f18ac
60. Elamin, M., Bede, P., Montuschi, A., Pender, N., Chio, A., and Hardiman, O. (2015). Predicting prognosis in amyotrophic lateral sclerosis: a simple algorithm. *J. Neurol.* 262, 1447–1454. doi: 10.1007/s00415-015- 7731-6
61. Elamin, M., Phukan, J., Bede, P., Jordan, N., Byrne, S., Pender, N., et al. (2011). Executive dysfunction is a negative prognostic indicator in patients with ALS without dementia. *Neurology* 76, 1263–1269. doi: 10.1212/wnl.0b013e318214359f
62. Elamin, M., Pinto-Grau, M., Burke, T., Bede, P., Rooney, J., O'Sullivan, M., et al. (2016). Identifying behavioural changes in ALS: validation of the beaumont behavioural inventory (BBI). *Amyotroph. Lateral Scler. Frontotemporal Degener.* 18, 68–73. doi: 10.1080/21678421.2016.1248976
63. Escorcio-Bezerra, M. L., Abrahao, A., Nunes, K. F., Braga, N. I. D. O., Oliveira, A. S. B., Zinman, L., et al. (2018). Motor unit number index and neurophysiological index as candidate biomarkers of presymptomatic motor neuron loss in amyotrophic lateral sclerosis. *Muscle Nerve* 58, 204–212. doi: 10.1002/mus.26087
64. Esteva, A., Kuprel, B., Novoa, R. A., Ko, J., Swetter, S. M., Blau, H. M., et al. (2017). Dermatologist-level classification of skin cancer with deep neural networks. *Nature* 542, 115–118. doi: 10.1038/nature21056
65. Fang, T., Khleifat, A. A., Meurgey, J.-H., Jones, A., Leigh, P. N., Bensimon, G., et al. (2018). Stage at which riluzole treatment prolongs survival in patients with amyotrophic lateral sclerosis: a retrospective analysis of data from a dose-ranging study. *Lancet Neurol.* 17, 416–422. doi: 10.1016/s1474-4422(18)30054-1
66. Fathi, D., Mohammadi, B., Dengler, R., Böselt, S., Petri, S., and Kollewe, K. (2016). Lower motor neuron involvement in ALS assessed by motor unit number index (MUNIX): long-term changes and reproducibility. *Clin. Neurophysiol.* 127, 1984–1988. doi: 10.1016/j.clinph.2015.12.023
67. Fawcett, T. (2004). Roc graphs: notes and practical considerations for researchers. *Mach. Learn.* 31, 1–38.
68. Ferraro, D., Consonni, D., Fini, N., Fasano, A., Giovane, C. D., and J. M. (2016). Amyotrophic lateral sclerosis: a comparison of two staging systems in a population-based study. *Eur. J. Neurol.* 23, 1426–1432. doi: 10.1111/ene.13053
Ferraro, P. M., Agosta, F., Riva, N., Copetti, M., Spinelli, E. G., Falzone, Y., et al. (2017). Multimodal structural MRI in the diagnosis of motor neuron diseases.
69. *Neuroimage Clin.* 16, 240–247. doi: 10.1016/j.nicl.2017.08.002
70. Filippini, N., Douaud, G., Mackay, C. E., Knight, S., Talbot, K., and Turner, M. R. (2010). Corpus callosum involvement is a consistent feature of amyotrophic lateral sclerosis. *Neurology* 75, 1645–1652. doi: 10.1212/wnl.0b013e3181fb84d1
Fodor, I. K. (2002). A survey of dimension reduction techniques. *Center Appl. Sci. Comput. Lawrence Livermore Natl Lab.* 9, 1–18.
71. Forbes, R. B. (2004). Unexpected decline in survival from amyotrophic lateral sclerosis/motor neurone disease. *J. Neurol. Neurosurg. Psychiatry* 75, 1753–1755. doi: 10.1136/jnnp.2003.024364
72. Fratello, M., Caiazzo, G., Trojsi, F., Russo, A., Tedeschi, G., Tagliaferri, R., et al. (2017). Multi-view ensemble classification of brain connectivity images for neurodegeneration type discrimination. *Neuroinformatics* 15, 199–213. doi: 10.1007/s12021-017-9324-2
73. Geifman, N., Kennedy, R. E., Schneider, L. S., Buchan, I., and Brinton, R. D. (2018). Data-driven identification of endophenotypes of alzheimer's disease progression: implications for clinical trials and therapeutic interventions. *Alzheimers Res. Ther.* 10:4. doi: 10.1186/s13195-017-0332-0
74. Gomeni, R., and Fava, M. (2013). Amyotrophic lateral sclerosis disease progression model. *Amyotroph. Lateral Scler. Frontotemporal Degener.* 15, 119–129. doi: 10.3109/21678421.2013.838970
75. Goodfellow, I., Bengio, Y., and Courville, A. (2017). *Deep Learning.* The MIT Press. Goodfellow, I., Pouget-Abadie, J., Mirza, M., Xu, B., Warde-Farley, D., Ozair, S., et al. (2014). "Generative adversarial nets," in *Advances in Neural Information Processing Systems* (Montreal, CA), 2672–2680.
76. Gordon, P. H., Cheng, B., Katz, I. B., Mitsumoto, H., and Rowland, L. P. (2009). Clinical features that distinguish PLS, upper motor neuron-dominant ALS, and typical ALS. *Neurology* 72, 1948–1952. doi: 10.1212/wnl.0b013e3181a8269b
77. Goutman, S. A. (2017). Diagnosis and clinical management of amyotrophic lateral sclerosis and other motor neuron disorders. *CONTINUUM: Lifelong Learn. Neurol.* 23, 1332–1359. doi: 10.1212/con.0000000000000535
78. Gresle, M. M., Liu, Y., Dagley, L. F., Haartsen, J., Pearson, F., Purcell, A. W., et al. (2014). Serum phosphorylated neurofilament-heavy chain levels in multiple sclerosis patients. *J. Neurol. Neurosurg. Psychiatry* 85, 1209–1213. doi: 10.1136/jnnp-2013-306789
79. Guyon, I., Nikravesh, M., Gunn, S., and Zadeh, L. A. (eds.) (2006). *Feature Extraction.* Berlin; Heidelberg: Springer.
80. Hardiman, O., Al-Chalabi, A., Chio, A., Corr, E. M., Logroscino, G., Robberecht, W., et al. (2017). Amyotrophic lateral sclerosis. *Nat. Rev. Dis. Primers* 3:17071. doi: 10.1038/nrdp.2017.71
81. Hastie, T. (2003). *Trees Bagging Random Forests and Boosting.* Standford: Stanford University.
82. Hastie, T., Tibshirani, R., and Friedman, J. (2009). *The Elements of Statistical Learning.* New York, NY: Springer.
83. Hayden, J. A., van der Windt, D. A., Cartwright, J. L., Côté, P., and Bombardier, C. (2013). Assessing bias in studies of prognostic factors. *Ann. Intern. Med.* 158:280. doi: 10.7326/0003-4819-158-4-201302190-00009
84. Hothorn, T., and Jung, H. H. (2014). RandomForest4life: a random forest for predicting ALS disease progression. *Amyotroph. Lateral Scler. Frontotemporal Degener.* 15, 444–452. doi: 10.3109/21678421.2014.893361
85. Hu, W. T., Seelaar, H., Josephs, K. A., Knopman, D. S., Boeve, B. F., Sorenson, E. J., et al. (2009). Survival profiles of patients with frontotemporal dementia and motor neuron disease. *Arch. Neurol.* 66, 1359–1364. doi: 10.1001/archneurol.2009.253
86. Huang, Z., Zhang, H., Boss, J., Goutman, S. A., Mukherjee, B., Dinov,
87. I. D., et al. (2017). Complete hazard ranking to analyze right- censored data: an ALS survival study. *PLoS Comput. Biol.* 13:e1005887. doi: 10.1371/journal.pcbi.1005887
88. Ihara, Y., Nobukuni, K., Takata, H., and Hayabara, T. (2005). Oxidative stress and metal content in blood and cerebrospinal fluid of amyotrophic lateral sclerosis patients with and without a cu, zn-superoxide dismutase mutation. *Neurol. Res.* 27, 105–108. doi: 10.1179/016164105x18430
89. Ince, P., Evans, J., Knopp, M., Forster, G., Hamdalla, H., Wharton, S., et al. (2003). Corticospinal tract degeneration in the progressive muscular atrophy variant of ALS. *Neurology* 60, 1252–1258. doi: 10.1212/01.wnl.0000058901.75728.4e
90. Jahandideh, S., Taylor, A. A., Beaulieu, D., Keymer, M., Meng, L., Bian, A., et al. (2017). Longitudinal modeling to predict vital capacity in amyotrophic lateral sclerosis. *Amyotroph. Lateral Scler. Frontotemporal Degener.* 19, 294–302. doi: 10.1080/21678421.2017.1418003
91. Jelinek, H., Abawajy, J., Kelarev, A., Chowdhury, M., and Stranieri, A. (2014). Decision trees and multi-level ensemble classifiers for neurological diagnostics. *Aust. J. Med. Sci.* 1, 1–12. doi: 10.3934/medsci2014.1.1
92. Johnston, M., Earll, L., Giles, M., Mcclenahan, R., Stevens, D., and Morrison, V. (1999). Mood as a predictor of disability and survival in patients newly diagnosed with ALS/MND. *Br. J. Health Psychol.* 4, 127–136. doi: 10.1348/135910799168524
93. Khoury, N., Attal, F., Amirat, Y., Oukhellou, L., and Mohammed, S. (2019). Data- driven based approach to aid parkinson's disease diagnosis. *Sensors* 19:242. doi: 10.3390/s19020242
94. Kiernan, M. C. (2018). Motor neuron disease in 2017: progress towards therapy in motor neuron disease. *Nat. Rev. Neurol.* 14, 65–66. doi: 10.1038/nrneurol.2017.186
95. Knibb, J. A., Keren, N., Kulka, A., Leigh, P. N., Martin, S., Shaw, C. E., et al. (2016). A clinical tool for predicting survival in ALS. *J. Neurol. Neurosurg. Psychiatry* 87, 1361–1367. doi: 10.1136/jnnp-2015-312908
96. Ko, K. D., El-Ghazawi, T., Kim, D., and Morizono, H. (2014). "Predicting the severity of motor neuron disease progression using electronic health record

data with a cloud computing big data approach," in *2014 IEEE Conference on Computational Intelligence in Bioinformatics and Computational Biology* (Honolulu, HI: IEEE), 1–6.
97. Kokic´, A. N., Stevic´, Z., Stojanovic´, S., Blagojevic´, D. P., Jones, D. R., Pavlovic´, S., et al. (2005). Biotransformation of nitric oxide in the cerebrospinal fluid of amyotrophic lateral sclerosis patients. *Redox Rep.* 10, 265–270. doi: 10.1179/135100005x70242
98. Kourou, K., Exarchos, T. P., Exarchos, K. P., Karamouzis, M. V., and Fotiadis, D. I. (2015). Machine learning applications in cancer prognosis and prediction.
99. *Comput. Struct. Biotechnol. J.* 13, 8–17. doi: 10.1016/j.csbj.2014.11.005 Küffner, R., Zach, N., Norel, R., Hawe, J., Schoenfeld, D., Wang, L., et al. (2014).
100. Crowdsourced analysis of clinical trial data to predict amyotrophic lateral sclerosis progression. *Nat. Biotechnol.* 33, 51–57. doi: 10.1038/nbt.3051
101. Larranaga, P., Calvo, B., Santana, R., Bielza, C., Galdiano, J., Inza, I., et al. (2006). Machine learning in bioinformatics. *Brief. Bioinformatics* 7, 86–112. doi: 10.1093/bib/bbk007
102. Lee, J. A., and Verleysen, M. (2007). *Nonlinear Dimensionality Reduction.* New York, NY: Springer.
103. Li, T., Howells, J., Lin, C., Garg, N., Kiernan, M., and Park, S. (2018). 8. predicting motor disorders from nerve excitability studies. *Clin. Neurophysiol.* 129:e4. doi: 10.1016/j.clinph.2017.12.021
104. Libbrecht, M. W., and Noble, W. S. (2015). Machine learning applications in genetics and genomics. *Nat. Rev. Genet.* 16, 321. doi: 10.1038/nrg3920
105. Lisboa, P. J., and Taktak, A. F. (2006). The use of artificial neural networks in decision support in cancer: a systematic review. *Neural Netw.* 19, 408–415. doi: 10.1016/j.neunet.2005.10.007
106. Litjens, G., Sánchez, C. I., Timofeeva, N., Hermsen, M., Nagtegaal, I., Kovacs, I., et al. (2016). Deep learning as a tool for increased accuracy and efficiency of histopathological diagnosis. *Sci. Rep.* 6:26286. doi: 10.1038/srep26286
107. Little, R. (2002). *Missing Data 2e.* John Wiley & Sons.
108. Lobo, J. M., Jiménez-Valverde, A., and Real, R. (2008). AUC: a misleading measure of the performance of predictive distribution models. *Global Ecol. Biogeogr.* 17, 145–151. doi: 10.1111/j.1466-8238.2007.00358.x
109. Louppe, G. (2014). Understanding random forests: from theory to practice. *arXiv preprint arXiv:1407.7502.*
110. Lu, H., Wang, H., and Yoon, S. W. (2019). A dynamic gradient boosting machine using genetic optimizer for practical breast cancer prognosis. *Expert Syst. Appl.* 116, 340–350. doi: 10.1016/j.eswa.2018.08.040
111. Lulé, D., Diekmann, V., Anders, S., Kassubek, J., Kübler, A., Ludolph, A. C., et al. (2007). Brain responses to emotional stimuli in patients with amyotrophic lateral sclerosis (ALS). *J. Neurol.* 254, 519–527. doi: 10.1007/s00415-006-0 409-3
112. Machts, J., Loewe, K., Kaufmann, J., Jakubiczka, S., Abdulla, S., Petri, S., et al. (2015). Basal ganglia pathology in ALS is associated with neuropsychological deficits. *Neurology* 85, 1301–1309. doi: 10.1212/wnl.0000000000
113. 002017
114. Majumder, V., Gregory, J. M., Barria, M. A., Green, A., and Pal, S. (2018). TDP-43 as a potential biomarker for amyotrophic lateral sclerosis: a systematic review and meta-analysis. *BMC Neurol.* 18:90. doi:10.1186/s12883-018-1091-7
115. Marek, K., Jennings, D., Lasch, S., Siderowf, A., Tanner, C., Simuni, T., et al. (2011). The parkinson progression marker initiative (PPMI). *Prog. Neurobiol.* 95, 629–635. doi: 10.1016/j.pneurobio.2011.09.005
116. Marin, B., Couratier, P., Arcuti, S., Copetti, M., Fontana, A., Nicol, M., et al. (2015). Stratification of ALS patients' survival: a population-based study. *J. Neurol.* 263, 100–111. doi: 10.1007/s00415-015-7940-z
117. Martinez-Murcia, F. J., Górriz, J. M., Ramírez, J., and Ortiz, A. (2016). A structural parametrization of the brain using hidden markov models- based paths in alzheimer's disease. *Int. J. Neural Syst.* 26:1650024. doi: 10.1142/s0129065716500246
118. Mathé, C., Sagot, M.-F., Schiex, T., and Rouzé, P. (2002). Current methods of gene prediction, their strengths and weaknesses. *Nucleic Acids Res.* 30, 4103–4117.
119. Matuz, T., Birbaumer, N., Hautzinger, M., and Kübler, A. (2015). Psychosocial adjustment to ALS: a longitudinal study. *Front. Psychol.* 6:1197. doi: 10.3389/fpsyg.2015.01197
120. Menke, R., Proudfoot, M., Talbot, K., and Turner, M. (2018). The two-year progression of structural and functional cerebral MRI in amyotrophic lateral sclerosis. *Neuroimage Clin.* 17, 953–961. doi: 10.1016/j.nicl.2017.12.025
121. Menke, R. A. L., Gray, E., Lu, C.-H., Kuhle, J., Talbot, K., Malaspina, A., et al. (2015). CSF neurofilament light chain reflects corticospinal tract degeneration in ALS. *Ann. Clin. Transl. Neurol.* 2, 748–755. doi: 10.1002/acn3.212
122. Miller, T. (2017). Explanation in artificial intelligence: insights from the social sciences. *arXiv preprint arxiv:1706.07269.*
123. Moon, T. (1996). The expectation-maximization algorithm. *IEEE Signal Process. Mag.* 13, 47–60.
124. Moons, K. G., Altman, D. G., Reitsma, J. B., Ioannidis, J. P., Macaskill, P., Steyerberg, E. W., et al. (2015). Transparent reporting of a multivariable prediction model for individual prognosis or diagnosis (TRIPOD): explanation and elaboration. *Ann. Intern. Med.* 162:W1. doi: 10.7326/m14-0698
125. Mora, G., and Chiò, A. (2015). "Disorders of upper and lower motor neurons," in *Prognosis of Neurological Diseases* (Milan: Springer), 261–272.
126. Moreau, C., Devos, D., Brunaud-Danel, V., Defebvre, L., Perez, T., Destee, A., et al. (2005). Elevated IL-6 and TNF- levels in patients with ALS: inflammation or hypoxia? *Neurology* 65, 1958–1960. doi: 10.1212/01.wnl.0000188907.97339.76
127. Mueller, S. G., Weiner, M. W., Thal, L. J., Petersen, R. C., Jack, C. R., Jagust, W., et al. (2005). Ways toward an early diagnosis in alzheimer's disease: the alzheimer's disease neuroimaging initiative (ADNI). *Alzheimers Dement.* 1, 55–66. doi: 10.1016/j.jalz.2005.06.003
128. Müller, H.-P., Turner, M. R., Grosskreutz, J., Abrahams, S., Bede, P., Govind, V., et al. (2016). A large-scale multicentre cerebral diffusion tensor imaging study in amyotrophic lateral sclerosis. *J. Neurol. Neurosurg. Psychiatry* 87, 570–579. doi: 10.1136/jnnp-2015-311952
129. NEALS Consortium (2018). *Northeastern Amyotrophic Lateral Sclerosis Consortium.* Available online at: https://www.neals.org/.
130. Neary, D., Snowden, J., and Mann, D. (2000). Cognitive change in motor neurone disease/amyotrophic lateral sclerosis (MND/ALS). *J. Neurol. Sci.* 180, 15–20. doi: 10.1016/s0022-510x(00)00425-1
131. Nelwamondo, F. V., Mohamed, S., and Marwala, T. (2007). Missing data: a comparison of neural network and expectation maximization techniques. *Curr. Sci.* 93, 1514–1521.
132. Neumann, M., Sampathu, D. M., Kwong, L. K., Truax, A. C., Micsenyi, M. C., Chou, T. T., et al. (2006). Ubiquitinated TDP-43 in frontotemporal lobar degeneration and amyotrophic lateral sclerosis. *Science* 314, 130–133. doi: 10.1126/science.1134108
133. Neuroimaging Society in ALS (2018). *Neuroimaging Society in Amyotrophic Lateral Sclerosis.* Available online at: https://nisals.net/.
134. Nie, D., Trullo, R., Lian, J., Petitjean, C., Ruan, S., Wang, Q., et al. (2017). "Medical image synthesis with context-aware generative adversarial networks," in *Lecture Notes in Computer Science* (Quebec, CA: Springer International Publishing), 417–425.
135. Olney, R. K., Murphy, J., Forshew, D., Garwood, E., Miller, B. L., Langmore, S., et al. (2005). The effects of executive and behavioral dysfunction on the course of ALS. *Neurology* 65, 1774–1777. doi: 10.1212/01.wnl.0000188759.87240.8b
136. Ong, M.-L., Tan, P. F., and Holbrook, J. D. (2017). Predicting functional decline and survival in amyotrophic lateral sclerosis. *PLoS ONE* 12:e0174925. doi: 10.1371/journal.pone.0174925
137. Pannucci, C. J., and Wilkins, E. G. (2010). Identifying and avoiding bias in research. *Plastic Reconstruct. Surg.* 126, 619–625. doi: 10.1097/prs.0b013e3181de24bc Pestov, V. (2007). An axiomatic approach to intrinsic dimension of a dataset. *Neural Netw.* 21, 204–213. doi: 10.1016/j.neunet.2007.12.030
138. Pfohl, S. R., Kim, R. B., Coan, G. S., and Mitchell, C. S. (2018). Unraveling the complexity of amyotrophic lateral sclerosis survival prediction. *Front. Neuroinformatics* 12:36. doi: 10.3389/fninf.2018.00036
139. Phukan, J., Elamin, M., Bede, P., Jordan, N., Gallagher, L., Byrne, S., et al. (2011). The syndrome of cognitive impairment in amyotrophic lateral sclerosis: a population-based study. *J. Neurol. Neurosurg. Psychiatry* 83, 102–108. doi: 10.1136/jnnp-2011-300188
140. Prell, T., and Grosskreutz, J. (2013). The involvement of the cerebellum in amyotrophic lateral sclerosis. *Amyotroph. Lateral Scler. Frontotemporal Degener.* 14, 507–515. doi: 10.3109/21678421.2013.812661
141. Querin, G., Mendili, M.-M. E., Bede, P., Delphine, S., Lenglet, T., Marchand-Pauvert, V., et al. (2018). Multimodal spinal cord MRI offers accurate diagnostic classification in ALS. *J. Neurol. Neurosurg. Psychiatry* 89, 1220–1221. doi: 10.1136/jnnp-2017-317214
142. Rafiq, M. K., Lee, E., Bradburn, M., McDermott, C. J., and Shaw, P. J. (2016). Creatine kinase enzyme level correlates positively with serum creatinine and lean body mass, and is a prognostic factor for survival in amyotrophic lateral sclerosis. *Eur. J. Neurol.* 23, 1071–1078. doi: 10.1111/ene.12995
143. Rasmussen, C. E. (2005). *Gaussian Processes for Machine Learning.* MIT University Press Group Ltd.
144. Raudys, Š. (2001). *Statistical and Neural Classifiers.* London: Springer.
145. Ravits, J. (2014). Focality, stochasticity and neuroanatomic propagation in ALS pathogenesis. *Exp. Neurol.* 262, 121–126. doi: 10.1016/j.expneurol.2014.07.021

Reniers, W., Schrooten, M., Claeys, K. G., Tilkin, P., D'Hondt, A., Reijen, D. V., et al. (2017). Prognostic value of clinical and electrodiagnostic parameters at time of diagnosis in patients with amyotrophic lateral sclerosis. *Amyotroph. Lateral Scler. Frontotemporal Degener.* 18, 341–350. doi: 10.1080/21678421.2017.1288254

146. Renton, A. E., Chiò, A., and Traynor, B. J. (2013). State of play in amyotrophic lateral sclerosis genetics. *Nat. Neurosci.* 17, 17–23. doi: 10.1038/nn.3584

147. Roche, J. C., Rojas-Garcia, R., Scott, K. M., Scotton, W., Ellis, C. E., Burman, R., et al. (2012). A proposed staging system for amyotrophic lateral sclerosis. *Brain* 135, 847–852. doi: 10.1093/brain/awr351

148. Rokach, L. (2016). Decision forest: twenty years of research. *Inform. Fusion* 27, 111–125. doi: 10.1016/j.inffus.2015.06.005

149. Rong, P., Yunusova, Y., Wang, J., and Green, J. R. (2015). Predicting early bulbar decline in amyotrophic lateral sclerosis: a speech subsystem approach. *Behav. Neurol.* 2015, 1–11. doi: 10.1155/2015/183027

150. Rooney, J. P., Visser, A. E., D'Ovidio, F., Vermeulen, R., Beghi, E., Chio, A., et al. (2017). A case-control study of hormonal exposures as etiologic factors for ALS in women. *Neurology* 89, 1283–1290. doi: 10.1212/wnl.0000000000004390

151. Rosenbohm, A., , Peter, R. S., Erhardt, S., Lulé, D., Rothenbacher, D., Ludolph, A. C., et al. (2017). Epidemiology of amyotrophic lateral sclerosis in southern germany. *J. Neurol.* 264, 749–757. doi: 10.1007/s00415-017-8413-3

152. Rossi, D., Volanti, P., Brambilla, L., Colletti, T., Spataro, R., and Bella, V. L. (2018). CSF neurofilament proteins as diagnostic and prognostic biomarkers for amyotrophic lateral sclerosis. *J. Neurol.* 265, 510–521. doi: 10.1007/s00415-017-8730-6

153. Roweis, S., and Ghahramani, Z. (1999). A unifying review of linear gaussian models. *Neural Comput.* 11, 305–345. doi: 10.1162/089976699300016674

154. Rubin, D. B. (ed.) (1987). *Multiple Imputation for Nonresponse in Surveys.* John Wiley & Sons, Inc. Samet, H. (2006). *Foundations of Multidimensional and Metric Data Structures.* Oxford: Elsevier LTD.

155. Sammut, C., and Webb, G. I. (2017). *Encyclopedia of Machine Learning and Data Mining.* Springer Publishing Company, Incorporated.

156. Sarica, A., Cerasa, A., Valentino, P., Yeatman, J., Trotta, M., Barone, S., et al. (2016). The corticospinal tract profile in amyotrophic lateral sclerosis. *Hum. Brain Mapp.* 38, 727–739. doi: 10.1002/hbm.23412

157. Schapire, R. E. (2003). "The boosting approach to machine learning: an overview," in *Nonlinear Estimation and Classification* (New York, NY: Springer), 149–171.

158. Schiffman, P. L., and Belsh, J. M. (1993). Pulmonary function at diagnosis of amyotrophic lateral sclerosis. *Chest* 103, 508–513. doi:10.1378/chest.103.2.508

159. Schuster, C., Elamin, M., Hardiman, O., and Bede, P. (2015). Presymptomatic and longitudinal neuroimaging in neurodegeneration—from snapshots to motion picture: a systematic review. *J. Neurol. Neurosurg. Psychiatry* 86, 1089–1096. doi: 10.1136/jnnp-2014-309888

160. Schuster, C., Elamin, M., Hardiman, O., and Bede, P. (2016a). The segmental diffusivity profile of amyotrophic lateral sclerosis associated white matter degeneration. *Eur. J. Neurol.* 23, 1361–1371. doi: 10.1111/ene.13038

161. Schuster, C., Hardiman, O., and Bede, P. (2016b). Development of an automated MRI-based diagnostic protocol for amyotrophic lateral sclerosis using disease-specific pathognomonic features: a quantitative disease-state classification study. *PLoS ONE* 11:e0167331. doi: 10.1371/journal.pone.0167331

162. Schuster, C., Hardiman, O., and Bede, P. (2017). Survival prediction in amyotrophic lateral sclerosis based on MRI measures and clinical characteristics. *BMC Neurol.* 17:73. doi:10.1186/s12883-017-0854-x

163. Seibold, H., Zeileis, A., and Hothorn, T. (2017). Individual treatment effect prediction for amyotrophic lateral sclerosis patients. *Stat. Methods Med. Res.* 27, 3104–3125. doi: 10.1177/0962280217693034

164. Shaik, A. B., and Srinivasan, S. (2018). "A brief survey on random forest ensembles in classification model," in *International Conference on Innovative Computing and Communications* (Singapore: Springer), 253–260.

165. Simpson, E. P., Henry, Y. K., Henkel, J. S., Smith, R. G., and Appel, S. H. (2004). Increased lipid peroxidation in sera of ALS patients: a potential biomarker of disease burden. *Neurology* 62, 1758–1765. doi: 10.1212/wnl.62.10.1758

166. Srivastava, T., Darras, B. T., Wu, J. S., and Rutkove, S. B. (2012). Machine learning algorithms to classify spinal muscular atrophy subtypes. *Neurology* 79, 358–364. doi: 10.1212/wnl.0b013e3182604395

167. Steinacker, P., Feneberg, E., Weishaupt, J., Brettschneider, J., Tumani, H., Andersen, P. M., et al. (2015). Neurofilaments in the diagnosis of motoneuron diseases: a prospective study on 455 patients. *J. Neurol. Neurosurg. Psychiatry* 87, 12–20. doi: 10.1136/jnnp-2015-311387

168. Strong, M. J., Abrahams, S., Goldstein, L. H., Woolley, S., Mclaughlin, P., Snowden, J., et al. (2017). Amyotrophic lateral sclerosis - frontotemporal spectrum disorder (ALS-FTSD): Revised diagnostic criteria. *Amyotroph. Lateral Scler. Frontotemporal Degener.* 18, 153–174. doi: 10.1080/21678421.2016.1267768

169. Strong, M. J., Grace, G. M., Freedman, M., Lomen-Hoerth, C., Woolley, S., Goldstein, L. H., et al. (2009). Consensus criteria for the diagnosis of frontotemporal cognitive and behaviouralfba syndromes in amyotrophic lateral sclerosis. *Amyotroph. Lateral Scler.* 10, 131–146. doi: 10.1080/17482960802654364

170. Suzuki, K. (2017). Overview of deep learning in medical imaging. *Radiol. Phys. Technol.* 10, 257–273. doi: 10.1007/s12194-017-0406-5

171. Tabrizi, S. J., Reilmann, R., Roos, R. A., Durr, A., Leavitt, B., Owen, G., et al. (2012). Potential endpoints for clinical trials in premanifest and early huntington's disease in the track-hd study: analysis of 24 month observational data. *Lancet Neurol.* 11, 42–53. doi: 10.1016/s1474-4422(11)70263-0

172. Talman, P., Duong, T., Vucic, S., Mathers, S., Venkatesh, S., Henderson, R., et al. (2016). Identification and outcomes of clinical phenotypes in amyotrophic lateral sclerosis/motor neuron disease: Australian national motor neuron disease observational cohort. *BMJ Open* 6:e012054. doi: 10.1136/bmjopen-2016-012054

173. Taylor, A. A., Fournier, C., Polak, M., Wang, L., Zach, N., Keymer, M., et al. (2016). Predicting disease progression in amyotrophic lateral sclerosis. *Ann. Clin. Transl. Neurol.* 3, 866–875. doi: 10.1002/acn3.348

174. Taylor, J. P., Brown, R. H., and Cleveland, D. W. (2016). Decoding ALS: from genes to mechanism. *Nature* 539, 197–206. doi: 10.1038/nature 20413

175. Thakore, N. J., Lapin, B. R., Kinzy, T. G., and Pioro, E. P. (2018). Deconstructing progression of amyotrophic lateral sclerosis in stages: a markov modeling approach. *Amyotroph. Lateral Scler. Frontotemporal Degener.* 19, 483–494. doi: 10.1080/21678421.2018.1484925

176. Tohgi, H., Abe, T., Yamazaki, K., Murata, T., Ishizaki, E., and Isobe, C. (1999). Remarkable increase in cerebrospinal fluid 3-nitrotyrosine in patients with sporadic amyotrophic lateral sclerosis. *Ann. Neurol.* 46, 129–131.

177. Tortelli, R., Copetti, M., Panza, F., Cortese, R., Capozzo, R., D'/Errico, E., et al. (2015). Time to generalisation as a predictor of prognosis in amyotrophic lateral sclerosis: Table 1. *J. Neurol. Neurosurg. Psychiatry* 87, 678–679. doi: 10.1136/jnnp-2014-308478

178. Tortelli, R., Copetti, M., Ruggieri, M., Cortese, R., Capozzo, R., Leo, A., et al. (2014). Cerebrospinal fluid neurofilament light chain levels: marker of progression to generalized amyotrophic lateral sclerosis. *Eur. J. Neurol.* 22, 215–218. doi: 10.1111/ene.12421

179. Traynor, B. J., Codd, M. B., Corr, B., Forde, C., Frost, E., and Hardiman, O. (2000). Amyotrophic lateral sclerosis mimic syndromes. *Arch. Neurol.* 57:109. doi: 10.1001/archneur.57.1.109

180. Turner, M. R. (2018). Progress and new frontiers in biomarkers for amyotrophic lateral sclerosis. *Biomark. Med.* 12, 693–696. doi: 10.2217/bmm-20 18-0149

181. Turner, M. R., Grosskreutz, J., Kassubek, J., Abrahams, S., Agosta, F., Benatar, M., et al. (2011). Towards a neuroimaging biomarker for amyotrophic lateral sclerosis. *Lancet Neurol.* 10, 400–403. doi: 10.1016/s1474-4422(11)7 0049-7

182. Turner, M. R., Hardiman, O., Benatar, M., Brooks, B. R., Chio, A., de Carvalho, M., et al. (2013). Controversies and priorities in amyotrophic lateral sclerosis. *Lancet Neurol.* 12, 310–322. doi: 10.1016/s1474-4422(13)7 0036-x

183. Turner, M. R., Kiernan, M. C., Leigh, P. N., and Talbot, K. (2009). Biomarkers in amyotrophic lateral sclerosis. *Lancet Neurol.* 8, 94–109. doi: 10.1016/s1474-4422(08)70293-x

184. van Buuren, S. (2007). Multiple imputation of discrete and continuous data by fully conditional specification. *Stat. Methods Med. Res.* 16, 219–242. doi: 10.1177/0962280206074463

185. van der Burgh, H. K., Schmidt, R., Westeneng, H.-J., de Reus, M. A., van den Berg, L. H., and van den Heuvel, M. P. (2017). Deep learning predictions of survival based on MRI in amyotrophic lateral sclerosis. *Neuroimage Clin.* 13, 361–369. doi: 10.1016/j.nicl.2016.10.008

186. Vapnik, V. N. (2000). *The Nature of Statistical Learning Theory.* New York, NY: Springer.

187. Varghese, A., Sharma, A., Mishra, P., Vijayalakshmi, K., Harsha, H., Sathyaprabha, T. N., et al. (2013). Chitotriosidase - a putative biomarker for sporadic amyotrophic lateral sclerosis. *Clin. Proteomics* 10:19. doi: 10.1186/1559-0275-10-19

188. Visser, A. E., Rooney, J. P. K., D'Ovidio, F., Westeneng, H.-J., Vermeulen,

189. R. C. H., Beghi, E., et al. (2018). Multicentre, cross-cultural, population-based, case–control study of physical activity as risk factor for amyotrophic lateral sclerosis. *J. Neurol. Neurosurg. Psychiatry* 89, 797–803. doi: 10.1136/jnnp-2017-317724

190. Visser, J., van den Berg-Vos, R. M., Franssen, H., van den Berg, L. H., Wokke, J. H., de Jong, J. M. V., et al. (2007). Disease course and prognostic

factors of progressive muscular atrophy. *Arch. Neurol.* 64:522. doi: 10.1001/archneur.64.4.522

191. Wang, S., Peng, J., Ma, J., and Xu, J. (2016). Protein secondary structure prediction using deep convolutional neural fields. *Sci. Rep.* 6:18962. doi: 10.1038/srep18962
192. Welsh, R. C., Jelsone-Swain, L. M., and Foerster, B. R. (2013). The utility of independent component analysis and machine learning in the identification of the amyotrophic lateral sclerosis diseased brain. *Front. Hum. Neurosci.* 7:251. doi: 10.3389/fnhum.2013.00251
193. Westeneng, H.-J., Debray, T. P. A., Visser, A. E., van Eijk, R. P. A., Rooney, J. P. K., Calvo, A., et al. (2018). Prognosis for patients with amyotrophic lateral sclerosis: development and validation of a personalised prediction model. *Lancet Neurol.* 17, 423–433. doi: 10.1016/s1474-4422(18)30 089-9
194. Wolf, J., Safer, A., Wöhrle, J. C., Palm, F., Nix, W. A., Maschke, M., et al. (2015). Factors predicting survival in ALS patients - data from a population-based registry in rhineland-palatinate, germany. *Neuroepidemiology* 44, 149–155. doi: 10.1159/000381625
195. Zetterström, P., Andersen, P. M., Brännström, T., and Marklund, S. L. (2011). Misfolded superoxide dismutase-1 in CSF from amyotrophic lateral sclerosis patients. *J. Neurochem.* 117, 91–99. doi: 10.1111/j.1471-4159.2011.07177.x
196. Zhang, F., Chen, G., He, M., Dai, J., Shang, H., Gong, Q., et al. (2018). Altered white matter microarchitecture in amyotrophic lateral sclerosis: A voxel-based meta-analysis of diffusion tensor imaging. *Neuroimage Clin.* 19, 122–129. doi: 10.1016/j.nicl.2018.04.005
197. Zhang, J., Ma, K.-K., Er, M.-H., and Chong, V. (2004). "Tumor segmentation from magnetic resonance imaging by learning via one-class support vector machine," in *International Workshop on Advanced Image Technology (IWAIT '04)* (Singapore).
198. Zhang, Y., Zhang, B., Coenen, F., Xiao, J., and Lu, W. (2014). One-class kernel subspace ensemble for medical image classification. *EURASIP J. Adv. Signal Process.* 2014:17. doi: 10.1186/s13634 015 0271 2
199. Zhou, J.-Y., Afjehi-Sadat, L., Asress, S., Duong, D. M., Cudkowicz, M., Glass,
200. J. D., et al. (2010). Galectin-3 is a candidate biomarker for amyotrophic lateral sclerosis: discovery by a proteomics approach. *J. Proteome Res.* 9, 5133–5141. doi: 10.1021/pr100409r
201. Zoccolella, S., Beghi, E., Palagano, G., Fraddosio, A., Samarelli, V., Lamberti, P., et al. (2006). Predictors of delay in the diagnosis and clinical trial entry of amyotrophic lateral sclerosis patients: a population-based study. *J. Neurol. Sci.* 250, 45–49. doi: 10.1016/j.jns.2006.06.027

GLOSSARY

ALS : Amyotrophic Lateral Sclerosis
ALSbi : Behaviorally impaired ALS
ALSFRS : ALS Functional Rating Scale
ALSbi : behaviorally impaired ALS
ALSnci : ALS with no cognitive impairment
ALSci : ALS with cognitive impairment
ALSexec : ALS with executive dysfunction
AUC : Area Under the ROC Curve
AD : Axial Diffusivity
CNN : Convolutional Neural Network
CSF : Cerebrospinal fluid
CST : Corticospinal
DeepCNF : Deep Convolutional Neural Fields
DTI : Diffusion Tensor Imaging
FA : Fractional Anisotropy
FTD : Frontotemporal Dementia
GMM : Gaussian Mixture Model
KD : Kennedy's disease
k-NN : k-Nearest Neighbors
LMN : Lower Motor Neurons
MD : Mean Diffusivity
ML : Machine Learning
MND : Motor Neuron Disease
NN : Neural Network
PBP : Progressive Bulbar Palsy
PCA : Principal Component Analysis
PD : Parkinson's Disease
PLS : Primary Lateral Sclerosis
PMA : Progressive Muscular Atrophy
PRO-ACT : Pooled Resource Open-Access ALS Clinical Trials
RBP : RNA-Binding Protein
RD : Radial Diffusivity
RF : Random Forest
RMSE : Root Mean Squared Error
RNN : Recurrent Neural Network
ROC : Receiver Operating Curve
SFR : Sample to Feature Ratio
SMA : Spinal Muscular Atrophy
SVM : Support Vector Machine
t-SNE : t-distributed Stochastic Neighbor Embedding
UMN : Upper Motor Neurons

4

Emerging Magnetic Resonance Imaging Techniques and Analysis Methods in Amyotrophic Lateral Sclerosis

Andrew W. Barritt [1,2*], ***Matt C. Gabel*** [3], ***Mara Cercignani*** [1] ***and P. Nigel Leigh*** [2,3]

[1] Clinical Imaging Sciences Centre, Brighton and Sussex Medical School, Falmer, United Kingdom, [2] Hurstwood Park Neurological Centre, Haywards Heath, West Sussex, United Kingdom, [3] Department of Neuroscience, Trafford Centre for Biomedical Research, Brighton and Sussex Medical School, Falmer, United Kingdom

***Correspondence:**
Andrew W. Barritt
a.barritt@bsms.ac.uk

Objective markers of disease sensitive to the clinical activity, symptomatic progression, and underlying substrates of neurodegeneration are highly coveted in amyotrophic lateral sclerosis in order to more eloquently stratify the highly heterogeneous phenotype and facilitate the discovery of effective disease modifying treatments for patients. Magnetic resonance imaging (MRI) is a promising, non-invasive biomarker candidate whose acquisition techniques and analysis methods are undergoing constant evolution in the pursuit of parameters which more closely represent biologically-applicable tissue changes. Neurite Orientation Dispersion and Density Imaging (NODDI; a form of diffusion imaging), and quantitative Magnetization Transfer Imaging (qMTi) are two such emerging modalities which have each broadened the understanding of other neurological disorders and have the potential to provide new insights into structural alterations initiated by the disease process in ALS. Furthermore, novel neuroimaging data analysis approaches such as Event-Based Modeling (EBM) may be able to circumvent the requirement for longitudinal scanning as a means to comprehend the dynamic stages of neurodegeneration *in vivo*. Combining these and other innovative imaging protocols with more sophisticated techniques to analyse ever-increasing datasets holds the exciting prospect of transforming understanding of the biological processes and temporal evolution of the ALS syndrome, and can only benefit from multicentre collaboration across the entire ALS research community.

Keywords: motor neuron disease, MRI—magnetic resonance imaging, event-based model, quantitative magnetization transfer imaging, neurite orientation dispersion and density imaging (NODDI)

Neuroimaging modalities sensitive to the dynamics and patterns of tissue degeneration in amyotrophic lateral sclerosis (ALS) are required as objective biological markers of disease activity *in vivo*. Standard clinical assessment is usually adequate for diagnosis, however there is a pressing need for non-invasive neuroimaging biomarkers that may differentiate between the various phenotypes within the ALS syndrome, provide more accurate prognostic information, and monitor responses to therapeutic interventions. There is also a need for neuroimaging techniques which have the potential to interrogate the specific mechanisms of neurodegeneration, given that conventional MRI primarily aims to exclude alternative diagnoses (1). As such, it will be important to integrate new modalities of structural and functional imaging (including MRI and PET) with molecular biomarkers of neuronal damage, and indicators of neuroinflammation if the therapeutic impasse for more effective disease treatments is to be broken. Diffusion MRI, particularly diffusion tensor imaging (DTI), has been extensively researched in patients with ALS to infer structural alterations within the brain and spinal cord by virtue of the movement of water molecules induced by magnetic field gradients. Fractional anisotropy (FA) is consistently reduced, often alongside increased mean or radial diffusivity (MD or RD, respectively), within the corticospinal tracts (CSTs) (2–15) and body of the corpus callosum through which pass the fibers connecting hemispheric motor areas (3, 5–8, 10, 12, 16, 17). Indeed, DTI changes are perhaps most reliably encountered within the posterior limb of the internal capsule (18, 19) which forms a common conduit for several descending motor pathways including the CST, cortico-rubro-spinal, and cortico-reticulo-spinal connections (20). Additional areas within the frontal, temporal (11, 21, 22), and parietal areas (11, 23) have shown reduced FA, all of which is consistent with the multisystem motor and extra-motor regions involved clinically and neuropathologically (24–26). Nevertheless, establishing the precise substrate or substrates underlying these changes observed on MRI is not straightforward and may be complimented by novel magnetic resonance imaging techniques and emerging big data analysis methods.

NEURITE ORIENTATION DISPERSION AND DENSITY IMAGING (NODDI)

Diffusion MRI is sensitive to the motion of water molecules at microscopic level. Nevertheless the signal it measures is averaged across volumes of 1-2 mm^3 (the so-called "voxel"). For this reason, any interpretation of the signal and its origin requires some degree of "modeling." More than one model has been proposed and each typically incorporates slightly differing mathematical assumptions to interpret and model the signal, thus providing only indirect inferences on anatomical configurations. For instance, DTI assumes that water movement will obey Gaussian properties and is widely accepted to lose consistency when neuronal fibers bend or fan out within a voxel, or where otherwise aligned fiber tracts are crossing each other (5) which is common to areas such as the centrum semiovale and even regions of the foliated corpus callosum (27, 28). Moreover, a reduction in FA signifies changes in both neurite density and orientation dispersion without distinguishing their individual contributions (28, 29). Therefore, variations on the diffusion tensor model have been created in an attempt to address these limitations. One such model is neurite orientation dispersion and density imaging (NODDI).

NODDI requires acquisition over a longer time than DTI and compartmentalizes non-Gaussian water diffusion into three geometric spaces encompassing isotropic (or free), hindered anisotropic and restricted anisotropic components. These are known as V_{ISO}, V_{IC}, and V_{EC} and each broadly correspond to free water/CSF, intra-neurite water (of axons and dendrites), and extra-neurite water (but potentially including glial cells and neuronal somata), respectively (29–31). The NODDI parameters ISO, NDI (neurite density index), and ODI (orientation dispersion index; a marker of the geometric complexity of neurites) can then be derived, the latter two of which are considered to provide a more structurally useful breakdown of single FA values (29) (see **Figure 1**). NODDI is able to better delineate white from gray matter, in which normal white matter displays higher NDI and lower ODI with the reverse in gray matter (33), and differentiate between different gray matter structures although might be more susceptible to changes in field strength in these areas (31). Compared to DTI, NODDI indices, particularly ODI, have been shown to correlate with histological measures of orientation dispersion in the spinal cord and might also display more inter-subject variability with implications for the sample sizes required for group analyses (33, 34). However, this may not necessarily be an inaccuracy in modeling rather a more accurate depiction of tissue composition (31). In addition, regions which might be expected to demonstrate considerable axon density and higher NDI values might counterintuitively show higher ISO due to the larger diameter axons enabling more freedom of water movement (31, 34).

NODDI has been used to demonstrate tissue alterations associated with normal aging (35–37) and in a range of conditions including focal cortical dysplasia (38), stroke (39), Wilson's disease (40), multiple sclerosis (33), neurofibromatosis type 1 (38, 41), and neurodegenerative diseases. Reduction in NDI and ODI of the contralateral substantia nigra pars compacta has been shown to correlate negatively with clinical severity of Parkinson's disease (42) whereas in pre-manifest Huntington's disease reductions in NDI and ODI are seen in a range of white matter tracts with reduced NDI in the corpus callosum correlating positively with markers of severity (43). In patients with young onset Alzheimer's disease reduction in NDI and ODI is seen corrected for reduced thickness within several relevant cortical areas, with lower NDI values in patients scoring less well on cognitive tests (44), while in a rodent model NODDI indices correlate more consistently than DTI parameters with the burden of tau pathology harbored by the cortex, corpus callosum, and hippocampus (45).

Use of NODDI imaging in ALS has only recently been undertaken. Whole brain analysis in patients with manifest disease has demonstrated a significant NDI reduction throughout the intracranial CSTs up to the subcortical matter of the precentral gyri and across the corpus callosum, with increased ODI in the anterior limb of right internal capsule and increased ISO adjacent to the right lateral ventricle relative to healthy controls (46). NDI within the right corona radiata and precentral subcortical white matter was decreased to a greater extent in those patients with both limb and bulbar involvement compared to limb alone, and longer disease durations correlated with reduced ODI in the precentral gyri, dorsolateral prefrontal cortices, and precuneus. Furthermore, at the statistical threshold used, FA was reduced as expected within the CSTs but less extensively than NDI, and changes were not observed within the corpus callosum, implying NODDI may be more sensitive than DTI. Indeed, combined NODDI and DTI has also been performed in pre-manifest C9orf72 mutation carriers alongside first degree relatives not possessing the pathological repeat

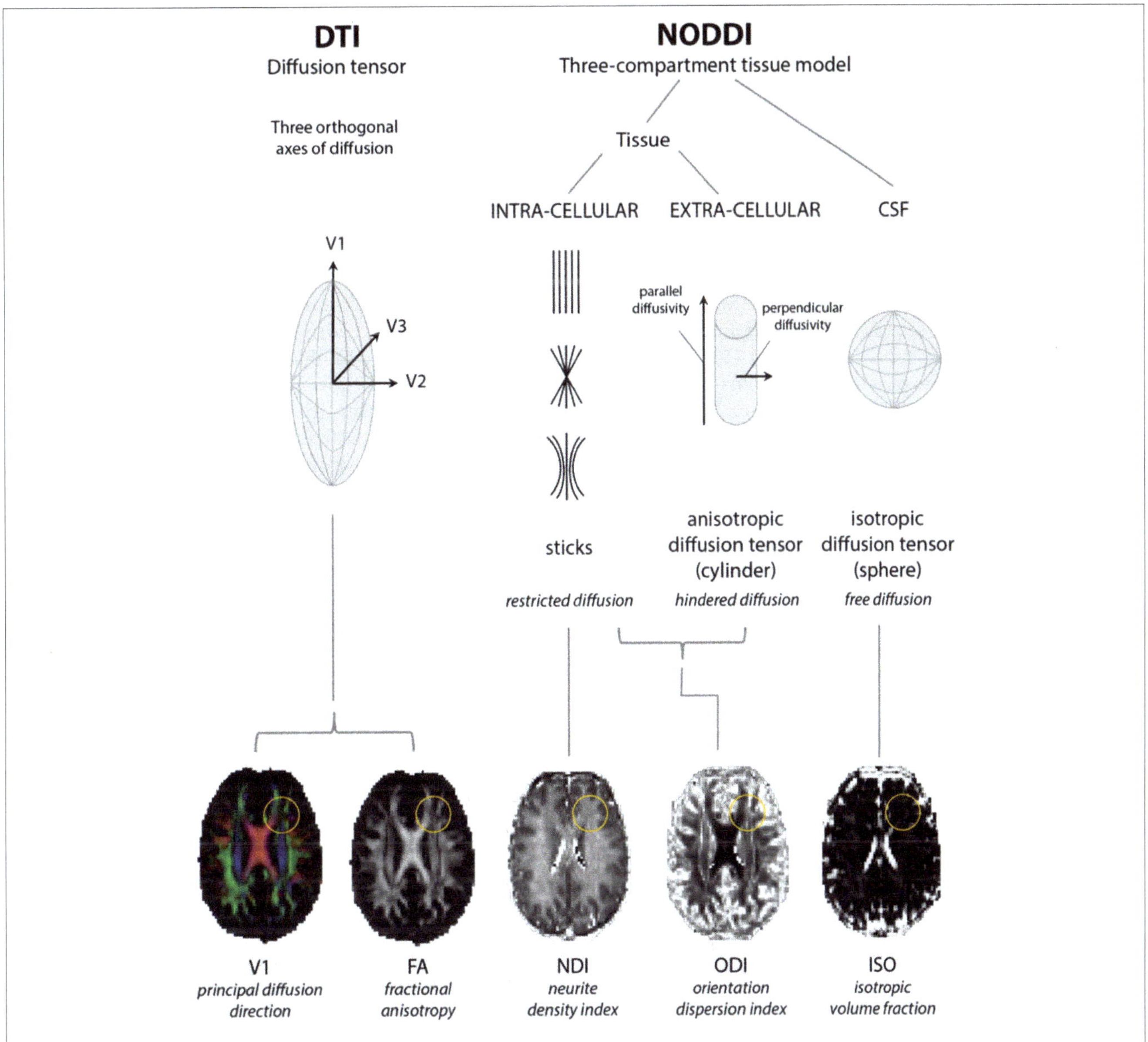

FIGURE 1 | Models of diffusion for neurite orientation dispersion and density imaging (NODDI) and diffusion tensor imaging (DTI). The diffusion tensor model of DTI is based upon three orthogonal axes of diffusion (V1, V2, and V3) yielding radial, axial, and mean diffusivity from which fractional anisotropy (FA) can be estimated. NODDI considers diffusion within three compartments: restricted diffusion in the intracellular compartment, hindered diffusion in the extracellular compartment, and free diffusion in cerebrospinal fluid (CSF), from which parameter maps representing neurite density (NDI), orientation dispersion (ODI), and isotropic fraction (ISO) indices can be estimated. Yellow circles highlight a region where changes in FA can be accompanied by changes in both NDI and ODI. Adapted from Rae et al. (32).

expansion (47). The effect size relating to detectable reductions of NDI within 7 of 11 white matter tracts, including the CSTs, is greater than that for DTI metrics (in this case increased axial diffusivity, RD, and MD rather than decreased FA) albeit statistically significant in just two. Therefore, the results appear to corroborate the implication that lowered FA (or increased diffusivity) in the CSTs and corpus callosum results from the loss of axon fibers rather than increased complexity or dispersion within tracts. Longitudinal NODDI scans have not yet been investigated although results from an ancillary imaging study to the Modifying Immune Response and Outcomes in ALS (MIROCALS) trial of low dose Interleukin-2 treatment are awaited.

In any case, neuroimaging techniques are constantly evolving with a raft of acronyms and employing different protocols aiming to reflect the true histological framework of gray and white matter. Although NODDI is considered non-inferior to other MRI modalities of high-angular resolution in this regard (48), it may be that acquisition protocols or MRI data modeling methods undertaken in NODDI, such as spherical (rather than linear) tensor encoding (49) along with tract-based (50), gray matter based (37), and gray matter surface based (51) spatial statistics are further refined in due course to overcome its own recognized limitations.

QUANTITATIVE MAGNETIZATION TRANSFER IMAGING (QMTI)

Magnetization transfer imaging, unlike the NODDI model of diffusion MRI, essentially utilizes a "two pool" model in which hydrogen protons are either free or bound to macromolecules (lipids and proteins) within the semisolid tissue. The latter protons do not directly contribute to the MRI signal and are "silent" in diffusion sequences (increased radial diffusivity with DTI is not specific for demyelination) (52), but can be indirectly probed thanks to their interaction with the free protons following off-frequency radiofrequency pulses. The exchange in magnetization between the two compartments allows the state of the semisolid pool (saturated) to affect that of the free protons, resulting in partial saturation and in a decrease of its overall magnetization (53). The magnetization transfer (MT) effect can thereby produce a qualitative magnetization transfer tissue contrast (MTC) image and is already clinically utilized as part of MR angiography and gadolinium-enhanced T1-weighted sequences, for instance. Indeed, MTC T1 images in patients with ALS have shown hyperintensity along the CST (54, 55) and CC (54) in a proportion of cases (and more conspicuously than FLAIR) (55) compared to control subjects which was significantly related to the degree of reduced FA in the same regions and presumed to reflect damage to the white matter tracts, although with no clear association with clinical rating scales or disease duration (54). Acquiring a proton-density image with and without a MT pulse renders it possible to semi-quantify the MT effect and produce a voxel-wise magnetization transfer ratio (MTR) to reflect changes in macromolecular integrity. Accordingly, reduced MTR within the brain has been reported within the CSTs (56), the precentral and other frontal and extramotor gyri (57, 58), in patients with ALS compared to healthy controls, and independently of gray matter atrophy as measured by voxel-base morphometry (57). Significantly reduced average MTR within the spinal cord has also been reported with respect to controls (59–61), accompanied by diminished cord cross-sectional area and average FA (60), and with a longitudinal decline between sequential scans (59). More recent segmentation of the cord into gray and white matter areas, and using a particular adjusted MT protocol called inhomogeneous MT, has demonstrated localized reductions in MTR to the CSTs and dorsal columns in addition to the anterior horns at several non-contiguous cervical levels (62). However, the MTC and MTR are dependent on a range of imaging variables and their biophysical basis is undefined (53).

The development of mathematical models able to describe the MT-weighted signal as a function of the saturating pulses has enabled more biologically applicable parameters to be derived from quantitative magnetization transfer imaging (qMTi), including the macromolecular pool fraction [f; modeled to essentially represent myelin content], forward exchange rate of magnetization transfer [k_f], and transverse relaxation time of the free pool [$T_2{}^F$]. Although qMTi is yet to be explored in patients with ALS, studies in multiple sclerosis (MS) have demonstrated reductions in f and k_f, and increased $T_2{}^F$ in acute inflammatory lesions with a subsequent return to baseline over several months (63). Compared to healthy controls, normal appearing white matter (NAWM) has reduced f, kf, and MTR (64), and reduced MTR in chronic MS plaques and has been shown to correlate with greater disability (65). Incidentally, reduced MTR in the context of MS is generally considered to be a marker of demyelination, although a small study subdivided NAWM according to distance from a T2 hyper-intense plaque and degree of MTR reduction and found that, whereas at the edge of plaques reduced MTR correlates with reduced myelin content reduced MTR in NAWM may be result from to swollen microglia and, perhaps, axons (66), thus highlighting the uncertainty of its interpretation. MTR in normal appearing gray matter is also reduced in patients with relapsing-remitting MS (67–69) and may also correlate with disability, although variable results are reported (68). Acute increases in kf (but without change in f or T2f) on qMTi have also been induced within the insula in the context of a systemic inflammatory stimulus comprising intramuscular injection of typhoid vaccination and are associated with increased levels of reported fatigue, in addition to a co-localized increase in glucose metabolism measured by FGD-PET (70). Although the mechanisms underlying changes in magnetization transfer parameters are likely to be very different between diseases, it is plausible that qMTi would be sensitive to structural alterations in ALS given the likely role for the immune system in its pathogenesis (71, 72).

MULTIMODAL MRI

Furthermore, it may be that performing simultaneous qMTi with several other MR neuroimaging sequences, such as diffusion and (resting state) functional MRI, will be most helpful in building a better understanding how both tissue structure and function are affected by the disease process and, ultimately, the difference between certain phenotypes to guide more personalized treatments. Indeed, this is exemplified by the estimations of the myelinated fiber "g-ratio," the axon diameter divided by the diameter of its ensheathing myelin, which is estimated to ideally be around 0.7 in the central nervous system (73). As diffusion MRI is insensitive to myelin, the combination of intraneurite and isotropic fractions from NODDI and the *f* value from qMTi is required to calculate the g-ratio across the brain. Following adolescence, white matter g-ratio tends to steadily increase with age inferring myelin reduction and knock on effects with respect to the velocity of neuronal conduction (74) and premature increases in the g-ratio are accordingly seen within MS plaques (75, 76). Although ALS is not primarily a demyelinating disease, new insights into the secondary effects of the neurodegenerative process may be revealed with these techniques and correlate with clinical measures.

EVENT-BASED MODELING

Aside from interpreting the deviations of imaging parameters in terms of current tissue configuration, collecting longitudinal

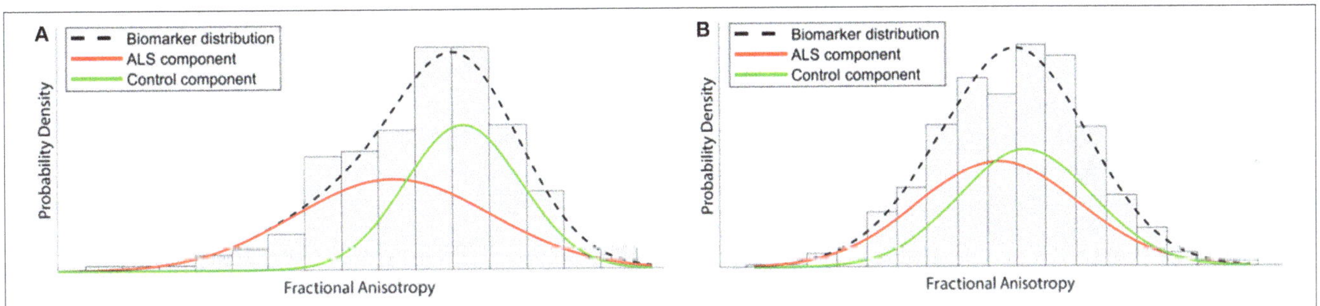

FIGURE 2 | Illustration of how the event-based model (EBM) aims to extract temporal information from a cross-sectional data set. Gaussian distributions of fractional anisotropy (FA) biomarker readings within a tract affected early in the course of the disease, such as the corticospinal tract, would be expected to demonstrate substantial separation between ALS and Control imaging data **(A)**. However, FA from another area affected at later stages demonstrates much less separation between distributions **(B)**. By exploiting and characterizing these differences across all biomarkers, the EBM attempts to order the change from "normal" to "diseased" across the entire disease course.

data is, at least conceptually, the most straightforward approach to understanding the temporal evolution of neurodegenerative pathology. However, patient tolerability for repeated MRI acquisition remains challenging in ALS, particularly, due to the rapid accumulation of symptoms and perhaps accounts for the relatively few studies conducted to date (5). Furthermore, it can be argued that participants who are included would be those harboring more slowly-progressing disease, and therefore may not be representative of the majority of patients with ALS.

Given these limitations, alternative methods such as "big data" analysis techniques and new modeling approaches have the potential to greatly increase our understanding of the mechanisms of disease progression. One such approach is the Event-Based Model (EBM) (77–79), a generative probabilistic model originally developed for use in Alzheimer's disease (AD) for which it has been validated in addition to Huntington's disease (80) and recently in ALS using oculomotor data (81). The EBM is designed to extract temporal information from cross-sectional data sets and, unlike traditional models of disease progression, does not rely on *a priori* staging of patients but instead extracts the event ordering directly from the data, thereby minimizing subjective bias.

The EBM defines a disease as a series of "events," where each event is the change of a biomarker reading from a "healthy" to a "diseased" state. Crucially, biomarker cut-off points are not determined beforehand, but are derived from the data during the modeling process. This not only reduces subjective bias, but also allows for much finer temporal characterization of disease progression than is possible under existing clinically-based staging systems. Healthy control data are used as a fixed reference, and each biomarker is modeled as a mixture of two Gaussian distributions (**Figure 2**). In order to perform temporal modeling, the EBM assumes that the disease progression is monotonic for individual biomarkers (i.e., the severity of disease burden can only increase). Thus, for biomarkers affected early on in the course of the disease, there will be larger differences between patient and control readings, while biomarkers that are affected late on will have smaller differences between patients and controls. Markov Chain Monte Carlo (MCMC) techniques can then be used to determine the most likely event order across the entire cohort (77).

As with any modeling approach, the EBM has strengths and weaknesses. The ability to extract fine-grained temporal information from cross-sectional data is exceptionally novel and valuable. Use of MCMC techniques also enables the model to quantify the positional variance of individual biomarkers across the cohort, thereby allowing a comparison of their relative importance and variability. In its current form, the EBM reveals aspects of disease progression that are common across the entire cohort (an "average" disease progression). The heterogeneity of ALS means that EBM analyses of stratified subgroups, based on genetic/prognostic factors, are an important future area for investigation.

The accuracy of the EBM output, as with any modeling process, will depend on the quality of the input biomarker data. As a consequence, ALS event-based modeling can require large quantities of data, particularly as individual mean cerebral CST FA values are known to have modest diagnostic power for ALS [found to have a pooled sensitivity and specificity of 0.68 and 0.73, respectively, in a meta-analysis (82)]. Current applications of the EBM to ALS data in progress include analysis of mean FA of white matter (WM) fiber bundles, modeling of patterns of cortical thinning, volumetric changes of brain structures, and oculomotor data. Future areas for development include the application of the EBM to multi-modal ALS biomarker data. Excitingly, the application of the EBM to higher order models of diffusion such as NODDI has the potential to give greater insight into ALS degeneration by simultaneously modeling the changes within ISO, NDI, and ODI parameters.

CONCLUSION

Ultimately, all modeling is an attempt to separate meaningful information from randomness. MRI techniques differentially model the signal to derive parameters that plausibly relate to tissue microstructure properties; these parameters can then be modeled further using the EBM to reveal patterns that exist within the data, but which still require human assessment and interpretation (as well as clinical and histological validation). Although the innovative imaging and data analysis techniques presented here constitute a selection of available methods or protocols, their use singly and in combination has the potential to transform our understanding of the biological processes and temporal evolution of ALS, which is likely to benefit further from multicenter collaboration across the entire ALS research community.

AUTHOR CONTRIBUTIONS

AWB and MCG performed a review of the literature and drafted the paper. MC and PNL provided specialized expertise and critical appraisal of the article for submission.

FUNDING

MCG was funded by the MND Association (MNDA Gabel/Oct16/966-799).

REFERENCES

1. Turner MR, Talbot K. Mimics and chameleons in motor neurone disease. *Pract Neurol.* (2013) 13:153–64. doi: 10.1136/practneurol-2013-000557
2. Blain CR, Williams VC, Johnston C, Stanton BR, Ganesalingam J, Jarosz JM, et al. A longitudinal study of diffusion tensor MRI in ALS. *Amyotroph Lateral Scler.* (2007) 8:348–55. doi: 10.1080/17482960701548139
3. Douaud G, Filippini N, Knight S, Talbot K, Turner MR. Integration of structural and functional magnetic resonance imaging in amyotrophic lateral sclerosis. *Brain* (2011) 134:3470–9. doi: 10.1093/brain/awr279
4. Huynh W, Simon NG, Grosskreutz J, Turner MR, Vucic S, Kiernan MC. Assessment of the upper motor neuron in amyotrophic lateral sclerosis. *Clin Neurophysiol.* (2016) 127:2643–60. doi: 10.1016/j.clinph.2016.04.025
5. Menke RA, Agosta F, Grosskreutz J, Filippi M, Turner MR. Neuroimaging endpoints in amyotrophic lateral sclerosis. *Neurotherapeutics* (2016) 14:11–23. doi: 10.1007/s13311-016-0484-9
6. Simon NG, Turner MR, Vucic S, Al-Chalabi A, Shefner J, Lomen-Hoerth C, et al. Quantifying disease progression in amyotrophic lateral sclerosis. *Ann Neurol.* (2014) 76:643–57. doi: 10.1002/ana.24273
7. Turner MR, Verstraete E. What does imaging reveal about the pathology of amyotrophic lateral sclerosis? *Curr Neurol Neurosci Rep.* (2015). 15:45. doi: 10.1007/s11910-015-0569-6
8. Verstraete E, Foerster BR. Neuroimaging as a new diagnostic modality in amyotrophic lateral sclerosis. *Neurotherapeutics* (2015) 12:403–16. doi: 10.1007/s13311-015-0347-9
9. Grolez G, Moreau C, Danel-Brunaud V, Delmaire C, Lopes R, Pradat PF, et al. The value of magnetic resonance imaging as a biomarker for amyotrophic lateral sclerosis: a systematic review. *BMC Neurol.* (2016) 16:155. doi: 10.1186/s12883-016-0672-6
10. Müller HP, Turner MR, Grosskreutz J, Abrahams S, Bede P, Govind V, et al. A large-scale multicentre cerebral diffusion tensor imaging study in amyotrophic lateral sclerosis. *J Neurol Neurosurg Psychiatry* (2016) 87:570–9. doi: 10.1136/jnnp-2015-311952
11. Sage CA, Peeters RR, Görner A, Robberecht W, Sunaert S. Quantitative diffusion tensor imaging in amyotrophic lateral sclerosis. *Neuroimage* (2007) 34:486–99. doi: 10.1016/j.neuroimage.2006.09.025
12. Iwata NK, Kwan JY, Danielian LE, Butman JA, Tovar-Moll F, Bayat E, et al. White matter alterations differ in primary lateral sclerosis and amyotrophic lateral sclerosis. *Brain* (2011) 134:2642–55. doi: 10.1093/brain/awr178
13. Iwata NK, Aoki S, Okabe S, Arai N, Terao Y, Kwak S, et al. Evaluation of corticospinal tracts in ALS with diffusion tensor MRI and brainstem stimulation. *Neurology* (2008) 70:528–32. doi: 10.1212/01.wnl.0000299186.72374.19
14. Stagg CJ, Knight S, Talbot K, Jenkinson M, Maudsley AA, Turner MR. Whole-brain magnetic resonance spectroscopic imaging measures are related to disability in ALS. *Neurology* (2013) 80:610–5. doi: 10.1212/WNL.0b013e318281ccec
15. Sarica A, Cerasa A, Valentino P, Yeatman J, Trotta M, Barone S, et al. The corticospinal tract profile in amyotrophic lateral sclerosis. *Hum Brain Mapp.* (2017) 38:727–39. doi: 10.1002/hbm.23412
16. Kollewe K, Körner S, Dengler R, Petri S, Mohammadi B. Magnetic resonance imaging in amyotrophic lateral sclerosis. *Neurol Res Int.* (2012) 2012:608501. doi: 10.1155/2012/608501
17. Agosta F, Pagani E, Rocca MA, Caputo D, Perini M, Salvi F, et al. Voxel-based morphometry study of brain volumetry and diffusivity in amyotrophic lateral sclerosis patients with mild disability. *Hum Brain Mapp.* (2007) 28:1430–8. doi: 10.1002/hbm.20364
18. Turner MR, Agosta F, Bede P, Govind V, Lulé D, Verstraete E. Neuroimaging in amyotrophic lateral sclerosis. *Biomark Med.* (2012) 6:319–37. doi: 10.2217/bmm.12.26
19. Li J, Pan P, Song W, Huang R, Chen K, Shang H. A meta-analysis of diffusion tensor imaging studies in amyotrophic lateral sclerosis. *Neurobiol Aging* (2012) 33:1833–8. doi: 10.1016/j.neurobiolaging.2011.04.007
20. Lindenberg R, Renga V, Zhu LL, Betzler F, Alsop D, Schlaug G. Structural integrity of corticospinal motor fibers predicts motor impairment in chronic stroke. *Neurology* (2010) 74:280–7. doi: 10.1212/WNL.0b013e3181ccc6d9
21. Sage CA, Van Hecke W, Peeters R, Sijbers J, Robberecht W, Parizel P, et al. Quantitative diffusion tensor imaging in amyotrophic lateral sclerosis: revisited. *Hum Brain Mapp.* (2009) 30:3657–75. doi: 10.1002/hbm.20794
22. Agosta F, Ferraro PM, Riva N, Spinelli EG, Chiò A, Canu E, et al. Structural brain correlates of cognitive and behavioral impairment in MND. *Hum Brain Mapp.* (2016) 37:1614–26. doi: 10.1002/hbm.23124
23. Senda J, Kato S, Kaga T, Ito M, Atsuta N, Nakamura T, et al. Progressive and widespread brain damage in ALS: MRI voxel-based morphometry and diffusion tensor imaging study. *Amyotroph Lateral Scler.* (2011) 12:59–69. doi: 10.3109/17482968.2010.517850
24. Brownell B, Oppenheimer DR, Hughes JT. The central nervous system in motor neurone disease. *J Neurol Neurosurg Psychiatry* (1970) 33:338–57.
25. Martin JE, Swash M. The pathology of motor neuron disease. In: Leigh PN, Swash M, editors. *Motor Neuron Disease: Biology and Management.* London: Springer-Verlag (1995). p. 93–118. doi: 10.1007/978-1-4471-1871-8_5
26. Smith, M.C. Nerve fibre degeneration in the brain in amyotrophic lateral sclerosis. *J Neurol Neurosurg Psychiatry* (1960) 23:269–82. doi: 10.1136/jnnp.23.4.269
27. Budde MD, Annese J. Quantification of anisotropy and fiber orientation in human brain histological sections. *Front Integr Neurosci.* (2013) 7:3. doi: 10.3389/fnint.2013.00003
28. Jones DK, Knösche TR, Turner R. White matter integrity, fiber count, and other fallacies: the do's and don'ts of diffusion MRI. *Neuroimage* (2013) 73:239–54. doi: 10.1016/j.neuroimage.2012.06.081
29. Zhang H, Schneider T, Wheeler-Kingshott CA, Alexander DC. NODDI: practical *in vivo* neurite orientation dispersion and density imaging of the human brain. *Neuroimage* (2012) 61:1000–16. doi: 10.1016/j.neuroimage.2012.03.072
30. Caverzasi E, Papinutto N, Castellano A, Zhu AH, Scifo P, Riva M, et al. Neurite orientation dispersion and density imaging color maps to characterize brain diffusion in neurologic disorders. *J Neuroimaging* (2016) 26:494–8. doi: 10.1111/jon.12359
31. Chung AW, Seunarine KK, Clark CA. NODDI reproducibility and variability with magnetic field strength: a comparison between 1.5 T and 3 T. *Hum Brain Mapp.* (2016) 37:4550–65. doi: 10.1002/hbm.23328
32. Rae CL, Davies G, Garfinkel SN, Gabel MC, Dowell NG, Cercignani M, et al. Deficits in neurite density underlie white matter structure abnormalities in first-episode psychosis. *Biol Psychiatry* (2017) 82:716–25. doi: 10.1016/j.biopsych.2017.02.008

33. Grussu F, Schneider T, Tur C, Yates RL, Tachrount M, Ianuş A, et al. Neurite dispersion: a new marker of multiple sclerosis spinal cord pathology? *Ann Clin Transl Neurol.* (2017) 4:663–79. doi: 10.1002/acn3.445
34. Grussu F, Schneider T, Zhang H, Alexander DC, Wheeler-Kingshott CA. Neurite orientation dispersion and density imaging of the healthy cervical spinal cord *in vivo*. *Neuroimage* (2015) 111:590–601. doi: 10.1016/j.neuroimage.2015.01.045
35. Billiet T, Vandenbulcke M, Mädler B, Peeters R, Dhollander T, Zhang H, et al. Age-related microstructural differences quantified using myelin water imaging and advanced diffusion MRI. *Neurobiol Aging* (2015) 36:2107–21. doi: 10.1016/j.neurobiolaging.2015.02.029
36. Merluzzi AP, Dean DC, Adluru N, Suryawanshi GS, Okonkwo OC, Oh JM, et al. Age-dependent differences in brain tissue microstructure assessed with neurite orientation dispersion and density imaging. *Neurobiol Aging* (2016) 43:79–88. doi: 10.1016/j.neurobiolaging.2016.03.026
37. Nazeri A, Chakravarty MM, Rotenberg DJ, Rajji TK, Rathi Y, Michailovich OV, et al. Functional consequences of neurite orientation dispersion and density in humans across the adult lifespan. *J Neurosci.* (2015) 35:1753–62. doi: 10.1523/JNEUROSCI.3979-14.2015
38. Winston GP, Micallef C, Symms MR, Alexander DC, Duncan JS, Zhang H. Advanced diffusion imaging sequences could aid assessing patients with focal cortical dysplasia and epilepsy. *Epilepsy Res.* (2014) 108:336–9. doi: 10.1016/j.eplepsyres.2013.11.004
39. Adluru G, Gur Y, Anderson JS, Richards LG, Adluru N, DiBella EV. Assessment of white matter microstructure in stroke patients using NODDI. *Conf Proc IEEE Eng Med Biol Soc.* (2014) 2014:742–5. doi: 10.1109/EMBC.2014.6943697
40. Song YK, Li XB, Huang XL, Zhao J, Zhou XX, Wang YL, et al. A study of neurite orientation dispersion and density imaging in wilson's disease. *J Magn Reson Imaging* (2018) 48:423–30. doi: 10.1002/jmri.25930
41. Billiet T, Mädler B, D'Arco F, Peeters R, Deprez S, Plasschaert E, et al. Characterizing the microstructural basis of "unidentified bright objects" in neurofibromatosis type 1: A combined *in vivo* multicomponent T2 relaxation and multi-shell diffusion MRI analysis. *Neuroimage Clin.* (2014) 4:649–58. doi: 10.1016/j.nicl.2014.04.005
42. Kamagata K, Hatano T, Okuzumi A, Motoi Y, Abe O, Shimoji K, et al. Neurite orientation dispersion and density imaging in the substantia nigra in idiopathic Parkinson disease. *Eur Radiol.* (2016) 26:2567–77. doi: 10.1007/s00330-015-4066-8
43. Zhang J, Gregory S, Scahill RI, Durr A, Thomas DL, Lehericy S, et al. *In vivo* characterization of white matter pathology in pre-manifest Huntington's disease. *Ann Neurol.* (2018) 84:497–504. doi: 10.1002/ana.25309
44. Parker TD, Slattery CF, Zhang J, Nicholas JM, Paterson RW, Foulkes AJM, et al. Cortical microstructure in young onset Alzheimer's disease using neurite orientation dispersion and density imaging. *Hum Brain Mapp.* (2018) 39:3005–17. doi: 10.1002/hbm.24056
45. Colgan N, Siow B, O'Callaghan JM, Harrison IF, Wells JA, Holmes HE, et al. Application of neurite orientation dispersion and density imaging (NODDI) to a tau pathology model of Alzheimer's disease. *Neuroimage* (2016) 125:739–44. doi: 10.1016/j.neuroimage.2015.10.043
46. Broad RJ, Gabel MC, Dowell NG, Schwartzman DJ, Seth AK, Zhang H, et al. Neurite orientation and dispersion density imaging (NODDI) detects cortical and corticospinal tract degeneration in ALS. *J Neurol Neurosurg Psychiatry* (2018). doi: 10.1136/jnnp-2018-318830. [Epub ahead of print].
47. Wen J, Zhang H, Alexander DC, Durrleman S, Routier A, Rinaldi D, et al. Neurite density is reduced in the presymptomatic phase of C9orf72 disease. *J Neurol Neurosurg Psychiatry* (2018). doi: 10.1136/jnnp-2018-318994. [Epub ahead of print].
48. Schilling KG, Janve V, Gao Y, Stepniewska I, Landman BA, Anderson AW. Histological validation of diffusion MRI fiber orientation distributions and dispersion. *Neuroimage* (2018) 165:200–21. doi: 10.1016/j.neuroimage.2017.10.046
49. Lampinen B, Szczepankiewicz F, Mårtensson J, van Westen D, Sundgren PC, Nilsson M. Neurite density imaging versus imaging of microscopic anisotropy in diffusion MRI: a model comparison using spherical tensor encoding. *Neuroimage* (2017) 147:517–31. doi: 10.1016/j.neuroimage.2016.11.053
50. Smith SM, Jenkinson M, Johansen-Berg H, Rueckert D, Nichols TE, Mackay CE, et al. Tract-based spatial statistics: voxelwise analysis of multi-subject diffusion data. *Neuroimage* (2006) 31:1487–505. doi: 10.1016/j.neuroimage.2006.02.024
51. Parvathaneni P, Rogers BP, Huo Y, Schilling KG, Hainline AE, Anderson AW, et al. Gray matter surface based spatial statistics (GS-BSS) in diffusion microstructure. *Med Image Comput Comput Assist Interv.* (2017) 10433:638–46. doi: 10.1007/978-3-319-66182-7_73
52. Cohen-Adad J. Microstructural imaging in the spinal cord and validation strategies. *Neuroimage* (2018) 182:169–83. doi: 10.1016/j.neuroimage.2018.04.009
53. Cercignani M, Dowell NG, Tofts P. *Quantitative MRI of the Brain : Principles of Physical Measurement.* Series in Medical Physics and Biomedical Engineering. CRC Press; Taylor & Francs Group (2018).
54. Carrara G, Carapelli C, Venturi F, Ferraris MM, Lequio L, Chiò A, et al. A distinct MR imaging phenotype in amyotrophic lateral sclerosis: correlation between T1 magnetization transfer contrast hyperintensity along the corticospinal tract and diffusion tensor imaging analysis. *AJNR Am J Neuroradiol.* (2012) 33:733–9. doi: 10.3174/ajnr.A2855
55. da Rocha AJ, Oliveira AS, Fonseca RB, Maia AC, Buainain RP, Lederman HM. Detection of corticospinal tract compromise in amyotrophic lateral sclerosis with brain MR imaging: relevance of the T1-weighted spin-echo magnetization transfer contrast sequence. *AJNR Am J Neuroradiol.* (2004) 25:1509–15.
56. Tanabe JL, Vermathen M, Miller R, Gelinas D, Weiner MW, Rooney WD. Reduced MTR in the corticospinal tract and normal T2 in amyotrophic lateral sclerosis. *Magn Reson Imaging* (1998) 16:1163–9. doi: 10.1016/S0730-725X(98)00129-5
57. Cosottini M, Cecchi P, Piazza S, Pesaresi I, Fabbri S, Diciotti S, et al. Mapping cortical degeneration in ALS with magnetization transfer ratio and voxel-based morphometry. *PLoS ONE* (2013) 8:e68279. doi: 10.1371/journal.pone.0068279
58. Cosottini M, Pesaresi I, Piazza S, Diciotti S, Belmonte G, Battaglini M, et al. Magnetization transfer imaging demonstrates a distributed pattern of microstructural changes of the cerebral cortex in amyotrophic lateral sclerosis. *AJNR Am J Neuroradiol.* (2011) 32:704–8. doi: 10.3174/ajnr.A2356
59. El Mendili MM, Cohen-Adad J, Pelegrini-Issac M, Rossignol S, Morizot-Koutlidis R, Marchand-Pauvert V, et al. Multi-parametric spinal cord MRI as potential progression marker in amyotrophic lateral sclerosis. *PLoS ONE* (2014) 9:e95516. doi: 10.1371/journal.pone.0095516
60. Querin G, El Mendili MM, Bede P, Delphine S, Lenglet T, Marchand-Pauvert V, et al. Multimodal spinal cord MRI offers accurate diagnostic classification in ALS. *J Neurol Neurosurg Psychiatry* (2018) 89:1220–1. doi: 10.1136/jnnp-2017-317214
61. Querin G, El Mendili MM, Lenglet T, Delphine S, Marchand-Pauvert V, Benali H, et al. Spinal cord multi-parametric magnetic resonance imaging for survival prediction in amyotrophic lateral sclerosis. *Eur J Neurol.* (2017) 24:1040–6. doi: 10.1111/ene.13329
62. Rasoanandrianina H, Grapperon AM, Taso M, Girard OM, Duhamel G, Guye M, et al. Region-specific impairment of the cervical spinal cord (SC) in amyotrophic lateral sclerosis: a preliminary study using SC templates and quantitative MRI (diffusion tensor imaging/inhomogeneous magnetization transfer). *NMR Biomed.* (2017) 30:e3801. doi: 10.1002/nbm.3801
63. Levesque IR, Giacomini PS, Narayanan S, Ribeiro LT, Sled JG, Arnold DL, et al. Quantitative magnetization transfer and myelin water imaging of the evolution of acute multiple sclerosis lesions. *Magn Reson Med.* (2010) 63:633–40. doi: 10.1002/mrm.22244
64. Liu Z, Pardini M, Yaldizli Ö, Sethi V, Muhlert N, Wheeler-Kingshott CA, et al. Magnetization transfer ratio measures in normal-appearing white matter show periventricular gradient abnormalities in multiple sclerosis. *Brain* (2015) 138:1239–46. doi: 10.1093/brain/awv065
65. Amann M, Papadopoulou A, Andelova M, Magon S, Mueller-Lenke N, Naegelin Y, et al. Magnetization transfer ratio in lesions rather than normal-appearing brain relates to disability in patients with multiple sclerosis. *J Neurol.* (2015) 262:1909–17. doi: 10.1007/s00415-015-7793-5
66. Moll NM, Rietsch AM, Thomas S, Ransohoff AJ, Lee JC, Fox R, et al. Multiple sclerosis normal-appearing white matter: pathology-imaging correlations. *Ann Neurol.* (2011) 70:764–73. doi: 10.1002/ana.22521
67. Davies GR, Altmann DR, Hadjiprocopis A, Rashid W, Chard DT, Griffin CM, et al. Increasing normal-appearing grey and white matter magnetisation

transfer ratio abnormality in early relapsing-remitting multiple sclerosis. *J Neurol.* (2005) 252:1037–44. doi: 10.1007/s00415-005-0808-x

68. Gracien RM, Jurcoane A, Wagner M, Reitz SC, Mayer C, Volz S, et al. Multimodal quantitative MRI assessment of cortical damage in relapsing-remitting multiple sclerosis. *J Magn Reson Imaging* (2016) 44:1600–7. doi: 10.1002/jmri.25297
69. Samson RS, Cardoso MJ, Muhlert N, Sethi V, Wheeler-Kingshott CA, Ron M, et al. Investigation of outer cortical magnetisation transfer ratio abnormalities in multiple sclerosis clinical subgroups. *Mult Scler.* (2014) 20:1322–30. doi: 10.1177/1352458514522537
70. Harrison NA, Cooper E, Dowell NG, Keramida G, Voon V, Critchley HD, et al. Quantitative magnetization transfer imaging as a biomarker for effects of systemic inflammation on the brain. *Biol Psychiatry* (2015) 78:49–57. doi: 10.1016/j.biopsych.2014.09.023
71. Schwartz M, Baruch K. Breaking peripheral immune tolerance to CNS antigens in neurodegenerative diseases: boosting autoimmunity to fight-off chronic neuroinflammation. *J Autoimmun.* (2014) 54:8–14. doi: 10.1016/j.jaut.2014.08.002
72. Zhao W, Beers DR, Appel SH. Immune-mediated mechanisms in the pathoprogression of amyotrophic lateral sclerosis. *J Neuroimmune Pharmacol.* (2013) 8:888–99. doi: 10.1007/s11481-013-9489-x
73. Chomiak T, Hu B. What is the optimal value of the g-ratio for myelinated fibers in the rat CNS? a theoretical approach. *PLoS ONE* (2009) 4:e7754. doi: 10.1371/journal.pone.0007754
74. Cercignani M, Giulietti G, Dowell NG, Gabel M, Broad R, Leigh PN, et al. Characterizing axonal myelination within the healthy population: a tract-by-tract mapping of effects of age and gender on the fiber g-ratio. *Neurobiol Aging* (2017) 49:109–18. doi: 10.1016/j.neurobiolaging.2016.09.016
75. Hagiwara A, Hori M, Yokoyama K, Nakazawa M, Ueda R, Horita M, et al. Analysis of white matter damage in patients with multiple sclerosis via a novel *in vivo* MR method for measuring myelin, axons, and G-Ratio. *AJNR Am J Neuroradiol.* (2017) 38:1934–40. doi: 10.3174/ajnr.A5312
76. Stikov N, Campbell JS, Stroh T, Lavelée M, Frey S, Novek J, et al. *In vivo* histology of the myelin g-ratio with magnetic resonance imaging. *Neuroimage* (2015) 118:397–405. doi: 10.1016/j.neuroimage.2015.05.023
77. Fonteijn HM, Clarkson MJ, Modat M, Barnes J, Lehmann M, Ourselin S, et al. An event-based disease progression model and its application to familial Alzheimer's disease. *Inf Process Med Imaging* (2011) 22:748–59. doi: 10.1007/978-3-642-22092-0_61
78. Oxtoby NP, Young AL, Cash DM, Benzinger TLS, Fagan AM, Morris JC, et al. Data-driven models of dominantly-inherited Alzheimer's disease progression. *Brain* (2018) 141:1529–44. doi: 10.1093/brain/awy050
79. Young AL, Oxtoby NP, Daga P, Cash DM, Fox NC, Ourselin S, et al. A data-driven model of biomarker changes in sporadic Alzheimer's disease. *Brain* (2014) 137:2564–77. doi: 10.1093/brain/awu176
80. Fonteijn HM, Modat M, Clarkson MJ, Barnes J, Lehmann M, Hobbs NZ, et al. An event-based model for disease progression and its application in familial Alzheimer's disease and Huntington's disease. *Neuroimage* (2012) 60:1880–9. doi: 10.1016/j.neuroimage.2012.01.062
81. Gabel MC, Schmidt DG, Leigh NP, Pinkhardt EH, Ludolph AC, Kassubek J, et al. *Event-Based Modelling Resembles the Sequential Development of Eye Movement Dysfunctions in Amyotrophic Lateral Sclerosis.* Berlin: Neurowoche (2018). Available online at: https://www.dgnkongress.org/
82. Foerster BR, Dwamena BA, Petrou M, Carlos RC, Callaghan BC, Pomper MG. Diagnostic accuracy using diffusion tensor imaging in the diagnosis of ALS: a meta-analysis. *Acad Radiol.* (2012) 19:1075–86. doi: 10.1016/j.acra.2012.04.012

5

Post-polio Syndrome: More than just a Lower Motor Neuron Disease

*Stacey Li Hi Shing, Rangariroyashe H. Chipika, Eoin Finegan, Deirdre Murray, Orla Hardiman and Peter Bede**

Computational Neuroimaging Group, Academic Unit of Neurology, Biomedical Sciences Institute, Trinity College Dublin, Dublin, Ireland

Correspondence:
Peter Bede
bedep@tcd.ie

Post-polio syndrome (PPS) is a neurological condition that affects polio survivors decades after their initial infection. Despite its high prevalence, the etiology of PPS remains elusive, mechanisms of progression are poorly understood, and the condition is notoriously under-researched. While motor dysfunction is a hallmark feature of the condition, generalized fatigue, sleep disturbance, decreased endurance, neuropsychological deficits, sensory symptoms, and chronic pain are also often reported and have considerable quality of life implications in PPS. The non-motor aspects of PPS are particularly challenging to evaluate, quantify, and treat. Generalized fatigue is one of the most distressing symptoms of PPS and is likely to be multifactorial due to weight-gain, respiratory compromise, poor sleep, and polypharmacy. No validated diagnostic, monitoring, or prognostic markers have been developed in PPS to date and the mainstay of therapy centers on symptomatic relief and individualized rehabilitation strategies such as energy conservation and muscle strengthening exercise regimes. Despite a number of large clinical trials in PPS, no effective disease-modifying pharmacological treatments are currently available.

Keywords: postpolio syndrome, PPS, polio, poliomyelitis, neuroimaging, biomarker, clinical trials, motor neuron disease

INTRODUCTION

Poliomyelitis was one of the most acutely debilitating infections of the twentieth century that affected millions in the 1940 and 1950s and more recently in India during an outbreak in 1988 (1). Following the introduction of the polio vaccine in the mid-1950s and early 1960s, there has been a dramatic decline in the number of new polio cases and it is estimated to be 99% eradicated today. Despite the enormous progress in the eradication of the polio virus, 15–20 million people across the world still suffer from the sequelae of the infection (2). A large proportion of polio survivors has been presenting with a constellation of new neurological symptoms that has been described as Post-Polio Syndrome (PPS). The description of PPS is attributed to Jean-Martin Charcot in 1875 but was only widely recognized by the medical community in the early 1980s (3). PPS is characterized by new neurological deficits after a long period of neurological stability, typically at least 15 years after the initial polio infection. PPS may manifest as new, persistent, and progressive muscle weakness, atrophy, limb fatigability, myalgia, arthralgia, and dysphagia, but also as generalized fatigue, which typically has a considerable impact on the patients' quality of life. The estimates of the percentage of polio patients affected by PPS are inconsistent, varying between 20 and 85% (4, 5) depending on the diagnostic criteria applied (2). As a result, despite the rarity of acute polio infection in the modern world, PPS is likely to persist for the next few decades. Despite its prevalence, post-polio syndrome remains surprisingly under-researched and poorly characterized. The purpose of this review is to provide a comprehensive overview of the aetiological, genetic, diagnostic, prognostic factors, and treatment modalities in PPS while highlighting key gaps that require further research.

METHODS

A literature search was performed on PubMed using the search term "post-polio syndrome," "postpolio syndrome" or "post-polio syndrome" alone and in combination with "epidemiology," "pathophysiology," "clinical features," "fatigue," "neurophysiology," "brain imaging," "electromyography," "inflammation," "diagnosis," "management," "clinical trial," "longitudinal," "cross-sectional," "case report," "autopsy," and "post mortem." Only articles written in English and published between January 1980 and May 2019 were selected for literature review. Identified publications were categorized into "academic" papers discussing pathophysiology, genetic susceptibility, biology, and "clinical" papers focusing on diagnostic criteria, management, rehabilitation, and clinical trials.

Abbreviations: 101-PNR, 101- point numeric rating; 10MWT, 10-meter walk test; 2MWT, 2-minute walk test; 6MWT, 6-minute walk test; ALS, Amyotrophic lateral sclerosis; BDI, Beck depression inventory; BiPAP, Bilevel positive airway pressure; CAS, cytokine analysis study; CBT, Cognitive behavioral therapy; CK, Creatine kinase; CMAP, Compound muscle action potential; CMV, Controlled mechanical ventilation; CSE, Clinical study extension; CSF, Cerebrospinal fluid; CSF-MC, cerebrospinal fluid mononuclear cells; ELISA, Enzyme-linked immunosorbent assay; EMG, Electromyography; ESS, Epworth sleepiness scale; FIS, Fatigue impact scale; FSS, Fatigue severity scale; FVC, forced vital capacity; HDsEMG, High density surface electromyography; HHD, hand-held dynamometry; IASP, International Association for the Study of Pain; IBM-FRS, Inclusion body myositis functional rating scale; IPAP, inspiratory positive airway pressure; KAFO, Knee ankle foot orthosis; LIC, lung insufflation capacity; LVR, Lung volume recruitment; MAF, Multidimensional assessment of fatigue; MD, Myotonic dystrophy; MEP, Maximal expiratory pressure; MFI-20, Multidimensional functional inventory; MFM scale, Motor function measurement scale; MIP, Maximal inspiratory pressure; MMPI, Minnesota multiphasic personality inventory; MRC, Medical Research Council Scale for muscle strength; MRI, Magnetic resonance imaging; MRS, Magnetic resonance spectroscopy; MUAP, Motor unit action potential; MV, Minute ventilation; MVA, Maximal voluntary activation; MVC, Maximal voluntary contraction; MVIC, Maximal isometric voluntary contraction; NHP, Nottingham health profile; NIPPV, Nasal intermittent positive pressure ventilation; NIV, Non-invasive ventilation; OSA, Obstructive sleep apnea; PASE, Physical activity of the elderly; PBMC, peripheral blood mononuclear cells; PCF, unassisted peak cough flow; PFS, Piper fatigue scale; PFT, Pulmonary function test; PLMS, Periodic limb movements of sleep; PPL, Polio problem list; PPS, Post-polio syndrome; PV, Polio virus; qMRI, quantitative magnetic resonance imaging; QMT, Quantitative motor test; rCT, randomized controlled trial; RDBPC, Randomized double-blind placebo controlled; REE, resting energy expenditure; RLS, Restless leg syndrome; RNA, Ribonucleic acid; RQ, respiratory quotient; RR, respiratory rate; RT-PCR, Reverse transcription polymerase chain reaction; rTMS, Repetitive transcranial magnetic stimulation; S-SFEMG, Single fiber electromyography stimulation; SF-36, 36-item short form survey; SFEMG, Single fiber electromyography; SFQ, Short fatigue questionnaire; SIP, Sickness impact profile; SIPP, Self-reported impairments in persons with late effects of polio; *SMN* gene, Survival motor neuron gene; SNIP, Sniff nasal inspiratory pressure; SSS test, Sit-stand-sit test; tDCS, Transcranial direct current stimulation; TQNE, Turf's quantitative neuromuscular examination; TUG test, Timed-Up-and-Go test; UW-SES, University of Washington self-efficacy scale; VAS, Visual analog scale; VAS-F, Visual analog scale for fatigue; VCO_2, carbon dioxide production; VO_2, oxygen consumption; WBV, Whole body vibration; WHOQOL-BREF, World Health Organization quality of life abbreviated scale.

RESULTS

Pathophysiology

During the acute poliomyelitis infection, 95% of those infected remain asymptomatic or only suffer flu-like symptoms while the remaining 5% succumb to the paralytic form of the disease. Acute poliomyelitis is typically spinal, affecting the limbs and respiratory musculature, but bulbar manifestations affecting speech and swallow are also well-documented. Polioenterovirus type 1 is the main cause of meningeal, spinal cord and brain inflammation as it can cross the blood-brain barrier independently from poliovirus receptors (6, 7). Ensuing anterior horn degeneration, and apoptosis post infection has been widely recognized as the hallmark feature of paralytic poliomyelitis. Following the acute phase, axonal sprouting takes place reinnervating the muscle of the affected regions (8, 9). Motor units gradually become abnormally enlarged, up to 7-fold their original size (10) rendering them metabolically unsustainable (11). This process can take up to three decades from the acute infection to the development of PPS symptoms (12). The concomitant denervation-reinnervation process is evidenced by electromyography (EMG) findings (13–17) and muscle histology showing small angulated fibers (18, 19) and muscle fiber type-grouping (15). Metabolic stress (11, 20), overuse (21, 22), physiological aging (20, 23), and persistent inflammation (24) are also thought to contribute to gradual motor unit failure. Motor units loss has been consistently correlated to functional decline in longitudinal studies (13, 14, 25, 26). Overuse of functioning muscle units is thought to induce detrimental structural alterations (27, 28). Cellular adaptation in the muscles, such as fiber alteration from type II (fast) to type I (slow) (28), changes in contractile properties (29–31), and muscle hypertrophy (9) are likely to contribute to muscular fatigue and myalgia in PPS. The persistence or reactivation of polio virus in polio survivors has also been suggested with conflicting reports. Two research studies (7, 32) have identified polio-virus (PV) genomic sequences in the CSF and peripheral leucocytes as well as high serum IgM anti-PV antibody titres, which were absent in stable polio survivors and in other neurodegenerative groups (33). Other studies however could not confirm these findings (34). An inflammatory or autoimmune basis to post-polio syndrome has also been proposed. This hypothesis originates from post mortem observations of inflammatory changes in the spinal cord of PPS patients (35, 36). The role of inflammation is also supported by *in vivo* evidence. Increased serum and CSF levels of pro-inflammatory cytokines and peptides such as TNF-α, IFN-γ were repeatedly observed in PPS (37–39). Furthermore, TNF-α and IFN-γ levels respond to IVIg therapy in PPS, and remain unchanged in controls (37, 38, 40). However, no correlations have been detected between symptom severity (38), rate of decline (37), and pro-inflammatory peptide levels. Skeletal muscle biopsies also exhibit inflammatory changes and increased expression of prostaglandin E2 synthetic pathway enzymes (41). Relatively limited evidence exists to support the autoimmune basis of PPS. One study identified high titres of PV antibodies concurrently with high levels of regulatory T cells (42), while another study (43) found normal levels of immune complexes in PPS patients. No specific anti-muscle or anti-neuronal autoantibodies have been associated with PPS (44). A genetic predisposition for PPS has also been investigated, but no conclusive risk profile has been identified to date. *SMN* gene deletion (45, 46) associated with spinal muscular atrophy (SMA) was not reported in PPS, but Fc-gamma receptor IIIA polymorphisms may play a role in the predisposition to PPS (47).

Neuropathology and Neuroimaging

Post-mortem studies are conflicting with regards to cerebral involvement in post-polio syndrome. Post-mortem studies (48) from 50 to 70 years ago suggest that polio virus preferentially affects the reticular formation, posterior hypothalamus, thalamus, putamen, caudate, locus co-eruleus, and substantia nigra which may account for the late-onset fatigue and attention deficit (49–52). Interestingly, cortical involvement is relatively selective and preferentially involves the precentral gyrus and pre-motor areas. A more recent case report (53) and a retrospective analysis of formalin-fixed central nervous system (CNS) tissue of a small cohort of patients (33) arrived at a different conclusion. They identified no cerebral involvement at all, but selective spinal cord pathology affecting the anterior roots with dorsal root sparing. These studies detected enterovirus RNA in spinal cord only. There have also been rare reports of polio patients developing ALS with characteristic histopathological findings (54, 55). Compared to other motor neuron diseases (56), there is a striking paucity of brain (57) and spinal cord imaging studies in PPS (58). Magnetic resonance imaging (MRI) has been used to evaluate volumetric changes (59) and to correlate anatomical changes to post mortem findings (48). The main focus of existing brain imaging studies in PPS was to explore the substrate of fatigue. Multiple hyperintensities were identified in the reticular formation, putamen and medial lemniscus in the majority of PPS patients (48) which is consistent with previous post mortem studies (49–52). A large study of 118 participants compared the brain volume profile of 42 PPS patients, 49 multiple sclerosis patients and 27 controls, and no statistically significant volume reductions were identified in PPS (59). No association was identified between fatigue and brain volumes. The majority of existing studies are cross-sectional which provide limited insights into progressive longitudinal alterations (60). There is an ongoing longitudinal, case-control study to characterize spinal cord alterations in PPS (61).

Diagnosis

Post-polio syndrome is a clinical diagnosis, supported by electrophysiological findings and possible mimics need to be reassuringly ruled out. An extensive work-up including laboratory tests, imaging studies, cerebrospinal fluid sampling, detailed electrophysiological evaluation, and muscle biopsies may be required to exclude alternative diagnoses. The diagnostic criteria for PPS was first proposed by Halstead in 1991 (62) and evolved over time to the current March of Dimes diagnostic criteria (63, 64) which include:

1. Prior paralytic poliomyelitis with evidence of motor neuron loss, as confirmed by history of the acute paralytic illness, signs of residual weakness and muscle atrophy on examination, or signs of denervation on EMG.
2. A period of partial or complete functional recovery after acute paralytic poliomyelitis, followed by an interval (usually 15 years or more) of stable neuromuscular function.
3. Gradual onset (rarely abrupt) progressive and persistent new muscle weakness or abnormal muscle fatigability (decreased endurance), with or without generalized fatigue, muscle atrophy, or muscle and joint pain. Onset may at times follow trauma, surgery, or a period of inactivity. Less commonly, bulbar dysfunction or respiratory weakness occurs.
4. Symptoms that persist for at least a year.
5. Exclusion of alternative neuromuscular, medical, and orthopedic problems as causes of symptoms.

PCR amplification of poliovirus RNA in the CSF is indicative of prior history of poliomyelitis (6, 7, 32) and the presence of pro-inflammatory cytokines may also be detected (39, 65). Proteomic CSF markers such as gelsolin, hemopexin, peptidylglycine alpha-amidating monooxygenase, glutathione synthetase, and kallikrein 6 have been proposed as diagnostic markers but supporting evidence from larger studies is lacking (4). On muscle biopsy, hypertrophic muscle fibers type I (66, 67), indicative of compensatory reinnervation and small angulated fibers, indicative of active denervation (19) may be observed. CSF sampling and muscle biopsy also allows the exclusion of other neuromuscular mimics. People with PPS typically undergo detailed spinal imaging to rule out alternative structural, neoplastic, compressive, or inflammatory spinal etiologies which could manifest in lower motor neuron dysfunction (58, 68–70). Electromyography (EMG) is an invaluable tool to assess suspected post-polio cases, as it allows the confirmation of a prior history of poliomyelitis while excluding differential diagnoses (71). A variety of EMG techniques have been used in post-polio research studies including single fiber EMG (SFEMG), high density surface EMG (HDsEMG) (72), and macro-EMG. Ongoing denervation can be detected on conventional EMG by the presence of fibrillation and fasciculation potentials and increased jitter on SFEMG in newly weakened muscles (73). Needle EMG can also readily detect sub-clinically affected muscles in PPS (74). EMG measures correlate well with muscle strength and endurance (75, 76). While EMG provides important insights, EMG measures don't differ significantly between those with PPS and stable polio (77) and thus EMG is not regarded as an electrodiagnostic tool to confirm PPS (73). PPS is therefore a clinical diagnosis supported by laboratory tests.

The Spectrum of Clinical Manifestations

Post-polio patients characteristically experience new onset muscle weakness, decreased endurance, muscle atrophy, myalgia, and fasciculations (78). Additional symptoms often include generalized fatigue, cold intolerance, dysarthria, dysphagia, and respiratory compromise (79, 80). New symptoms typically occur in previously affected areas but sub-clinically affected body regions can also get affected (74). Ambulatory difficulties often necessitate assistive devices, and may lead to increased fall risk (81). PPS is also associated with a wide range of non-motor symptoms. Frank sensory deficits may be detected and paraesthesias are often reported by PPS patients. Changes in sensory evoked potentials have been linked to cord atrophy on MRI (82). There have been consistent reports of cognitive deficits (83) in PPS including word finding difficulties (84), poor concentration, limited attention, memory impairment (85), and mood disturbances (86). The non-motor aspects of PPS are often under evaluated despite their considerable quality of life implications (87). Due to the combination of motor disability (88) and non-motor symptoms, many patients engage less in social activities (89) which may lead to social isolation. Generalized fatigue is one of the most distressing sequelae of PPS which is likely to be multifactorial due to muscle unit pathology, weight-gain, respiratory compromise, polypharmacy, and poor sleep (**Figure 1**). The identification of the key "fatigue-factors" in individual patients is indispensable for the effective pharmacological and non-pharmacological management of fatigue. Fatigue is thought to exhibit circadian variations throughout the day (90). Sleep disorders such as restless leg syndrome (RLS) (87, 91–94), sleep related breathing disturbances (95), obstructive sleep apnoea (OSA) (96), excessive daytime somnolence (EDS), and periodic limb movement in sleep (PLMS) (97) are not only often reported in PPS but they are likely to play an important role in the pathogenesis of fatigue in PPS (98, 99). Fatigue is thought to be more severe in PPS with RLS, and correlate to the severity of RLS (87). The simultaneous onset of RLS and PPS symptoms (91) and the positive response to pramipexole in an uncontrolled trial by Kumru et al. (93) have been interpreted as a pathophysiological link between RLS and PPS (98). The putative link between RLS and neuroimmunological alterations (100, 101) may also suggest shared pathophysiological processes between PPS and RLS (99). Furthermore, a higher incidence of cauda equina syndrome (102) and renal impairment (103) has also been reported in PPS but the association between these syndromes remains to be elucidated.

Progression, Assessment, and Monitoring

The majority of longitudinal studies (14, 25, 104–107) detect progressive muscle weakness, which contributes to deteriorating gait performance (107) and declining mobility (105). Quantifying the rate of decline in PPS is challenging and no reliable functional predictors have been validated. Male gender is thought to be a negative prognostic indicator (108), but PPS is more common in females (12). Most PPS patients who participated in research studies have lived with PPS for over 13 years suggesting that PPS is a relatively slowly progressive condition. There have also been however sporadic reports of rapidly progressive and life-threatening forms of PPS (109), which raises the question of occasional misdiagnoses or a link between PPS and amyotrophic lateral sclerosis (ALS) (54). The severity of PPS-associate disability is typically evaluated clinically but a number of rating scales and questionnaires have been developed and validated for both clinical and research use. In addition to mobility and dexterity, these instruments evaluate the non-motor aspects of the condition such as fatigue, pain, sleeping disturbances, and mood (110). Clinical tests used to assess motor disability include the 6-min walking test (6MWT) (111) at self-preferred speed, the 2-min walking test (2MWT) at maximal speed (112), Timed-Up-and-Go test (TUG) (113), 10 meters walking test (10MWT), Sit-Stand-Sit test (SSS) (114). Muscle strength is typically appraised by manual muscle testing using the MRC scale, or more objectively using a dynamometer during maximal isokinetic and isometric voluntary contraction. Endurance is measured using isometric contraction peak torque, isometric endurance, tension time index (TTI) or recovery of torque after endurance test (76). Quantitative muscle mass assessment can be performed using ultrasound parameters such as muscle echo intensity and muscle thickness which are non-invasive tools for disease monitoring (115). The most commonly used instruments to assess non-motor domains include the Fatigue Severity Scale (FSS) (116), Fatigue Impact Scale (FIS), Piper Fatigue Scale (PFS), Short Fatigue Questionnaire (SFQ), Nottingham Health Profile (NHP), Physical activity scale for the elderly (PASE) (117), Polio Problem List (PPL), Visual analog scale (VAS) (118), Multidimensional Fatigue Inventory (MFI-20) (119), World Health Organization quality of life abbreviated scale (WHOQOL-BREF) (120), University of Washington Self-Efficacy Scale (UW-SES) (121), Sickness Impact Profile (SIP), 36-item Short Form Health Survey (SF-36) (112). Sleep disturbances (97) and respiratory function can be formally assessed through polysomnography and pulmonary function tests (PFT) (122, 123). RLS is typically diagnosed clinically (124) and most commonly evaluated using the validated international RLS rating scale (IRLS) (87, 93, 125). Maximal inspiratory and expiratory pressures (MIP and MEP), sniff nasal inspiratory pressure (SNIP) (126), and arterial blood gases are validate markers of respiratory function in PPS.

Non-pharmacological Interventions

The effective management of the heterogeneous symptoms of PPS requires individualized care in a multidisciplinary setting (127). Expert input from physiotherapists, occupational therapists, speech and language therapists, respiratory physicians, podiatrists, psychologists, dieticians, pain specialists, social workers, nurse specialists, and orthotists are needed to meet the multifaceted care and support needs of PPS patients (128). Individualized lifestyle modifications and energy conservation strategies are indispensable in the effective management of PPS (129). PPS-specific training regimens alternating active intervals and rest have been developed to improve cardiorespiratory fitness, conserve energy during routine activities, and maintain independence (130). Isokinetic, isometric, resistance, and endurance training are thought to improve muscle strength and endurance without further muscle unit degeneration (131–140). Combining aerobic and flexibility training is also thought to improve QoL. Supervised training is advised in those with significant disability (141). Training in a warm environment may have longer lasting effects than training in colder temperatures (142). Patients with arthralgia may benefit from dynamic water exercises (143) as well as exercising in a group setting (144). Deconditioning of the cardiorespiratory system (145) may limit the effectiveness of aerobic training in PPS (146), therefore

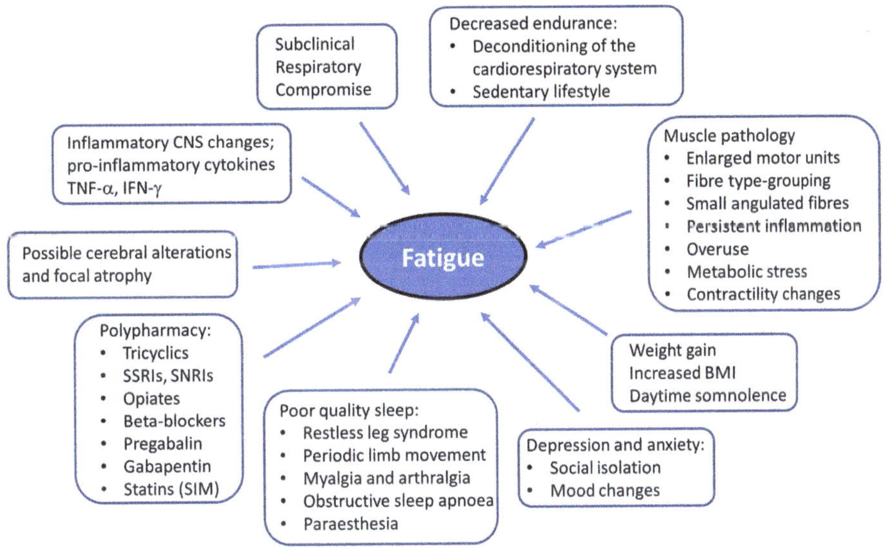

FIGURE 1 | Putative factors in the etiology of generalized fatigue in post-polio syndrome. RLS, Restless leg syndrome; PLMS, periodic limb movement in sleep; CNS, Central nervous system.

aerobic regimens must be carefully tailored to individual fitness levels (147). While some studies show improved endurance following mid- to high-intensity aerobic exercises (139, 140), a recent study (148) highlights that high-intensity aerobic exercise may not be beneficial in PPS patients with fatigue. Due to the heterogeneity of disability profiles in PPS, individualized training regimes and exercises that don't rely on anti-gravity strength are particularly important (148–150). Home-based arm ergometry for example is a well-tolerated and safe form of aerobic exercise (149, 150). Whole body vibration (WBV) has been proposed as an alternative to exercise in PPS (151) and improved mobility was reported in a small study (152), but no improvement was noted in muscle strength or gait performance (153). Orthoses are commonly prescribed for PPS patients to improve mobility and reduce pain. New powered-type Knee Ankle Foot Orthosis (KAFOs) offer limited benefits on gait symmetry or walking speeds but were shown to improve base support, swing time, stance-phase, and knee flexion during swing phase (154). The emergence of novel, light-weight materials such as carbon fiber (155) and the biomechanical analysis of individual walking patterns have helped to optimize orthosis-design for patients. The use of MIG3 Bioceramics fabrics for example had beneficial effects on pain and periodic limb movement (156). Other lifestyle modification such as weight loss, smoking cessation, increased physical activity, and modification to daily activities have all been beneficial to patients with PPS (22). There are sporadic reports that anodal transcranial direct current stimulation (tDCS) of premotor regions (157), repetitive transcranial magnetic stimulation (rTMS) of the left prefrontal cortex (158) and static magnetic fields (159) may ameliorate fatigue, improve sleep, reduce pain, and even improve motor functions in PPS, but these studies have not been replicated. PPS patients with bulbar involvement require expert phonatory and swallowing assessments by a speech-and-language therapist (160) and careful follow-up. Instrumental modalities such as ultrasonography and videofluoroscopy (161) and clinical instruments (162) can be used to detect progressive bulbar dysfunction and appraise the risk aspiration. Compensatory swallowing techniques, dietician input for food consistency alterations, individualized speech therapy, and laryngeal muscle training may be helpful in PPS patients with bulbar involvement (163). PPS patients who suffer from respiratory compromise and sleep related breathing disorders benefit from lung volume recruitment (LVR) (164) and non-invasive ventilation (NIV) such as Bi-PAP (165) or nasal intermittent positive-pressure ventilators (NIPPV) (166). Invasive ventilatory support with a tracheostomy is seldom required in PPS (167).

Addressing the non-physical aspects of PPS; mitigating psychological responses, emotional reactions, frustration, and fear of falling are equally important aspects of multidisciplinary care (168). Despite its positive effects on self-esteem (169), cognitive behavioral therapy (CBT) is not superior to standard multidisciplinary care in the treatment of fatigue (170–172). Psychotherapy is primarily aimed at reducing anxiety, improving depressive symptoms (173), alleviating pain (174, 175), and enhancing subjective well-being (176). Hope-oriented psychotherapy and encouraging participation in work (177) promote resilience in polio survivors and is associated with improved social functioning (178), satisfaction with social roles, improved quality of life, and superior mental health (179). Peer-support groups are also instrumental in buffering the impact of a functional impairment on psychosocial well-being (180). Furthermore, a reduction of physical demands at work and ergonomic adaptations at the workplace not only help PPS patients to maintain their occupational activities but enjoy their work (181). Rehabilitation nurses also play an important role in

TABLE 1 | Pharmaceutical and non-pharmaceutical clinical trials in post-polio syndrome; study characteristics and key outcomes.

References	Study Design/selection criteria of PPS patients	Number of follow-up time points	Follow-up interval (months)	Number of participants receiving drug/placebo	Assessment tools used	Key study findings
PREDNISONE						
Dinsmore et al. (183)	RDBPC/U	3	3	7/7	MRC scale, MVIC using electronic strain gauge tensiometer, fatigue on a 0–3 scale	- Short-lived improvement in muscle strength - No improvement in fatigue - Not recommended
AMANTADINE						
Stein et al. (184)	RDBPC/S (fatigue)	2	2	10/13	FSS, VAS-F, MMPI, BDI, somatization scale, reaction time evaluation	- Not superior to placebo for fatigue
PYRIDOSTIGMINE						
Trojan et al. (185)	RDBPC/S(fatigue/muscle weakness)	6	at 6 weeks, 10 weeks, and 6 months	43/42	SF-36, modified TQNE, MVIC by electronic strain gauge, Hare Fatigue Symptom Scale, FSS, IGF-1 serum levels	- Very weak muscles became slightly stronger - IGF-1 increased in compliant patients - No clear benefits on QoL, muscle strength, and fatigue
Horemans et al. (186)	RDBPC/S (fatigue and muscle weakness)	5	0.75	31/31	NHP, FSS, 2MWT at comfortable pace, time to walk 75 m at fastest speed, ambulatory activity monitor, MVC by chair dynamometer, MVA by interpolated stimulation; muscle fatigability by sEMG during 30 s sustained isometric contraction at 40% of MVC, NMJ defects by jitter on S-SFEMG	- No significant effects on fatigue - Significant effects on walking distance - Little effects on walking duration, muscle strength, MVA - Limited benefits in physical performance
MODAFINIL						
Chan et al. (187)	RDBPC cross-over/S (fatigue)	12	0.25	7/7 Cross-over 7/7	PFS, ESS, aural digit spans, reaction time	- Not effective in fatigue
Vasconcelos et al. (188)	RDBPC cross-over/ S (fatigue)	2	1.5	18/18 Cross-over 18/15	FSS, VAS-F, FIS; SF-36	- Not superior to placebo in fatigue and QoL improvement
CO-ENZYME Q10						
Skough et al. (189)	Parallel RDBPC/S(ability to perform resistance training)	2	3	7/7	Sit-stand-sit test (SSS); Timed up and go (TUG) test, 6MWT, dynamometer, bloods for CK, LD	- No change in CK or LD - No additional effects of the Co-enzyme Q10 supplementation during resistance training
Peel et al. (190)	Parallel RDBPC/S (fatigue)	2	2	54/49	MAF (revised Piper Fatigue Scale), FSS	- Not effective in fatigue
LAMOTRIGINE						
On et al. (191)	RDBPC/S (ambulatory with lower limb involvement only)	3	0.5	15/15	VAS, NHP, FSS	- Superior to placebo for pain, fatigue, and QoL as detected in VAS, NHP, FSS

(Continued)

TABLE 1 | Continued

References	Study Design/selection criteria of PPS patients	Number of follow-up time points	Follow-up interval (months)	Number of participants receiving drug/placebo	Assessment tools used	Key study findings
INTRAVENOUS IMMUNOGLOBULIN (IVIg)						
Gonzalez et al. (38)	Controlled open-label/U	2	1.5-2	16PPS; 26OND/0	CSF for CSF-MC, PB for PBMC, real-time quantitative RT-PCR for relative quantitation of mRNA	- Significant decrease of CSF-MC expression of TNF-α and IFN-γ not seen in PBMC expression of cytokines
Kaponides et al. (192)	Uncontrolled open-label/S (ambulatory, BMI < 28)	3	at 2 and 6 months	14/0	Dynamic dynamometer, 6MWT, SF-36	- No significant effect on muscle strength and physical performance
Gonzalez et al. (193)	RDBPC/U	2	3	67/68	Dynamometer, SF-36, 6MWT, TUG, PASE, sway, sleep quality, VAS, MFI-20	- Positive changes in muscle strength, physical activity, and those with significant pain - No change on QoL, fatigue sleep quality, "better" limb muscles or mild pain
Farbu et al. (40)	RDBPC/U	5	3	10/10	MAF (revised Piper Fatigue Scale), FSS, CSF, and PB for expression of cytokines (TNF-α, IFN-γ, IL-6, IL-1β, IFN-β, IL-10) using ELISA	- Positive effects on pain after 3 months - No effects on muscle strength and fatigue - TNF-α increased in CSF
Werhagen et al. (194)	Uncontrolled open-label/S (pain)	2	6	45/0	Neurological examination, sensory testing, soft tissue palpation, and joint assessment, VAS, pain classified according to IASP	- Better results on pain in younger, those with more pronounced paresis, had acute polio <10 yo
Östlund et al. (195)	Uncontrolled open-label/S(fatigue, muscle weakness)	2	6	113/0	SF-36, PASE, VAS	- Likely responders include those with pain intensity above VAS of 20 mm, younger than 65 yo, and paresis in lower extremities
Gonzalez et al. (65)	RDBPC and controlled quantitative cytokine study/U	2	12	CSE: 20/21 CAS: 20/30	CSE: SF-36, 6MWT, VAS CAS: CSF and PB for cytokines (TNF, IL-23, IFN-γ, TGF-β, IL-10, IL-13) using RT-PCR	- Improvement in QoL but not in pain and walking ability compared to placebo - Decline in CSF IFN-γ and IL-23, TNF, and increase in IL-10 and IL-13 - No changes in PB cytokine levels
Bertolasi et al. (196)	RDBPC/U	3	2	24/26	SF-36, MRC scale, dynamometer, 6MWT, VAS, 101-PNR, FSS	- Improvement in QoL; mental activity subscale - No effects on gait, muscle strength, fatigue, and pain
L-CITRULLINE						
Schmidt et al. (197)	RDBPC/U	5	6	15/15	6MWT, MFM scale, qMRI, MRS, bloods for muscle necrosis (CK), oxidative stress (8OHDG, 4-HNE), nitrosative stress(nitrotyrosine, cGMP), mitochondrial-related	- Ongoing clinical trial

(Continued)

TABLE 1 | Continued

References	Study Design/selection criteria of PPS patients	Number of follow-up time points	Follow-up interval (months)	Number of participants receiving drug/placebo	Assessment tools used	Key study findings
					genes (*Citratsynthase, Cytochrome C oxidase subunit 1, Succinate dehydrogenase subunit A)*, QMT using HHD, SIPP,IBM-FRS,WHOQOL-BREF	
RESPIRATORY SUPPORT						
Kaminska et al. (164)	Feasibility/S(restrictive respiratory defects)	2	3	7ALS, 7PPS, 5MD	SF-36, SIP, standard spirometry (FVC, FVC% predicted, LIC, LIC-FVC difference, PCF, MIP, MEP)	- LVR Feasible - Encouraging effects on respiratory mechanics - LIC increased
Gillis-Haegerstrand et al. (165)	Randomized comparative/S(using VCV)	2	30 min	8	BP, oxygen saturation, ABG, indirect calorimetry (SaO_2, VO_2, VCO_2, REE, RQ, RR, IPAP)	- BiPAP PSV decreases oxygen cost of breathing in PPS with respiratory failure without decreasing ventilation efficiency. - Significant $PaCO_2$ decrease using this ventilation modality. - Maintains adequate ventilation in PPS patient with resp. failure
Barle et al. (167)	Comparative /S (nocturnal invasive CMV)	7	30 min	9	BP, oxygen saturation, ABG, indirect calorimetry (SaO_2, VO_2, VCO_2, REE, RQ, MV,RR, IPAP)	- Invasive BiPAP reduces oxygen cost of breathing in long-standing tracheotomized PPS compared to CMV.
EXERCISE PROGRAM						
Murray et al. (149)	Assessor blinded rCT/U	2	2 months	26/29	6-MAT, PASIPD, 6MWT, FSS, SF-MPQ-2, QMA, exercise log	- Home-based ergometry is a well-tolerated form of aerobic exercise - No improvement of physical fitness, fatigue, activity - Slight decrease in BP in interventional group
PRAMIPEXOLE						
Kumru et al. (93)	Uncontrolled open label/U	3	At 0, 2 months and 6 months	16/0	RLS severity scale	- Significant decrease of RLS severity detected on RLS rating scale - Maintenance of improvement of RLS with pramipexole at 6 months follow-up

rCT, randomized controlled trial; S, selected (i.e., fatigued); U, unselected; RDBPC, Randomized double-blind placebo controlled.

the setting of realistic health goals, encouraging resiliency, and providing emotional support (182).

Pharmacological Trials

Several randomized controlled clinical trials (RCT) were conducted in PPS (**Table 1**). High-dose prednisone (183), amantadine (184), and modafinil (187, 188) showed no superiority to placebo in the management of fatigue. Prednisone therapy, showed a short-lived improvement in muscular strength but no meaningful functional improvement (183). The evidence for the benefit of pyridostigmine therapy remains conflicting. Some studies (185) identified no benefit on muscle function while others reported a slight improvement in walking performance (186). Co-enzyme Q10 supplements are thought to have no effect on muscle strength, endurance or fatigue in PPS (189, 190). A small RCT of lamotrigine, demonstrated improvements in VAS, NHP, and FSS suggesting that it may be beneficial to treat pain and fatigue and improve quality of life (191). Given the inflammatory and autoimmune hypothesis of PPS pathogenesis, intravenous immunoglobulin has been extensively investigated for its potential therapeutic effects. Its benefit with regards to pain, muscle strength, physical functioning, and quality of life is inconsistent. Improved pain control and overall vitality (192, 196) seem to be the main benefit of intravenous immunoglobulin (IVIg) treatment. Two small uncontrolled trials (38, 194) and two larger RCTs (40, 65) arrived to similar conclusions with regards to pain control and improvement in serum and CSF inflammatory markers. The main indicators for response to IVIg include severe pain, fatigue, <65 years of age, and paresis mainly affecting the lower extremities (194, 195, 198). Studies are somewhat conflicting on its effect on muscle strength (65, 193). These findings however encourage further large RCTs to establish the target PPS cohort for IVIg treatment, treatment intervals, and dose optimisation. A single-center, double-blind RCT trial of L-citrulline (197) is currently underway to investigate its effect on muscle metabolism and function. It is at clinical phase IIa and has proven to be of beneficial in muscular dystrophies in improving endurance in both aerobic and anaerobic exercise. The symptomatic management of non-motor symptoms in PPS also has considerable quality of life benefits. Restless leg syndrome in PPS often responds to dopamine agonists such as pramipexole (93, 199). The use of analgesics and antidepressants such as amitryptiline, duloxetine, and codeine may decrease physical discomfort and improve mood but need careful monitoring as they may worsen fatigue and lead to poor concentration. Adverse reactions to certain anesthetic agents are well-documented in PPS. Post-anesthesia fatigue, somnolence, and weakness are well-recognized, and fatal outcomes due to respiratory arrest have also been reported (200, 201). The diagnosis of PPS needs to be carefully discussed with the anaesthesiologists, so the appropriate muscle relaxants and anesthetics can be used, and patients should be advised of the possibility of a prolonged post-operative phase (202).

CONCLUSIONS

Despite being one of the most devastating neurodegenerative conditions in the world, surprisingly limited research is undertaken in post-polio syndrome. Its pathogenesis remains elusive, no sensitive diagnostic tools have been developed, and validated prognostic and monitoring markers are lacking. Non-motor symptoms of PPS have considerable quality of life implications and are notoriously challenging to manage. The etiology of fatigue in PPS is yet to be elucidated and successful individualized management strategies are needed to maintain mobility, independence, and patient autonomy. There is striking a paucity of neuroimaging studies in PPS that could provide anatomical insights into the substrate of extra-motor symptoms. Ultimately, the characterization of PPS-associated pathology may help research efforts in other motor neuron diseases.

AUTHOR CONTRIBUTIONS

The manuscript was drafted by SL and PB. The manuscript was edited, adjusted, and reviewed for intellectual content by RC, EF, DM, and OH.

ACKNOWLEDGMENTS

Peter Bede and the Computational Neuroimaging Group are supported by the Health Research Board (HRB–Ireland; HRB EIA-2017-019), the Andrew Lydon Scholarship, the Irish Institute of Clinical Neuroscience (IICN)–Novartis Ireland Research Grant, the Iris O'Brien Foundation, and the Research Motor Neuron (RMN–Ireland) Foundation.

REFERENCES

1. Cousins S. Accounting for polio survivors in the post-polio world. *Lancet.* (2017) 389:1503–4. doi: 10.1016/S0140-6736(17)30999-6
2. Gonzalez H, Olsson T, Borg K. Management of postpolio syndrome. *Lancet Neurol.* (2010) 9:634–42. doi: 10.1016/S1474-4422(10)70095-8
3. Gawne AC, Halstead LS. Post-polio syndrome: historical perspective, epidemiology and clinical presentation. *NeuroRehabilitation.* (1997) 8:73–81. doi: 10.1016/S1053-8135(96)00212-0
4. Trojan DA, Cashman NR. Post-poliomyelitis syndrome. *Muscle Nerve.* (2005) 31:6–19. doi: 10.1002/mus.20259
5. Farbu E, Gilhus NE, Barnes MP, Borg K, de Visser M, Driessen A, et al. EFNS guideline on diagnosis and management of post-polio syndrome. Report of an EFNS task force. *Eur J Neurol.* (2006) 13:795–801. doi: 10.1111/j.1468-1331.2006.01385.x
6. Baj A, Colombo M, Headley JL, McFarlane JR, Liethof MA, Toniolo A. Post-poliomyelitis syndrome as a possible viral disease. *Int J Infect Dis.* (2015) 35:107–16. doi: 10.1016/j.ijid.2015.04.018
7. Leon-Monzon ME, Dalakas MC. Detection of poliovirus antibodies and poliovirus genome in patients with the post-polio syndrome. *Ann N Y Acad Sci.* (1995) 753:208–18. doi: 10.1111/j.1749-6632.1995.tb27547.x
8. Luciano CA, Sivakumar K, Spector SA, Dalakas MC. Electrophysiologic and histologic studies in clinically unaffected muscles of patients with prior paralytic poliomyelitis. *Muscle Nerve.* (1996) 19:1413–20. doi: 10.1002/(SICI)1097-4598(199611)19:11<1413::AID-MUS5>3.0.CO;2-F

9. Luciano CA, Sivakumar K, Spector SA, Dalakas MC. Reinnervation in clinically unaffected muscles of patients with prior paralytic poliomyelitis. Correlation between macroelectromyography and histology. *Ann N Y Acad Sci.* (1995) 753:394–6. doi: 10.1111/j.1749-6632.1995.tb27570.x
10. Cashman NR, Trojan DA. Correlation of electrophysiology with pathology, pathogenesis, and anticholinesterase therapy in post-polio syndrome. *Ann N Y Acad Sci.* (1995) 753:138–50. doi: 10.1111/j.1749-6632.1995.tb27540.x
11. Wiechers DO, Hubbell SL. Late changes in the motor unit after acute poliomyelitis. *Muscle Nerve.* (1981) 4:524–8. doi: 10.1002/mus.880040610
12. Bertolasi L, Danese A, Monaco S, Turri M, Borg K, Werhagen L. Polio patients in Northern Italy, a 50 year follow-up. *Open Neurol J.* (2016) 10:77–82. doi: 10.2174/1874205X01610010077
13. Ivanyi B, Ongerboer de Visser BW, Nelemans PJ, de Visser M. Macro EMG follow-up study in post-poliomyelitis patients. *J Neurol.* (1994) 242:37–40. doi: 10.1007/BF00920572
14. Bickerstaffe A, van Dijk JP, Beelen A, Zwarts MJ, Nollet F. Loss of motor unit size and quadriceps strength over 10 years in post-polio syndrome. *Clin Neurophysiol.* (2014) 125:1255–60. doi: 10.1016/j.clinph.2013.11.003
15. Maselli RA, Cashman NR, Wollman RL, Salazar-Grueso EF, Roos R. Neuromuscular transmission as a function of motor unit size in patients with prior poliomyelitis. *Muscle Nerve.* (1992) 15:648–55. doi: 10.1002/mus.880150603
16. Sandberg A, Stalberg E. Changes in macro electromyography over time in patients with a history of polio: a comparison of 2 muscles. *Arch Phys Med Rehabil.* (2004) 85:1174–82. doi: 10.1016/j.apmr.2003.08.101
17. Sandberg A, Nandedkar SD, Stalberg E. Macro electromyography and motor unit number index in the tibialis anterior muscle: differences and similarities in characterizing motor unit properties in prior polio. *Muscle Nerve.* (2011) 43:335–41. doi: 10.1002/mus.21878
18. Emeryk B, Rowinska-Marcinska K, Ryniewicz B, Hausmanowa-Petrusewicz I. Disintegration of the motor unit in post-polio syndrome. Part II. Electrophysiological findings in patients with post-polio syndrome. *Electromyogr Clin Neurophysiol.* (1990) 30:451–8.
19. Jubelt B, Cashman NR. Neurological manifestations of the post-polio syndrome. *Critic Rev Neurobiol.* (1987) 3:199–220.
20. Gordon T, Hegedus J, Tam SL. Adaptive and maladaptive motor axonal sprouting in aging and motoneuron disease. *Neurol Res.* (2004) 26:174–85. doi: 10.1179/016164104225013806
21. Perry J, Barnes G, Gronley JK. The postpolio syndrome. An overuse phenomenon. *Clin Orthop Relat Res.* (1988) 1988:145–62. doi: 10.1097/00003086-198808000-00018
22. Perry J, Fontaine JD, Mulroy S. Findings in post-poliomyelitis syndrome. Weakness of muscles of the calf as a source of late pain and fatigue of muscles of the thigh after poliomyelitis. *J Bone Joint Surg Am Vol.* (1995) 77:1148–53. doi: 10.2106/00004623-199508000-00002
23. Trojan DA, Cashman NR, Shapiro S, Tansey CM, Esdaile JM. Predictive factors for post-poliomyelitis syndrome. *Arch Phys Med Rehabil.* (1994) 75:770–7.
24. Dalakas MC. Pathogenetic mechanisms of post-polio syndrome: morphological, electrophysiological, virological, and immunological correlations. *Ann N Y Acad Sci.* (1995) 753:167–85. doi: 10.1111/j.1749-6632.1995.tb27543.x
25. Daube JR, Sorenson EJ, Windebank AJ. Prospective 15-year study of neuromuscular function in a cohort of patients with prior poliomyelitis. *Suppl Clin Neurophysiol.* (2009) 60:197–201. doi: 10.1016/S1567-424X(08)00020-2
26. Sorenson EJ, Daube JR, Windebank AJ. A 15-year follow-up of neuromuscular function in patients with prior poliomyelitis. *Neurology.* (2005) 64:1070–2. doi: 10.1212/01.WNL.0000154604.97992.4A
27. Grimby G, Hedberg M, Henning GB. Changes in muscle morphology, strength and enzymes in a 4-5-year follow-up of subjects with poliomyelitis sequelae. *Scand J Rehabil Med.* (1994) 26:121–30.
28. Borg K, Borg J, Edstrom L, Grimby L. Effects of excessive use of remaining muscle fibers in prior polio and LV lesion. *Muscle Nerve.* (1988) 11:1219–30. doi: 10.1002/mus.880111206
29. Larsson L, Li X, Tollback A, Grimby L. Contractile properties in single muscle fibres from chronically overused motor units in relation to motoneuron firing properties in prior polio patients. *J Neurol Sci.* (1995) 132:182–92. doi: 10.1016/0022-510X(95)00138-R
30. Borg J, Borg K, Edstrom L, Grimby L, Henriksson J, Larsson L, et al. Motoneuron and muscle fiber properties of remaining motor units in weak tibialis anterior muscles in prior polio. *Ann N Y Acad Sci.* (1995) 753:335–42. doi: 10.1111/j.1749-6632.1995.tb27559.x
31. Borg K, Henriksson J. Prior poliomyelitis-reduced capillary supply and metabolic enzyme content in hypertrophic slow-twitch (type I) muscle fibres. *J Neurol Neurosurg Psychiatry.* (1991) 54:236–40. doi: 10.1136/jnnp.54.3.236
32. Julien J, Leparc-Goffart I, Lina B, Fuchs F, Foray S, Janatova I, et al. Postpolio syndrome: poliovirus persistence is involved in the pathogenesis. *J Neurol.* (1999) 246:472–6. doi: 10.1007/s004150050386
33. Muir P, Nicholson F, Spencer GT, Ajetunmobi JF, Starkey WG, Khan M, et al. Enterovirus infection of the central nervous system of humans: lack of association with chronic neurological disease. *J Gen Virol.* (1996) 77 (Pt 7):1469–76. doi: 10.1099/0022-1317-77-7-1469
34. Melchers W, de Visser M, Jongen P, van Loon A, Nibbeling R, Oostvogel P, et al. The postpolio syndrome: no evidence for poliovirus persistence. *Ann Neurol.* (1992) 32:728–32. doi: 10.1002/ana.410320605
35. Kaminski HJ, Tresser N, Hogan RE, Martin E. Pathological analysis of spinal cords from survivors of poliomyelitis. *Ann N Y Acad Sci.* (1995) 753:390–3. doi: 10.1111/j.1749-6632.1995.tb27569.x
36. Sharief MK, Hentges R, Ciardi M. Intrathecal immune response in patients with the post-polio syndrome. *N Engl J Med.* (1991) 325:749–55. doi: 10.1056/NEJM199109123251101
37. Bickerstaffe A, Beelen A, Lutter R, Nollet F. Elevated plasma inflammatory mediators in post-polio syndrome: no association with long-term functional decline. *J Neuroimmunol.* (2015) 289:162–7. doi: 10.1016/j.jneuroim.2015.10.019
38. Gonzalez H, Khademi M, Andersson M, Piehl F, Wallstrom E, Borg K, et al. Prior poliomyelitis-IVIg treatment reduces proinflammatory cytokine production. *J Neuroimmunol.* (2004) 150:139–44. doi: 10.1016/j.jneuroim.2004.01.010
39. Gonzalez H, Khademi M, Andersson M, Wallstrom E, Borg K, Olsson T. Prior poliomyelitis-evidence of cytokine production in the central nervous system. *J Neurol Sci.* (2002) 205:9–13. doi: 10.1016/S0022-510X(02)00316-7
40. Farbu E, Rekand T, Vik-Mo E, Lygren H, Gilhus NE, Aarli JA. Post-polio syndrome patients treated with intravenous immunoglobulin: a double-blinded randomized controlled pilot study. *Eur J Neurol.* (2007) 14:60–5. doi: 10.1111/j.1468-1331.2006.01552.x
41. Melin E, Lindroos E, Lundberg IE, Borg K, Korotkova M. Elevated expression of prostaglandin E2 synthetic pathway in skeletal muscle of prior polio patients. *J Rehabil Med.* (2014) 46:67–72. doi: 10.2340/16501977-1230
42. Wahid R. *Regulatory T Cells as a Biomarker of Post-polio Syndrome.* (2008). Available online at: http://www.post-polio.org/edu/pphnews/pph24-2p1-5.pdf
43. Melin E, Sohrabian A, Ronnelid J, Borg K. Normal serum levels of immune complexes in postpolio patients. *Results Immunol.* (2014) 4:54–7. doi: 10.1016/j.rinim.2014.06.001
44. Farbu E, Rekand T, Tysnes OB, Aarli JA, Gilhus NE, Vedeler CA. GM1 antibodies in post-polio syndrome and previous paralytic polio. *J Neuroimmunol.* (2003) 139:141–4. doi: 10.1016/S0165-5728(03)00123-1
45. Bartholdi D, Gonzalez H, Borg K, Melki J. Absence of SMN gene deletion in post-polio syndrome. *Neuromuscul Disord.* (2000) 10:99. doi: 10.1016/S0960-8966(99)00076-0
46. Querin G, El Mendili MM, Lenglet T, Behin A, Stojkovic T, Salachas F, et al. The spinal and cerebral profile of adult spinal-muscular atrophy: a multimodal imaging study. *NeuroImage Clin.* (2019) 21:101618. doi: 10.1016/j.nicl.2018.101618
47. Rekand T, Langeland N, Aarli JA, Vedeler CA. Fcgamma receptor IIIA polymorphism as a risk factor for acute poliomyelitis. *J Infect Dis.* (2002) 186:1840–3. doi: 10.1086/345769
48. Bruno RL, Cohen JM, Galski T, Frick NM. The neuroanatomy of post-polio fatigue. *Arch Phys Med Rehabil.* (1994) 75:498–504.
49. Bodian D. Histopathologic basis of clinical findings in poliomyelitis. *Am J Med.* (1949) 6:563–78. doi: 10.1016/0002-9343(49)90130-8

50. Barnhart M, Rhines R. Distribution of lesions of the brain stem in poliomyelitis. *Arch Neurol Psychiatry.* (1948) 59:368–77. doi: 10.1001/archneurpsyc.1948.02300380097008
51. Matzke HA, Baker AB. Poliomyelitis. IV. A study of the midbrain. *AMA Arch Neurol Psychiatry.* (1951) 65:1–15. doi: 10.1001/archneurpsyc.1951.02320010007001
52. Luhan JA. Epidemic poliomyelitis; some pathologic observations on human material. *Arch Pathol (Chic).* (1946) 42:245–60.
53. Miller DC. Post-polio syndrome spinal cord pathology. Case report with immunopathology. *Ann N Y Acad Sci.* (1995) 753:186–93. doi: 10.1111/j.1749-6632.1995.tb27544.x
54. Casula M, Steentjes K, Aronica E, van Geel BM, Troost D. Concomitant CNS pathology in a patient with amyotropic lateral sclerosis following poliomyelitis in childhood. *Clin Neuropathol.* (2011) 30:111–7. doi: 10.5414/NPP30111
55. Shimada A, Lange DJ, Hays AP. Amyotrophic lateral sclerosis in an adult following acute paralytic poliomyelitis in early childhood. *Acta Neuropathol.* (1999) 97:317–21. doi: 10.1007/s004010050991
56. Bede P, Hardiman O. Lessons of ALS imaging: pitfalls and future directions — a critical review. *NeuroImage Clin.* (2014) 4:436–43. doi: 10.1016/j.nicl.2014.02.011
57. Bede P, Querin G, Pradat PF. The changing landscape of motor neuron disease imaging: the transition from descriptive studies to precision clinical tools. *Curr Opin Neurol.* (2018) 31:431–8. doi: 10.1097/WCO.0000000000000569
58. El Mendili MM, Querin G, Bede P, Pradat PF. Spinal cord imaging in amyotrophic lateral sclerosis: historical concepts-novel techniques. *Front Neurol.* (2019) 10:350. doi: 10.3389/fneur.2019.00350
59. Trojan DA, Narayanan S, Francis SJ, Caramanos Z, Robinson A, Cardoso M, et al. Brain volume and fatigue in patients with postpoliomyelitis syndrome. *PMR.* (2014) 6:215–20. doi: 10.1016/j.pmrj.2013.09.009
60. Schuster C, Elamin M, Hardiman O, Bede P. Presymptomatic and longitudinal neuroimaging in neurodegeneration–from snapshots to motion picture: a systematic review. *J Neurol Neurosurg Psychiatry.* (2015) 86:1089–96. doi: 10.1136/jnnp-2014-309888
61. *Spinal Cord Gray Matter Imaging in Post Polio Syndrome.* (2018). Available online at: https://ClinicalTrials.gov/show/NCT03561623
62. Halstead LS. Assessment and differential diagnosis for post-polio syndrome. *Orthopedics.* (1991) 14:1209–17.
63. March of Dimes. *Post-polio Syndrome: Identifying Best Practices in Diagnosis and Care.* (2001). Available online at: http://www.post-polio.org/edu/pps.html
64. Farbu E. Update on current and emerging treatment options for post-polio syndrome. *Ther Clin Risk Manag.* (2010) 6:307–13. doi: 10.2147/TCRM.S4440
65. Gonzalez H, Khademi M, Borg K, Olsson T. Intravenous immunoglobulin treatment of the post-polio syndrome: sustained effects on quality of life variables and cytokine expression after one year follow up. *J Neuroinflamm.* (2012) 9:167. doi: 10.1186/1742-2094-9-167
66. Dalakas MC. Morphologic changes in the muscles of patients with postpoliomyelitis neuromuscular symptoms. *Neurology.* (1988) 38:99–104. doi: 10.1212/WNL.38.1.99
67. Grimby G, Einarsson G, Hedberg M, Aniansson A. Muscle adaptive changes in post-polio subjects. *Scand J Rehabil Med.* (1989) 21:19–26.
68. Bede P, Walsh R, Fagan AJ, Hardiman O. "Sand-watch" spinal cord: a case of inferior cervical spinal cord atrophy. *J Neurol.* (2013) 261:235–7. doi: 10.1007/s00415-013-7193-7
69. Lebouteux MV, Franques J, Guillevin R, Delmont E, Lenglet T, Bede P, et al. Revisiting the spectrum of lower motor neuron diseases with snake eyes appearance on magnetic resonance imaging. *Eur J Neurol.* (2014) 21:1233–41. doi: 10.1111/ene.12465
70. Bede P, Bokde AL, Byrne SC, Elamin M, Walsh RJ, Hardiman O. Waterskier's Hirayama syndrome. *J Neurol.* (2011) 258:2078–9. doi: 10.1007/s00415-011-6046-5
71. Sandberg A, Stalberg E. How to interpret normal electromyographic findings in patients with an alleged history of polio. *J Rehabil Med.* (2004) 36:169–76. doi: 10.1080/16501970410025135
72. Roeleveld K, Sandberg A, Stalberg EV, Stegeman DF. Motor unit size estimation of enlarged motor units with surface electromyography. *Muscle Nerve.* (1998) 21:878–86. doi: 10.1002/(SICI)1097-4598(199807)21:7<878::AID-MUS5>3.0.CO;2-3
73. Trojan DA, Gendron D, Cashman NR. Electrophysiology and electrodiagnosis of the post-polio motor unit. *Orthopedics.* (1991) 14:1353–61.
74. On AY, Sungur U. Patients with post-polio syndrome are more likely to have subclinical involvement as compared to polio survivors without new symptoms. *Ann Indian Acad Neurol.* (2016) 19:44–7. doi: 10.4103/0972-2327.167705
75. Rodriquez AA, Agre JC. Electrophysiologic study of the quadriceps muscles during fatiguing exercise and recovery: a comparison of symptomatic and asymptomatic postpolio patients and controls. *Arch Phys Med Rehabil.* (1991) 72:993–7.
76. Rodriquez AA, Agre JC, Franke TM. Electromyographic and neuromuscular variables in unstable postpolio subjects, stable postpolio subjects, and control subjects. *Arch Phys Med Rehabil.* (1997) 78:986–91. doi: 10.1016/S0003-9993(97)90062-9
77. Cashman NR, Maselli R, Wollmann RL, Roos R, Simon R, Antel JP. Late denervation in patients with antecedent paralytic poliomyelitis. *N Engl J Med.* (1987) 317:7–12. doi: 10.1056/NEJM198707023170102
78. Grabljevec K, Burger H, Kersevan K, Valencic V, Marincek C. Strength and endurance of knee extensors in subjects after paralytic poliomyelitis. *Disabil Rehabil.* (2005) 27:791–9. doi: 10.1080/09638280400020623
79. Soderholm S, Lehtinen A, Valtonen K, Ylinen A. Dysphagia and dysphonia among persons with post-polio syndrome - a challenge in neurorehabilitation. *Acta Neurol Scand.* (2010) 122:343–9. doi: 10.1111/j.1600-0404.2009.01315.x
80. Driscoll BP, Gracco C, Coelho C, Goldstein J, Oshima K, Tierney E, et al. Laryngeal function in postpolio patients. *Laryngoscope.* (1995) 105:35–41. doi: 10.1288/00005537-199501000-00010
81. Bertolasi L, Acler M, dall'Ora E, Gajofatto A, Frasson E, Tocco P, et al. Risk factors for post-polio syndrome among an Italian population: a case-control study. *Neurol Sci.* (2012) 33:1271–5. doi: 10.1007/s10072-012-0931-2
82. Prokhorenko OA, Vasconcelos OM, Lupu VD, Campbell WW, Jabbari B. Sensory physiology assessed by evoked potentials in survivors of poliomyelitis. *Muscle Nerve.* (2008) 38:1266–71. doi: 10.1002/mus.21093
83. Bruno RL, Galski T, DeLuca J. The neuropsychology of post-polio fatigue. *Arch Phys Med Rehabil.* (1993) 74:1061–5. doi: 10.1016/0003-9993(93)90062-F
84. Bruno RL, Zimmerman JR. Word finding difficulty as a post-polio sequelae. *Am J Phys Med Rehabil.* (2000) 79:343–8. doi: 10.1097/00002060-200007000-00005
85. Hazendonk KM, Crowe SF. A neuropsychological study of the postpolio syndrome: support for depression without neuropsychological impairment. *Neuropsychiatry Neuropsychol Behav Neurol.* (2000) 13:112–8.
86. Bruno RL, Sapolsky R, Zimmerman JR, Frick NM. Pathophysiology of a central cause of post-polio fatigue. *Ann N Y Acad Sci.* (1995) 753:257–75. doi: 10.1111/j.1749-6632.1995.tb27552.x
87. Romigi A, Pierantozzi M, Placidi F, Evangelista E, Albanese M, Liguori C, et al. Restless legs syndrome and post polio syndrome: a case-control study. *Eur J Neurol.* (2015) 22:472–8. doi: 10.1111/ene.12593
88. Murray D, Hardiman O, Meldrum D. Assessment of subjective and motor fatigue in Polio survivors, attending a Postpolio clinic, comparison with healthy controls and an exploration of clinical correlates. *Physiother Theory Pract.* (2014) 30:229–35. doi: 10.3109/09593985.2013.862890
89. Duncan A, Batliwalla Z. Growing older with post-polio syndrome: social and quality-of-life implications. *SAGE Open Med.* (2018) 6:2050312118793563. doi: 10.1177/2050312118793563
90. Viana CF, Pradella-Hallinan M, Quadros AA, Marin LF, Oliveira AS. Circadian variation of fatigue in both patients with paralytic poliomyelitis and post-polio syndrome. *Arq Neuropsiquiatr.* (2013) 71:442–5. doi: 10.1590/0004-282X20130059
91. Marin LF, Carvalho LBC, Prado LBF, Oliveira ASB, Prado GF. Restless legs syndrome is highly prevalent in patients with post-polio syndrome. *Sleep Med.* (2017) 37:147–50. doi: 10.1016/j.sleep.2017.06.025

92. Marin LF, Carvalho LB, Prado LB, Quadros AA, Oliveira AS, Prado GF. Restless legs syndrome in post-polio syndrome: a series of 10 patients with demographic, clinical and laboratorial findings. *Parkinsonism Relat Disord.* (2011) 17:563–4. doi: 10.1016/j.parkreldis.2011.02.011
93. Kumru H, Portell E, Barrio M, Santamaria J. Restless legs syndrome in patients with sequelae of poliomyelitis. *Parkinsonism Relat Disord.* (2014) 20:1056–8. doi: 10.1016/j.parkreldis.2014.06.014
94. De Grandis E, Mir P, Edwards MJ, Bhatia KP. Restless legs may be associated with the post-polio syndrome. *Parkinsonism Relat Disord.* (2009) 15:74–5. doi: 10.1016/j.parkreldis.2008.02.005
95. Hsu AA, Staats BA. "Postpolio" sequelae and sleep-related disordered breathing. *Mayo Clin Proc.* (1998) 73:216–24. doi: 10.4065/73.3.216
96. Dolmage TE, Avendano MA, Goldstein RS. Respiratory function during wakefulness and sleep among survivors of respiratory and non-respiratory poliomyelitis. *Eur Respir J.* (1992) 5:864–70.
97. Araujo MA, Silva TM, Moreira GA, Pradella-Hallinan M, Tufik S, Oliveira AS. Sleep disorders frequency in post-polio syndrome patients caused by periodic limb movements. *Arq Neuropsiquiatr.* (2010) 68:35–8. doi: 10.1590/S0004-282X2010000100008
98. Romigi A, Maestri M. Circadian fatigue or unrecognized restless legs syndrome? The post-polio syndrome model. *Front Neurol.* (2014) 5:115. doi: 10.3389/fneur.2014.00115
99. Romigi A, Placidi F, Evangelista E, Desiato MT. Circadian variation of fatigue in paralytic poliomyelitis and postpolio syndrome: just fatigue or masked restless legs syndrome? *Arq Neuropsiquiatr.* (2014) 72:475–6. doi: 10.1590/0004-282X20140046
100. Romigi A, Franco V, Placidi F, Liguori C, Rastelli E, Vitrani G, et al. Comparative sleep disturbances in myotonic dystrophy types 1 and 2. *Curr Neurol Neurosci Rep.* (2018) 18:102. doi: 10.1007/s11910-018-0903-x
101. Weinstock LB, Walters AS, Paueksakon P. Restless legs syndrome–theoretical roles of inflammatory and immune mechanisms. *Sleep Med Rev.* (2012) 16:341–54. doi: 10.1016/j.smrv.2011.09.003
102. Tseng WC, Wu ZF, Liaw WJ, Hwa SY, Hung NK. A patient with postpolio syndrome developed cauda equina syndrome after neuraxial anesthesia: a case report. *J Clin Anesthesia.* (2017) 37:49–51. doi: 10.1016/j.jclinane.2016.09.032
103. Leming MK, Breyer MJ. Renal failure in a patient with postpolio syndrome and a normal creatinine level. *Am J Emergency Med.* (2012) 30:247.e1-3. doi: 10.1016/j.ajem.2010.07.026
104. Willen C, Thoren-Jonsson AL, Grimby G, Sunnerhagen KS. Disability in a 4-year follow-up study of people with post-polio syndrome. *J Rehabil Med.* (2007) 39:175–80. doi: 10.2340/16501977-0034
105. Bickerstaffe A, Beelen A, Nollet F. Change in physical mobility over 10 years in post-polio syndrome. *Neuromuscul Disord.* (2015) 25:225–30. doi: 10.1016/j.nmd.2014.11.015
106. Klein MG, Whyte J, Keenan MA, Esquenazi A, Polansky M. Changes in strength over time among polio survivors. *Arch Phys Med Rehabil.* (2000) 81:1059–64. doi: 10.1053/apmr.2000.3890
107. Flansbjer UB, Lexell J, Brogardh C. Predictors of changes in gait performance over four years in persons with late effects of polio. *NeuroRehabilitation.* (2017) 41:403–11. doi: 10.3233/NRE-162057
108. Flansbjer UB, Brogardh C, Horstmann V, Lexell J. Men with late effects of polio decline more than women in lower limb muscle strength: a 4-year longitudinal study. *PMR.* (2015) 7:1127–36. doi: 10.1016/j.pmrj.2015.05.005
109. Kosaka T, Kuroha Y, Tada M, Hasegawa A, Tani T, Matsubara N, et al. A fatal neuromuscular disease in an adult patient after poliomyelitis in early childhood: consideration of the pathology of post-polio syndrome. *Neuropathology.* (2013) 33:93–101. doi: 10.1111/j.1440-1789.2012.01327.x
110. Nollet F, Trojan DA. *Finding causes of and managing fatigue in PPS.* (2009). Available online at: https://www.cvppsg.org/wp-content/uploads/2012/02/findingcausesmanagingfatiguepps.pdf
111. Skough K, Broman L, Borg K. Test-retest reliability of the 6-min walk test in patients with postpolio syndrome. *Int J Rehabil Res.* (2013) 36:140–5. doi: 10.1097/MRR.0b013e32835b669b
112. Stolwijk-Swuste JM, Beelen A, Lankhorst GJ, Nollet F, group Cs. SF36 physical functioning scale and 2-minute walk test advocated as core qualifiers to evaluate physical functioning in patients with late-onset sequelae of poliomyelitis. *J Rehabil Med.* (2008) 40:387–94. doi: 10.2340/16501977-0188
113. Podsiadlo D, Richardson S. The timed "Up & Go": a test of basic functional mobility for frail elderly persons. *J Am Geriatr Soc.* (1991) 39:142–8. doi: 10.1111/j.1532-5415.1991.tb01616.x
114. Whitney SL, Wrisley DM, Marchetti GF, Gee MA, Redfern MS, Furman JM. Clinical measurement of sit-to-stand performance in people with balance disorders: validity of data for the Five-Times-Sit-to-Stand Test. *Phys Ther.* (2005) 85:1034–45.
115. Bickerstaffe A, Beelen A, Zwarts MJ, Nollet F, van Dijk JP. Quantitative muscle ultrasound and quadriceps strength in patients with post-polio syndrome. *Muscle Nerve.* (2015) 51:24–9. doi: 10.1002/mus.24272
116. Koopman FS, Brehm MA, Heerkens YF, Nollet F, Beelen A. Measuring fatigue in polio survivors: content comparison and reliability of the Fatigue Severity Scale and the Checklist Individual Strength. *J Rehabil Med.* (2014) 46:761–7. doi: 10.2340/16501977-1838
117. Washburn RA, McAuley E, Katula J, Mihalko SL, Boileau RA. The physical activity scale for the elderly (PASE): evidence for validity. *J Clin Epidemiol.* (1999) 52:643–51. doi: 10.1016/S0895-4356(99)00049-9
118. Ostlund G, Wahlin A, Sunnerhagen KS, Borg K. Post polio syndrome: fatigued patients a specific subgroup? *J Rehabil Med.* (2011) 43:39–45. doi: 10.2340/16501977-0634
119. Dencker A, Sunnerhagen KS, Taft C, Lundgren-Nilsson A. Multidimensional fatigue inventory and post-polio syndrome - a Rasch analysis. *Health Qual Life Outcomes.* (2015) 13:20. doi: 10.1186/s12955-015-0213-9
120. Pomeroy IM, Tennant A, Young CA. Rasch analysis of the WHOQOL-BREF in post polio syndrome. *J Rehabil Med.* (2013) 45:873–80. doi: 10.2340/16501977-1186
121. Chung H, Kim J, Park R, Bamer AM, Bocell FD, Amtmann D. Testing the measurement invariance of the University of Washington Self-Efficacy Scale short form across four diagnostic subgroups. *Qual Life Res.* (2016) 25:2559–64. doi: 10.1007/s11136-016-1300-z
122. Silva TM, Moreira GA, Quadros AA, Pradella-Hallinan M, Tufik S, Oliveira AS. Analysis of sleep characteristics in post-polio syndrome patients. *Arq Neuropsiquiatr.* (2010) 68:535–40. doi: 10.1590/S0004-282X2010000400011
123. Orsini M, Lopes AJ, Guimaraes FS, Freitas MR, Nascimento OJ, Anna Mde SJ, et al. Currents issues in cardiorespiratory care of patients with post-polio syndrome. *Arq Neuropsiquiatr.* (2016) 74:574–9. doi: 10.1590/0004-282X20160072
124. Allen RP, Picchietti DL, Garcia-Borreguero D, Ondo WG, Walters AS, Winkelman JW, et al. Restless legs syndrome/Willis-Ekbom disease diagnostic criteria: updated International Restless Legs Syndrome Study Group (IRLSSG) consensus criteria–history, rationale, description, and significance. *Sleep Med.* (2014) 15:860–73. doi: 10.1016/j.sleep.2014.03.025
125. Walters AS, LeBrocq C, Dhar A, Hening W, Rosen R, Allen RP, et al. Validation of the International Restless Legs Syndrome Study Group rating scale for restless legs syndrome. *Sleep Med.* (2003) 4:121–32. doi: 10.1016/S1389-9457(02)00258-7
126. Soliman MG, Higgins SE, El-Kabir DR, Davidson AC, Williams AJ, Howard RS. Non-invasive assessment of respiratory muscle strength in patients with previous poliomyelitis. *Respir Med.* (2005) 99:1217–22. doi: 10.1016/j.rmed.2005.02.035
127. Natterlund B, Ahlstrom G. Problem-focused coping and satisfaction with activities of daily living in individuals with muscular dystrophy and postpolio syndrome. *Scand J Caring Sci.* (1999) 13:26–32. doi: 10.1111/j.1471-6712.1999.tb00511.x
128. Saeki S, Takemura J, Matsushima Y, Chisaka H, Hachisuka K. Workplace disability management in postpolio syndrome. *J Occup Rehabil.* (2001) 11:299–307. doi: 10.1023/A:1013352710035
129. Davidson AC, Auyeung V, Luff R, Holland M, Hodgkiss A, Weinman J. Prolonged benefit in post-polio syndrome from comprehensive rehabilitation: a pilot study. *Disabil Rehabil.* (2009) 31:309–17. doi: 10.1080/09638280801973206
130. Agre JC, Rodriquez AA. Intermittent isometric activity: its effect on muscle fatigue in postpolio subjects. *Arch Phys Med Rehabil.* (1991) 72:971–5.
131. Agre JC, Rodriquez AA, Franke TM, Swiggum ER, Harmon RL, Curt JT. Low-intensity, alternate-day exercise improves muscle performance without apparent adverse effect in postpolio patients. *Am J Phys Med Rehabil.* (1996) 75:50–8. doi: 10.1097/00002060-199601000-00014

132. Dean E, Ross J. Effect of modified aerobic training on movement energetics in polio survivors. *Orthopedics.* (1991) 14:1243–6.
133. Ernstoff B, Wetterqvist H, Kvist H, Grimby G. Endurance training effect on individuals with postpoliomyelitis. *Arch Phys Med Rehabil.* (1996) 77:843–8. doi: 10.1016/S0003-9993(96)90268-3
134. Chan KM, Amirjani N, Sumrain M, Clarke A, Strohschein FJ. Randomized controlled trial of strength training in post-polio patients. *Muscle Nerve.* (2003) 27:332–8. doi: 10.1002/mus.10327
135. Fillyaw MJ, Badger GJ, Goodwin GD, Bradley WG, Fries TJ, Shukla A. The effects of long-term non-fatiguing resistance exercise in subjects with post-polio syndrome. *Orthopedics.* (1991) 14:1253–6.
136. Feldman RM, Soskolne CL. The use of nonfatiguing strengthening exercises in post-polio syndrome. *Birth Defects Original Article Ser.* (1987) 23:335–41.
137. Spector SA, Gordon PL, Feuerstein IM, Sivakumar K, Hurley BF, Dalakas MC. Strength gains without muscle injury after strength training in patients with postpolio muscular atrophy. *Muscle Nerve.* (1996) 19:1282–90. doi: 10.1002/(SICI)1097-4598(199610)19:10<1282::AID-MUS5>3.0.CO;2-A
138. Agre JC, Rodriquez AA, Franke TM. Strength, endurance, and work capacity after muscle strengthening exercise in postpolio subjects. *Arch Phys Med Rehabil.* (1997) 78:681–6. doi: 10.1016/S0003-9993(97)90073-3
139. Kriz JL, Jones DR, Speier JL, Canine JK, Owen RR, Serfass RC. Cardiorespiratory responses to upper extremity aerobic training by postpolio subjects. *Arch Phys Med Rehabil.* (1992) 73:49–54.
140. Jones DR, Speier J, Canine K, Owen R, Stull GA. Cardiorespiratory responses to aerobic training by patients with postpoliomyelitis sequelae. *JAMA.* (1989) 261:3255–8. doi: 10.1001/jama.261.22.3255
141. Oncu J, Durmaz B, Karapolat H. Short-term effects of aerobic exercise on functional capacity, fatigue, and quality of life in patients with post-polio syndrome. *Clin Rehabil.* (2009) 23:155–63. doi: 10.1177/0269215508098893
142. Strumse YA, Stanghelle JK, Utne L, Ahlvin P, Svendsby EK. Treatment of patients with postpolio syndrome in a warm climate. *Disabil Rehabil.* (2003) 25:77–84. doi: 10.1080/dre.25.2.77.84
143. Willen C, Sunnerhagen KS, Grimby G. Dynamic water exercise in individuals with late poliomyelitis. *Arch Phys Med Rehabil.* (2001) 82:66–72. doi: 10.1053/apmr.2001.9626
144. Willen C, Scherman MH. Group training in a pool causes ripples on the water: experiences by persons with late effects of polio. *J Rehabil Med.* (2002) 34:191–7. doi: 10.1080/16501970213232
145. Stanghelle JK, Festvag L, Aksnes AK. Pulmonary function and symptom-limited exercise stress testing in subjects with late sequelae of poliomyelitis. *Scand J Rehabil Med.* (1993) 25:125–9.
146. Kilmer DD. Response to aerobic exercise training in humans with neuromuscular disease. *Am J Phys Med Rehabil.* (2002) 81(11 Suppl):S148–50. doi: 10.1097/00002060-200211001-00015
147. Voorn EL, Gerrits KH, Koopman FS, Nollet F, Beelen A. Determining the anaerobic threshold in postpolio syndrome: comparison with current guidelines for training intensity prescription. *Arch Phys Med Rehabil.* (2014) 95:935–40. doi: 10.1016/j.apmr.2014.01.015
148. Voorn EL, Koopman FS, Brehm MA, Beelen A, de Haan A, Gerrits KH, et al. Aerobic exercise training in post-polio syndrome: process evaluation of a randomized controlled trial. *PLoS ONE.* (2016) 11:e0159280. doi: 10.1371/journal.pone.0159280
149. Murray D, Hardiman O, Campion A, Vance R, Horgan F, Meldrum D. The effects of a home-based arm ergometry exercise programme on physical fitness, fatigue and activity in Polio survivors: a randomised controlled trial. *Clin Rehabil.* (2017) 31:913–25. doi: 10.1177/0269215516661225
150. Murray D, Meldrum D, Moloney R, Campion A, Horgan F, Hardiman O. The effects of a home-based arm ergometry exercise programme on physical fitness, fatigue and activity in polio survivors: protocol for a randomised controlled trial. *BMC Neurol.* (2012) 12:157. doi: 10.1186/1471-2377-12-157
151. Da Silva CP, Szot CL, deSa N. Whole body vibration on people with sequelae of polio. Physiother *Theory Pract.* (2018) 2018:1–11. doi: 10.1080/09593985.2018.1454559
152. Da Silva CP. Whole body vibration methods with survivors of polio. *J Vis Exp.* (2018) 2018:140. doi: 10.3791/58449
153. Brogardh C, Flansbjer UB, Lexell J. No effects of whole-body vibration training on muscle strength and gait performance in persons with late effects of polio: a pilot study. *Arch Phys Med Rehabil.* (2010) 91:1474–7. doi: 10.1016/j.apmr.2010.06.024
154. Arazpour M, Ahmadi F, Bahramizadeh M, Samadian M, Mousavi ME, Bani MA, et al. Evaluation of gait symmetry in poliomyelitis subjects: comparison of a conventional knee-ankle-foot orthosis and a new powered knee-ankle-foot orthosis. *Prosthet Orthot Int.* (2016) 40:689–95. doi: 10.1177/0309364615596063
155. Heim M, Yaacobi E, Azaria M. A pilot study to determine the efficiency of lightweight carbon fibre orthoses in the management of patients suffering from post-poliomyelitis syndrome. *Clin Rehabil.* (1997) 11:302–5. doi: 10.1177/026921559701100406
156. Silva TM, Moreira GA, Quadros AA, Pradella-Hallinan M, Tufik S, Oliveira AS. Effects of the use of MIG3 bioceramics fabrics use–long infrared emitter–in pain, intolerance to cold and periodic limb movements in post-polio syndrome. *Arq Neuropsiquiatr.* (2009) 67:1049–53. doi: 10.1590/S0004-282X2009000600016
157. Acler M, Bocci T, Valenti D, Turri M, Priori A, Bertolasi L. Transcranial direct current stimulation (tDCS) for sleep disturbances and fatigue in patients with post-polio syndrome. *Restor Neurol Neurosci.* (2013) 31:661–8. doi: 10.3233/RNN-130321
158. Pastuszak Z, Piusinska-Macoch R, Stepien A, Czernicki Z. Repetitive transcranial magnetic stimulation in treatment of post polio syndrome. *Neurol Neurochir Pol.* (2018) 52:281–4. doi: 10.1016/j.pjnns.2017.10.013
159. Vallbona C, Hazlewood CF, Jurida G. Response of pain to static magnetic fields in postpolio patients: a double-blind pilot study. *Arch Phys Med Rehabil.* (1997) 78:1200–3. doi: 10.1016/S0003-9993(97)90332-4
160. Sonies BC. Dysphagia and post-polio syndrome: past, present, and future. *Semin Neurol.* (1996) 16:365–70. doi: 10.1055/s-2008-1040995
161. Sonies BC, Dalakas MC. Dysphagia in patients with the post-polio syndrome. *N Engl J Med.* (1991) 324:1162–7. doi: 10.1056/NEJM199104253241703
162. Yunusova Y, Plowman EK, Green JR, Barnett C, Bede P. Clinical measures of bulbar dysfunction in ALS. *Front Neurol.* (2019) 10:106. doi: 10.3389/fneur.2019.00106
163. Silbergleit AK, Waring WP, Sullivan MJ, Maynard FM. Evaluation, treatment, and follow-up results of post polio patients with dysphagia. *Otolaryngol Head Neck Surg.* (1991) 104:333–8. doi: 10.1177/019459989110400308
164. Kaminska M, Browman F, Trojan DA, Genge A, Benedetti A, Petrof BJ. Feasibility of lung volume recruitment in early neuromuscular weakness: a comparison between amyotrophic lateral sclerosis, myotonic dystrophy, and postpolio syndrome. *PMR.* (2015) 7:677–84. doi: 10.1016/j.pmrj.2015.04.001
165. Gillis-Haegerstrand C, Markstrom A, Barle H. Bi-level positive airway pressure ventilation maintains adequate ventilation in post-polio patients with respiratory failure. *Acta Anaesthesiol Scand.* (2006) 50:580–5. doi: 10.1111/j.1399-6576.2006.001015.x
166. Bach JR, Alba AS, Shin D. Management alternatives for post-polio respiratory insufficiency. Assisted ventilation by nasal or oral-nasal interface. *Am J Phys Med Rehabil.* (1989) 68:264–71. doi: 10.1097/00002060-198912000-00002
167. Barle H, Soderberg P, Haegerstrand C, Markstrom A. Bi-level positive airway pressure ventilation reduces the oxygen cost of breathing in long-standing post-polio patients on invasive home mechanical ventilation. *Acta Anaesthesiol Scand.* (2005) 49:197–202. doi: 10.1111/j.1399-6576.2004.00566.x
168. Brogardh C, Lexell J, Hammarlund CS. Experiences of falls and strategies to manage the consequences of falls in persons with late effects of polio: a qualitative study. *J Rehabil Med.* (2017) 49:652–8. doi: 10.2340/16501977-2262
169. Bakker M, Schipper K, Koopman FS, Nollet F, Abma TA. Experiences and perspectives of patients with post-polio syndrome and therapists with exercise and cognitive behavioural therapy. *BMC Neurol.* (2016) 16:23. doi: 10.1186/s12883-016-0544-0
170. Koopman FS, Beelen A, Gerrits KH, Bleijenberg G, Abma TA, de Visser M, et al. Exercise therapy and cognitive behavioural therapy to improve fatigue, daily activity performance and quality of life in postpoliomyelitis syndrome: the protocol of the FACTS-2-PPS trial. *BMC Neurol.* (2010) 10:8. doi: 10.1186/1471-2377-10-8
171. Koopman FS, Brehm MA, Beelen A, Voet N, Bleijenberg G, Geurts A, et al. Cognitive behavioural therapy for reducing fatigue in post-polio syndrome

and in facioscapulohumeral dystrophy: a comparison. *J Rehabil Med.* (2017) 49:585–90. doi: 10.2340/16501977-2247
172. Koopman FS, Voorn EL, Beelen A, Bleijenberg G, de Visser M, Brehm MA, et al. No reduction of severe fatigue in patients with postpolio syndrome by exercise therapy or cognitive behavioral therapy: results of an RCT. *Neurorehabil Neural Repair.* (2016) 30:402–10. doi: 10.1177/1545968315600271
173. Battalio SL, Glette M, Alschuler KN, Jensen MP. Anxiety, depression, and function in individuals with chronic physical conditions: a longitudinal analysis. *Rehabil Psychol.* (2018) 63:532–41. doi: 10.1037/rep0000231
174. Muller R, Gertz KJ, Molton IR, Terrill AL, Bombardier CH, Ehde DM, et al. Effects of a tailored positive psychology intervention on well-being and pain in individuals with chronic pain and a physical disability: a feasibility trial. *Clin J Pain.* (2016) 32:32–44. doi: 10.1097/AJP.0000000000000225
175. Hirsh AT, Kupper AE, Carter GT, Jensen MP. Psychosocial factors and adjustment to pain in individuals with postpolio syndrome. *Am J Phys Med Rehabil.* (2010) 89:213–24. doi: 10.1097/PHM.0b013e3181c9f9a1
176. Furrer A, Michel G, Terrill AL, Jensen MP, Muller R. Modeling subjective well-being in individuals with chronic pain and a physical disability: the role of pain control and pain catastrophizing. *Disabil Rehabil.* (2017) 2017:1–10. doi: 10.1080/09638288.2017.1390614
177. Shiri S, Gartsman I, Meiner Z, Schwartz I. Long-standing poliomyelitis and psychological health. *Disabil Rehabil.* (2015) 37:2233–7. doi: 10.3109/09638288.2015.1019007
178. Silverman AM, Molton IR, Alschuler KN, Ehde DM, Jensen MP. Resilience predicts functional outcomes in people aging with disability: a longitudinal investigation. *Arch Phys Med Rehabil.* (2015) 96:1262–8. doi: 10.1016/j.apmr.2015.02.023
179. Battalio SL, Silverman AM, Ehde DM, Amtmann D, Edwards KA, Jensen MP. Resilience and function in adults with physical disabilities: an observational study. *Arch Phys Med Rehabil.* (2017) 98:1158–64. doi: 10.1016/j.apmr.2016.11.012
180. Silverman AM, Molton IR, Smith AE, Jensen MP, Cohen GL. Solace in solidarity: disability friendship networks buffer well-being. *Rehabil Psychol.* (2017) 62:525–33. doi: 10.1037/rep0000128
181. Ten Katen K, Beelen A, Nollet F, Frings-Dresen MH, Sluiter JK. Overcoming barriers to work participation for patients with postpoliomyelitis syndrome. *Disabil Rehabil.* (2011) 33:522–9. doi: 10.3109/09638288.2010.503257
182. Pierini D, Stuifbergen AK. Psychological resilience and depressive symptoms in older adults diagnosed with post-polio syndrome. *Rehabil Nurs.* (2010) 35:167–75. doi: 10.1002/j.2048-7940.2010.tb00043.x
183. Dinsmore S, Dambrosia J, Dalakas MC. A double-blind, placebo-controlled trial of high-dose prednisone for the treatment of post-poliomyelitis syndrome. *Ann N Y Acad Sci.* (1995) 753:303–13. doi: 10.1111/j.1749-6632.1995.tb27556.x
184. Stein DP, Dambrosia JM, Dalakas MC. A double-blind, placebo-controlled trial of amantadine for the treatment of fatigue in patients with the post-polio syndrome. *Ann N Y Acad Sci.* (1995) 753:296–302. doi: 10.1111/j.1749-6632.1995.tb27555.x
185. Trojan DA, Collet JP, Shapiro S, Jubelt B, Miller RG, Agre JC, et al. A multicenter, randomized, double-blinded trial of pyridostigmine in postpolio syndrome. *Neurology.* (1999) 53:1225–33. doi: 10.1212/WNL.53.6.1225
186. Horemans HL, Nollet F, Beelen A, Drost G, Stegeman DF, Zwarts MJ, et al. Pyridostigmine in postpolio syndrome: no decline in fatigue and limited functional improvement. *J Neurol Neurosurg Psychiatry.* (2003) 74:1655–61. doi: 10.1136/jnnp.74.12.1655
187. Chan KM, Strohschein FJ, Rydz D, Allidina A, Shuaib A, Westbury CF. Randomized controlled trial of modafinil for the treatment of fatigue in postpolio patients. *Muscle Nerve.* (2006) 33:138–41. doi: 10.1002/mus.20437
188. Vasconcelos OM, Prokhorenko OA, Salajegheh MK, Kelley KF, Livornese K, Olsen CH, et al. Modafinil for treatment of fatigue in post-polio syndrome: a randomized controlled trial. *Neurology.* (2007) 68:1680–6. doi: 10.1212/01.wnl.0000261912.53959.b4
189. Skough K, Krossen C, Heiwe S, Theorell H, Borg K. Effects of resistance training in combination with coenzyme Q10 supplementation in patients with post-polio: a pilot study. *J Rehabil Med.* (2008) 40:773–5. doi: 10.2340/16501977-0245
190. Peel MM, Cooke M, Lewis-Peel HJ, Lea RA, Moyle W. A randomized controlled trial of coenzyme Q10 for fatigue in the late-onset sequelae of poliomyelitis. *Complement Ther Med.* (2015) 23:789–93. doi: 10.1016/j.ctim.2015.09.002
191. On AY, Oncu J, Uludag B, Ertekin C. Effects of lamotrigine on the symptoms and life qualities of patients with post polio syndrome: a randomized, controlled study. *NeuroRehabilitation.* (2005) 20:245–51.
192. Kaponides G, Gonzalez H, Olsson T, Borg K. Effect of intravenous immunoglobulin in patients with post-polio syndrome – an uncontrolled pilot study. *J Rehabil Med.* (2006) 38:138–40. doi: 10.1080/16501970500441625
193. Gonzalez H, Sunnerhagen KS, Sjoberg I, Kaponides G, Olsson T, Borg K. Intravenous immunoglobulin for post-polio syndrome: a randomised controlled trial. *Lancet Neurol.* (2006) 5:493–500. doi: 10.1016/S1474-4422(06)70447-1
194. Werhagen L, Borg K. Effect of intravenous immunoglobulin on pain in patients with post-polio syndrome. *J Rehabil Med.* (2011) 43:1038–40. doi: 10.2340/16501977-0884
195. Ostlund G, Broman L, Werhagen L, Borg K. IVIG treatment in post-polio patients: evaluation of responders. *J Neurol.* (2012) 259:2571–8. doi: 10.1007/s00415-012-6538-y
196. Bertolasi L, Frasson E, Turri M, Gajofatto A, Bordignon M, Zanolin E, et al. A randomized controlled trial of IV immunoglobulin in patients with postpolio syndrome. *J Neurol Sci.* (2013) 330:94–9. doi: 10.1016/j.jns.2013.04.016
197. Schmidt S, Gocheva V, Zumbrunn T, Rubino-Nacht D, Bonati U, Fischer D, et al. Treatment with L-citrulline in patients with post-polio syndrome: study protocol for a single-center, randomised, placebo-controlled, double-blind trial. *Trials.* (2017) 18:116. doi: 10.1186/s13063-017-1829-3
198. Ostlund G, Broman L, Werhagen L, Borg K. Immunoglobulin treatment in post-polio syndrome: identification of responders and non-responders. *J Rehabil Med.* (2015) 47:727–33. doi: 10.2340/16501977-1985
199. Scholz H, Trenkwalder C, Kohnen R, Riemann D, Kriston L, Hornyak M. Dopamine agonists for restless legs syndrome. *Cochrane Database Syst Rev.* (2011) 2011:CD006009. doi: 10.1002/14651858.CD006009.pub2
200. Schwartz A, Bosch LM. Anesthetic implications of postpolio syndrome: new concerns for an old disease. *AANA J.* (2012) 80:356–61.
201. Spencer GT, Reynolds F. Postoperative respiratory arrest in a post poliomyelitis patient. *Anaesthesia.* (2003) 58:609–10; author reply 10. doi: 10.1046/j.1365-2044.2003.03207_14.x
202. Wheeler D. Anesthetic considerations for patients with postpolio syndrome: a case report. *AANA J.* (2011) 79:408–10.

6

Spinal Cord Imaging in Amyotrophic Lateral Sclerosis: Historical Concepts—Novel Techniques

Mohamed Mounir El Mendili[1,2], *Giorgia Querin*[2,3], *Peter Bede*[2,3,4†] *and Pierre-François Pradat*[2,3*†]

[1] Department of Neurology, Icahn School of Medicine at Mount Sinai, New York, NY, United States, [2] Biomedical Imaging Laboratory (LIB), Sorbonne University, CNRS, INSERM, Paris, France, [3] Department of Neurology, Pitié-Salpêtrière University Hospital (APHP), Paris, France, [4] Computational Neuroimaging Group, Trinity College Dublin, Dublin, Ireland

***Correspondence:**
Pierre-François Pradat
pierre-francois.pradat@psl.aphp.fr

† These authors have contributed equally as co-senior authors

Amyotrophic lateral sclerosis (ALS) is the most common adult onset motor neuron disease with no effective disease modifying therapies at present. Spinal cord degeneration is a hallmark feature of ALS, highlighted in the earliest descriptions of the disease by Lockhart Clarke and Jean-Martin Charcot. The anterior horns and corticospinal tracts are invariably affected in ALS, but up to recently it has been notoriously challenging to detect and characterize spinal pathology *in vivo*. With recent technological advances, spinal imaging now offers unique opportunities to appraise lower motor neuron degeneration, sensory involvement, metabolic alterations, and interneuron pathology in ALS. Quantitative spinal imaging in ALS has now been used in cross-sectional and longitudinal study designs, applied to presymptomatic mutation carriers, and utilized in machine learning applications. Despite its enormous clinical and academic potential, a number of physiological, technological, and methodological challenges limit the routine use of computational spinal imaging in ALS. In this review, we provide a comprehensive overview of emerging spinal cord imaging methods and discuss their advantages, drawbacks, and biomarker potential in clinical applications, clinical trial settings, monitoring, and prognostic roles.

Keywords: ALS (Amyotrophic lateral sclerosis), MRI—magnetic resonance imaging, MND, spinal cord, neuroimaging

INTRODUCTION

Amyotrophic lateral sclerosis (ALS) is a relentlessly progressive neurodegenerative disorder. Anterior horn pathology and corticospinal tract degeneration has been identified as a core feature of ALS since the earliest descriptions of the condition (1, 2). Despite repeated attempts to detect and characterize spinal cord pathology *in vivo* (3), technological constraints have traditionally precluded reliable quantitative spinal imaging in ALS. Due to the plethora of methodological challenges, such as the small cross-sectional area of the human spinal cord, respiratory, and cardiac movement effects, the overwhelming majority of imaging studies have focused on cerebral alterations in ALS (4).

The diagnosis of ALS is primarily clinical and requires the careful exclusion of ALS-mimics (5). Given the heterogeneity of clinical presentations and the prevalence of atypical phenotypes, diagnostic delay in ALS is not uncommon, and the average period between symptom onset and definite diagnosis is ~12 months worldwide (6). The median survival from symptom onset ranges from 20 to 48 months (7–9). Progression rates in ALS show considerable variation, and prognosis depends on age at onset, region of onset, co-morbid cognitive impairment, nutritional status, and certain genotypes are associated with faster progression (10–16). Given the considerable clinical, cognitive, and genetic heterogeneity of ALS, there is an unmet need for early diagnostic biomarkers to aid patient stratification into specific phenotypes (17). Clinical trials of ALS continue to rely on survival, functional scores and respiratory measures as outcome measures despite the potential of candidate imaging markers (18).

Magnetic resonance imaging (MRI) not only contributed to the characterization of ALS-associated cerebral changes, it has also contributed important pathophysiological insights, such as the role of inflammation (19), patterns of spread (20, 21), inhibitory dysfunction (22, 23), and network-wise propagation (24, 25). In addition to describing unifying disease-associated signatures, imaging studies of ALS have gradually characterized the features of specific genotypes (26, 27), phenotypes (28, 29), the substrate of cognitive and extra-pyramidal impairments (30), as well as presymptomatic (31) and longitudinal changes (32). Despite the momentous advances however, the overwhelming majority of imaging studies in ALS remain cerebral, overlooking a disease-defining site of ALS pathology; the spinal cord (3).

SPINAL CORD IMAGING

One of the key challenges of spinal cord imaging stems from its elongated dimensions, small cross-sectional area in the axial plane coupled with long sagittal and coronal expansion (33). Furthermore, the cord is surrounded by tissues that have very different magnetic susceptibility profiles and is it subject to both direct (cardiac and respiratory) and fluid-mediated [cerebrospinal fluid (CSF)] movement effects. The main challenges of quantitative spinal cord imaging include (i) partial volume effects, (ii) an inhomogeneous magnetic field environment, and (iii) physiological and patient motion (34).

Abbreviations: 1H-MRS, proton spectroscopy; A-P, anterior-posterior; AD, axial diffusivity; ALS, Amyotrophic lateral sclerosis; ALSFRS-R, revised ALS functional scale; Cho, choline; CNR, contrast-to-noise ratio; Cr, creatine; CSA, cross-sectional area; CSF, cerebrospinal flood; CST, corticospinal tract; DTI, diffusion tensor imaging; FA, fractional anisotropy; fMRI, functional MRI; ihMT, Inhomogeneous magnetization transfer; LMN, lower motor neuron; MD, mean diffusivity; MRI, Magnetic resonance imaging; MRS, Magnetic resonance spectroscopy; MT, Magnetization transfer; MTR, Magnetization transfer ratio; Myo, myo-Inositol; NAA, N-Acetyl Aspartate; NODDI, neurite orientation dispersion and density imaging; RD, radial diffusivity; RL, right-left; SNR, signal-to-noise ratio; TMS, transracial magnetic stimulation; SOD1, superoxide dismutase 1 gene; SOD1+, presymptomatic superoxide dismutase 1 gene.

METHODOLOGICAL CHALLENGES

Partial Volume Effects

Partial volume refers to scenarios where different tissues contribute to the same voxel. In spinal cord imaging this occurs when a voxel is at the CSF/white matter, white matter/gray matter, CSF/vascular, white matter/vascular interfaces. Signals from different tissue densities with different amounts of spins contribute to the total MR signal in these voxels, which results in indistinct tissue-boundaries. Partial volume effects can be reduced by increasing the spatial resolution, but this in turn results in lower signal-to-noise (SNR) and contrast-to-noise ratios (CNR). Magnetic fields strengths of three or seven Tesla compared to conventional 1.5 Tesla platforms (35–38), higher number of phased-array coils with parallel imaging (35, 38, 39), and corrections for physiological motion improves spatial resolution, SNR, and CNR (35, 38, 39).

Physiological and Patient Motion

Due to its proximity to the lungs and the heart, almost the entire spinal cord undergoes repetitive displacement due to respiration, CSF, and cardiac pulsation (40–43). The movement of the human spinal cord linearly increases caudally with distance from the head. The available literature suggest that physiological anterior-posterior (A-P) cord movement (0.60 ± 0.34 mm) exceeds those observed in superior-inferior (SI) (0.4 ± 0.1 mm) and right-left (RL) direction (0.17 ± 0.09 mm) (44, 45). Spinal imaging is also susceptible to movement artifacts from swallowing and patient movements during long MR acquisitions which can create ghosting artifacts (42, 46). By "gating" the acquisition, i.e., synchronizing with the respiratory or cardiac cycles, the effect of periodical movements can be significantly reduced (38, 39, 47). Motion artifacts can also be reduced using "saturation bands" that cover the esophagus, chest, and abdomen, by attenuating signals from moving structures so that it does not corrupt the signal from the spinal cord itself. Velocity compensating gradient sequences and signal averaging across multiple phases of motion can also be applied to minimize motion artifacts. Reducing acquisition time by using fast sequences, i.e., fast-spin-echo, parallel imaging that increases acquisition speed by factors from 1.5 to 3, i.e., SENSitivity Encoding/GeneRalized Autocalibration Partial Parallel Acquisition-type reconstructions, partial Fourier imaging, reducing the size of the phase-encoded direction, and decreasing the k-space matrix size effectively reduce both physiological and subject motion effects (48–53). MRI compatible cervical collars, which minimize involuntary neck movements, may also reduce movement artifacts (46). Co-registration of all data when dealing with multiple series acquisition, e.g., diffusion tensor imaging (DTI) and functional MRI (fMRI), can also be performed to limit the inconsistency in derived maps (54, 55).

Inhomogeneous Magnetic Field Environment

The spinal canal is surrounded by bones, ligaments, disks, arteries, and venous plexi. Its proximity to the esophagus, mediastinum, and the lungs, each containing various amounts of air, create a challenging scanning environment. Adipose tissue, bone, and air have different magnetic susceptibility profiles, and respiration-induced B0 field fluctuations (43) also contribute to the inhomogeneity of the magnetic field around the spinal cord, resulting in geometric distortions and signal intensity loss (56). To some extent, these artifacts can be counteracted with "shimming." Shimming aims at compensating for field inhomogeneities by creating an auxiliary magnetic field via shim coils (57). While shimming improves overall field homogeneity, it is limited to smooth variations across larger regions and cannot fully compensate for small, and localized field variations, such as those observed at cartilaginous discs between the vertebral bodies. Echo planar imaging sequences, such as DTI, are particularly sensitive to geometric distortions around vertebral disks. In addition to shimming, parallel imaging, and careful slices positioning may reduce magnetic field inhomogeneity, i.e., slices centered in the middle of each vertebral body and perpendicular to the spinal cord (38, 47, 58). The specific geometry of the magnetic field inhomogeneities should be considered in order to correct for its effect (59–61).

SPINAL CORD IMAGING IN ALS

The role of conventional spinal MRI in ALS is to rule of alternative structural, inflammatory or neoplastic pathologies which may result in a combination of upper and lower motor neuron involvement mimicking ALS (62). Compressive myelopathies and radiculopathies are relatively common and early, predominantly lower limb presentations of ALS are sometimes attributed to these radiological findings resulting in laminectomies and other invasive procedures (63, 64). Conventional, clinical spinal sequences are typically only qualitatively interpreted without specific measurements. The majority of clinical spinal scans in ALS are reported as normal, but non-specific signs such as high signal along the corticospinal tracts are occasionally observed on T2-weighted imaging (65–67).

In sharp contrast with clinical sequences, advanced quantitative spinal protocols allow for the detailed and quantitative characterization of spinal gray and white matter integrity (38, 47, 58, 68). These protocols provide high resolution, high SNR, and high CNR images compared to standard clinical sequences. Furthermore, purpose-designed spinal protocols are based on mathematical MR signal modeling (e.g., diffusion-based methods, quantitative magnetization transfer, and MR spectroscopy) and the derived outputs can be quantitatively interpreted to provide accurate, motion-corrected white, and gray matter metrics.

Cord Morphometry

Gross axonal and gray matter loss have traditionally been estimated by measuring spinal cord cross-sectional areas at specific levels and interpreted as a proxy of atrophy in the context of reference normative values (69–72). The "cross-sectional approach" consists of estimating a mean cord cross-sectional area over a representative number of slices at a given vertebral level (70, 71, 73, 74), which can be relatively easily calculated from conventional MR sequences such as T1- or T2-weighted images. A variety of indexes, such as A-P dimension, L-R width, and radial distance can be derived from the cross-sectional area (CSA) approach. These measures reflect on different aspects of pathology, such as global vs. regional, lateral vs. anterior tissue loss, and are often interpreted as predominantly motor or sensory involvement (70, 75). More specific gray and white matter measures can be derived from higher resolution images followed by tissue-type segmentation methods (72, 76, 77). Novel quantitative approaches, such as tensor based morphometry and surface based-morphometry permit a more fine-grained characterization of cord topography and the definition of disease-associated signatures (74, 78). Recent studies demonstrated that spinal cord atrophy, especially gray matter atrophy, correlates with disability and disease progression and may be predictive of respiratory failure and of survival in ALS (58, 70, 72, 73, 79). The main findings of structural spinal cord studies are summarized in **Table 1**.

Diffusion Weighted Imaging

Diffusion weighted imaging (DWI) relies on the evaluation of water diffusion in CNS tissues and is primarily used to characterize white matter integrity (90, 91). DWI-derived metrics, such as axial diffusivity (AD), mean diffusivity (MD), fractional anisotropy (FA), radial diffusivity (RD) enable the quantitative characterization of white matter integrity. Novel high-directional approaches, such as high-angular resolution diffusion imaging (92), q-ball imaging (93), diffusion kurtosis imaging (94), diffusion basis spectrum imaging (DBSI) (95) are particularly well-suited to assess the integrity of crossing-fibers (96, 97). Emerging diffusion techniques such as neurite orientation dispersion and density imaging (NODDI) (98) help to estimate the microstructural attributes of dendrites and axons (99). While in ALS NODDI has been primarily used in cerebral studies in ALS (100, 101), it also has been also piloted in spinal applications (90, 102). Specific DTI indices (AD, RD) have been associated with specific pathological processes, such as axonal (103, 104) vs. myelin-related (105, 106) degeneration, but this interpretation is likely to be simplistic, as DTI measures are affected by axonal density, axonal diameter, myelin thickness and fiber orientation, fiber coherence, and acquisition parameters. DTI has been extensively used to study cerebral changes in ALS and describe phenotype-associated (107), genotype-specific (27), presymptomatic (32), and longitudinal white matter changes in the brain (81). In contrast to the plethora of cerebral DTI studies, relatively few spinal DTI studies have been published in ALS to date (58, 69, 73, 80–82, 85). These have consistently highlighted both motor and sensory tract alterations (**Table 1**).

Magnetization Transfer Imaging

Hydrogen nuclei linked to macromolecules such as the proteins and lipids of the myelin sheet have an extremely short T2 signal. While these macromolecules are not directly detectable by standard MRI sequences, magnetization transfer (MT) imaging enables the characterization of these structures. Macromolecular spins can be saturated using an off-resonance RF pulse, then the magnetization transfer between bound and free pools

TABLE 1 | Quantitative spinal imaging studies in ALS, ALS, amyotrophic lateral sclerosis; ALSFRS-r, the revised ALS functional scale; FA, fractional anisotropy; CSA, cross-sectional area; CST, corticospinal tract; FVC, force vital capacity; ihMT, inhomogeneous magnetization transfer; ihMTR, inhomogeneous magnetization transfer ratio; MD, mean diffusivity; MT, magnetization transfer; MTR, magnetization transfer ratio; MMT, manual muscle testing; SC, spinal cord; SOD1, superoxide dismutase 1 gene.

Author year of publication (references)	Patient cohort *n*	Controls *n*	Spinal imaging technique	Spinal cord region evaluated	Main findings
Valsasina et al. (80)	28 Sporadic ALS	20	CSA/DTI	Cervical spinal cord	Decreased FA and CSA decreased in ALS. Strong correlation between FA and the ALSFRS and moderate correlation between spinal and brain FA
Agosta et al. (81)	17/17 at baseline/follow-up (9 months) Sporadic ALS	20	CSA/DTI	Cervical spinal cord	Longitudinal FA, MD, and CSA changes detected. Brain CST diffusivity measurements are stable over time and do not correlate with cord measures
Nair et al. (82)	14 Sporadic ALS	15	DTI	C2-C6 vertebral levels	Reduced FA and RD in ALS. FA and RD correlate with finger and foot tapping rates. RD correlates with FVC and ALSFRS-R
Carew et al. (31)	23 sporadic ALS, 24 presymptomatic SOD1carriers	29	1H-MRS	C2 vertebral level	Reduced NAA/Cr and NAA/Myo ratios in both SOD1+ and sporadic ALS. Reduced Myo/Cr in SOD1+ subjects but not in sporadic ALS. Reduced NAA/Cho in sporadic ALS but not in SOD1+ subjects
Carew et al. (83)	14 Sporadic ALS	16	1H-MRS	C2 vertebral level	Reduced NAA/Cr and NAA/Myo ratios in ALS. NAA/Myo and NAA/Cho reductions correlate with FVC
Ikeda et al. (84)	19 Sporadic ALS	20	1H-MRS	C2 vertebral level	Reduced NAA/Cr and NAA/Myo ratios in ALS. NAA/Cr and NAA/Myo correlate with ALSFRS and FVC. NAA/Cr, NAA/m-Ins, and m-Ins/Cr are markedly altered in patients with C2 denervation and neurogenic changes
Cohen-Adad et al. (69)	27 sporadic ALS, 2 SOD1-linked familial ALS	21	CSA/DTI/ MT	C2-T2 vertebral levels	Altered DTI and MT metrics in the lateral and dorsal columns. FA correlates with ALSFRS-r. Segmental cord atrophy is associated with disability. FA profile of the cervical cord is suggestive of retrograde CST degeneration i.e., "dying back"
Branco et al. (70)	25 Sporadic ALS	43	CSA	C2 vertebral level	Decreased CSA in ALS. CSA correlates with disease duration, ALSFRS-r, and ALS severity scale
El Mendili et al. (73)	29 at baseline, 14 at follow-up	–	CSA/DTI/ MT	C2-T2 vertebral levels	CSA correlates with MMT. At follow-up, CSA predicts upper limb ALSFSR-R subscores, and FA predicts lower limb disability. CSA and MTR decrease between baseline and follow-up
Wang et al. (85)	24 Sporadic ALS	16	DTI	C2-C4 vertebral levels	CST FA and ADC changes in ALS. No difference in FA or ADC between patients with "definite" and "probable" ALS. No correlations between DTI parameters and modified Norris or ALSFRS-r scores
Iglesias et al. (86)	21 Sporadic ALS	21	DTI	Cervical spinal cord	Abnormal DTI metrics indicate decreased integrity of ascending sensory fibers. Significant correlation between DTI metrics and the depression of the peripheral afferent volley. The combination of SEP and DTI reveals sub-clinical sensory deficits in 85% ALS patients
Rasoanandrianina et al. (58)	10 Sporadic ALS	20	CSA/DTI/MT/ihMT	Cervical spinal cord	Spinal GM and WM atrophy in ALS. GM atrophy correlates with UMN scores. FA and MTR decrease in the CST. Axial diffusivity and ihMT decreased in the CST and dorsal columns. CSA correlates with the ALSFRS-r and spinal ALSFRS-R subscores. DTI and MT/ihMT metrics correlate with disease duration and MRC scores
de Albuquerque et al. (87)	27 at baseline, 27 at follow-up 8 months apart	27	CSA/DTI	C2 vertebral level	Longitudinal reduction in CSA. Cord area reduction correlates with change in ALSFRS-r

(Continued)

TABLE 1 | Continued

Author year of publication (References)	Patient cohort *n*	Controls *n*	Spinal imaging technique	Spinal cord region evaluated	Main findings
Querin et al. (79)	49 sporadic ALS	–	CSA/DTI/MT	C2-T2 vertebral levels	Spinal MRI parameters are more predictive of survival than clinical variables (ALSFRS-R, MMT, and disease duration)
Paquin et al. (72)	27 sporadic, 2 SOD1-linked familial ALS	22	CSA	C3-C6 vertebral levels	Spinal gray matter metrics are more sensitive to discriminate ALS patients from controls than overall cord CSA. Gray matter and spinal cord CSA correlates with ALSFRS-r and MMT arm scores. ALSFRS-r prediction improves when including a combination of gray and white matter CSA
Querin et al. (76)	60 sporadic ALS	45	CSA/DTI/MT	Cervical spinal cord	Random forest classification algorithm leads to good diagnostic performance distinguishing patients with ALS from controls with a sensitivity of 88% and specificity of 85%. The highest discrimination ability was achieved by evaluating RD, followed by FA, and CSA at the C5 spinal level
Piaggio et al. (88)	23 Sporadic ALS	18	CSA	Level of the Foramen magnum	Spinal cord area at the foramen magnum is significantly lower in ALS patients than in control subjects and is significantly correlated to ALSFRS-r. Spinal cord CSA at the foramen magnum correlates with disability in ALS independently of cerebral measures
Grolez et al. (89)	40 at baseline, 40 at follow-up 3 months apart	21	SC volume	Cervical spinal cord	Longitudinal change in cervical spinal cord volume is predictive of slow vital capacity decline and is also associated with survival

can be measured (108). Magnetization transfer occurs by means of cross relaxation processes, such as dipole-dipole interactions and chemical exchange. Magnetization transfer ratio (MTR) is calculated as the percentage difference of MT images with macromolecules signal saturation and one without. MTR enables inferences on myelin content, axonal count, and density as shown by three MS histological studies, and has been used extensively to assess demyelination, remyelination, and degeneration in MS (109–111). Conversely, relatively few studies have used cerebral MT imaging in ALS, and the majority of these focused on corticospinal tract alterations (112–115). Relatively few studies evaluated spinal MT changes in ALS, but they have shown progressive reduction overt time and correlation with muscle weakness (58, 69, 73). The key findings of spinal MT imaging studies in ALS and associated technical challenges are summarized in **Tables 1, 2**.

Inhomogeneous Magnetization Transfer Imaging

Inhomogeneous magnetization transfer (ihMT) imaging is a novel method (116, 117), which allows the unprecedented characterization of myelin integrity, by isolating key myelin components from the broader macromolecular pool. ihMT shows unparalleled potential to detect and quantify demyelination (118) and may be adapted to spinal applications. ihMT imaging has already been applied to ALS cohorts and demonstrated significant correlation with muscle strength and disability profiles (58).

MR Spectroscopy

Magnetic resonance spectroscopy (MRS) is well-established, non-invasive imaging tool which provides neurochemical insights based on the concentration and relaxation profile of specific metabolites in cerebral and spinal tissues. MRS has been extensively used in cerebral studies of ALS (119), used to assess the therapeutic effect of Riluzole (120, 121), and also used to study brainstem metabolic alterations (122). Cross-sectional and longitudinal (123), single voxel and whole brain multi-voxel studies have both contributed to our understanding of ALS pathophysiology (124). The main targets of proton spectroscopy (1H-MRS) include the following metabolites; N-Acetyl Aspartate (NAA), creatine (Cr), choline (Cho), and myo-Inositol (Myo). These metabolites are typically associated with neuronal integrity/viability (NAA), tissue energy metabolism (Cr), membrane integrity (Cho), and glial function (Myo). (125). Relatively few studies have used 1H-MRS to characterize metabolic changes at the spinal level, and the majority of these studies focused on multiple sclerosis (126, 127) MRS however seems particularly applicable to ALS cohorts, where it promises the characterization of presymptomatic changes and by including both the upper and lower motor components of the motor system, it has led to particularly significant clinico-radiological correlations (31, 83, 84). For the contribution of MRS studies to

TABLE 2 | The advantages and methodological challenges associated with specific spinal imaging techniques.

Imaging technique	Advantages of specific techniques in ALS	Challenges and correction strategies
Diffusion-weighted imaging	Evaluation of specific white matter bundles; motor; and sensory white matter tracts integrity. Availability of multiple derived diffusivity metrics reflecting on various histological aspects of white matter integrity; AD, MD, RD, FA. Emerging high angular resolution diffusion techniques to assess crossing fiber integrity. Derived metrics can be interpreted in comparative, longitudinal, correlation, and machine learning analyses	Motion artifacts: - Gating the acquisition (DWI, CSA, and volume estimation, fMRI, 1H-MRS) - Saturation bands (all modalities) - Velocity compensating gradient sequences (DWI) - Signal averaging across multiple phases of motion (DWI, fMRI, 1H-MRS) - Fast sequences (DWI) - MRI compatible cervical collar (DWI, CSA, and volume estimation, fMRI, 1H-MRS) - Co-registration of all data (DWI, fMRI) - Non-linear co-registration between T1 with and without magnetization transfer saturation pulse (MTR, ihMT) Magnetic field inhomogeneities: - Shimming (all modalities) - Parallel imaging (all modalities) - Corrections for gradients nonlinearity induced geometric distortion (DWI, MT, ihMT, CSA, and volume estimation, fMRI) - Corrections for breathing induced B0 field fluctuations (DWI, fMRI, CSA) Partial volume effect (all modalities) - Higher magnet field strength - Higher number of phased-array coils with parallel imaging - Multi-channel image acquisition - Limiting physiological motion
Magnetization transfer imaging	Evaluation of both white and gray matter integrity. Sensitive detection and measurement of demyelination. Derived metrics can be evaluated at individual and group-level statistical analyses	
Inhomogeneous magnetization transfer imaging	Applicability to both gray and white matter tissue components, superior sensitivity to detect demyelination	
Cross-sectional area and volume estimation	Automated segmentation pipelines enable the estimation of overall cord cross-sectional area and gray and white matter components separately. Gray matter components correlate with clinical and electrophysiological lower motor neuron (LMN) measures, therefore may be regarded an imaging proxy of LMN integrity	
1H-MR spectroscopyd	MRS provides a number of metrics which reflect on focal neuronal integrity (NAA), energy metabolism (Cr), membrane integrity (Cho), and glial function (Myo). MRS readily captures segmental metabolic alterations in symptomatic and presymptomatic ALS cohorts	
Functional MRI	As an emerging technique spinal fMRI has the potential to detect segmental cord activation during motor tasks and at rest	

ALS, amyotrophic lateral sclerosis; ALSFRS-r, revised ALS functional scale; FA, fractional anisotropy; CST, corticospinal tract; FVC, force vital capacity; MD, mean diffusivity; MMT, manual muscle testing.

ALS research and specific methodological considerations please see **Tables 1, 2**.

Functional MRI

Functional MRI (fMRI) detects local variations in blood oxygenation level-dependent MR signal at rest and during activation paradigms (128). FMRI has been extensively applied to ALS cohorts to describe network changes and assess altered activation patterns when performing motor or cognitive tasks (129–131). Following decades of successful cerebral studies, the first spinal fMRI studies have now been published (55, 132). Emerging spinal cord fMRI studies in healthy controls provide proof of feasibility and the first studies using spinal fMRI in neurological conditions are underway (133).

THE CONTRIBUTION OF SPINAL IMAGING TO ALS RESEARCH

Evidence for Motor Involvement in ALS

Quantitative spinal MRI studies in ALS have consistently detected corticospinal tract and anterior horns degeneration and changes correlated with functional disability (36, 58, 80, 82, 85). Segmental spinal cord atrophy was not only linked to muscle weakness (58, 70, 88), but also to electrophysiological markers such as transracial magnetic stimulation (TMS) and motor evoked potentials (69). Two studies have demonstrated that both white and gray matter atrophy contributes to global cord atrophy in ALS (58, 72), but a recent study indicates that cord atrophy in ALS may be predominantly driven by anterior horn degeneration (72), confirming the role of spinal MRI as a putative LMN marker. DTI and MTR indices of the corticospinal tract (CST) correlated with TMS facilitation motor thresholds, a functional parameter that reflects pyramidal tract integrity.

Longitudinal Spinal Cord Changes in ALS

In contrast to the plethora of longitudinal cerebral studies in ALS (21), relatively few longitudinal spinal studies are available to demonstrate that spinal MRI metrics can track subtle progressive changes over time (73, 81, 87, 89). These longitudinal studies captured decreasing CST MTR and progressive cord atrophy (73, 87) While some longitudinal studies also captured progressive DTI alterations (81), other studies did not (73). Some studies suggest that CSA estimates may be more reliable markers of longitudinal cord pathology than MTR or DTI metrics (73, 87). Progressive cord atrophy not only mirrors clinical progression, but early cervical cord atrophy is thought to predict respiratory dysfunction in ALS (89, 134). Furthermore, spinal MRI metrics may be superior predictive indicators of survival than clinical measures (79). Given the scarcity of longitudinal spinal imaging studies in ALS, it remains to be established which imaging metrics capture early ALS-associated changes, therefore may be used in diagnostic applications, and which metrics can track changes in the later stages making them suitable as monitoring markers.

Evidence for Sensory Involvement in ALS

Several spinal MRI studies (58, 69) have captured dorsal column degeneration using DTI, MT, and ihMT imaging, and one study demonstrated progressive sensory tract degeneration over time (135). Dorsal column pathology can be detected relatively soon after symptoms onset, which suggests that sensory involvement is a core and relatively early feature of ALS. Combined spinal DTI and neurophysiology studies have also confirmed considerable sensory pathway degeneration in ALS patients without sensory symptoms (86). The combined MRI-neurophysiology approach revealed sub-clinical sensory deficits in 85% of ALS patients. These findings suggest that sensory dysfunction may have been underestimated by previous studies and that sensory afferent pathways may be affected early in the course of ALS and are important facets of ALS pathogenesis (69, 86). In contrast to longitudinal cerebral studies (4, 32), longitudinal spinal studies suggest that dorsal column metrics (73), and CST DTI indices (87) may be relatively constant (135).

Evidence for Spinal Metabolic Alterations in ALS

1H-MRS studies in ALS have shown reduced NAA/Cr and NAA/Myo ratios at the C2 vertebral level (31, 83, 84). One spinal MRS study captured reduced NAA/Myo and NAA/Cr ratios in presymptomatic superoxide dismutase 1 gene (SOD1+) carriers (31). In addition to group-level differences in symptomatic and presymptomatic ALS cohorts, NAA/Myo and NAA/Cho reductions correlate with force vital capacity (FVC) and revised ALS functional scale (ALSFRS-r) and inversely correlated to the rates of decline (31, 83, 84).

FUTURE DIRECTIONS

Existing spinal studies in ALS indicate that it is possible to detect disease-specific imaging signatures at a group level, and emerging machine-learning studies (76) have demonstrated that it may be possible to classify individual scans into "ALS" and "Healthy" groups. Despite the pioneering studies however, it is clear that spinal imaging lags behind cerebral imaging. Cerebral imaging has shown that phenotype and genotype specific patterns can be detected, multi-time point longitudinal studies have shown divergent rates of gray and white matter degeneration, studies have been validated by post mortem examination and robust multi-site studies have also been published (136). It is likely that improved coil designs with higher number of phased-array elements, new generation scanners with higher gradients optimized for advanced diffusion-weighted imaging, ultra-high filed platforms with superior spatial resolution, and SNR, spinal imaging will contribute unprecedented insights in ALS. It is conceivable that spinal imaging will contribute to the longstanding debate about dying back and dying forward, and ALS being a primarily spinal vs. cerebral disease. Spinal imaging provides a unique opportunity to appraise both lower and upper motor neuron degeneration. It is also likely that imaging sequences currently primarily used in cerebral imaging in ALS such as resting state fMRI, task-based fMRI, quantitative susceptibility weighted imaging, presymptomatic imaging, texture analyses, and post mortem imaging will filter down to spinal applications. Data-sharing initiatives, cross-platform harmonization, inclusion of upper motor neuron (UMN) and lower motor neuron (LMN) predominant ALS cohorts, correlations with advanced neurophysiological techniques are trends of ALS imaging which is likely to be adopted in spinal studies. One of the key ambitions of multiparametric spinal imaging is to overcome the methodological challenges of thoracic and lumbar imaging.

CONCLUSIONS

The momentous advances in spinal imaging in ALS suggest the spinal metrics may soon be used as validated diagnostic, monitoring, and prognostic markers, contributing both to individualized patient care and pharmacological trials.

AUTHOR CONTRIBUTIONS

ME, GQ, PB, and P-FP contributed equally to the conceptualization, drafting, and revision of the manuscript.

FUNDING

Peter Bede is supported by the Health Research Board (HRB—Ireland; HRB EIA-2017-019), the Iris O'Brien Foundation, the Irish Institute of Clinical Neuroscience IICN—Novartis Ireland Research Grant, and the Research Motor Neuron (RMN-Ireland) Foundation. P-FP is supported by the French Association for Myopathies (AFM-Telethon), the Institute for Research in Brain and Spinal Cord (IRME) the French Association for Research in ALS (ARSLA) and the Target ALS Foundation.

REFERENCES

1. Clarke JL, Jackson JH. On a case of muscular atrophy, with disease of the spinal cord and medulla oblongata. *Med Chir Trans.* (1867) 50:489–98. doi: 10.1177/095952876705000122
2. Charcot J, Joffroy A. Deux cas d'atrophie musculaire progressive avec lésions de la substance grise et de faisceaux antérolatéraux de la moelle épinière. *Arch Physiol Norm Pathol.* (1869) 1:354–7.
3. Bede P, Bokde AL, Byrne S, Elamin M, Fagan AJ, Hardiman O. Spinal cord markers in ALS: diagnostic and biomarker considerations. *Amyotroph Lateral Scler.* (2012) 13:407–15. doi: 10.3109/17482968.2011.649760
4. Bede P, Querin G, Pradat PF. The changing landscape of motor neuron disease imaging: the transition from descriptive studies to precision clinical tools. *Curr Opin Neurol.* (2018) 31:431–8. doi: 10.1097/WCO.0000000000000569
5. Andersen PM, Abrahams S, Borasio GD, de Carvalho M, Chio A, Van Damme P, et al. EFNS guidelines on the clinical management of amyotrophic lateral sclerosis (MALS)–revised report of an EFNS task force. *Eur J Neurol.* (2012) 19:360–75. doi: 10.1111/j.1468-1331.2011.03501.x

6. Mitchell JD, Callagher P, Gardham J, Mitchell C, Dixon M, Addison-Jones R, et al. Timelines in the diagnostic evaluation of people with suspected amyotrophic lateral sclerosis (ALS)/motor neuron disease (MND)–a 20-year review: can we do better? *Amyotroph Lateral Scler.* (2010) 11:537–41. doi: 10.3109/17482968.2010.495158
7. Marin B, Boumediene F, Logroscino G, Couratier P, Babron MC, Leutenegger AL, et al. Variation in worldwide incidence of amyotrophic lateral sclerosis: a meta-analysis. *Int J Epidemiol.* (2017) 46:57–74. doi: 10.1093/ije/dyw061
8. Chio A, Logroscino G, Traynor BJ, Collins J, Simeone JC, Goldstein LA, et al. Global epidemiology of amyotrophic lateral sclerosis: a systematic review of the published literature. *Neuroepidemiology.* (2013) 41:118–30. doi: 10.1159/000351153
9. Gordon PH, Salachas F, Bruneteau G, Pradat PF, Lacomblez L, Gonzalez-Bermejo J, et al. Improving survival in a large French ALS center cohort. *J Neurol.* (2012) 259:1788–92. doi: 10.1007/s00415-011-6403-4
10. Elamin M, Phukan J, Bede P, Jordan N, Byrne S, Pender N, et al. Executive dysfunction is a negative prognostic indicator in patients with ALS without dementia. *Neurology.* (2011) 76:1263–9. doi: 10.1212/WNL.0b013e318214359f
11. Byrne S, Elamin M, Bede P, Shatunov A, Walsh C, Corr B, et al. Cognitive and clinical characteristics of patients with amyotrophic lateral sclerosis carrying a C9orf72 repeat expansion: a population-based cohort study. *Lancet Neurol.* (2012) 11:232–40. doi: 10.1007/978-0-387-88555-1
12. Westeneng HJ, Debray TPA, Visser AE, van Eijk RPA, Rooney JPK, Calvo A, et al. Prognosis for patients with amyotrophic lateral sclerosis: development and validation of a personalised prediction model. *Lancet Neurol.* (2018) 17:423–33. doi: 10.1016/S1474-4422(18)30089-9
13. Chio A, Logroscino G, Hardiman O, Swingler R, Mitchell D, Beghi E, et al. Prognostic factors in ALS: a critical review. *Amyotroph Lateral Scler.* (2009) 10:310–23. doi: 10.3109/17482960802566824
14. Pupillo E, Messina P, Logroscino G, Beghi E. Long-term survival in amyotrophic lateral sclerosis: a population-based study. *Ann Neurol.* (2014) 75:287–97. doi: 10.1002/ana.24096
15. Yunusova Y, Plowman EK, Green JR, Barnett C, Bede P. Clinical measures of bulbar dysfunction in ALS. *Front Neurol.* (2019) 10:106. doi: 10.3389/fneur.2019.00106
16. Christidi F, Karavasilis E, Rentzos M, Kelekis N, Evdokimidis I, Bede P. Clinical and radiological markers of extra-motor deficits in amyotrophic lateral sclerosis. *Front Neurol.* (2018) 9:1005. doi: 10.3389/fneur.2018.01005
17. Pradat PF, Dib M. Biomarkers in amyotrophic lateral sclerosis: facts and future horizons. *Mol Diagn Ther.* (2009) 13:115–25. doi: 10.1007/BF03256320
18. Mitsumoto H, Brooks BR, Silani V. Clinical trials in amyotrophic lateral sclerosis: why so many negative trials and how can trials be improved? *Lancet Neurol.* (2014) 13:1127–38. doi: 10.1016/S1474-4422(14)70129-2
19. Evans MC, Couch Y, Sibson N, Turner MR. Inflammation and neurovascular changes in amyotrophic lateral sclerosis. *Mol Cell Neurosci.* (2013) 53:34–41. doi: 10.1016/j.mcn.2012.10.008
20. Bede P, Hardiman O. Longitudinal structural changes in ALS: a three time-point imaging study of white and gray matter degeneration. *Amyotroph Lateral Scler Frontotemporal Degener.* (2018) 19:232–41. doi: 10.1080/21678421.2017.1407795
21. Menke RAL, Proudfoot M, Talbot K, Turner MR. The two-year progression of structural and functional cerebral MRI in amyotrophic lateral sclerosis. *Neuroimage Clin.* (2018) 17:953–61. doi: 10.1016/j.nicl.2017.12.025
22. Goodin DS, Rowley HA, Olney RK. Magnetic resonance imaging in amyotrophic lateral sclerosis. *Ann Neurol.* (1988) 23:418–20. doi: 10.1002/ana.410230424
23. Bede P, Hardiman O. Lessons of ALS imaging: pitfalls and future directions - a critical review. *Neuroimage Clin.* (2014) 4:436–43. doi: 10.1016/j.nicl.2014.02.011
24. Verstraete E, van den Heuvel MP, Veldink JH, Blanken N, Mandl RC, Hulshoff Pol HE, et al. Motor network degeneration in amyotrophic lateral sclerosis: a structural and functional connectivity study. *PLoS ONE.* (2010) 5:e13664. doi: 10.1371/journal.pone.0013664
25. Bede P, Omer T, Finegan E, Chipika RH, Iyer PM, Doherty MA, et al. Connectivity-based characterisation of subcortical grey matter pathology in frontotemporal dementia and ALS: a multimodal neuroimaging study. *Brain Imaging Behav.* (2018) 12:1696–707. doi: 10.1007/s11682-018-9837-9
26. Turner MR, Hammers A, Al-Chalabi A, Shaw CE, Andersen PM, Brooks DJ, et al. Distinct cerebral lesions in sporadic and 'D90A' SOD1 ALS: studies with [11C]flumazenil PET. *Brain.* (2005) 128:1323–9. doi: 10.1093/brain/awh509
27. Bede P, Bokde ALW, Byrne S, Elamin M, McLaughlin RL, Kenna K, et al. Multiparametric MRI study of ALS stratified for the C9orf72 genotype. *Neurology.* (2013) 81:361–9. doi: 10.1093/med/9780199696277.003.0005
28. Lomen-Hoerth C. Clinical phenomenology and neuroimaging correlates in ALS-FTD. *J Mol Neurosci.* (2011) 45:656–62. doi: 10.1007/s12031-011-9636-x
29. Bede P, Bokde A, Elamin M, Byrne S, McLaughlin RL, Jordan N, et al. Grey matter correlates of clinical variables in amyotrophic lateral sclerosis (ALS): a neuroimaging study of ALS motor phenotype heterogeneity and cortical focality. *J Neurol Neurosurg Psychiatry.* (2013) 84:766–73. doi: 10.1136/jnnp-2012-302674
30. Feron M, Couillandre A, Mseddi E, Termoz N, Abidi M, Bardinet E, et al. Extrapyramidal deficits in ALS: a combined biomechanical and neuroimaging study. *J Neurol.* (2018) 265:2125–36. doi: 10.1007/s00415-018-8964-y
31. Carew JD, Nair G, Andersen PM, Wuu J, Gronka S, Hu X, et al. Presymptomatic spinal cord neurometabolic findings in SOD1-positive people at risk for familial ALS. *Neurology.* (2011) 77:1370–5. doi: 10.1212/WNL.0b013e318231526a
32. Schuster C, Elamin M, Hardiman O, Bede P. Presymptomatic and longitudinal neuroimaging in neurodegeneration–from snapshots to motion picture: a systematic review. *J Neurol Neurosurg Psychiatry.* (2015) 86:1089–96. doi: 10.1136/jnnp-2014-309888
33. Fradet L, Arnoux PJ, Ranjeva JP, Petit Y, Callot V. Morphometrics of the entire human spinal cord and spinal canal measured from *in vivo* high-resolution anatomical magnetic resonance imaging. *Spine.* (2014) 39:E262–9. doi: 10.1097/BRS.0000000000000125
34. Stroman PW, Wheeler-Kingshott C, Bacon M, Schwab JM, Bosma R, Brooks J, et al. The current state-of-the-art of spinal cord imaging: methods. *Neuroimage.* (2014) 84:1070–81. doi: 10.1016/j.neuroimage.2013.04.124
35. Zhao W, Cohen-Adad J, Polimeni JR, Keil B, Guerin B, Setsompop K, et al. Nineteen-channel receive array and four-channel transmit array coil for cervical spinal cord imaging at 7T. *Magn Reson Med.* (2014) 72:291–300. doi: 10.1002/mrm.24911
36. Cohen-Adad J, Zhao W, Keil B, Ratai EM, Triantafyllou C, Lawson R, et al. 7-T MRI of the spinal cord can detect lateral corticospinal tract abnormality in amyotrophic lateral sclerosis. *Muscle Nerve.* (2013) 47:760–2. doi: 10.1002/mus.23720
37. Atassi N, Xu M, Triantafyllou C, Keil B, Lawson R, Cernasov P, et al. Ultra high-field (7tesla) magnetic resonance spectroscopy in amyotrophic lateral sclerosis. *PLoS ONE.* (2017) 12:e0177680. doi: 10.1371/journal.pone.0177680
38. Massire A, Rasoanandrianina H, Taso M, Guye M, Ranjeva JP, Feiweier T, et al. Feasibility of single-shot multi-level multi-angle diffusion tensor imaging of the human cervical spinal cord at 7T. *Magn Reson Med.* (2018) 80:947–57. doi: 10.1002/mrm.27087
39. Taso M, Le Troter A, Sdika M, Ranjeva JP, Guye M, Bernard M, et al. Construction of an *in vivo* human spinal cord atlas based on high-resolution MR images at cervical and thoracic levels: preliminary results. *MAGMA.* (2014) 27:257–67. doi: 10.1007/s10334-013-0403-6
40. Kharbanda HS, Alsop DC, Anderson AW, Filardo G, Hackney DB. Effects of cord motion on diffusion imaging of the spinal cord. *Magn Reson Med.* (2006) 56:334–9. doi: 10.1002/mrm.20959
41. Clark CA, Werring DJ, Miller DH. Diffusion imaging of the spinal cord *in vivo*: estimation of the principal diffusivities and application to multiple sclerosis. *Magn Reson Med.* (2000) 43:133–8. doi: 10.1002/(SICI)1522-2594(200001)43:1<133::AID-MRM16>3.0.CO;2-X
42. Verma T, Cohen-Adad J. Effect of respiration on the B0 field in the human spinal cord at 3T. *Magn Reson Med.* (2014) 72:1629–36. doi: 10.1002/mrm.25075
43. Vannesjo SJ, Miller KL, Clare S, Tracey I. Spatiotemporal characterization of breathing-induced B0 field fluctuations in the cervical spinal cord at 7T. *Neuroimage.* (2018) 167:191–202. doi: 10.1016/j.neuroimage.2017.11.031

44. Figley CR, Stroman PW. Investigation of human cervical and upper thoracic spinal cord motion: implications for imaging spinal cord structure and function. *Magn Reson Med.* (2007) 58:185–9. doi: 10.1002/mrm.21260
45. Mikulis DJ, Wood ML, Zerdoner OA, Poncelet BP. Oscillatory motion of the normal cervical spinal cord. *Radiology.* (1994) 192:117–21. doi: 10.1148/radiology.192.1.8208922
46. Yiannakas MC, Kearney H, Samson RS, Chard DT, Ciccarelli O, Miller DH, et al. Feasibility of grey matter and white matter segmentation of the upper cervical cord *in vivo*: a pilot study with application to magnetisation transfer measurements. *Neuroimage.* (2012) 63:1054–9. doi: 10.1016/j.neuroimage.2012.07.048
47. Cohen-Adad J, El Mendili MM, Lehericy S, Pradat PF, Blancho S, Rossignol S, et al. Demyelination and degeneration in the injured human spinal cord detected with diffusion and magnetization transfer MRI. *Neuroimage.* (2011) 55:1024–33. doi: 10.1016/j.neuroimage.2010.11.089
48. Jaermann T, Crelier G, Pruessmann KP, Golay X, Netsch T, van Muiswinkel AM, et al. SENSE-DTI at 3 T. *Magn Reson Med.* (2004) 51:230–6. doi: 10.1002/mrm.10707
49. Glockner JF, Hu HH, Stanley DW, Angelos L, King K. Parallel MR imaging: a user's guide. *Radiographics.* (2005) 25:1279–97. doi: 10.1148/rg.255045202
50. Noebauer-Huhmann IM, Glaser C, Dietrich O, Wallner CP, Klinger W, Imhof H, et al. MR imaging of the cervical spine: assessment of image quality with parallel imaging compared to non-accelerated MR measurements. *Eur Radiol.* (2007) 17:1147–55. doi: 10.1007/s00330-006-0411-2
51. Fruehwald-Pallamar J, Szomolanyi P, Fakhrai N, Lunzer A, Weber M, Thurnher MM, et al. Parallel imaging of the cervical spine at 3T: optimized trade-off between speed and image quality. *AJNR Am J Neuroradiol.* (2012) 33:1867–74. doi: 10.3174/ajnr.A3101
52. Samson RS, Levy S, Schneider T, Smith AK, Smith SA, Cohen-Adad J, et al. ZOOM or Non-ZOOM? assessing spinal cord diffusion tensor imaging protocols for multi-centre studies. *PLoS ONE.* (2016) 11:e0155557. doi: 10.1371/journal.pone.0155557
53. Yokohama T, Iwasaki M, Oura D, Furuya S, Okuaki T. The reliability of reduced field-of-view DTI for highly accurate quantitative assessment of cervical spinal cord tracts. *Magn Reson Med Sci.* (2018) 18:36–43. doi: 10.2463/mrms.mp.2017-0078
54. Mohammadi S, Freund P, Feiweier T, Curt A, Weiskopf N. The impact of post-processing on spinal cord diffusion tensor imaging. *Neuroimage.* (2013) 70:377–85. doi: 10.1016/j.neuroimage.2012.12.058
55. Vahdat S, Lungu O, Cohen-Adad J, Marchand-Pauvert V, Benali H, Doyon J. Simultaneous brain-cervical cord fMRI reveals intrinsic spinal cord plasticity during motor sequence learning. *PLoS Biol.* (2015) 13:e1002186. doi: 10.1371/journal.pbio.1002186
56. Andre JB, Bammer R. Advanced diffusion-weighted magnetic resonance imaging techniques of the human spinal cord. *Top Magn Reson Imaging.* (2010) 21:367–78. doi: 10.1097/RMR.0b013e31823e65a1
57. Romeo F, Hoult DI. Magnet field profiling: analysis and correcting coil design. *Magn Reson Med.* (1984) 1:44–65. doi: 10.1002/mrm.1910010107
58. Rasoanandrianina H, Grapperon AM, Taso M, Girard OM, Duhamel G, Guye M, et al. Region-specific impairment of the cervical spinal cord (SC) in amyotrophic lateral sclerosis: a preliminary study using SC templates and quantitative MRI (diffusion tensor imaging/inhomogeneous magnetization transfer). *NMR Biomed.* (2017) 30:e3801. doi: 10.1002/nbm.3801
59. Zeng H, Constable RT. Image distortion correction in EPI: comparison of field mapping with point spread function mapping. *Magn Reson Med.* (2002) 48:137–46. doi: 10.1002/mrm.10200
60. Samson RS, Ciccarelli O, Kachramanoglou C, Brightman L, Lutti A, Thomas DL, et al. Tissue- and column-specific measurements from multi-parameter mapping of the human cervical spinal cord at 3 T. *NMR Biomed.* (2013) 26:1823–30. doi: 10.1002/nbm.3022
61. Papinutto N, Bakshi R, Bischof A, Calabresi PA, Caverzasi E, Constable RT, et al. Gradient nonlinearity effects on upper cervical spinal cord area measurement from 3D T1 -weighted brain MRI acquisitions. *Magn Reson Med.* (2018) 79:1595–601. doi: 10.1002/mrm.26776
62. Bede P, Bokde AL, Byrne SC, Elamin M, Walsh RJ, Hardiman O. Waterskier's Hirayama syndrome. *J Neurol.* (2011) 258:2078–9. doi: 10.1007/s00415-011-6046-5
63. Belsh JM, Schiffman PL. The Amyotrophic Lateral Sclerosis (ALS) patient perspective on misdiagnosis and its repercussions. *J Neurol Sci.* (1996) 139:110–6. doi: 10.1016/0022-510X(96)00088-3
64. Traynor BJ, Codd MB, Corr B, Forde C, Frost E, Hardiman O. amyotrophic lateral sclerosis mimic syndromes: a population-based study. *Arch Neurol.* (2000) 57:109–13. doi: 10.1001/archneur.57.1.109
65. Rocha AJ, Maia Junior AC. Is magnetic resonance imaging a plausible biomarker for upper motor neuron degeneration in amyotrophic lateral sclerosis/primary lateral sclerosis or merely a useful paraclinical tool to exclude mimic syndromes? a critical review of imaging applicability in clinical routine. *Arq Neuropsiquiatr.* (2012) 70:532–9. doi: 10.1590/S0004-282X2012000700012
66. Lebouteux MV, Franques J, Guillevin R, Delmont E, Lenglet T, Bede P, et al. Revisiting the spectrum of lower motor neuron diseases with snake eyes appearance on magnetic resonance imaging. *Eur J Neurol.* (2014) 21:1233–41. doi: 10.1111/ene.12465
67. Turner MR, Talbot K. Mimics and chameleons in motor neurone disease. *Pract Neurol.* (2013) 13:153–64. doi: 10.1136/practneurol-2013-000557
68. Taso M, Girard OM, Duhamel G, Le Troter A, Feiweier T, Guye M, et al. Tract-specific and age-related variations of the spinal cord microstructure: a multi-parametric MRI study using diffusion tensor imaging (DTI) and inhomogeneous magnetization transfer (ihMT). *NMR Biomed.* (2016) 29:817–32. doi: 10.1002/nbm.3530
69. Cohen-Adad J, El Mendili MM, Morizot-Koutlidis R, Lehericy S, Meininger V, Blancho S, et al. Involvement of spinal sensory pathway in ALS and specificity of cord atrophy to lower motor neuron degeneration. *Amyotroph Lateral Scler Frontotemporal Degener.* (2013) 14:30–8. doi: 10.3109/17482968.2012.701308
70. Branco LM, De Albuquerque M, De Andrade HM, Bergo FP, Nucci A, Franca MC Jr. Spinal cord atrophy correlates with disease duration and severity in amyotrophic lateral sclerosis. *Amyotroph Lateral Scler Frontotemporal Degener.* (2014) 15:93–7. doi: 10.3109/21678421.2013.852589
71. El Mendili MM, Chen R, Tiret B, Villard N, Trunet S, Pelegrini-Issac M, et al. Fast and accurate semi-automated segmentation method of spinal cord MR images at 3T applied to the construction of a cervical spinal cord template. *PLoS ONE.* (2015) 10:e0122224. doi: 10.1371/journal.pone.0122224
72. Paquin ME, El Mendili MM, Gros C, Dupont SM, Cohen-Adad J, Pradat PF. Spinal cord gray matter atrophy in amyotrophic lateral sclerosis. *AJNR Am J Neuroradiol.* (2018) 39:184–92. doi: 10.3174/ajnr.A5427
73. El Mendili MM, Cohen-Adad J, Pelegrini-Issac M, Rossignol S, Morizot-Koutlidis R, Marchand-Pauvert V, et al. Multi-parametric spinal cord MRI as potential progression marker in amyotrophic lateral sclerosis. *PLoS ONE.* (2014) 9:e95516. doi: 10.1371/journal.pone.0095516
74. El Mendili MM, Lenglet T, Stojkovic T, Behin A, Guimaraes-Costa R, Salachas F, et al. Cervical spinal cord atrophy profile in adult SMN1-linked SMA. *PLoS ONE.* (2016) 11:e0152439. doi: 10.1371/journal.pone.0152439
75. Lundell H, Barthelemy D, Skimminge A, Dyrby TB, Biering-Sorensen F, Nielsen JB. Independent spinal cord atrophy measures correlate to motor and sensory deficits in individuals with spinal cord injury. *Spinal Cord.* (2011) 49:70–5. doi: 10.1038/sc.2010.87
76. Querin G, El Mendili MM, Bede P, Delphine S, Lenglet T, Marchand-Pauvert V, et al. Multimodal spinal cord MRI offers accurate diagnostic classification in ALS. *J Neurol Neurosurg Psychiatry.* (2018) 89:1220–1221. doi: 10.1136/jnnp-2017-317214
77. De Leener B, Levy S, Dupont SM, Fonov VS, Stikov N, Louis Collins D, et al. SCT: Spinal Cord Toolbox, an open-source software for processing spinal cord MRI data. *Neuroimage.* (2017) 145:24–43. doi: 10.1016/j.neuroimage.2016.10.009
78. Taso M, Le Troter A, Sdika M, Cohen-Adad J, Arnoux PJ, Guye M, et al. A reliable spatially normalized template of the human spinal cord–Applications to automated white matter/gray matter segmentation and tensor-based morphometry (TBM) mapping of gray matter alterations occurring with age. *Neuroimage.* (2015) 117:20–8. doi: 10.1016/j.neuroimage.2015.05.034
79. Querin G, El Mendili MM, Lenglet T, Delphine S, Marchand-Pauvert V, Benali H, et al. Spinal cord multi-parametric magnetic resonance imaging

for survival prediction in amyotrophic lateral sclerosis. *Eur J Neurol.* (2017) 24:1040–6. doi: 10.1111/ene.13329

80. Valsasina P, Agosta F, Benedetti B, Caputo D, Perini M, Salvi F, et al. Diffusion anisotropy of the cervical cord is strictly associated with disability in amyotrophic lateral sclerosis. *J Neurol Neurosurg Psychiatry.* (2007) 78:480–4. doi: 10.1136/jnnp.2006.100032
81. Agosta F, Rocca MA, Valsasina P, Sala S, Caputo D, Perini M, et al. A longitudinal diffusion tensor MRI study of the cervical cord and brain in amyotrophic lateral sclerosis patients. *J Neurol Neurosurg Psychiatry.* (2009) 80:53–5. doi: 10.1136/jnnp.2008.154252
82. Nair G, Carew JD, Usher S, Lu D, Hu XP, Benatar M. Diffusion tensor imaging reveals regional differences in the cervical spinal cord in amyotrophic lateral sclerosis. *Neuroimage.* (2010) 53:576–83. doi: 10.1016/j.neuroimage.2010.06.060
83. Carew JD, Nair G, Pineda-Alonso N, Usher S, Hu X, Benatar M. Magnetic resonance spectroscopy of the cervical cord in amyotrophic lateral sclerosis. *Amyotroph Lateral Scler.* (2011) 12:185–91. doi: 10.3109/17482968.2010.515223
84. Ikeda K, Murata K, Kawase Y, Kawabe K, Kano O, Yoshii Y, et al. Relationship between cervical cord 1H-magnetic resonance spectroscopy and clinoco-electromyographic profile in amyotrophic lateral sclerosis. *Muscle Nerve.* (2013) 47:61–7. doi: 10.1002/mus.23467
85. Wang Y, Liu L, Ma L, Huang X, Lou X, Wang Y, et al. Preliminary study on cervical spinal cord in patients with amyotrophic lateral sclerosis using MR diffusion tensor imaging. *Acad Radiol.* (2014) 21:590–6. doi: 10.1016/j.acra.2014.01.014
86. Iglesias C, Sangari S, El Mendili MM, Benali H, Marchand-Pauvert V, Pradat PF. Electrophysiological and spinal imaging evidences for sensory dysfunction in amyotrophic lateral sclerosis. *BMJ Open.* (2015) 5:e007659. doi: 10.1136/bmjopen-2015-007659
87. de Albuquerque M, Branco LM, Rezende TJ, de Andrade HM, Nucci A, Franca MC, Jr. Longitudinal evaluation of cerebral and spinal cord damage in amyotrophic lateral sclerosis. *Neuroimage Clin.* (2017) 14:269–76. doi: 10.1016/j.nicl.2017.01.024
88. Piaggio N, Pardini M, Roccatagliata L, Scialo C, Cabona C, Bonzano L, et al. Cord cross-sectional area at foramen magnum as a correlate of disability in amyotrophic lateral sclerosis. *Eur Radiol Exp.* (2018) 2:13. doi: 10.1186/s41747-018-0045-6
89. Grolez G, Kyheng M, Lopes R, Moreau C, Timmerman K, Auger F, et al. MRI of the cervical spinal cord predicts respiratory dysfunction in ALS. *Sci Rep.* (2018) 8:1828. doi: 10.1038/s41598-018-19938-2
90. Cohen Y, Anaby D, Morozov D. Diffusion MRI of the spinal cord: from structural studies to pathology. *NMR Biomed.* (2017) 30:e3592. doi: 10.1002/nbm.3592
91. Novikov DS, Fieremans E, Jespersen SN, Kiselev VG. Quantifying brain microstructure with diffusion MRI: theory and parameter estimation. *NMR Biomed.* 2018:e3998. doi: 10.1002/nbm.3998
92. Tuch DS, Reese TG, Wiegell MR, Makris N, Belliveau JW, Wedeen VJ. High angular resolution diffusion imaging reveals intravoxel white matter fiber heterogeneity. *Magn Reson Med.* (2002) 48:577–82. doi: 10.1002/mrm.10268
93. Tuch DS, Reese TG, Wiegell MR, Wedeen VJ. Diffusion MRI of complex neural architecture. *Neuron.* (2003) 40:885–95. doi: 10.1016/S0896-6273(03)00758-X
94. Jensen JH, Helpern JA, Ramani A, Lu H, Kaczynski K. Diffusional kurtosis imaging: the quantification of non-gaussian water diffusion by means of magnetic resonance imaging. *Magn Reson Med.* (2005) 53:1432–40. doi: 10.1002/mrm.20508
95. Wang Y, Wang Q, Haldar JP, Yeh FC, Xie M, Sun P, et al. Quantification of increased cellularity during inflammatory demyelination. *Brain.* (2011) 134:3590–601. doi: 10.1093/brain/awr307
96. Cohen-Adad J, Descoteaux M, Rossignol S, Hoge RD, Deriche R, Benali H. Detection of multiple pathways in the spinal cord using q-ball imaging. *Neuroimage.* (2008) 42:739–49. doi: 10.1016/j.neuroimage.2008.04.243
97. Trojsi F, Caiazzo G, Di Nardo F, Fratello M, Santangelo G, Siciliano M, et al. High angular resolution diffusion imaging abnormalities in the early stages of amyotrophic lateral sclerosis. *J Neurol Sci.* (2017) 380:215–22. doi: 10.1016/j.jns.2017.07.039
98. Zhang H, Schneider T, Wheeler-Kingshott CA, Alexander DC. NODDI: practical *in vivo* neurite orientation dispersion and density imaging of the human brain. *Neuroimage.* (2012) 61:1000–16. doi: 10.1016/j.neuroimage.2012.03.072
99. Barritt AW, Gabel MC, Cercignani M, Leigh PN. Emerging magnetic resonance imaging techniques and analysis methods in amyotrophic lateral sclerosis. *Front Neurol.* (2018) 9:1065. doi: 10.3389/fneur.2018.01065
100. Broad RJ, Gabel MC, Dowell NG, Schwartzman DJ, Seth AK, Zhang H, et al. Neurite orientation and dispersion density imaging (NODDI) detects cortical and corticospinal tract degeneration in ALS. *J Neurol Neurosurg Psychiatry.* (2018) doi: 10.1136/jnnp-2018-318830. [Epub ahead of print].
101. Wen J, Zhang H, Alexander DC, Durrleman S, Routier A, Rinaldi D, et al. Neurite density is reduced in the presymptomatic phase of C9orf72 disease. *J Neurol Neurosurg Psychiatry.* (2018). doi: 10.1136/jnnp-2018-318994. [Epub ahead of print].
102. By S, Xu J, Box BA, Bagnato FR, Smith SA. Application and evaluation of NODDI in the cervical spinal cord of multiple sclerosis patients. *Neuroimage Clin.* (2017) 15:333–42. doi: 10.1016/j.nicl.2017.05.010
103. Budde MD, Xie M, Cross AH, Song SK. Axial diffusivity is the primary correlate of axonal injury in the experimental autoimmune encephalomyelitis spinal cord: a quantitative pixelwise analysis. *J Neurosci.* (2009) 29:2805–13. doi: 10.1523/JNEUROSCI.4605-08.2009
104. Sun SW, Liang HF, Trinkaus K, Cross AH, Armstrong RC, Song SK. Noninvasive detection of cuprizone induced axonal damage and demyelination in the mouse corpus callosum. *Magn Reson Med.* (2006) 55:302–8. doi: 10.1002/mrm.20774
105. Song SK, Sun SW, Ramsbottom MJ, Chang C, Russell J, Cross AH. Dysmyelination revealed through MRI as increased radial (but unchanged axial) diffusion of water. *Neuroimage.* (2002) 17:1429–36. doi: 10.1006/nimg.2002.1267
106. Song SK, Yoshino J, Le TQ, Lin SJ, Sun SW, Cross AH, et al. Demyelination increases radial diffusivity in corpus callosum of mouse brain. *Neuroimage.* (2005) 26:132–40. doi: 10.1016/j.neuroimage.2005.01.028
107. Bede P, Elamin M, Byrne S, McLaughlin RL, Kenna K, Vajda A, et al. Patterns of cerebral and cerebellar white matter degeneration in ALS. *J Neurol Neurosurg Psychiatry.* (2015) 86:468–70. doi: 10.1136/jnnp-2014-308172
108. Sled JG. Modelling and interpretation of magnetization transfer imaging in the brain. *Neuroimage.* (2018) 182:128–35. doi: 10.1016/j.neuroimage.2017.11.065
109. Schmierer K, Scaravilli F, Altmann DR, Barker GJ, Miller DH. Magnetization transfer ratio and myelin in postmortem multiple sclerosis brain. *Ann Neurol.* (2004) 56:407–15. doi: 10.1002/ana.20202
110. Schmierer K, Tozer DJ, Scaravilli F, Altmann DR, Barker GJ, Tofts PS, et al. Quantitative magnetization transfer imaging in postmortem multiple sclerosis brain. *J Magn Reson Imaging.* (2007) 26:41–51. doi: 10.1002/jmri.20984
111. Mottershead JP, Schmierer K, Clemence M, Thornton JS, Scaravilli F, Barker GJ, et al. High field MRI correlates of myelin content and axonal density in multiple sclerosis–a post-mortem study of the spinal cord. *J Neurol.* (2003) 250:1293–301. doi: 10.1007/s00415-003-0192-3
112. Borsodi F, Culea V, Langkammer C, Khalil M, Pirpamer L, Quasthoff S, et al. Multimodal assessment of white matter tracts in amyotrophic lateral sclerosis. *PLoS ONE.* (2017) 12:e0178371. doi: 10.1371/journal.pone.0178371
113. Carrara G, Carapelli C, Venturi F, Ferraris MM, Lequio L, Chio A, et al. A distinct MR imaging phenotype in amyotrophic lateral sclerosis: correlation between T1 magnetization transfer contrast hyperintensity along the corticospinal tract and diffusion tensor imaging analysis. *AJNR Am J Neuroradiol.* (2012) 33:733–9. doi: 10.3174/ajnr.A2855
114. Tanabe JL, Vermathen M, Miller R, Gelinas D, Weiner MW, Rooney WD. Reduced MTR in the corticospinal tract and normal T2 in amyotrophic lateral sclerosis. *Magn Reson Imaging.* (1998) 16:1163–9. doi: 10.1016/S0730-725X(98)00129-5
115. Kato Y, Matsumura K, Kinosada Y, Narita Y, Kuzuhara S, Nakagawa T. Detection of pyramidal tract lesions in amyotrophic lateral sclerosis with magnetization-transfer measurements. *AJNR Am J Neuroradiol.* (1997) 18:1541–7.
116. Girard OM, Callot V, Prevost VH, Robert B, Taso M, Ribeiro G, et al. Magnetization transfer from inhomogeneously broadened lines (ihMT):

improved imaging strategy for spinal cord applications. *Magn Reson Med.* (2017) 77:581–91. doi: 10.1002/mrm.26134

117. Varma G, Girard OM, Prevost VH, Grant AK, Duhamel G, Alsop DC. Interpretation of magnetization transfer from inhomogeneously broadened lines (ihMT) in tissues as a dipolar order effect within motion restricted molecules. *J Magn Reson.* (2015) 260:67–76. doi: 10.1016/j.jmr.2015.08.024
118. Van Obberghen E, McHinda S, le Troter A, Prevost VH, Viout P, Guye M, et al. Evaluation of the sensitivity of Inhomogeneous Magnetization Transfer (ihMT) MRI for multiple sclerosis. *AJNR Am J Neuroradiol.* (2018) 39:634–41. doi: 10.3174/ajnr.A5563
119. Pioro EP, Antel JP, Cashman NR, Arnold DL. Detection of cortical neuron loss in motor neuron disease by proton magnetic resonance spectroscopic imaging *in vivo*. *Neurology.* (1994) 44:1933–8. doi: 10.1212/WNL.44.10.1933
120. Kalra S, Cashman NR, Genge A, Arnold DL. Recovery of N-acetylaspartate in corticomotor neurons of patients with ALS after riluzole therapy. *Neuroreport.* (1998) 9:1757–61. doi: 10.1097/00001756-199806010-00016
121. Kalra S, Tai P, Genge A, Arnold DL. Rapid improvement in cortical neuronal integrity in amyotrophic lateral sclerosis detected by proton magnetic resonance spectroscopic imaging. *J Neurol.* (2006) 253:1060–3. doi: 10.1007/s00415-006-0162-7
122. Pioro EP, Majors AW, Mitsumoto H, Nelson DR, Ng TC. 1H-MRS evidence of neurodegeneration and excess glutamate + glutamine in ALS medulla. *Neurology.* (1999) 53:71–9. doi: 10.1212/WNL.53.1.71
123. Rule RR, Suhy J, Schuff N, Gelinas DF, Miller RG, Weiner MW. Reduced NAA in motor and non-motor brain regions in amyotrophic lateral sclerosis: a cross-sectional and longitudinal study. *Amyotroph Lateral Scler Other Motor Neuron Disord.* (2004) 5:141–9. doi: 10.1080/14660820410017109
124. Verma G, Woo JH, Chawla S, Wang S, Sheriff S, Elman LB, et al. Whole-brain analysis of amyotrophic lateral sclerosis by using echo-planar spectroscopic imaging. *Radiology.* (2013) 267:851–7. doi: 10.1148/radiol.13121148
125. Hock A, Henning A, Boesiger P, Kollias SS. (1)H-MR spectroscopy in the human spinal cord. *AJNR Am J Neuroradiol.* (2013) 34:1682–9. doi: 10.3174/ajnr.A3342
126. Marliani AF, Clementi V, Albini Riccioli L, Agati R, Carpenzano M, Salvi F, et al. Quantitative cervical spinal cord 3T proton MR spectroscopy in multiple sclerosis. *AJNR Am J Neuroradiol.* (2010) 31:180–4. doi: 10.3174/ajnr.A1738
127. Wyss PO, Hock A, Kollias S. The application of human spinal cord magnetic resonance spectroscopy to clinical studies: a review. *Semin Ultrasound CT MR.* (2017) 38:153–62. doi: 10.1053/j.sult.2016.07.005
128. Proudfoot M, Bede P, Turner MR. Imaging cerebral activity in amyotrophic lateral sclerosis. *Front Neurol.* (2018) 9:1148. doi: 10.3389/fneur.2018.01148
129. Abrahams S, Goldstein LH, Simmons A, Brammer M, Williams SCR, Giampietro V, et al. Word retrieval in amyotrophic lateral sclerosis: a functional magnetic resonance imaging study. *Brain.* (2004) 127:1507–17. doi: 10.1093/brain/awh170
130. Agosta F, Valsasina P, Absinta M, Riva N, Sala S, Prelle A, et al. Sensorimotor functional connectivity changes in amyotrophic lateral sclerosis. *Cereb Cortex.* (2011) 21:2291–8. doi: 10.1093/cercor/bhr002
131. Kollewe K, Munte TF, Samii A, Dengler R, Petri S, Mohammadi B. Patterns of cortical activity differ in ALS patients with limb and/or bulbar involvement depending on motor tasks. *J Neurol.* (2011) 258:804–10. doi: 10.1007/s00415-010-5842-7
132. Kong Y, Eippert F, Beckmann CF, Andersson J, Finsterbusch J, Buchel C, et al. Intrinsically organized resting state networks in the human spinal cord. *Proc Natl Acad Sci USA.* (2014) 111:18067–72. doi: 10.1073/pnas.1414293111
133. Powers JM, Ioachim G, Stroman PW. Ten key insights into the use of spinal cord fMRI. *Brain Sci.* (2018) 8:E173. doi: 10.3390/brainsci8090173
134. Gil J, Funalot B, Verschueren A, Danel-Brunaud V, Camu W, Vandenberghe N, et al. Causes of death amongst French patients with amyotrophic lateral sclerosis: a prospective study. *Eur J Neurol.* (2008) 15:1245–51. doi: 10.1111/j.1468-1331.2008.02307.x
135. El Mendili MM. *Analysis of the Structural Integrity of the Spinal Cord in Motor Neuron Diseases Using a Multi-Parametric MRI Approach.* Doctoral dissertation, Université Pierre et Marie Curie-Paris VI (2016).
136. Muller HP, Turner MR, Grosskreutz J, Abrahams S, Bede P, Govind V, et al. A large-scale multicentre cerebral diffusion tensor imaging study in amyotrophic lateral sclerosis. *J Neurol Neurosurg Psychiatry.* (2016) 87:570–9. doi: 10.1136/jnnp-2015-311952

7

Functional Biomarkers for Amyotrophic Lateral Sclerosis

William Huynh [1,2], Thanuja Dharmadasa [1], Steve Vucic [3] and Matthew C. Kiernan [1,4]*

[1] Brain and Mind Centre, University of Sydney, Sydney, NSW, Australia, [2] Prince of Wales Clinical School, University of New South Wales, Sydney, NSW, Australia, [3] Western Clinical School, University of Sydney, Sydney, NSW, Australia, [4] Institute of Clinical Neurosciences, Royal Prince Alfred Hospital, Sydney, NSW, Australia

***Correspondence:**
William Huynh
william.huynh@sydney.edu.au

The clinical diagnosis of amyotrophic lateral sclerosis (ALS) relies on determination of progressive dysfunction of both cortical as well as spinal and bulbar motor neurons. However, the variable mix of upper and lower motor neuron signs result in the clinical heterogeneity of patients with ALS, resulting frequently in delay of diagnosis as well as difficulty in monitoring disease progression and treatment outcomes particularly in a clinical trial setting. As such, the present review provides an overview of recently developed novel non-invasive electrophysiological techniques that may serve as biomarkers to assess UMN and LMN dysfunction in ALS patients.

Keywords: amyotrophic lateral sclerosis, motor neuron disease, neurophysiological biomarkers, transcranial magnetic stimulation, cortical excitability

INTRODUCTION

Amyotrophic lateral sclerosis (ALS) is a rapidly progressive neurodegenerative disease that was first described in the 1869 by Jean-Martin Charcot (1–3) although earlier detailed clinicopathological descriptions of a case of ALS, was published by Radcliffe and Clarke (4). Charcot postulated the importance of the upper motor neuron in its pathogenesis (3) and its associated degeneration of motor cortical Betz cells that has become a well-recognized pathological feature (5, 6). The diagnosis of classical amyotrophic lateral sclerosis (ALS) relies on the clinical identification of progressive dysfunction in both the cortical ("upper", UMN) and spinal ("lower", LMN) motor neurons involving multiple body regions, much of which is encompassed within the El Escorial criteria (7, 8). The clinical heterogeneity of ALS is a result of the variable mix of UMN and LMN signs (9), hence contributing to delay in diagnosis and difficulty in monitoring disease progression as well as treatment outcomes particularly in a clinical trial setting (6). As such, there is a critical need to devise objective biomarkers of disease progression in ALS that may facilitate both improvement in diagnosis as well as to provide meaningful outcome measures to monitor treatment (10).

The present review will provide an overview of recently developed neurophysiological biomarkers, with emphases on novel non-invasive electrophysiological techniques used to assess UMN and LMN dysfunction in ALS patients.

Biomarkers of UMN Dysfunction

An important component in the diagnosis of ALS relies on clinical features of UMN involvement in the presence of progressive LMN weakness (11), but often these signs of UMN impairment may be underappreciated in a limb that is concurrently affected by LMN loss especially in early stages of ALS (6, 12, 13). Upper motor neuron signs may initially be absent in approximately 7–10% of ALS patients (6, 14). As such, objective UMN biomarkers may be critical for the diagnosis of ALS, as potential mimicking disorders such as multifocal motor neuropathy, Kennedy's disease and adult-onset spinal muscular atrophy (SMA), may present as pure LMN syndromes (6, 15, 16). Autopsy reports have also demonstrated UMN degeneration in 50–75% of patients with clinically pure LMN syndromes (5, 17, 18).

Transcranial Magnetic Stimulation

Since its original description more than 3 decades ago (19), Transcranial magnetic stimulation (TMS) has undergone significant evolution as a non-invasive technique for cortical stimulation, providing valuable insight into the functional integrity of brain pathways. Its main application has been in the investigation of complex neuronal networks of the primary motor cortex (M1), which is influenced by both inhibitory and excitatory mechanisms (20). Transcranial magnetic stimulation (TMS) biomarkers of cortical hyperexcitability appear to be useful biomakers of UMN dysfunction in ALS (21). In addition, TMS have provided insights into the underlying pathophysiological mechanisms in ALS, thereby allowing for the development of diagnostic and prognostic biomarkers in ALS (21).

The TMS technique utilizes a transient magnetic field to induce an electric current in the cortex (22). This magnetic field is generated through a stimulating coil held over a subject's head, which painlessly and non-invasively penetrates the skull without attenuation (**Figure 1**). Depending on stimulation intensity and coil type, the electromagnetic force can stimulate neurons at a depth of 1.5–3.0 cm beneath the scalp (23). There have been several theoretical models postulated to explain the exact effect of this electromagnetic field on biological tissue, with studies in both animals and humans conferring that TMS generates a corticomotoneuronal volley composed of direct (D) and indirect (I) waves occurs at intervals of 1.5–2.5 ms (24). Direct waves are thought to represent the activation of corticospinal axons and are only recruited at high intensities or with the TMS coil positioned such that induces currents in a lateral-medial direction. Indirect waves seem to be activated at lower intensities and are mediated by a more complex interaction between cortical excitatory and inhibitory neurons (25). TMS delivered over the primary motor cortex (M1) is thought to activate pyramidal neurons (Betz cells) trans-synaptically via I-waves (26), but the exact neural circuitries evoked remain to be determined. These complex neural circuits are critically dependent on both excitatory and inhibitory interneuronal systems, facilitated by cellular receptor and neurotransmitter interactions (27). Excitation is primarily mediated by glutamate/NMDA receptor interaction, while inhibition is facilitated by γ-aminobutyric acid (GABA)/$GABA_{A/B}$ receptor action (28).

Cortical hyperexcitability in ALS is heralded by reduced short-interval intracortical inhibition and CSP duration, in addition to increased intracortical facilitation and motor evoked potential amplitude (12, 29, 30). Furthermore, significant bilateral TMS abnormalities was observed in ALS patients at an early disease stage (31), consistent with previous studies that have reported functional abnormalities of the motor cortex as an early and specific feature of ALS, and preceding the onset of LMN dysfunction (6, 12, 29, 30, 32–34). More recent studies have demonstrated changes in TMS parameters indicative of cortical hyperexcitability, were more prominent over the dominant motor cortex and in particular, contralateral to the site of disease onset, suggesting a vulnerability of the dominant motor cortical neurons and supporting the importance of cortical processes in the pathophysiology of ALS as postulated first by Menon et al. (31).

Single-Pulse TMS

The resting motor threshold (RMT) is a reflection of the ease with which corticomotoneurons are excited, hence the corticomotoneuronal membrane excitability, as well as the density of UMN projections onto motor neurons (35). Through the α-amino-3-hydroxy-5-methyl-4-isoxazoleproprionic acid (AMPA) receptors, RMT is influenced by the glutamatergic neurotransmitter system, such that excessive glutamate activity reduces RMT, and is susceptible to modulation by sodium channel blockers (28, 36). In ALS, the RMT is reduced early in the disease (indicative of cortical hyperexcitability) followed by progressive increase and eventual inexcitability with disease progression (32, 37–39). As motor threshold is modulated by glutamate activity (28), the reduced motor threshold supports the notion that cortical hyperexcitability being an early feature of ALS contributing to the ensuing lower motor neuron degeneration (21). The motor cortex is found to be inexcitable in approximately 20% of ALS patients and appears to be a late finding. In contrast, motor cortex inexcitability is a relatively frequent fidning in patients exhibiting the pure UMN phenotype termed primary lateral sclerosis [PLS] (40).

The central motor conduction time (CMCT) time is defined by the time interval between stimulation of the motor cortex and arrival of the corticospinal volleys at the spinal motor neurons, and is inferred from the motor evoked potential (MEP) onset latency (21). Prolongation of CMCT is an invariable finding in ALS being documented in 16–100% across different series (5, 21, 37, 41–44). In patients without clinically predominant UMN phenotypes, prolongation of CMCTs occurs in 50–71% of patients (41, 44). Although the mechanisms underlying CMCT prolongation are presently not fully elucidated, an increase in desynchronization of corticomotoneuronal volleys resulting from degeneration of the fastest conducting corticomotoneuronal fibers has been suggested (45, 46). Large discrepancies in sensitivity of this parameter reported by previous studies are likely attributable to technique-dependent variations associated with CMCT calculations.

The cortical silent period (CSP) refers to the interruption of voluntary electromyography activity in a target muscle after motor cortex stimulation (47), and the mechanisms that underly the CSP are complex but thought to be mediated primarily by the activation of inhibitory neurons acting via GABA-B receptors within the cortex (21, 48). The CSP duration has been consistently reduced in patients across all ALS phenotypes (21, 30, 32, 34, 43, 49–51). The decrease in CSP duration in ALS patients likely represent a combination of degeneration of

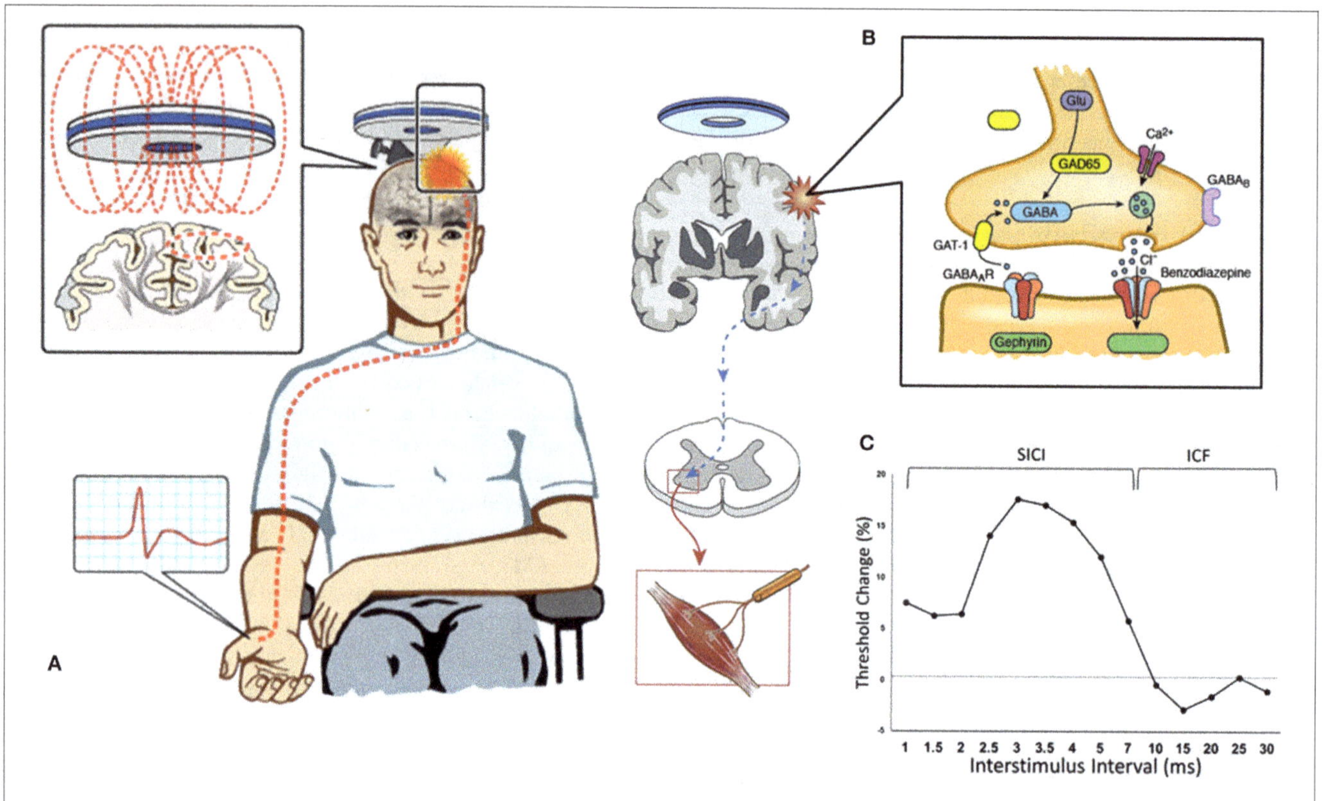

FIGURE 1 | Paired-pulse threshold tracking transcranial magnetic stimulation (TMS). **(A)** TMS coil placed over the vertex activates the primary motor cortex and the response (motor evoked potential, MEP) is recorded from the contralateral abductor pollicis brevis muscle. **(B)** TMS parameters are mediated by a complex interplay between intraneural circuits and cortical output cells, with cortical interneurons mediating inhibition by activation of GABAergic synapses leading to influx of chloride anions (Cl^-) and hyperpolarization of post-synaptic neurons. **(C)** Change in stimulus intensity required to achieve a target MEP of 0.2 mV (±20%) is used to quantify SICI (which is recorded with interstimulus intervals between 1–7 ms) and ICF (between 10–30 ms).

inhibitory interneurons as well as GABAB-mediated receptor inhibition dysfunction (21).

Paired-Pulse TMS

In the paired-pulse paradigm, a conditioning stimulus (CS) precedes and is utilized to modulate the effect of a second test stimulus (TS). By varying the time interval between the paired pulses (the interstimulus interval, ISI) a number of parameters can be determined, using either a constant stimulus method [in which the CS and TS are kept at a constant level and MEP amplitude is evaluated (52)] or the threshold-tracking (TT) TMS protocol (53). TT-TMS was developed to overcome the marked MEP amplitude variability seen when utilizing the earlier protocol and uses a fixed MEP response which is tracked by a varying TS (53, 54). By applying a subthreshold (set at 70% RMT) conditioning stimulus at predetermined time intervals prior to a suprathreshold test stimulus, the threshold-tracking TMS technique allows the short-interval intracortical inhibition (SICI) and intracortical facilitation (ICF) to be investigated (53, 55) (**Figure 1**).

Reduction or absence of SICI, which is a biomarker of cortical interneuronal inhibitory GABAergic function, has been established as an early feature of ALS (**Figures 2A,B**), correlating with biomarkers of peripheral neurodegeneration and at times preceding the onset of LMN dysfunction in sporadic ALS cohorts [(31, 53), etc]. Although there were no significant differences in the degree of reduction observed between the sides of the motor cortices, there was a trend for more changes observed over the dominant motor cortex, particularly contralateral to the side of disease onset (31). The changes were also similar regardless of the severity of LMN dysfunction, or site of onset (bulbar or limb) (12, 21, 32, 56).

The reduction in SICI has been a widely reported feature present in both familial and sporadic forms of ALS with the alterations observed as an early feature (21, 30, 34, 57–62). Further to this, longitudinal assessments of asymptomatic SOD-1 mutation carriers have identified cortical hyperexcitability developing prior to the clinical onset of ALS, therefore suggesting that cortical hyperexcitability underlies the process of neurodegeneration in familial ALS (34).

The use of threshold-tracking TMS may be able to uncover UMN involvement in ALS phenotypes without clinically evident UMN signs such as the flail limb variant of ALS or progressive muscular atrophy (PMA). Moreover, this technique was able to reliably distinguish between ALS and other neurological mimic conditions including multifocal motor neuropathy, spinal muscular atrophy, Kennedy's disease, peripheral nerve hyperexcitability disorders, Hirayama disease,

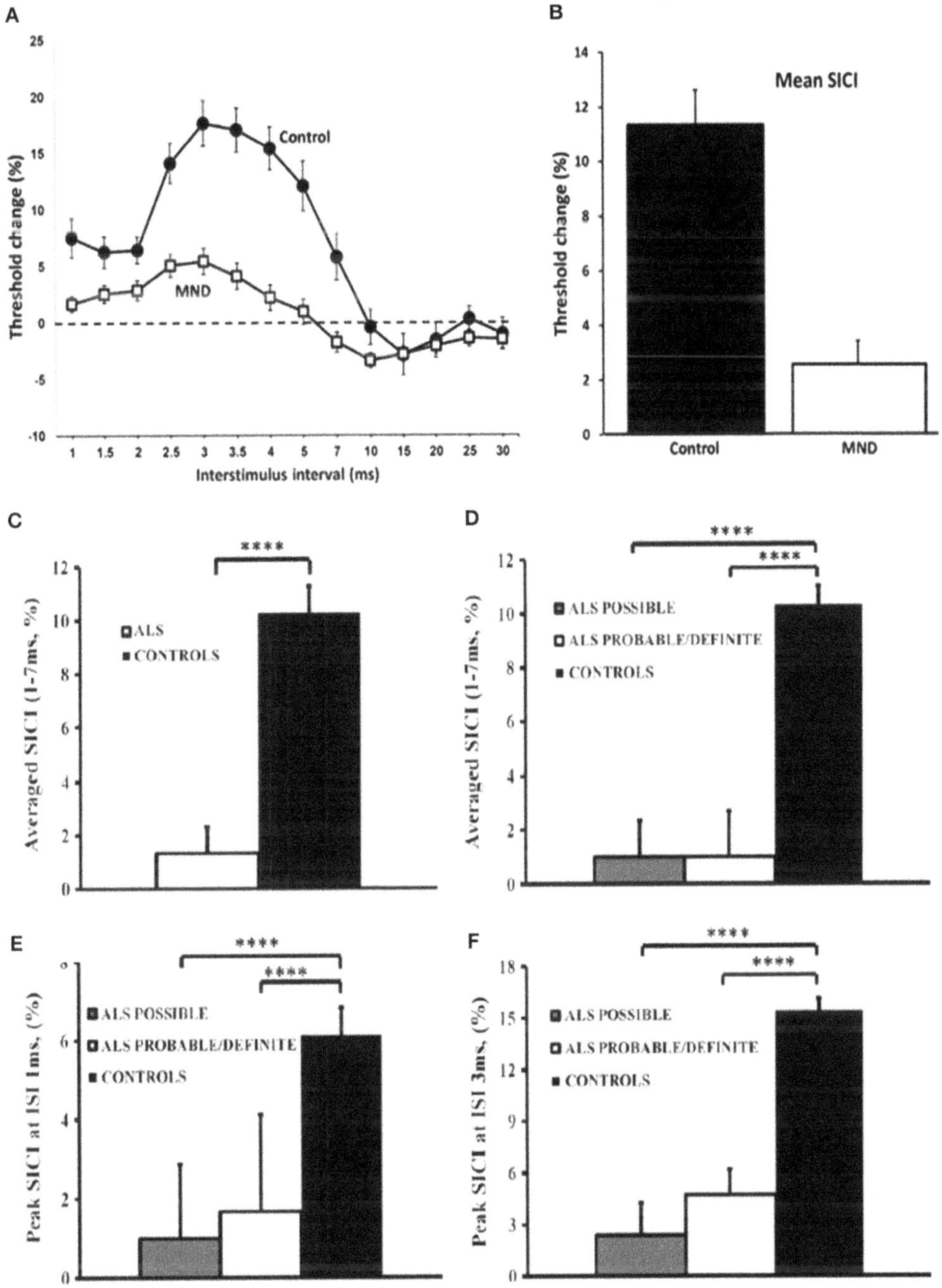

FIGURE 2 | Cortical excitability in motor neuron disease (MND). Paired-pulse subthreshold conditioning transcranial magnetic stimulation demonstrating **(A)** reduction in short-interval intracortical inhibition (SICI, above dotted line) and intracortical facilitation (ICF, below dotted line) and **(B)** significant reductions in averaged SICI (between interstimulus intervals of 1–7 ms) in MND patients compared with controls **(C)** Averaged short-interval intracortical inhibition (SICI), between interstimulus interval (ISI) 1–7 ms, was significantly reduced in amyotrophic lateral sclerosis (ALS). **(D)** The reduction of averaged SICI was comparable in Awaji subgroups. Peak SICI at ISI **(E)** 1 ms, and **(F)** 3 ms was significantly reduced in Awaji subgroups.

CIDP, lead neuropathy, hereditary spastic paraparesis, as well as hereditary motor neuropathy with pyramidal features (63–68).

SICI abnormalities using the threshold-tracking technique, appear to be the most robust diagnostic parameter that is indicative of UMN dysfunction in ALS patients (12, 29, 69). Using either an abnormal SICI or an inexcitable cortex, this TMS method demonstrated a sensitivity of approximately 73% and a specificity of 81% (69). Moreover, an absent SICI was associated with a 97% sensitivity (33). TMS abnormalities were observed in 77% of patients with ALS, with frequency of abnormalities that were similar across all Awaji diagnostic groups, using the established cut-off SICI of <5.5% (63) resulting in 88% of Awaji-criteria possible patients being reclassified as Awaji-criteria probable or definite (12). More specifically, an abnormally reduced SICI was demonstrated in 56% of Awaji-criteria possible patients (12) (**Figures 2C–F**).

More recent studies have also documented increasing cortical hyperexcitability with advancing disease indicating that intracortical inhibitory neurons become progressively dysfunctional in ALS (**Figure 3A**) (70). Reduced SICI was also reported to be an independent prognostic biomarker in ALS patients within the first 2 years of disease onset (71) (**Figure 3B**). Separately, SICI was shown to partially normalize with treatment by riluzole (72), an anti-glutamatergic agent exhibiting modest clinical effectiveness in ALS (73, 74). Paralleling the clinical efficacy Riluzole, the modulating effects last about 3 months (75), and may be related to overexpression of efflux pumps located at the blood brain barrier during the disease course (76). Regardless of the underlying mechanisms, studies of riluzole have suggested a utility of threshold-tracking TMS in assessing biological effectiveness of compounds at an early stage of drug development. Taken together, these results suggest that non-invasive *in vivo* monitoring of cortical function and particularly, SICI may also be an effective biomarker used to monitor the effects of novel therapeutics in a clinical trial setting.

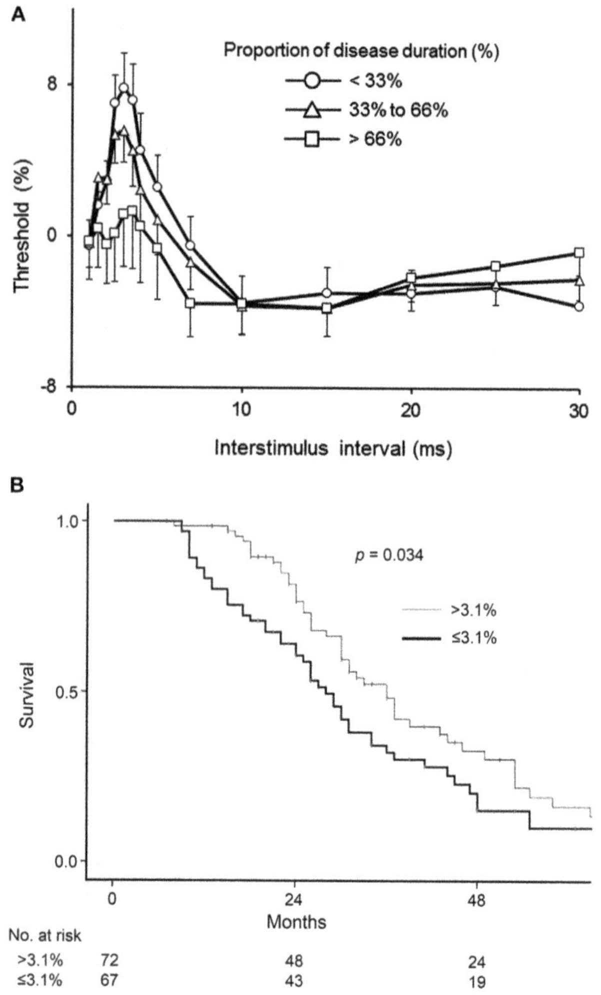

FIGURE 3 | (A) Cortical excitability changes with disease progression. Patients were divided into three groups according to disease stage. The duration of the illness from onset to death was normalized between zero and one and expressed as a percentage (%), with data averaged by proportion of disease duration. Early stage (Circle) was defined as the proportion of disease duration <33%, mid (Triangle) was 33–66%, and late (Square) was >66%. ALSFRS-R of patients in early stage was 42.3 ± 0.6, that in mid was 40.2 ± 0.7, and that in late was 34.8 ± 2.0. SICI at ISI 1–7 ms decreased with disease progression. Data are given as mean ± SE. Reproduced with permission license no. 4456860473754 (70). **(B)** Kaplan-Meier plots of survival probabilities according to averaged short-interval intracortical inhibition (SICI) values. Amyotrophic lateral sclerosis patients with a disease duration under 2 years were divided into 2 groups according to values in average SICI, interstimulus interval 1–7 ms. Patients with SICI ≤3.1% demonstrated reduced survival compared to patients with SICI >3.1% ($p = 0.034$). Estimated median survival was 28 months in patients with reduced SICI and 36 months in patients with higher SICI.

Biomarkers of LMN Dysfunction

Objective assessment of LMN dysfunction, utilizing neurophysiological techniques, appear to be more sensitive than clinical assessments (77, 78). Conventional neurophysiological techniques, such as nerve conduction studies which measure the compound muscle action potential (CMAP) amplitude, may be relatively insensitive in assessing LMN degeneration due to the process of reinnervation (79).

Estimation of Motor Unit Numbers

As such, various methods to approximate the number of motor units innervating individual muscles, including motor unit number estimation (MUNE), and motor unit number index (MUNIX), may potentially represent valuable biomarkers of LMN degeneration. Since the development of the first MUNE technique in 1971 (80), there have been numerous other MUNE techniques introduced (81–85). The basic principle of MUNE techniques is the dividing of the maximal CMAP amplitude by the average surface-recorded motor unit potential (86). The original MUNE technique utilized incremental stimulation whereby the stimulus intensity at one point on the nerve was gradually increased from subthreshold until 10 increments in the motor response was recorded, but this technique relied on the assumption that the smallest recorded potential using the surface electrode over a target muscle following minimal stimulation represented a single motor unit potential (**Figure 4A**). Consequently, the variance in the result MUNE was considerable and resulted not uncommonly in artificially lower MUNE counts (86, 88).

The motor unit index (MUNIX) technique is a method designed to express the number of functioning motor units within a muscle as an index, instead of providing a direct measure of their absolute numbers. It is based on patients performing a voluntary contraction at various intensity levels and surface interference patterns being captured and decomposed to obtain

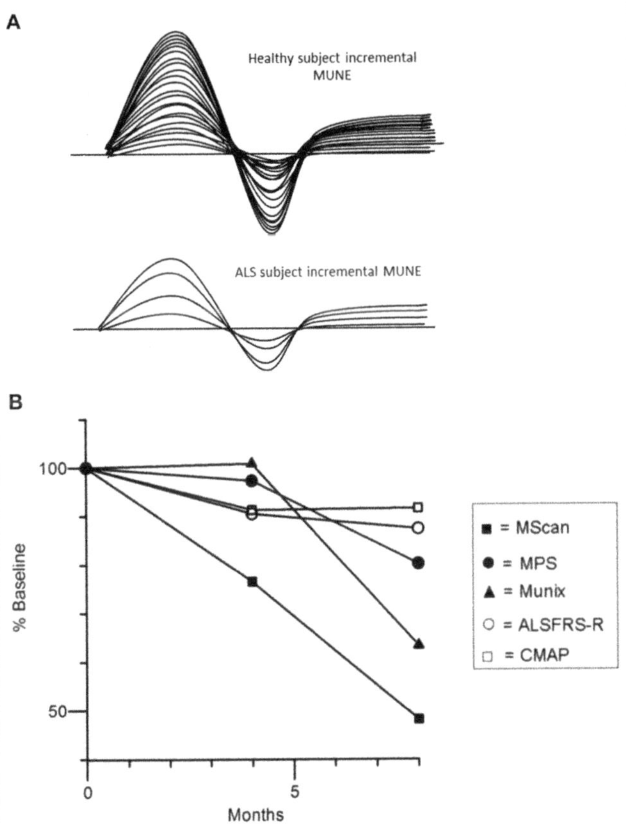

FIGURE 4 | (A) Incremental MUNE in healthy and ALS subjects, demonstrating a large number of "steps" with increasing stimulus intensity consistent with a large number of functioning motor units within measured muscle, whilst there were only four steps in the ALS subject indicating only four functional motor units remaining in muscle. **(B)** Percentage changes in MUNE values (geometric means) and mean ALSFRS-R and CMAP amplitude at 4 and 8 months.

a normalized motor unit size, which is then in turn divided into the maximal CMAP value to obtain the MUNIX (86, 89, 90).

Recent studies using different MUNE methods have demonstrated potential utility for assessing disease progression in ALS patients as reflected by a progressive linear decline in MUNE counts (87, 91–94). Interestingly, a recently developed MUNE technique, termed MScan, appeared to be the most sensitive MUNE method in detecting ALS disease progression (**Figure 4B**) (87). Additionally, MUNIX was able to detect disease progression in presymptomatic muscles in ALS (95, 96), and changes longitudinally in these muscle groups appeared more sensitive to those changes in the revised ALS Functional Rating Scale (ALSFRS-R) (93).

Neurophysiological Index

The neurophysiological index (NI) is a potential electrophysiological biomarker in assessing lower motor neuron loss in ALS (97). Using a simple formula, The NI has the advantage of using routine CMAP amplitude, F-wave frequency, and distal motor latency of the ulnar-nerve innervated abductor digit minimi (ADM) muscle and is more sensitive than the CMAP amplitude alone in demonstrating longitudinal lower motor neuron loss in ALS. NI was able to detect motor neuron loss in muscles of the presymptomatic limb in ALS patients as well as successfully tracking disease progression, demonstrating continued loss of functional motor units during this presymptomatic period, when weakness, atrophy, or fasciculations were not detectable to both patients and evaluating clinicians (78). The validation of NI as a clinically meaningful parameter in disease progression of ALS patients was also demonstrated longitudinally in the symptomatic muscles of patients that correlated with their ALSFRS-R decline (97, 98). Additionally, NI was able to detect deterioration that occurred over a short period of 4 weeks in ALS patients, hence enabling the utility of this index in a clinical trial setting (77). NI has favorable reproducibility and low intraindividual variability but amongst its limitations, the index is only restricted to the ADM muscle (which is less affected compared to other intrinsic hand muscles such as the APB and FDI, in keeping with the split hand pattern of wasting and weakness) (99) and requires persistent F-waves (that can be frequently absent in ALS) (78).

Split-Hand Index

The split-hand sign is documented as an early and specific clinical feature in patients with ALS that is not characteristic in other commonly encountered clinical mimics (99, 100). It refers to the preferential wasting and weakness of the thenar complex muscles (APB and FDI) with relative preservation of the hypothenar muscle, ADM (99), and appeared to have a cortical origin with the corticomotoneuronal input to the thenar complex in ALS patients preferentially affected (101, 102). This clinical observation provided an opportunity to develop a simple neurophysiological biomarker to aid the diagnosis of ALS using conventional nerve conduction studies. The split-hand index (SI) was derived by multiplying the CMAP amplitude of the APB muscle by the FDI CMAP amplitude and then dividing the product by the ADM CMAP amplitude. It was demonstrated that a reduction in the split-hand index was consistent across ALS phenotypes but appeared most pronounced in those with limb-onset, and that a cut-off value ≤ 5.2 reliably differentiated between ALS and other neurological disorders (103).

Electrical Impedance Myography

Electrical impedance myography (EIM) is a novel non-invasive form of testing to provide quantitative information on neuromuscular disorders that may be useful and reliable in assessing longitudinally the severity of a disease process (104–107). EIM utilizes a small, high-frequency electrical current applied across two electrodes positioned over a muscle, and the resulting surface voltages are measured between a second pair of electrodes, from which the resistive and capacitive properties of the tissue are obtained (86, 105). The advantage is that this technique does not rely on inherent electrical activity of the tissue (which conventional neurophysiological techniques do), but rather on how the tissue impacts the applied current, rendering the technique sensitive to structural and compositional changes in muscle such as denervation, reinnervation, myofiber atrophy and fat replacement within the muscle that occur in ALS (104). EIM values have been shown to correlate with standard clinical approaches including handheld dynamometry and MUNE (106, 107), and may be able to provide more than a five-fold reduction in sample size requirements for ALS clinical therapeutic trials over standard outcome measures such as the ALS functional rating scale-revised (ALSFRS-R) (108). Although EIM can detect changes early in the disease course of ALS as well as in clinically unaffected muscle groups (105), a limitation of EIM is that identified changes may not be able to differentiate ALS from other neuromuscular conditions (109, 110).

CONCLUSION

Amyotrophic lateral sclerosis remains a devastating neurodegenerative disorder with a poor prognosis, much of which is attributable to frequent delays in diagnosis, an incomplete understanding of the underlying pathophysiological mechanisms, and the current lack of effective disease-modifying treatment available. As such, there is a critical need to devise accurate and reliable biomarkers to address the above shortfalls in current ALS management. The current review has presented recent developments in novel neurophysiological biomarkers that are able to effectively interrogate upper and lower motor neuron dysfunction and characterize their change over time with disease progression, thereby exhibiting the potential to improve diagnosis, as well as facilitating in the prognosis and monitoring of the effects of future therapeutic agents in a clinical trial setting.

AUTHOR CONTRIBUTIONS

WH drafted manuscript and made all necessary edits and revisions as well as obtained required copyright permissions for figures. TD, SV, and MK revised and edited manuscript.

FUNDING

This work was supported by funding to ForeFront, a collaborative research group dedicated to the study of frontotemporal dementia and motor neuron disease, from the National Health and Medical Research Council (NHMRC) (1132524, 1095127, 1060992). WH was supported by the Beryl Bayley Fellowship of Motor Neuron Disease Research Institute of Australia. MK is a NHMRC Practitioner Fellow (#1156093).

REFERENCES

1. Simon NG, Huynh W, Vucic S, Talbot K, Kiernan MC. Motor neuron disease: current management and future prospects. *Intern Med J.* (2015) 45:1005–13. doi: 10.1111/imj.12874
2. Cleveland DW, Rothstein JD. From Charcot to Lou Gehrig: deciphering selective motor neuron death in ALS. *Nat Rev Neurosci.* (2001) 2:806–19. doi: 10.1038/35097565
3. Charcot J, Joffroy A. Deus cas d'atrophie musculaire progressive avec lesions de la substance grise et des faisceaux antéro-latérale. *Arch Physiol.* (1869) 2:354–67.
4. Radcliffe CB, Clarke JL. An important case of paralysis and muscular atrophy, with disease of the nervous centres. *Br Foreign Med Chir Rev.* (1862) 30:215–25.
5. Kaufmann P, Pullman SL, Shungu DC, Chan S, Hays AP, Del Bene ML, et al. Objective tests for upper motor neuron involvement in amyotrophic lateral sclerosis (ALS). *Neurology* (2004) 62:1753–7. doi: 10.1212/01.WNL.0000125182.17874.59
6. Huynh W, Simon NG, Grosskreutz J, Turner MR, Vucic S, Kiernan MC. Assessment of the upper motor neuron in amyotrophic lateral sclerosis. *Clin Neurophysiol.* (2016) 127:2643–60. doi: 10.1016/j.clinph.2016.04.025
7. Brooks BR. El Escorial World Federation of Neurology criteria for the diagnosis of amyotrophic lateral sclerosis. Subcommittee on Motor Neuron Diseases/Amyotrophic Lateral Sclerosis of the World Federation of Neurology Research Group on Neuromuscular Diseases and the El Escorial "Clinical limits of amyotrophic lateral sclerosis" workshop contributors. *J Neurol Sci.* (1994) 124:S96–107.
8. Brooks BR, Miller RG, Swash M, Munsat TL, World Federation of Neurology Research Group on Motor Neuron Diseases. El Escorial revisited: revised criteria for the diagnosis of amyotrophic lateral sclerosis. *Amyotroph Lateral Scler Other Motor Neuron Disord.* (2000) 1:293–9. doi: 10.1080/146608200300079536
9. Sabatelli M, Zollino M, Luigetti M, Grande AD, Lattante S, Marangi G, et al. Uncovering amyotrophic lateral sclerosis phenotypes: clinical features and long-term follow-up of upper motor neuron-dominant ALS. *Amyotroph Lateral Scler.* (2011) 12:278–82. doi: 10.3109/17482968.2011.580849
10. Kiernan M, Vucic S, Cheah B, Turner M, Eisen A, Hardiman O, et al. Amyotrophic lateral sclerosis. *Lancet* (2011) 277:942–55. doi: 10.1016/S0140-6736(10)61156-7
11. De Carvalho M. Testing upper motor neuron function in amyotrophic lateral sclerosis: the most difficult task of neurophysiology. *Brain* (2012) 135:2581–2. doi: 10.1093/brain/aws228
12. Geevasinga N, Menon P, Yiannikas C, Kiernan MC, Vucic S. Diagnostic utility of cortical excitability studies in amyotrophic lateral sclerosis. *Eur J Neurol.* (2014) 21:1451–7. doi: 10.1111/ene.12422
13. Swash M. Why are upper motor neuron signs difficult to elicit in amyotrophic lateral sclerosis? *J Neurol Neurosurg Psychiatr.* (2012) 83:659–62. doi: 10.1136/jnnp-2012-302315
14. Rocha AJ, Maia Junior AC. Is magnetic resonance imaging a plausible biomarker for upper motor neuron degeneration in amyotrophic lateral sclerosis/primary lateral sclerosis or merely a useful paraclinical tool to exclude mimic syndromes? A critical review of imaging applicability in clinical routine. *Arq Neuropsiquiatr.* (2012) 70:532–9. doi: 10.1590/S0004-282X2012000700012
15. Simon NG, Turner MR, Vucic S, Al-Chalabi A, Shefner J, Lomen-Hoerth C, et al. Quantifying disease progression in amyotrophic lateral sclerosis. *Ann Neurol.* (2014) 76:643–57. doi: 10.1002/ana.24273
16. Turner MR, Hardiman O, Benatar M, Brooks BR, Chio A, De Carvalho M, et al. Controversies and priorities in amyotrophic lateral sclerosis. *Lancet Neurol.* (2013) 12:310–22. doi: 10.1016/S1474-4422(13)70036-X
17. Ince PG, Evans J, Knopp M, Forster G, Hamdalla HH, Wharton SB, et al. Corticospinal tract degeneration in the progressive muscular atrophy variant of ALS. *Neurology* (2003) 60:1252–8. doi: 10.1212/01.WNL.0000058901.75728.4E
18. Lawyer T Jr, Netsky MG. Amyotrophic lateral sclerosis. *AMA Arch Neurol Psychiatr.* (1953) 69:171–92. doi: 10.1001/archneurpsyc.1953.02320260029002
19. Barker A, Jalinous R, Freeston I. Non-invasive magnetic stimulation of human motor cortex. *Lancet* (1985) 1:1106–7. doi: 10.1016/S0140-6736(85)92413-4
20. Vucic S, Kiernan M. Transcranial magnetic stimulation for the assessment of neurodegenerative disease. *Neurotherapeutics* (2017) 14:91–106. doi: 10.1007/s13311-016-0487-6

21. Vucic S, Kiernan MC. Utility of transcranial magnetic stimulation in delineating amyotrophic lateral sclerosis pathophysiology. *Handb Clin Neurol.* (2013) 116:561–75. doi: 10.1016/B978-0-444-53497-2.00045-0
22. Rossini P, Burke D, Chen R, Cohen L, Daskalakis Z, Di Lorio R, et al. Non-invasive electrical and magnetic stimulation of the brain, spinal cord, roots and peripheral nerves: basic principles and procedures for routine clinical and research application. An updated report from an IFCN Committee. *Clin Neurophysiol.* (2015) 126:1071–107. doi: 10.1016/j.clinph.2015.02.001
23. Roth B, Basser P. A model of the stimulation of a nerve fiber by electromagnetic induction. *IEEE Trans Biomed Eng.* (1990) 37:588–97. doi: 10.1109/10.55662
24. Di Lazzaro V, Oliviero A, Profice P, Saturno E, Pilato F, Insola A, et al. Comparison of descending volleys evoked by transcranial magnetic and electric stimulation in conscious humans. *Electroencephalogr Clin Neurophysiol.* (1998) 109:5. doi: 10.1016/S0924-980X(98)00038-1
25. Di Lazzaro V, Profice P, Ranieri F, Capone F, Dileone M, Oliviero A, et al. I-wave origin and modulation. *Brain Stimul.* (2012) 5:512–25. doi: 10.1016/j.brs.2011.07.008
26. Chen R, Cros D, Curra A, Di Lazzaro V, Lefaucheur J, Magistris M, et al. The clinical diagnostic utility of transcranial magnetic stimulation: report of an IFCN committee. *Clin Neurophysiol.* (2008) 119:504–32. doi: 10.1016/j.clinph.2007.10.014
27. Robinson D. Implications of neural networks for how we think about brain function. *Behav Brain Sci.* (1992) 13:644–55.
28. Ziemann U, Reis J, Schwenkreis P, Rosanova M, Strafella A, Badawy R, et al. TMS and drugs revisited (2014). *Clin Neurophysiol.* (2015) 126:1847–68. doi: 10.1016/j.clinph.2014.08.028
29. Menon P, Kiernan MC, Vucic S. Cortical hyperexcitability precedes lower motor neuron dysfunction in ALS. *Clin Neurophysiol.* (2015) 126:803–9. doi: 10.1016/j.clinph.2014.04.023
30. Vucic S, Kiernan MC. Novel threshold tracking techniques suggest that cortical hyperexcitability is an early feature of motor neuron disease. *Brain* (2006) 129:2436–46. doi: 10.1093/brain/awl172
31. Menon P, Geevasinga N, Van Den Bos M, Yiannikas C, Kiernan MC, Vucic S. Cortical hyperexcitability and disease spread in amyotrophic lateral sclerosis. *Eur J Neurol.* (2017) 24:816–24. doi: 10.1111/ene.13295
32. Grieve SM, Menon P, Korgaonkar MS, Gomes L, Foster S, Kiernan MC, et al. Potential structural and functional biomarkers of upper motor neuron dysfunction in ALS. *Amyotroph Lateral Scler Frontotemporal Degener.* (2015) 17:85–92. doi: 10.3109/21678421.2015.1074707
33. Vucic S, Ziemann U, Eisen A, Hallett M, Kiernan MC. Transcranial magnetic stimulation and amyotrophic lateral sclerosis: pathophysiological insights. *J Neurol Neurosurg Psychiatr.* (2013) 84:1161–70. doi: 10.1136/jnnp-2012-304019
34. Vucic S, Nicholson GA, Kiernan MC. Cortical hyperexcitability may precede the onset of familial amyotrophic lateral sclerosis. *Brain* (2008) 131:1540–50. doi: 10.1093/brain/awn071
35. Rossini PM, Berardelli A, Deuschl G, Hallett M, Maertens De Noordhout AM, Paulus W, et al. Applications of magnetic cortical stimulation. The International Federation of Clinical Neurophysiology. *Electroencephalogr Clin Neurophysiol Suppl.* (1999) 52:171–85.
36. Di Lazzaro V, Oliviero A, Profice P, Pennisi MA, Pilato F, Zito G, et al. Ketamine increases human motor cortex excitability to transcranial magnetic stimulation. *J Physiol.* (2003) 547:485–96. doi: 10.1113/jphysiol.2002.030486
37. Triggs WJ, Menkes D, Onorato J, Yan RS, Young MS, Newell K, et al. Transcranial magnetic stimulation identifies upper motor neuron involvement in motor neuron disease. *Neurology* (1999) 53:605–11. doi: 10.1212/WNL.53.3.605
38. Mills KR, Nithi KA. Corticomotor threshold is reduced in early sporadic amyotrophic lateral sclerosis. *Muscle Nerve* (1997) 20:1137–41.
39. Eisen A, Pant B, Stewart H. Cortical excitability in amyotrophic lateral sclerosis: a clue to pathogenesis. *Can J Neurol Sci.* (1993) 20:11–6. doi: 10.1017/S031716710004734X
40. Geevasinga N, Menon P, Sue CM, Kumar KR, Ng K, Yiannikas C, et al. Cortical excitability changes distinguish the motor neuron disease phenotypes from hereditary spastic paraplegia. *Eur J Neurol.* (2015) 22:826–31, e57–8. doi: 10.1111/ene.12669
41. Miscio G, Pisano F, Mora G, Mazzini L. Motor neuron disease: usefulness of transcranial magnetic stimulation in improving the diagnosis. *Clin Neurophysiol.* (1999) 110:975–81. doi: 10.1016/S1388-2457(99)00030-9
42. Mills KR, Nithi KA. Peripheral and central motor conduction in amyotrophic lateral sclerosis. *J Neurol Sci.* (1998) 159:82–7. doi: 10.1016/S0022-510X(98)00148-8
43. Pouget J, Trefouret S, Attarian S. Transcranial magnetic stimulation (TMS): compared sensitivity of different motor response parameters in ALS. *Amyotroph Lateral Scler Other Motor Neuron Disord.* (2000) 1:S45–9. doi: 10.1080/14660820052415817
44. Schulte-Mattler WJ, Muller T, Zierz S. Transcranial magnetic stimulation compared with upper motor neuron signs in patients with amyotrophic lateral sclerosis. *J Neurol Sci.* (1999) 170:51–6. doi: 10.1016/S0022-510X(99)00201-4
45. Eisen A, Entezari-Taher M, Stewart H. Cortical projections to spinal motoneurons: changes with aging and amyotrophic lateral sclerosis. *Neurology* (1996) 46:1396–404. doi: 10.1212/WNL.46.5.1396
46. Kohara N, Kaji R, Kojima Y, Mills KR, Fujii H, Hamano T, et al. Abnormal excitability of the corticospinal pathway in patients with amyotrophic lateral sclerosis: a single motor unit study using transcranial magnetic stimulation. *Electroencephalogr Clin Neurophysiol.* (1996) 101:32–41. doi: 10.1016/0013-4694(95)00166-2
47. Cantello R, Gianelli M, Civardi C, Mutani R. Magnetic brain stimulation: the silent period after the motor evoked potential. *Neurology* (1992) 42:1951–9. doi: 10.1212/WNL.42.10.1951
48. Ziemann U, Netz J, Szelenyi A, Homberg V. Spinal and supraspinal mechanisms contribute to the silent period in the contracting soleus muscle after transcranial magnetic stimulation of human motor cortex. *Neurosci Lett.* (1993) 156:167–71. doi: 10.1016/0304-3940(93)90464-V
49. Desiato MT, Caramia MD. Towards a neurophysiological marker of amyotrophic lateral sclerosis as revealed by changes in cortical excitability. *Electroencephalogr Clin Neurophysiol.* (1997) 105:1–7. doi: 10.1016/S0924-980X(96)96582-0
50. Uozumi T, Tsuji S, Murai Y. Motor potentials evoked by magnetic stimulation of the motor cortex in normal subjects and patients with motor disorders. *Electroencephalogr Clin Neurophysiol.* (1991) 81:251–6. doi: 10.1016/0168-5597(91)90010-U
51. Prout AJ, Eisen AA. The cortical silent period and amyotrophic lateral sclerosis. *Muscle Nerve* (1994) 17:217–23. doi: 10.1002/mus.880170213
52. Ziemann U, Rothwell J, Ridding M. Interaction between intracortical inhibition and facilitation in human mortor cortex. *J Physiol.* (1996) 496:873–81. doi: 10.1113/jphysiol.1996.sp021734
53. Vucic S, Howells J, Trevillion L, Kiernan M. Assessment of cortical excitability using threshold tracking techniques. *Muscle Nerve* (2006) 33:477–86. doi: 10.1002/mus.20481
54. Kiers L, Cros D, Chiappa KH, Fang J. Variability of motor potentials evoked by transcranial magnetic stimulation. *Electroencephalogr Clin Neurophysiol.* (1993) 89:415–23. doi: 10.1016/0168-5597(93)90115-6
55. Kujirai T, Caramia MD, Rothwell JC, Day BL, Thompson PD, Ferbert A, et al. Corticocortical inhibition in human motor cortex. *J Physiol.* (1993) 471:501–19. doi: 10.1113/jphysiol.1993.sp019912
56. Turner MR, Kiernan MC, Leigh PN, Talbot K. Biomarkers in amyotrophic lateral sclerosis. *Lancet Neurol.* (2009) 8:94–109. doi: 10.1016/S1474-4422(08)70293-X
57. Vucic S, Winhammar JM, Rowe DB, Kiernan MC. Corticomotoneuronal function in asymptomatic SOD-1 mutation carriers. *Clin Neurophysiol.* (2010) 121:1781–5. doi: 10.1016/j.clinph.2010.02.164
58. Zanette G, Tamburin S, Manganotti P, Refatti N, Forgione A, Rizzuto N. Different mechanisms contribute to motor cortex hyperexcitability in amyotrophic lateral sclerosis. *Clin Neurophysiol.* (2002) 113:1688–97. doi: 10.1016/S1388-2457(02)00288-2
59. Ziemann U, Winter M, Reimers CD, Reimers K, Tergau F, Paulus W. Impaired motor cortex inhibition in patients with amyotrophic lateral sclerosis. Evidence from paired transcranial magnetic stimulation. *Neurology* (1997) 49:1292–8. doi: 10.1212/WNL.49.5.1292

60. Yokota T, Yoshino A, Inaba A, Saito Y. Double cortical stimulation in amyotrophic lateral sclerosis. *J Neurol Neurosurg Psychiatr.* (1996) 61:596–600. doi: 10.1136/jnnp.61.6.596
61. Hanajima R, Ugawa Y, Terao Y, Ogata K, Kanazawa I. Ipsilateral cortico-cortical inhibition of the motor cortex in various neurological disorders. *J Neurol Sci.* (1996) 140:109–16. doi: 10.1016/0022-510X(96)00100-1
62. Geevasinga N, Menon P, Nicholson GA, Ng K, Howells J, Kril JJ, et al. Cortical function in asymptomatic carriers and patients with C9orf72 Amyotrophic Lateral Sclerosis. *JAMA Neurol.* (2015) 72:1268–74. doi: 10.1001/jamaneurol.2015.1872
63. Vucic S, Cheah BC, Yiannikas C, Kiernan MC. Cortical excitability distinguishes ALS from mimic disorders. *Clin Neurophysiol.* (2011) 122:1860–6. doi: 10.1016/j.clinph.2010.12.062
64. Vucic S, Cheah BC, Yiannikas C, Vincent A, Kiernan MC. Corticomotoneuronal function and hyperexcitability in acquired neuromyotonia. *Brain* (2010) 133:2727–33. doi: 10.1093/brain/awq188
65. Vucic S, Kiernan MC. Cortical excitability testing distinguishes Kennedy's disease from amyotrophic lateral sclerosis. *Clin Neurophysiol.* (2008) 119:1088–96. doi: 10.1016/j.clinph.2008.01.011
66. Vucic S, Nicholson GA, Kiernan MC. Cortical excitability in hereditary motor neuronopathy with pyramidal signs: comparison with ALS. *J Neurol Neurosurg Psychiatr.* (2010) 81:97–100. doi: 10.1136/jnnp.2008.157537
67. Farrar MA, Vucic S, Johnston HM, Kiernan MC. Corticomotoneuronal integrity and adaptation in spinal muscular atrophy. *Arch Neurol.* (2012) 69:467–73. doi: 10.1001/archneurol.2011.1697
68. Matamala JM, Geevasinga N, Huynh W, Dharmadasa T, Howells J, Simon NG, et al. Cortical function and corticomotoneuronal adaptation in monomelic amyotrophy. *Clin Neurophysiol.* (2017) 128:1488–95. doi: 10.1016/j.clinph.2017.05.005
69. Menon P, Geevasinga N, Yiannikas C, Howells J, Kiernan MC, Vucic S. Sensitivity and specificity of threshold tracking transcranial magnetic stimulation for diagnosis of amyotrophic lateral sclerosis: a prospective study. *Lancet Neurol.* (2015) 14:478–84. doi: 10.1016/S1474-4422(15)00014-9
70. Shibuya K, Simon NG, Geevasinga N, Menon P, Howells J, Park SB, et al. The evolution of motor cortical dysfunction in amyotrophic lateral sclerosis. *Clin Neurophysiol.* (2017) 128:1075–82. doi: 10.1016/j.clinph.2017.03.004
71. Shibuya K, Park SB, Geevasinga N, Menon P, Howells J, Simon NG, et al. Motor cortical function determines prognosis in sporadic ALS. *Neurology* (2016) 87:513–20. doi: 10.1212/WNL.0000000000002912
72. Vucic S, Lin CS-Y, Cheah BC, Murray J, Menon P, Krishnan AV, et al. Riluzole exerts central and peripheral modulating effects in amyotrophic lateral sclerosis. *Brain* (2013) 136:1361–70. doi: 10.1093/brain/awt085
73. Lacomblez L, Bensimon G, Leigh PN, Guillet P, Meininger V. Dose-ranging study of riluzole in amyotrophic lateral sclerosis. Amyotrophic Lateral Sclerosis/Riluzole Study Group II. *Lancet* (1996) 347:1425–31. doi: 10.1016/S0140-6736(96)91680-3
74. Bensimon G, Lacomblez L, Meininger V. A controlled trial of riluzole in amyotrophic lateral sclerosis. ALS/Riluzole Study Group. *N Engl J Med.* (1994) 330:585–91. doi: 10.1056/NEJM199403033300901
75. Geevasinga N, Menon P, Ng K, Van Den Bos M, Byth K, Kiernan MC, et al. Riluzole exerts transient modulating effects on cortical and axonal hyperexcitability in ALS. *Amyotroph Lateral Scler Frontotemporal Degener.* (2016) 17:1–9. doi: 10.1080/21678421.2016.1188961
76. Kuo MT. Redox regulation of multidrug resistance in cancer chemotherapy: molecular mechanisms and therapeutic opportunities. *Antioxid Redox Signal.* (2009) 11:99–133. doi: 10.1089/ars.2008.2095
77. Cheah BC, Vucic S, Krishnan AV, Boland RA, Kiernan MC. Neurophysiological index as a biomarker for ALS progression: validity of mixed effects models. *Amyotroph Lateral Scler.* (2011) 12:33–8. doi: 10.3109/17482968.2010.531742
78. Escorcio-Bezerra ML, Abrahao A, Nunes KF, De Oliveira Braga NI, Oliveira ASB, Zinman L, et al. Motor unit number index and neurophysiological index as candidate biomarkers of presymptomatic motor neuron loss in amyotrophic lateral sclerosis. *Muscle Nerve* (2018) 58:204–12. doi: 10.1002/mus.26087
79. Felice KJ. A longitudinal study comparing thenar motor unit number estimates to other quantitative tests in patients with amyotrophic lateral sclerosis. *Muscle Nerve* (1997) 20:179–85.
80. McComas AJ, Fawcett PR, Campbell MJ, Sica RE. Electrophysiological estimation of the number of motor units within a human muscle. *J Neurol Neurosurg Psychiatr.* (1971) 34:121–31. doi: 10.1136/jnnp.34.2.121
81. Boe SG, Stashuk DW, Doherty TJ. Motor unit number estimation by decomposition-enhanced spike-triggered averaging: control data, test-retest reliability, and contractile level effects. *Muscle Nerve* (2004) 29:693–9. doi: 10.1002/mus.20031
82. Stashuk DW, Doherty TJ, Kassam A, Brown WF. Motor unit number estimates based on the automated analysis of F-responses. *Muscle Nerve* (1994) 17:881–90. doi: 10.1002/mus.880170807
83. Doherty TJ, Brown WF. The estimated numbers and relative sizes of thenar motor units as selected by multiple point stimulation in young and older adults. *Muscle Nerve* (1993) 16:355–66. doi: 10.1002/mus.880160404
84. Shefner JM. Motor unit number estimation in human neurological diseases and animal models. *Clin Neurophysiol.* (2001) 112:955–64. doi: 10.1016/S1388-2457(01)00520-X
85. Shefner JM, Cudkowicz ME, Brown RH Jr. Comparison of incremental with multipoint MUNE methods in transgenic ALS mice. *Muscle Nerve* (2002) 25:39–42. doi: 10.1002/mus.10000
86. Vucic S, Rutkove SB. Neurophysiological biomarkers in amyotrophic lateral sclerosis. *Curr Opin Neurol.* (2018) 31:640–7. doi: 10.1097/WCO.0000000000000593
87. Jacobsen AB, Bostock H, Tankisi H. Following disease progression in motor neuron disorders with 3 MUNE methods. *Muscle Nerve* (2018). doi: 10.1002/mus.26304. [Epub ahead of print].
88. Swash M. MUNIX in the clinic in ALS: MUNE comes of age. *Clin Neurophysiol.* (2017) 128:482–3. doi: 10.1016/j.clinph.2016.12.021
89. Nandedkar SD, Nandedkar DS, Barkhaus PE, Stalberg EV. Motor unit number index (MUNIX). *IEEE Trans Biomed Eng.* (2004) 51:2209–11. doi: 10.1109/TBME.2004.834281
90. Nandedkar SD, Barkhaus PE, Stalberg EV. Motor unit number index (MUNIX): principle, method, and findings in healthy subjects and in patients with motor neuron disease. *Muscle Nerve* (2010) 42:798–807. doi: 10.1002/mus.21824
91. Gooch CL, Shefner JM. ALS surrogate markers. MUNE. *Amyotroph Lateral Scler Other Motor Neuron Disord.* (2004) 5:104–7. doi: 10.1080/17434470410019889
92. Shefner JM, Watson ML, Simionescu L, Caress JB, Burns TM, Maragakis NJ, et al. Multipoint incremental motor unit number estimation as an outcome measure in ALS. *Neurology* (2011) 77:235–41. doi: 10.1212/WNL.0b013e318225aabf
93. Neuwirth C, Barkhaus PE, Burkhardt C, Castro J, Czell D, De Carvalho M, et al. Motor Unit Number Index (MUNIX) detects motor neuron loss in pre-symptomatic muscles in Amyotrophic Lateral Sclerosis. *Clin Neurophysiol.* (2017) 128:495–500. doi: 10.1016/j.clinph.2016.11.026
94. Neuwirth C, Barkhaus PE, Burkhardt C, Castro J, Czell D, De Carvalho M, et al. Tracking motor neuron loss in a set of six muscles in amyotrophic lateral sclerosis using the Motor Unit Number Index (MUNIX): a 15-month longitudinal multicentre trial. *J Neurol Neurosurg Psychiatr.* (2015) 86:1172–9. doi: 10.1136/jnnp-2015-310509
95. Fukada K, Matsui T, Furuta M, Hirozawa D, Matsui M, Kajiyama Y, et al. The Motor Unit Number Index of Subclinical Abnormality in Amyotrophic Lateral Sclerosis. *J Clin Neurophysiol.* (2016) 33:564–8. doi: 10.1097/WNP.0000000000000296
96. Escorcio-Bezerra ML, Abrahao A, De Castro I, Chieia MAT, De Azevedo LA, Pinheiro DS, et al. MUNIX: reproducibility and clinical correlations in Amyotrophic Lateral Sclerosis. *Clin Neurophysiol.* (2016) 127:2979–84. doi: 10.1016/j.clinph.2016.06.011
97. Swash M, De Carvalho M. The Neurophysiological Index in ALS. *Amyotroph Lateral Scler Other Motor Neuron Disord.* (2004) 5:108–10. doi: 10.1080/17434470410020067
98. De Carvalho M, Scotto M, Lopes A, Swash M. Quantitating progression in ALS. *Neurology* (2005) 64:1783–5. doi: 10.1212/01.WNL.0000162036.76024.AB

99. Wilbourn AJ. The "split hand syndrome". *Muscle Nerve* (2000) 23:138. doi: 10.1002/(sici)1097-4598(200001)23:1<138::aid-mus22<3.0.co;2-7
100. Kuwabara S, Sonoo M, Komori T, Shimizu T, Hirashima F, Inaba A, et al. Dissociated small hand muscle atrophy in amyotrophic lateral sclerosis: frequency, extent, and specificity. *Muscle Nerve* (2008) 37:426–30. doi: 10.1002/mus.20949
101. Weber M, Eisen A, Stewart H, Hirota N. The split hand in ALS has a cortical basis. *J Neurol Sci.* (2000) 180:66–70. doi: 10.1016/S0022-510X(00)00430-5
102. Menon P, Kiernan MC, Vucic S. Cortical dysfunction underlies the development of the split-hand in amyotrophic lateral sclerosis. *PLoS ONE* (2014) 9:e87124. doi: 10.1371/journal.pone.0087124
103. Menon P, Kiernan MC, Yiannikas C, Stroud J, Vucic S. Split-hand index for the diagnosis of amyotrophic lateral sclerosis. *Clin Neurophysiol.* (2013) 124:410–6. doi: 10.1016/j.clinph.2012.07.025
104. Rutkove SB, Partida RA, Esper GJ, Aaron R, Shiffman CA. Electrode position and size in electrical impedance myography. *Clin Neurophysiol.* (2005) 116:290–9. doi: 10.1016/j.clinph.2004.09.002
105. Rutkove SB, Aaron R, Shiffman CA. Localized bioimpedance analysis in the evaluation of neuromuscular disease. *Muscle Nerve* (2002) 25:390–7. doi: 10.1002/mus.10048
106. Rutkove SB, Gregas MC, Darras BT. Electrical impedance myography in spinal muscular atrophy: a longitudinal study. *Muscle Nerve* (2012) 45:642–7. doi: 10.1002/mus.23233
107. Rutkove SB, Caress JB, Cartwright MS, Burns TM, Warder J, David WS, et al. Electrical impedance myography as a biomarker to assess ALS progression. *Amyotroph Lateral Scler.* (2012) 13:439–45. doi: 10.3109/17482968.2012.688837
108. Shefner JM, Rutkove SB, Caress JB, Benatar M, David WS, Cartwright MC, et al. Reducing sample size requirements for future ALS clinical trials with a dedicated electrical impedance myography system. *Amyotroph Lateral Scler Frontotemporal Degener.* (2018) 19:555–61. doi: 10.1080/21678421.2018.1510008
109. Rutkove S. Electrical impedance myography as a biomarker for ALS. *Lancet Neurol.* (2009) 8:226–7. doi: 10.1016/S1474-4422(09)70030-4
110. Esper GJ, Shiffman CA, Aaron R, Lee KS, Rutkove SB. Assessing neuromuscular disease with multifrequency electrical impedance myography. *Muscle Nerve* (2006) 34:595–602. doi: 10.1002/mus.20626

8

A Role for GDNF and Soluble APP as Biomarkers of Amyotrophic Lateral Sclerosis Pathophysiology

Serena Stanga[1]*, Liliana Brambilla[2], Bernadette Tasiaux[1], Anh H. Dang[3], Adrian Ivanoiu[4], Jean-Noël Octave[1], Daniela Rossi[2†], Vincent van Pesch[3,4†] and Pascal Kienlen-Campard[1]*

[1] Alzheimer Research Group, Institute of Neuroscience, Université Catholique de Louvain, Brussels, Belgium, [2] Laboratory for Research on Neurodegenerative Disorders, Istituti Clinici Scientifici Maugeri SpA SB - IRCCS, Pavia, Italy, [3] Unité de Neurochimie, Institute of Neuroscience, Université Catholique de Louvain, Brussels, Belgium, [4] Neurology Department, Cliniques Universitaires Saint-Luc, Brussels, Belgium

****Correspondence:***
Serena Stanga
serena.stanga@uclouvain.be
Pascal Kienlen-Campard
pascal.kienlen-campard@uclouvain.be

† These authors have contributed equally to this work.

The current inability of clinical criteria to accurately identify the “at-risk group” for Amyotrophic Lateral Sclerosis (ALS) development as well as its unknown etiology are fueling the interest in biomarkers aimed at completing clinical approaches for the diagnosis. The Glial cell line-derived neurotrophic factor (GDNF) is a diffusible peptide critically involved in neuronal differentiation and survival. GDNF is largely studied in various neurological and neuromuscular diseases, with a great interest in the peripheral nervous system (PNS). The recent discovery of Amyloid Precursor Protein (APP)-dependent GDNF regulation driving neuro-muscular junctions’ formation in APP null transgenic mice, prompts to study whether neurodegeneration relies on loss or gain of APP function and suggests that it could affect peripheral processes. Here, we explored a brand-new aspect of the loss of trophic support in ALS by measuring GDNF, APP, soluble APP fragments and Aβ peptides levels in $SOD1^{WT}$ or $SOD1^{G93A}$ transgenic mouse models of ALS and in human biological fluids [i.e. serum and cerebrospinal fluid (CSF)] from ALS patients and control subjects. Our results show that both GDNF and soluble APP fragments levels are altered at the onset of motor deficits in mice and that their levels are also modified in patient samples. This study indicates that both GDNF and soluble APPα represent possible biomarkers for ALS.

Keywords: biomarker, neurodegeneration, glial cell line-derived neurotrophic factor (GDNF), amyloid precursor protein (APP), amyotrophic lateral sclerosis (ALS)

INTRODUCTION

Amyotrophic lateral sclerosis (ALS) is a neurodegenerative disease characterized by the selective and progressive loss of motor neurons from the motor cortex, brain stem, and spinal cord leading to muscle atrophy, irreversible paralysis and eventually death within 3–5 years from symptom onset as a result of respiratory failure. Most patients are aged between 50 and 75 years at diagnosis and ALS is mostly sporadic with 90% of the cases occurring without a family history of the disease. Although the disease is considered a rare type of motor neuron neurodegeneration, by 2040 it has been estimated that around 400,000 patients will be diagnosed with ALS worldwide (1). Currently approved treatments for the disease, i.e. Riluzole and Edaravone, extend survival by few months and only mildly improve motor function. The inefficacy of the available treatments may be attributed to the fact that ALS is a heterogeneous disease. Furthermore, the process of diagnosis is often delayed, mainly because many parameters need to meet diagnostic criteria.

Understanding the pathophysiology of both familial and sporadic ALS and finding specific biomarkers to accelerate diagnosis could help in developing more effective treatments. Trophic factors have been largely studied as potential therapeutic targets for ALS because of their essential role in neuronal development, motor neuron maintenance and survival (2). Difficulties for growth factor-based therapies relate to the fact that therapeutic intervention mostly occurs after the diagnosis, thereby resulting as ineffective in counteracting the already ongoing neurodegenerative process. In this regard, trophic factors' levels would rather be useful as biomarkers for diagnosis and/or prognosis.

Interestingly, aside from their synthesis in the local spinal/muscular microenvironment, trophic factors play important roles in the nourishing feedback during which originating neurons receive trophic input from their target tissues (3). In ALS, it has been proposed that the failure of muscle cells to release neurotrophic factors that maintain the favorable physiological context for spinal motor neurons may lead to the loss of that neuronal cell population (4).

The glial cell line-derived neurotrophic factor (GDNF) is one of the factors produced by muscles and Schwann cells. The absence of GDNF alters the location of developing spinal motor neurons that innervate the limbs (5) and selectively affects the innervation of intrafusal muscle spindles in mice (6). Interestingly, the overexpression of this factor in muscle during development causes a hyperinnervation of neuromuscular junctions (7), while GDNF heterozygous mice (+/−) exhibit locomotor deficiencies (8), suggesting that GDNF dosage plays a key role in neuromuscular function. When GDNF is administered directly in muscles, it preserves the muscle-nerve synapse and promotes motor neuron function and survival in a familial rat model of ALS (9). Furthermore, overexpression of GDNF in muscle extends lifespan in ALS mice (10). Interestingly, GDNF can be retrogradely transported along motor neuronal axons (11), thereby enabling to explore the relevance of the intramuscular delivery route to act on both somas and nerve endings.

Recently, we demonstrated that the Amyloid Precursor Protein (APP) controls GDNF transcription in mouse embryonic fibroblasts (MEFs) and muscles with an important impact on muscular trophy and on the formation of neuromuscular contacts (12). Together with others, our study suggests that defects in APP function might be directly related not only to Alzheimer's disease (AD), but also to other neurodegenerative diseases involving muscle denervation, such as ALS. Indeed, APP is upregulated in muscle from mouse models of familial ALS as well as from patients with ALS, where APP upregulation correlates with clinical symptoms (13, 14).

In this study, we investigated in parallel the expression levels of GDNF and APP and its metabolites in muscles from non-transgenic mice and transgenic mice overexpressing the wild-type human isoform of the Cu/Zn superoxide dismutase 1 ($SOD1^{WT}$) enzyme or the mutant $SOD1^{G93A}$ protein, the latter animals recapitulating much of the pathophysiology of ALS. We analyzed APP processing by measuring the levels of its soluble non-amyloidogenic fragments (sAPPα and sAPPβ) and amyloid-β (Aβ peptides), together with GDNF levels, in cerebrospinal fluid (CSF) and serum from ALS patients and healthy controls.

We found that both GDNF and APP levels are increased in hindlimbs muscles of the transgenic $SOD1^{G93A}$ mouse model of ALS at the onset of motor deficits. Alterations in GDNF and sAPPα levels have been observed also in human biological fluids from patients with a moderate and fast progression of the disease. More precisely, GDNF levels are importantly decreased in the serum of ALS patients while sAPPα levels are increased in the same fluid, compared to healthy controls.

Altogether, our results suggest that both GDNF and sAPPα, which are clearly involved in neuromuscular pathologies, represent possible biomarkers for ALS pathophysiology.

MATERIALS AND METHODS

Mouse Models and Genotyping

Transgenic mice expressing human $SOD1^{WT}$ [B6SJL-Tg(SOD1) 2Gur/J-002298] or $SOD1^{G93A}$ [B6SJL-TgN(SOD1-G93A) 1Gur/J-002726] were purchased from The Jackson Laboratories. Animal care and handling were performed according to the European Council Directive 2010/63/EU and to the Italian and Belgian Animal Welfare Act for the use and care of laboratory animals and approved by the Animal Ethics Committee of the Universite Catholique of Louvain.

Genotyping and Tissue Processing

Genomic DNA was extracted from mouse tail biopsies and used as DNA template in genotyping PCR analysis. Offspring positive for the $SOD1^{G93A}$ transgene were identified using the following primers: SOD1, forward 5′-CATCAGCCCTAATCC ATCTGA-3′ and reverse 5′-CGCGACTAACAATCAAAGTGA-3′ as described in Brambilla et al. (15). Hindlimbs muscles (gastrocnemius and tibialis anterior) from transgenic mice were snap frozen in liquid nitrogen and stored at −80°C until further use (RNA isolation for RT-qPCR and Western blotting).

RNA Preparation, RT-PCR, and Quantitative PCR

RNAs were extracted from tissues in TRIzol Reagent and reverse transcribed using an iScript cDNA Synthesis Kit (Bio-Rad). Real-time quantitative PCR (qPCR) analysis was performed on 2ng cDNA template by using iQ SYBR Green Supermix in an iCycler IQ Multicolor Real-Time PCR Detection System (Bio-Rad). qPCR conditions were typically 95°C for 30 s, followed by 40 cycles of 30 s at 95°C, 45 s at 60°C, and 15 s at 79°C and ended by 71 cycles of 30 s at 60°C. The relative changes in the target gene: glyceraldehyde 3-phosphate dehydrogenase mRNA ratio were determined by the $2^{(-\Delta\Delta Ct)}$ calculation.

The sequences for qPCR primers are the following: GDNF, forward 5′-TTAATGTCCAACTGGGGGTCT-3′ and reverse 5′-GCCGAGGGAGTGGTCTTC-3′; and glyceraldehyde 3-phosphate dehydrogenase, forward 5′-ACCCAGAAGACTGTG GATGG-3′ and reverse 5′-ACACATTGGGGGTAGGAACA-3′.

Western Blotting

Muscles were homogenized in 10 volumes of lysis buffer [50 mM Tris (pH 7.5), 150 mM NaCl, 0.05 mM EDTA, 1% Triton X-100, and 0.1% sodium dodecyl sulfate] with Complete Protease Inhibitor Cocktail on ice using a Ultraturax homogenizer 3 × 10 s for each sample and in between 30 s (or more) on ice to cool down. After 1h at 4°C with continuous rotation, samples were centrifuged at 10,000 g for 10 min at 4°C and the supernatants were collected. Protein concentration was determined by the BCA Protein Assay Kit (Bio-Rad). A total of 15 μg protein was heated for 10 min at 70°C in loading buffer (lysis buffer containing 0.5 M DTT and staining NuPAGE blue), loaded and separated onto NuPAGE4–12% Bis-TrisGel, and then transferred for 2 h at 30 V onto PVDF membranes. After blocking (5% nonfat milk in PBS-Tween 0.05%), membranes were incubated overnight at 4°C with the primary antibodies, washed, and incubated with the secondary antibody coupled to peroxidase prior to ECL detection (GEHealthcare). ECL signals were quantified with a GelQuantNET software. Primary antibodies included anti-APP Y188 (1:5,000) or $GAPDH_2$ (1:25,000) in 5% nonfat milk in PBS-Tween 0.05%. Secondary antibody included anti-rabbit (1:10,000).

Study Group and Sampling

Venous serum samples and CSF were obtained from a group of subjects consisting of 7 patients with sporadic ALS and 7 healthy age-matched controls (CTR); clinical and demographic features are summarized in **Table 1**. All the subjects were examined by a senior neurologist and diagnosis of ALS was made according to the El Escorial criteria (16). ALS was diagnosed based upon symptom evaluation, neurological examination, laboratory and brain and/or spinal cord magnetic resonance imaging. Disease progression rates have been calculated as the ratio between the functional scale and disease duration in months; < 0.5 is considered slow; 0.5–1: moderate and >1: fast progression.

Control subjects were individuals with subjective complaints but with no diagnosis of neurological or psychiatric disease. None of the subjects selected in this study was affected by neoplastic or autoimmune disease when the blood and CSF samples were taken.

The patients had undergone a lumbar puncture and blood sampling in the Neurology department of the Cliniques Universitaires Saint-Luc (Brussels, Belgium) as part of the routine diagnostic procedure. Patients admitted to this hospital sign an internal regulatory document, stating that left-overs from biological samples used for routine diagnostic procedures can be used for retrospective academic studies, without an additional informed consent (ethics committee approval 2007/10SEP/233). Haemorrhagic CSF samples were excluded. CSF sample collection and storage were carried out in accordance with the consensus protocol proposed by Teunissen et al. (17). For serum studies, blood samples were collected in S-Monovette® 7.5 ml Serum Z tube (ref. 01-1601, Sarstedt). Both blood and CSF were centrifuged at 3600 rpm for 6 min. Serum and cell-free CSF were respectively aliquoted and stored at −80°C for later analysis.

GDNF, sAPP, and Aβ Measurements

Secreted GDNF levels were quantified in serum and CSF from the study group by ELISA following the manufacturer's instructions (Promega). sAPPα and β and Aβ38, Aβ40, and Aβ42 peptides were quantified using a sAPPα/sAPPβ multiplex and an Aβ multiplex electro-chemiluminescence immunoassay ECLIA (Meso Scale Discovery), respectively. sAPPα and β and Aβ were quantified according to the manufacturer's instructions.

Statistical Analysis

The number of samples in each experimental condition is indicated in the figure legends. Data were analyzed using GraphPad Prism software (GraphPad Software, La Jolla, CA, USA) by unpaired Student's t-test (2 experimental conditions) or by ANOVA followed by Bonferroni's multiple comparison tests (>2 experimental conditions).

RESULTS

We analyzed GDNF mRNA levels in hindlimbs muscles from non-transgenic (NTg) or transgenic $SOD1^{WT}$ and $SOD1^{G93A}$ mice at 30 (asymptomatic stage), ~100 (onset of motor deficits) and ~130 days of age (symptomatic stage) (**Figure 1**). GDNF mRNA levels remained below the detection limit at the asymptomatic stage in all the mouse genotypes (data not shown). A significant increase in GDNF mRNA levels in $SOD1^{G93A}$ mice vs. NTg and $SOD1^{WT}$ mice was observed only at the onset of motor deficits at 100 days (**Figure 1A**), and diminished thereafter.

In the same tissues, we measured by Western blotting APP levels, which showed a significant increase in its expression in $SOD1^{G93A}$ mice at the onset of motor deficits. More specifically, we found a 3.5-fold increase in APP levels in the hindlimb muscles at 100 days of age in $SOD1^{G93A}$ mice compared to both NTg and $SOD1^{WT}$ mice (**Figures 1B,C**). To note, the maturation profile of APP was also sharply pronounced at this stage (APP appearing as a doublet). This increase in APP expression levels was not detectable in animals aged 30 days or 130 days. By contrast, in NTg or $SOD1^{WT}$ APP levels remained low and constant throughout the lifespan (**Figures 1B,C**).

Since ALS transgenic mouse models mimic the clinical situation observed in patients, we analyzed both GDNF and soluble APP fragments in biological fluids from controls subjects and ALS patients. Group characteristics of study population are shown in **Table 1**. The mean age of the control group was 58.6 ± 9.9 years (range 43–75 years) and that of ALS group was 64.1 ± 13.5 years (range 38–81 years). There was no significant statistical difference between the groups ($p = 0.398$). The mean duration of disease in ALS patients was 13.4 ± 15.7 months; the mean ALSFRS-R and the Progression rate calculated at the diagnosis were 41.7 ± 3 and 9.9 ± 15.1 respectively, indicating that ALS patients were all fast progressors, with one intermediate and no slow progressors.

We measured GDNF concentration in CSF and serum from healthy subjects and ALS patients to follow their expression in biological fluids reflecting the biochemical changes ongoing in the brain and in the peripheral tissues, respectively. The median

TABLE 1 | Demographic and clinical variables of the study group.

Patients	Age range at collection (years)	Onset	L.O.I. until diagnosis (months)	ALSFRS-R score	Progression rate (point/month)
Control 1	56–61	NA	NA	NA	NA
Control 2	60–65	NA	NA	NA	NA
Control 3	40–45	NA	NA	NA	NA
Control 4	60–65	NA	NA	NA	NA
Control 5	70–75	NA	NA	NA	NA
Control 6	50–55	NA	NA	NA	NA
Control 7	50–55	NA	NA	NA	NA
ALS 1	56–61	Bulbar	1	44	44
ALS 2	36–41	Bulbar + hemiparesis	6	43	7.2
ALS 3	66–71	Paraparesis	48	38	0.8
ALS 4	60–65	Bulbar + hemiparesis	8	37	4.6
ALS 5	70–75	Paraparesis	11	43	3.9
ALS 6	70–75	Bulbar	12	42	3.5
ALS 7	80–85	Paraparesis	8	45	5.6

L.O.I., Length of Illness; ALSFRS-R, ALS Functional Rating Scale-Revised; NA, Not applicable. Both the ALSFRS-R and the Progression rate were calculated at the diagnosis. The references for the Progression Rate are: slow < 0.5, intermediate 0.5–1.0, fast >1.0.

of GDNF levels in CSF was higher in ALS patients (33.1 ± 20.5 pg/ml) compared to CTR (21.2 ± 4.3 pg/ml), but the statistical significance was reached only in serum, where ALS patients showed clearly lower levels of GDNF when compared to CTR (107.3 ± 37.7 pg/ml vs. 198.1 ± 41 pg/ml, respectively). These results (**Figures 2A,B**) were consistent with the decrease in GDNF expression oberserved in $SOD1^{G93A}$ mouse muscles at the advanced stage (**Figure 1A**). APP holoprotein cannot be tracked in extracellular media. In order to analyse a potential correlation with the amount of soluble APP levels in subjects' biological fluids and GDNF levels, we measured by ECLIA the soluble non-amyloidogenic fragments of APP: sAPPα and β, both in CSF and serum (**Figures 3A–D**) and their ratio (**Figures 3E,F**) that provides additional information about the equilibrium between non-amyloidogenic and amyloidogenic APP processing. Interestingly, the levels of sAPPα were increased only in serum of ALS patients compared to controls. No differences were observed in CSF. To note, neither sAPPβ levels nor sAPPα/β ratio was affected in serum or CSF of patients with ALS. Concerning the levels of Aβ38, Aβ40, and Aβ42, in both CTR and ALS patients, Aβ peptides were detectable only in CSF (**Figure 4A**), while in serum Aβ levels were very low (**Figure 4B**). No significant differences were observed in Aβ42/Aβ40 ratio (**Figure 4C**).

DISCUSSION

The lack of clinical criteria to accurately identify the "at-risk group" for ALS development together with the unknown etiology of the disease are fueling the interest in biomarkers aimed at completing clinical approaches for the diagnosis and suitable as new therapeutic targets. In this study, we explored specifically if the loss of trophic support in neurodegenerative diseases could provide *bona fide* biomarkers for ALS. We measured GDNF, APP as well as soluble APP fragments and Aβ peptides levels, in mouse models of ALS and in human biological fluids (i.e., serum and CSF) from patients and control subjects.

Glial cell line-derived neurotrophic factor is a diffusible peptide critically involved in neuronal differentiation and survival and it has been identified in an unbiased proteomic assay as potential AD biomarker (18, 19). It has been evaluated for symptomatic treatment of Parkinson's disease (PD) (20), and shown to be able to reverse some aspects of aging in monkeys (21). Importantly, GDNF is particularly involved in the pathophysiology of various neurological and neuromuscular diseases, with a great interest in the peripheral nervous system (PNS). GDNF has been reported to preserve motor neurons from dying by using neural progenitor cells delivery (22) or muscle-derived GDNF (23), suggesting that therapies targeting GDNF could be efficient to cope with ALS. Here, we have reported a clear alteration of GDNF levels both in muscles from ALS mouse models and serum from ALS patients. We found an increase in GDNF levels in muscle from mice expressing the mutant isoform of $SOD1^{G93A}$ at the onset of symptoms (100 days). Other groups observed an increased expression of GDNF mRNA in skeletal muscle from patients (24–26). The increment in GDNF mRNA levels in SOD1G93A mice is concomitant to the onset of ALS symptoms (denervation) but it is temporary. As it has been demonstrated in patients; GDNF levels increase contemporary to denervation aiming to promote potential reinnervation, but the reaction may be transient. We believe that the decrease in GDNF mRNA levels observed at day 130 might be due to the reduction in the total number of muscle fibers, the low number of fibers in acute stages of neurogenic atrophy and replacement of muscle fibers by connective tissue occurring in later stages of the disease. The fact that a similar reduction in GDNF mRNA levels is detected in SOD1wt mice can be explained by the presence of motor neuron pathology and skeletal muscle atrophy also in these animals (27, 28).

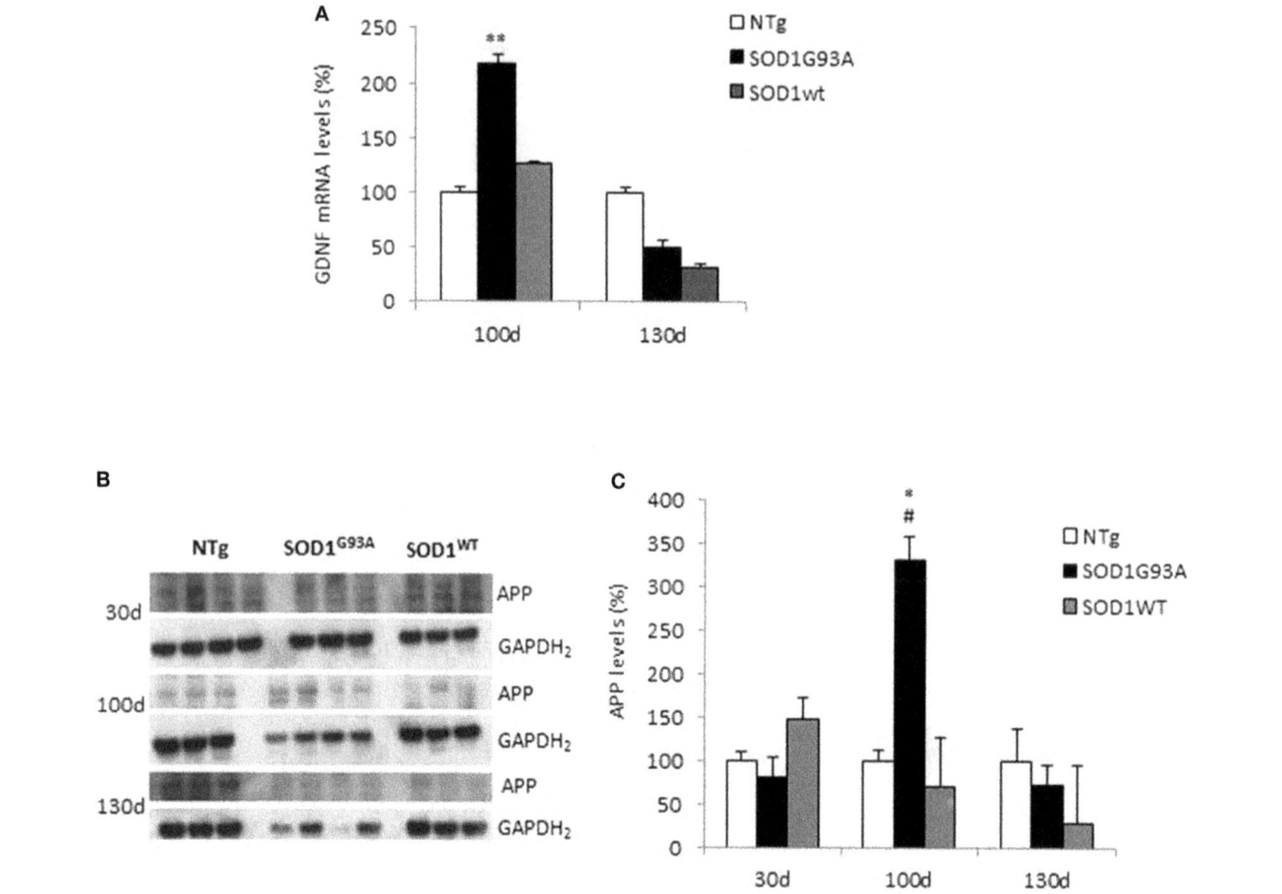

FIGURE 1 | GDNF and APP levels in non-transgenic and SOD1 transgenic mice models. **(A)** GDNF mRNA levels were analyzed in hindlimbs muscles from non-transgenic (NTg), $SOD1^{WT}$ and $SOD1^{G93A}$ mice at ~100 (onset of motor deficits) and ~130 days of age (symptomatic stage). Values (mean ± SEM) are expressed as percentage of age-matched NTg mice. $^{**}P < 0.01$, ANOVA followed by Bonferroni *post-hoc* test, n = 3–4 mice per genotype and age. **(B)** APP levels were analyzed by Western blotting in the same muscles' lysates at 100 and 130 days, plus at 30 days (asymptomatic stage) in NTg, $SOD1^{WT}$ and $SOD1^{G93A}$ mice; $GAPDH_2$ was used as a loading control probe. Quantifications are shown in **(C)**. Values (mean ± SEM) are expressed as percentage of expression level of age-matched NTg mice. $^{*}P < 0.05$ and $^{\#}P < 0.05$ vs. 100-day-old genotype-matched mice NTg and $SOD1^{WT}$; ANOVA followed by Bonferroni *post-hoc* test, n = 3–4 mice per genotype and age.

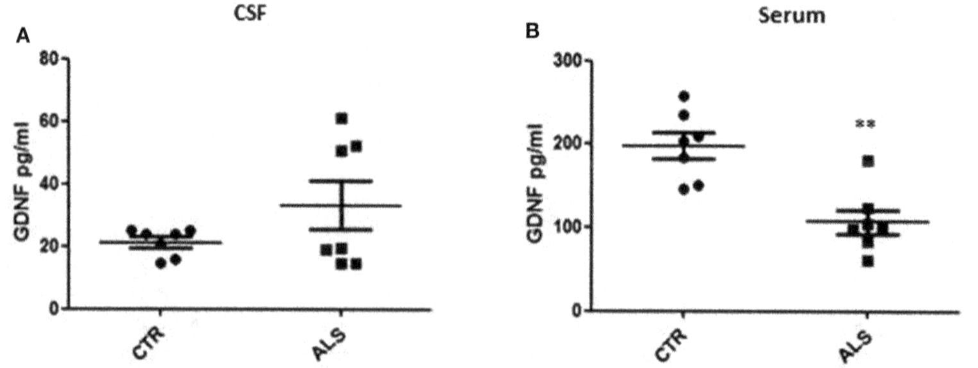

FIGURE 2 | GDNF levels in biological fluids from CTR subjects and ALS patients. GDNF levels were quantified by ELISA in the CSF **(A)** and serum **(B)** of controls without neurological disease and ALS patients. Values are given in picograms per milliliter (pg/ml). Each dot corresponds to one subject studied; the horizontal bar indicates the mean in each group. $^{**}P < 0.001$, Student's t-test (n = 7/group).

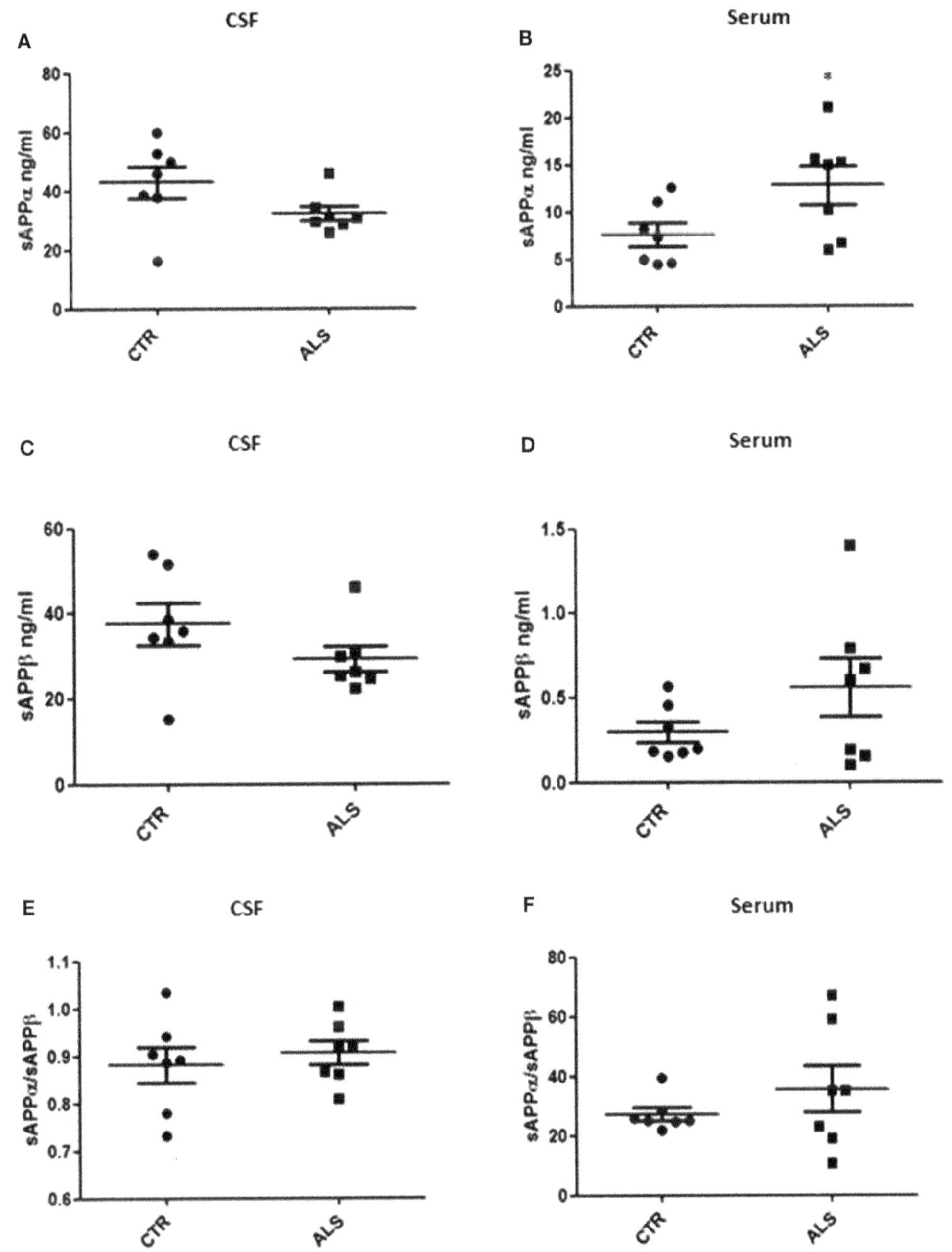

FIGURE 3 | CSF and serum sAPPα, β and their ratio in CTR and ALS patients. sAPP α levels **(A,B)** and sAPP β **(C,D)** were quantified by ECLIA in the CSF and serum of controls without neurological disease and ALS patients. sAPP α / sAPP β ratio have been showed for both CSF **(E)** and Serum **(F)**. Values are given in nanograms per milliliter (ng/ml). Each dot corresponds to one subject studied; the horizontal bar indicates the mean in each group. $^{*}P < 0.05$, Student's t-test ($n = 7$/group).

All together, these findings suggest that GDNF is importantly synthetized by muscles to sustain the increased demand for trophic factors by motor neurons, which are prone to degenerate in ALS. Interestingly, we observed also a significant increment in APP levels in mice expressing the mutant isoform of $SOD1^{G93A}$ at the stage of disease onset (100 days). This is in line with previously published work (13, 14). We recently found that APP controls GDNF transcription in muscles, supporting the neuromuscular phenotype observed in APP knock-out (KO) mice (12). This result suggests that changes in APP expression observed herein and in muscles of patients with ALS (14), could directly affect muscular GDNF expression and release. Thus, APP could not only be a biomarker of ALS progression, but it could be involved in the pathways controlling trophic supply that are impaired in the ALS pathology.

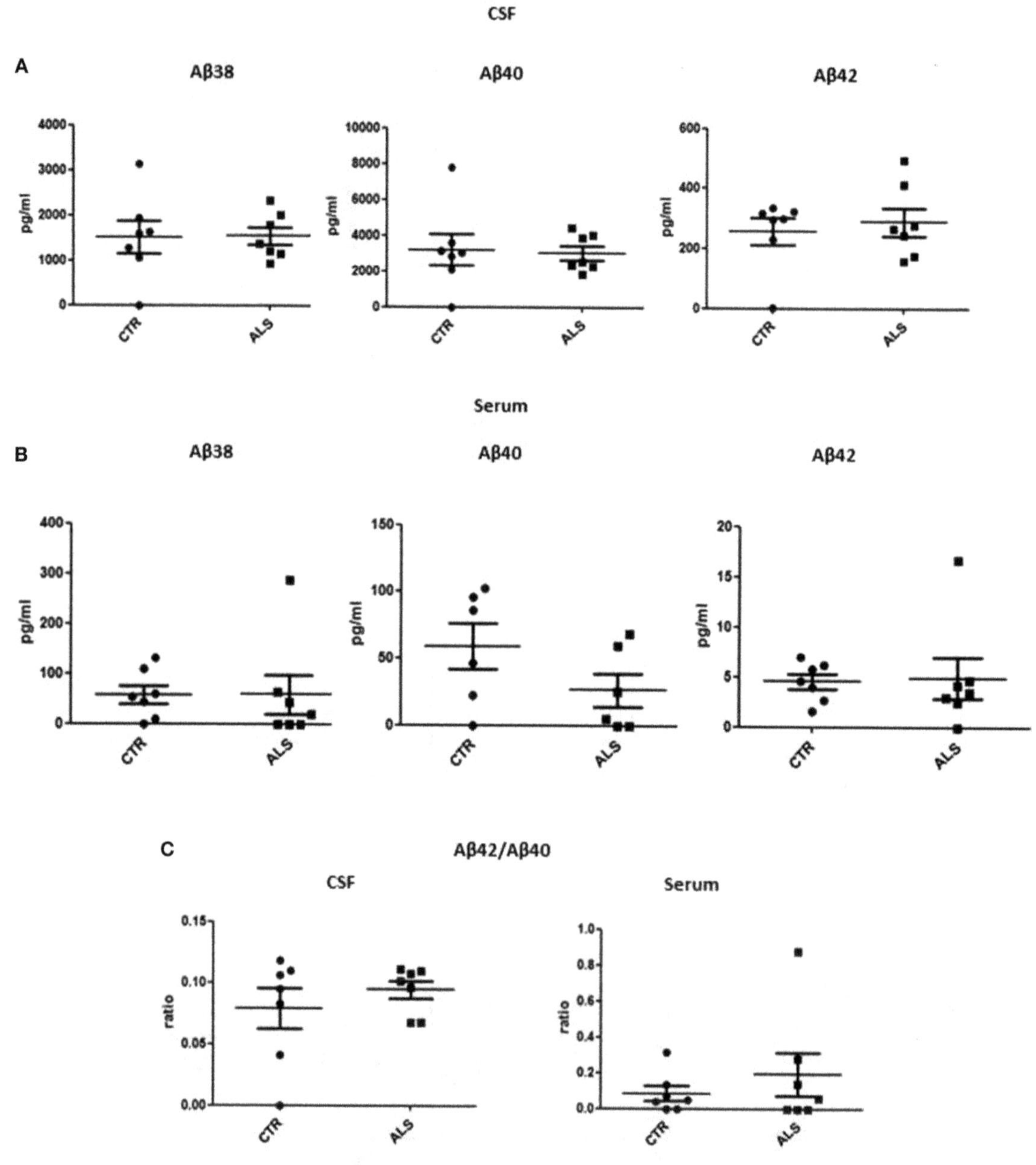

FIGURE 4 | CSF and serum Aβ38, Aβ40, and Aβ42 and Aβ42/Aβ40 ratio in CTR and ALS patients. Soluble monomeric Aβ38, Aβ40, and Aβ42 were quantified by ECLIA in the CSF **(A)** and serum **(B)** of controls without neurological disease and ALS patients. **(C)** Aβ42/Aβ40 ratio have been showed for both CSF and Serum. Values are given in nanograms per milliliter (ng/ml). Each dot corresponds to one subject studied ($n = 7$/group); the horizontal bar indicates the mean in each group.

In human samples, we observed significant and clear-cut results in serum while we measured only tendencies of impairment for both GDNF and APP metabolites in CSF. More specifically, we recorded a trend of GDNF levels to increase in the CSF of only 3 over 7 ALS patients, while a uniform and significant decrease in serum from ALS patients was detected. Our results indicate that peripheral GDNF (serum) is decreased as consequence to the fact that the regulatory system of GDNF production, likely involving APP, is no more functional and therefore reflected by a decrease of GDNF in serum. This is a peripheral process since central GDNF (CSF) is not significantly affected in the pathology. In parallel, we studied APP metabolite levels in the patient samples and we observed a trend to decrease of sAPPα levels in the CSF of ALS patients and a significant increase in sAPPα levels in serum from patients. Interestingly, sAPPα has been suggested to have potent neuroprotective capacities (29). Alterations in sAPPα levels in peripheral fluids from patients could indicate that peripheral mechanisms involving APP-dependent GDNF regulation may be implicated in the disease. Same observations, though not statistically significant, hold true for sAPPβ while no differences have been detected neither in sAPPα/sAPPβ ratio nor in Aβ levels.

Aβ levels are one of the most extensively evaluated markers of sporadic AD, since GDNF was identified as potential AD biomarker (18, 19), could we suggest it as a general biomarker of neurodegenerative diseases? The question is open. What is clear is that in AD Aβ levels are importantly high, while in ALS there are no alterations compared to age-matched control subjects at any stage of the disease. This suggests that very likely, APP and GDNF are linked in different neurodegenerative diseases but the mechanistic aspects are peculiar to the specific disease and still need to be decipher.

It is at this stage difficult to make clear-cut correlations between GDNF and APP soluble fragments in human samples because of the reduced number of ALS patients enrolled in the study, the variability existing between them and especially because of the peculiarity of disease history. Large scale studies on bigger cohorts would be useful to elaborate on the observations we made here. Clearly, both GDNF and soluble sAPPα levels are altered in fluids from patients with intermediate and fast progression of the disease, indicating that GDNF and soluble APP are biomarkers of ALS pathophysiology. The unequivocal observations in mouse muscles and serum from patients strongly suggest that changes in APP and GDNF levels result from peripheral processes. Assessing biomarkers in blood has the great advantage of minimal invasiveness when compared to measurement in CSF samples.

Changes in GDNF and sAPPα in serum go in opposite directions leaving open the following question: is APP-dependant GDNF expression involved in ALS progression, or are they independent biomarkers? The correlation between APP-related and GDNF changes, and their contribution to ALS pathways need to be fully elucidated, in order to consider them as possible targets for therapeutic approaches.

In conclusion, we suggest that the combined analysis of GDNF and sAPPα that we propose as possible predictive peripheral biomarkers for ALS, could help for the comprehension of the etiopathogenesis and the improved precision of the diagnosis of ALS.

AUTHOR CONTRIBUTIONS

SS and PK-C designed the research study. SS conducted experiments, LB, BT, and AD offered technical help. VvP enrolled subjects and conducted the clinical diagnosis. SS wrote the paper with fundamental input of J-NO, DR, and P-KC. All the authors analyzed data, read and approved the final manuscript.

FUNDING

This work was supported by a grant of the Foundation for Research on Alzheimer's disease (PK-C), by the Interuniversity Attraction Pole Programme-Belgian Sate-Belgian Science Policy (IAP-P7/16 and IAP-P7/13) to J-NO and PK-C, by the Action de Recherche Concertée (ARC 14/19-059) to PK-C.

ACKNOWLEDGMENTS

We are grateful to Giulia Guidotti (Laboratory for Research on Neurodegenerative Disorders, Istituti Clinici Scientifici Maugeri SpA SB, Pavia, Italy) for the helpful technical assistance.

REFERENCES

1. Hardiman O, van den Berg LH, Kiernan MC. Clinical diagnosis and management of amyotrophic lateral sclerosis. *Nat Rev Neurol.* (2011) **7**:639–49. doi: 10.1038/nrneurol.2011.153
2. Ekestern E. Neurotrophic factors and amyotrophic lateral sclerosis. *Neurodegener Dis.* (2004) **1**:88–100. doi: 10.1159/000080049
3. Tovar-Y-Romo LB, Ramírez-Jarquín UN, Lazo-Gómez R, Tapia R. Trophic factors as modulators of motor neuron physiology and survival: implications for ALS therapy. *Front Cell Neurosci.* (2014) **8**:61. doi: 10.3389/fncel.2014.00061
4. Loeffler JP, Picchiarelli G, Dupuis L, Gonzalez De Aguilar JL. The role of skeletal muscle in amyotrophic lateral sclerosis. *Brain Pathol.* (2016) **26**:227–36. doi: 10.1111/bpa.12350
5. Kramer ER, Knott L, Su F, Dessaud E, Krull CE, Helmbacher F et al. Cooperation between GDNF/Ret and ephrinA/EphA4 signals for motor-axon pathway selection in the limb. *Neuron* (2006) **50**:35–47. doi: 10.1016/j.neuron.2006.02.020
6. Gould TW, Yonemura S, Oppenheim RW, Ohmori S, Enomoto H. The neurotrophic effects of glial cell line-derived neurotrophic factor on spinal motoneurons are restricted to fusimotor subtypes. *J Neurosci.* (2008) **28**:2131–46. doi: 10.1523/JNEUROSCI.5185-07.2008
7. Nguyen QT, Parsadanian AS, Snider WD, Lichtman JW. Hyperinnervation of neuromuscular junctions caused by GDNF overexpression in muscle. *Science* (1998) **279**:1725–9. doi: 10.1126/science.279.5357.1725
8. Littrell OM, Pomerleau F, Huettl P, Surgener S, McGinty JF, Middaugh LD, et al. Enhanced dopamine transporter activity in middle-aged Gdnf heterozygous mice. *Neurobiol Aging* (2012) **33**:427.e1–14. doi: 10.1016/j.neurobiolaging.2010.10.013
9. Suzuki M, McHugh J, Tork C, Shelley B, Hayes A, Bellantuono I, et al. Direct muscle delivery of GDNF with human mesenchymal stem cells improves motor neuron survival and function in a rat model of familial ALS. *Mol Ther.* (2008) **16**:2002–10. doi: 10.1038/mt.2008.197
10. Mohajeri MH, Figlewicz DA, Bohn MC. Intramuscular grafts of myoblasts genetically modified to secrete glial cell line-derived neurotrophic factor prevent motoneuron loss and disease progression in a mouse model of familial amyotrophic lateral sclerosis. *Hum Gene Ther.* (1999) **10**:1853–66. doi: 10.1089/10430349950017536
11. Leitner ML, Molliver DC, Osborne PA, Vejsada R, Golden JP, Lampe PA, et al. Analysis of the retrograde transport of glial cell line-derived neurotrophic factor (GDNF), neurturin, and persephin suggests that *in vivo* signaling for the GDNF family is GFRalpha coreceptor-specific. *J Neurosci.* (1999) **19**:9322–31. doi: 10.1523/JNEUROSCI.19-21-09322.1999
12. Stanga S, Zanou N, Audouard E, Tasiaux B, Contino S, Vandermeulen G, et al. APP-dependent glial cell line-derived neurotrophic factor gene expression drives neuromuscular junction formation. *FASEB J.* (2016) **30**:1696–711. doi: 10.1096/fj.15-278739
13. Bryson JB, Hobbs C, Parsons MJ, Bosch KD, Pandraud A, Walsh FS, et al. Amyloid precursor protein (APP) contributes to pathology in the SOD1(G93A) mouse model of amyotrophic lateral sclerosis. *Hum Mol Genet.* (2012) **21**:3871–82. doi: 10.1093/hmg/dds215
14. Koistinen H, Prinjha R, Soden P, Harper A, Banner SJ, Pradat PF, et al. Elevated levels of amyloid precursor protein in muscle of patients with amyotrophic

lateral sclerosis and a mouse model of the disease. *Muscle Nerve* (2006) **34**:444–450. doi: 10.1002/mus.20612
15. Brambilla L, Guidotti G, Martorana F, Iyer AM, Aronica E, Valori CF, et al. Disruption of the astrocytic TNFR1-GDNF axis accelerates motor neuron degeneration and disease progression in amyotrophic lateral sclerosis. *Hum Mol Genet.* (2016) **25**:3080–95. doi: 10.1093/hmg/ddw161
16. Brooks BR, Miller RG, Swash M, Munsat TL. World federation of neurology group on motor neuron diseases. el escorial revisited: revised criteria for the diagnosis of amyotrophic lateral sclerosis. *Amyotroph Lateral Scler Other Motor Neuron Disord.* (2000) **1**:293–9. doi: 10.1080/146608200300079536
17. Teunissen CE, Petzold A, Bennett JL, Berven FS, Brundin L, Comabella M, et al. A consensus protocol for the standardization of cerebrospinal fluid collection and biobanking. *Neurology* (2009) **73**:1914–22. doi: 10.1212/WNL.0b013e3181c47cc2
18. Ray S, Britschgi M, Herbert C, Takeda-Uchimura Y, Boxer A, Blennow K, et al. Classification and prediction of clinical Alzheimer's diagnosis based on plasma signaling proteins. *Nat Med.* (2007) **13**:1359–62. doi: 10.1038/nm1653
19. Straten G, Eschweiler GW, Maetzler W, Laske C, Leyhe T. Glial cell-line derived neurotrophic factor (GDNF) concentrations in cerebrospinal fluid and serum of patients with early Alzheimer's disease and normal controls. *J Alzheimers Dis.* (2009) **18**:331–7. doi: 10.3233/JAD-2009-1146
20. Taylor H, Barua N, Bienemann A, Wyatt M, Castrique E, Foster R, et al. Clearance and toxicity of recombinant methionyl human glial cell line-derived neurotrophic factor (r-metHu GDNF) following acute convection-enhanced delivery into the striatum. *PLoS ONE* (2013) **8**:e56186. doi: 10.1371/journal.pone.0056186
21. Ai Y, Markesbery W, Zhang Z, Grondin R, Elseberry D, Gerhardt GA, et al. Intraputamenal infusion of GDNF in aged rhesus monkeys: distribution and dopaminergic effects. *J Comp Neurol.* (2003) **461**:250–61. doi: 10.1002/cne.10689
22. Suzuki M, McHugh J, Tork C, Shelley B, Klein SM, Aebischer P, et al. GDNF secreting human neural progenitor cells protect dying motor neurons, but not their projection to muscle, in a rat model of familial ALS. *PLoS ONE* (2007) **2**:e689. doi: 10.1371/journal.pone.0000689
23. Li W, Brakefield D, Pan Y, Hunter D, Myckatyn TM, Parsadanian A. Muscle-derived but not centrally derived transgene GDNF is neuroprotective in G93A-SOD1 mouse model of ALS. *Exp Neurol.* (2007) **203**:457–71. doi: 10.1016/j.expneurol.2006.08.028
24. Grundström E, Askmark H, Lindeberg J, Nygren I, Ebendal T, Aquilonius SM. Increased expression of glial cell line-derived neurotrophic factor mRNA in muscle biopsies from patients with amyotrophic lateral sclerosis. *J Neurol Sci.* (1999) **162**:169–73. doi: 10.1016/S0022-510X(98)00333-5
25. Lie DC, Weis J. GDNF expression is increased in denervated human skeletal muscle. *Neurosci Lett.* (1998) **250**:87–90. doi: 10.1016/S0304-3940(98)00434-0
26. Yamamoto M, Mitsuma N, Inukai A, Ito Y, Li M, Mitsuma T, et al. Expression of GDNF and GDNFR-alpha mRNAs in muscles of patients with motor neuron diseases. *Neurochem Res.* (1999) **24**:785–90. doi: 10.1023/A:1020739831778
27. Jaarsma D, Haasdijk ED, Grashorn JA, Hawkins R, van Duijn W, Verspaget HW, et al. Human Cu/Zn superoxide dismutase (SOD1) overexpression in mice causes mitochondrial vacuolization, axonal degeneration, and premature motoneuron death and accelerates motoneuron disease in mice expressing a familial amyotrophic lateral sclerosis mutant SOD1. *Neurobiol Dis.* (2000) **7**:623–43. doi: 10.1006/nbdi.2000.0299
28. Wong M, and Martin LJ. Skeletal muscle-restricted expression of human SOD1 causes motor neuron degeneration in transgenic mice. *Hum Mol Genet.* (2010) **19**:2284–302. doi: 10.1093/hmg/ddq106
29. Chasseigneaux S, and Allinquant B. Functions of Aβ, sAPPα and sAPPβ : similarities and differences. *J Neurochem.* (2012) **120** (Suppl. 1):99–108. doi: 10.1111/j.1471-4159.2011.07584.x.2011.07584.x

9

Diagnostic and Prognostic Performance of Neurofilaments in ALS

Koen Poesen [1,2]* *and Philip Van Damme* [3,4]*

[1] Department of Neurosciences, Laboratory for Molecular Neurobiomarker Research, KU Leuven, Leuven, Belgium, [2] Laboratory Medicine, University Hospitals Leuven, Leuven, Belgium, [3] Laboratory of Neurobiology, Department of Neurosciences, KU Leuven and Center for Brain & Disease Research VIB Leuven, Leuven, Belgium, [4] Department of Neurology, Neuromuscular Reference Centre, University Hospitals Leuven, Leuven, Belgium

***Correspondence:**
Koen Poesen
koen.poesen@uzleuven.be
Philip Van Damme
philip.vandamme@uzleuven.be

There is a need for biomarkers for amyotrophic lateral sclerosis (ALS), to support the diagnosis of the disease, to predict disease progression and to track disease activity and treatment responses. Over the last decade multiple studies have investigated the potential of neurofilament levels, both in cerebrospinal fluid and blood, as biomarker for ALS. The most widely studied neurofilament subunits are neurofilament light chain (NfL) and phosphorylated neurofilament heavy chain (pNfH). Neurofilament levels are reflecting neuronal injury and therefore potentially of value in ALS and other neurological disorders. In this mini-review, we summarize and discuss the available evidence about neurofilaments as diagnostic and prognostic biomarker for human ALS.

Keywords: amyotrophic lateral sclerosis, frontotemporal dementia, neurofilament, cerebrospinal fluid, serum, plasma, NfL, pNfH

INTRODUCTION

Amyotrophic lateral sclerosis (ALS) is a neurodegenerative disorder primarily affecting the motor system network, giving rise to progressive muscle weakness in the limbs, the bulbar region, but also of the respiratory muscles. Survival is typically between 2 and 5 years after disease onset, but in about 15% of patients a slower disease progression is present (1). The most important extramotor manifestations of the disease include behavioral changes, executive dysfunction and language problems, reminiscent of frontotemporal dementia.

As of today, the diagnosis of ALS remains based on clinical judgement and requires a combination of signs of upper and lower motor neuron involvement in a patients with progressive muscle weakness, without alternative explanation for the presenting symptoms and signs (2). Despite efforts to make the diagnostic criteria more sensitive (3, 4), the diagnostic delay remains about 10–12 months after symptom onset (5). The current clinical criteria also do not discriminate between different subtypes of ALS, although they may have very different disease trajectories. Combinations of clinical parameters allow to predict disease progression and survival in ALS patients, but they do not reflect the underlying biological processes (6).

Biomarkers, which reflect hallmarks of the disease, may not only aid in the diagnostic algorithm of ALS, but could also be of value in defining homogeneous subgroups of patients. Potentially, they could also be helpful to track disease progression and treatment responses (7). Neurofilaments (NF) have been studied extensively in different neurological conditions, and are considered to be useful as marker of acute and chronic neuronal injury (8). Neurofilaments are intermediate filaments of 10 nm in neurons, composed of heteropolymers of different subunits, neurofilament light chain (NfL), neurofilament medium chain (NfM), and neurofilament heavy chain (NfH) (9). Phosphorylation and O-glycosylation are believed to be important for NF assembly (9) and especially NfM and NfH undergo these posttranslational modifications. NF are highly expressed in neurons, provide structural support for neurons and determine axon caliber and conduction velocity (10). Mutations in the genes encoding NfH and NfL can cause the inherited neuropathy Charcot-Marie-Tooth disease (11), inframe deletions or insertions in the side arm domain or C-terminal tail domain of NfH have also been linked to ALS (12). Neurofilamentous abnormalities and elevated NF levels are not restricted to ALS. However, NF have been implicated in the pathogenesis of ALS for more than 2 decades (13). In post mortem spinal cord of ALS patients, accumulations of NF are seen in the perikaryon and axons of motor neurons (14) and motor neurons display reduced NfL mRNA levels (15). Overexpression of NfH causes a motor axonopathy with NF inclusions in mice, which can be rescued by NfL overexpression (16), suggesting that an imbalance between the relative expression levels of the different NF subunits may be important. In line with this hypothesis, reducing the NfL levels and overexpression of NfH levels in the SOD1 mouse model of ALS, increased the lifespan of these animals (17, 18). In this model of ALS, the degeneration of motor neurons is accompanied by a progressive rise in blood NF levels, and these levels have been shown to be able to capture treatment responses (19, 20).

In this review, we will give an overview of the current knowledge about the diagnostic and prognostic value of NF levels in cerebrospinal fluid and blood for human ALS.

AVAILABLE METHODS TO MEASURE NEUROFILAMENTS LEVELS

Numerous studies employed in house developed assays or commercial "for research use only" ELISAs for NF measurements (20–27). Although the precision and recovery profile of such kits was acceptable (**Table 1**), the analytical sensitivity in terms of limit of detection and limit of quantification was insufficient to precisely detect NF levels in CSF of controls or in blood of most patients with ALS (30). Using the same antibodies against NfL, novel technologies including electrochemiluminescence (ECL) and Single Molecule Array (SIMOA) enabled to precisely and sensitively quantify NfL in CSF and blood (22, 29, 40). Furthermore, an improved ELISA assay allowed to accurately quantify pNfH in blood and CSF of patients with ALS (39).

DIAGNOSTIC VALUE OF NEUROFILAMENTS

It is already known for more than 2 decades that NF levels are roughly 5–10 times higher in ALS patients compared to healthy controls (41). Numerous studies since then, have shown that NF levels are increased in patients with ALS, not only in CSF, but also in serum or plasma (42). As NFs are produced by neurons, the serum/plasma levels are 10 fold lower compared to CSF levels.

Several studies showed that NfL and pNfH are elevated in CSF and serum/plasma in patients with ALS (20, 23, 30–32, 35, 37–39, 43–55). There is a good correlation between NF levels in CSF and in blood, and this is the case for NfL and pNfH (34, 39, 40). Nevertheless, the diagnostic performance was found to be better in CSF compared to blood (39, 54). Most studies compared ALS patients to healthy controls, only few studies tested the diagnostic performance in comparison to ALS mimicking disorders (23, 30, 31, 39). The sensitivity and specificity for ALS was better for pNfH than for NfL in studies comparing both neurofilament subunits (23, 32, 39). Even though there is considerable elevation in NF in some of the ALS mimicking disorders, the diagnostic accuracy to detect ALS is still good. The diagnostic performance of NfL and pNfH assays is shown in **Table 1**. One study suggested that the discrimination from disease controls improved by using the CSF pNfH/complement C3 ratio (24). For implementation in the routine clinical practice, assay standardization, and characterization, and independent validation of the cut-offs are required. Indeed, the development of reference methods for NF measurements, e.g., by means of mass spectrometry (56, 57), and of certified reference materials for traceability of the calibrators and to demonstrate commutability among the different assays should be encouraged (58). Independent evaluation of the performance characteristics of the NF assays enables the public availability of data on the analytical quality of the different commercially available assays. Furthermore, automation of immunoassay facilitates single measurements with similar precision profiles as duplicate measurements in manually performed ELISAs, the former significantly reducing the implementation costs for patients (59). As the range of NF levels in ALS mimicking disorders is rather wide, the robustness of reported cut-offs might be challenged by the rather low number of ALS mimicking disorders included in most studies (23, 39). Multicenter studies are warranted to establish universally applicable cut-offs for NF.

Importantly, the increase in NF is already measurable early in the disease course (23, 31, 40). A recent study showed that NfL levels increase already several months prior to symptom onset in *SOD1* mutation carriers (60). NFs are elevated in sporadic and familial ALS patients, although slightly lower in confirmed *SOD1* cases (43) and higher in *C9orf72* positive patients (51).

The neuroanatomical correlate of elevated NF levels in ALS is not entirely clear. Both NfL and pNFH correlate with the extent of clinical upper and lower motor neuron involvement (23), although pNfH levels correlate better with lower motor neuron involvement and NfL levels better with upper motor neuron involvement (23, 34). An imaging study revealed that NfL levels in CSF correlate with the extent of corticospinal tract involvement on DTI (48).

TABLE 1 | Analytical and diagnostic performance of NfL and pNfH assays.

NfL	Capture antibody epitope	Calibrator	Analytical performance					Diagnostic performance (ALS vs. mimics)					
			LOD	LOQ	CV_{wr}	CV_{rr}	Recovery	Sens	Spec	PPV	NPV	LR+	LR-
			pg/mL		%	%	%	%	%	%	%		
Gothenburg (Blennow lab) ELISA (21)	Core domain (aa 93-396) of full length recombinant NfL (Origene)	Not disclosed	-	78[a,b]	8[a,b]	13[a,b]	80 - 109[a,c]	Not addressed					
NF-light ELISA (22) (Uman Diagnostics)	Core domain (aa 92–396) (NF-L mAb 47:3 and NF-L mAb 2:1 having nonsterical overlapping epitopes) (28)	Purified bovine spinal cord NfL (Progen Biotechnik GmbH)	–	78(29),c,e	1.5 [a,c]	17.4[a,c]	-	78(23),c 77(30),c 89(31),c 96.2c,(32)	85 88 89 56.3	92 95 - -	64 56 - -	3.9 - - -	- - - -
Simoa NF-light digital immunoassay (29) (Quanterix)			0.038[a,o]	0.62(29),c,e	6.6	17.0	118.5[c,o] 90.7[d,o]	100d,(31) 85.5d,(33)	84 77.3	- 91.4	- 65.4	- -	- -
NFL ECL assay (29)			-	15.6[c,e]	9.2 3.6[p]	14.8 6.6 [p]	-	79(34),d	84-90[f]	98	34	-	-
pNfH													
Nijmegen pNfH ELISA (35)	Low to highly phosphorylated NFH (Anti-SMI35 (or 03-44) Ab via Sternberger Monoclonals Incorporatedand later on via Covance Research Products) (36) Cross-reacting for 7.8% with NFM (25)	Bovine NFHp35 standard (ICN, Burlingame, CA)						72[c]	80 [c]	-	-	-	-
London pNfH ELISA (25)		HPLC-purified bovine NfH (Affiniti Research	200[c,g]		10.6 [c] 7.9c,(26)	23[c] 9.76[h]- 14.08l,c,(26)	119(26)		CSF levels of NfHSMI35 were five times higher in patients with ALS (1.7 ng/mL) than in controls (37)				
pNfH ECL assay (38)		Bovine NfH (USBiological)	(0.6) 24 [g]		4.8[c]	8.4[c]	84.5-93.2[c]	-	-	-	-	-	-
Gainesville pNfH ELISA (26, 27)	220 kDa Form of NFH isolated from bovine Spinal cord [affinity purified chicken anti pNfH via EnCor Biotechnology (Alachua, Florida)], no obvious Reacting with of NFM or other lower molecular weight material (27)	In house purified bovine NfH	400[g]		2.96 [c,h,]	6.67[c,h,j]	-	-	-	-	-	-	-
Euroimmun pNfH ELISA		Purified bovine pNfH (EnCor Biotechnology Inc., Gainesville, Florida, USA)	69[c,n]	150[c,n]	5.50[a,o] 6.90 [c,n]	5.95[a,o] 9.17 [c,n]	-	92.9c,(39) 100c,m,(32) 71.8d,(39)	96.0 68.8 85.2	98.7 - 93.8	80.0 - 48.9	23.3 - 4.8	- - -

(Continued)

TABLE 1 | Continued

NfL	Capture antibody epitope	Calibrator	Analytical performance					Diagnostic performance (ALS vs. mimics)					
			LOD	LOQ	CV_{wr}	CV_{rr}	Recovery	Sens	Spec	PPV	NPV	LR+	LR-
			pg/mL		%	%	%	%	%	%	%		
Jacksonville pNfH ELISA (20)	Bovine pNfH purified from spinal cord (purified AH1 monoclonal antibody)	Bovine pNhH purified from spinal cord	31.25[g,k]			8.5-12.5[l]	-	First paper to show higher levels of plasma pNfH in ALS than in healthy controls					
Biovendor pNfH ELISA (24)	Not publically available		23.5[g,o]	-	4.5[a,b,o]	-	98.8[c,o] 95.8[d,o]	84.4[c,m] 83[c,(30)] 90.7[c,(23)]	93.5[c,m] 80 88.0	- 93 95.8	- 62 75.9	- - 7.6	- - -

a, protocol not (fully) disclosed/available; b, matrix not disclosed; c, in CSF; d, in serum; e, value below lowest calibrator reaching accuracy of 80-120% and CV% ≤ 20% (which is most closely related to the definition of LOQ); f, <6 m and >6 m disease duration, respectively; g, signal of blank + 3 times the standard deviation, considered as limit of blank within current review; h, high pNfH sample; i, low pNfH sample; j, 9 consecutive days for 12 samples; k, serially diluted bovine pNfH; l, standards run 16 times on each of 7 days; m, in disease controls also including ALS mimics; n, in house data (not published) via the "Verification of Performance for Precision and Trueness; Approved Guideline-Second Edition". CLSI document EP15-A2.; o, manufacturer's data - p, low NfL levels ranging from 9.91 pg/mL to 72.8 pg/mL. aa, amino acids; CVwr, within-run or intra assay coefficient of variance; CVrr, between-run or inter assay coefficient of variance; ECL, Electrochemiluminescence; ELISA, Enzyme-Linked Immunosorbent Assay; LOD, limit of detection; LOQ, limit of quantification; LR, likelihood ratio for abnormal (+) or normal (-) result; NFM, neurofilament medium chain; NPV, negative predictive value; PPV, positive predictive value; sens, sensitivity; spec, specificity.

PROGNOSTIC VALUE OF NEUROFILAMENTS

The levels of both NfL and pNfH have been shown to correlate with parameters of disease severity, such as the decline on the ALS functional rating scale-revised or ALSFRS-R (23, 30, 34). They also predict survival of ALS patients, with higher NF levels being unfavorable. In Cox regression analyses both NfL and pNfH have been shown to be independent predictors of survival, when taking other prognostic factors into account (30, 34, 45, 61). Patients with very long survival typically have low levels of NFs (23, 53). The predictive value of NFs is present when using both CSF and blood samples. As higher NF levels are associated with a faster disease progression in typical ALS patients, NF levels could theoretically be used to stratify patients in clinical trials. However, data on this topic are currently lacking.

The difference in disease progression between different clinical subtypes of ALS is not always reflected in NF levels. Patients with *C9orf72* ALS have been reported to have higher pNfH CSF levels (51), but further studies on NF levels are needed in different motor neuron disease subtypes. In patients with primary lateral sclerosis (PLS), the levels can also be increased, but mostly to a lesser extent (30, 31, 34). ALS patients with cognitive/behavioral impairment or comorbid FTD have a worse outcome (62, 63), but if this is reflected in NF levels requires further study (64). The unfavorable outcome of patients with bulbar onset or respiratory onset ALS may not be reflected in NF levels.

VALUE OF NEUROFILAMENTS TO TRACK TREATMENT RESPONSE?

NFs may not only have value to help with the diagnosis and prediction of disease severity in ALS, they may also become of value to track the response to treatments. As marker of neuronal injury it is anticipated that neuroprotective treatments would result in lower NF levels. For ALS, there are no studies in patients that report a treatment response on NF levels at present. Whether the effect of riluzole on survival can be captured by measuring NF levels remains unknown. On the other hand, a recent study using rodent mutant SOD1 models, showed a clear survival benefit of treatment with antisense oligonucleotides, which was accompanied by a reduction in serum pNfH levels (65). In addition, in other neurological disorders, such as multiple sclerosis, NFs levels reflect the effect of disease-modifying therapies (66).

In patients with ALS, it is know that NFs levels are relatively stable during the course of the disease in many patients (51, 67). However, there is some evidence that the levels may increase during the first phase of the disease (53). This is backed up by data from a recent study in *SOD1* mutation carriers, which showed that the levels slowly increase up to 12 months prior to symptom onset and can continue to rise the months following symptom onset (60). The NF levels also correlate with the number of body regions affected by ALS and the ALS progression rate (23, 34), suggesting that they reflect the extent and rate of motor neuron degeneration. Several cross-sectional studies have reported a negative correlation of NF levels with survival (30, 34, 53). This may suggest that the levels drop slightly in later disease stages, although there certainly is a bias introduced by the enrichment for patients with a longer survival at later time points. Longitudinal sampling shows a tendency to lower levels upon follow up, especially in fast-progressing patients (67).

CONCLUSION

Evidence is emerging that NF levels can become valuable biomarker for ALS, both for diagnosing ALS, for predicting outcome, and potentially for the monitoring of treatment effects. The CSF pNfH level seems to be the most accurate diagnostic marker, but both pNfH and NfL serum or plasma measurements perform good to predict survival and disease progression. Further research is needed to establish the value of NF levels for stratification and for disease monitoring in clinical trials.

AUTHOR CONTRIBUTIONS

All authors listed have made a substantial, direct and intellectual contribution to the work, and approved it for publication.

ACKNOWLEDGMENTS

PV is supported by grants from KU Leuven (C14/17/107), Opening the Future Fund (KU Leuven), the Interuniversity Attraction Poles (IUAP) program P7/16 of the Belgian Federal Science Policy Office, the Alzheimer Research Foundation (SAO-FRA), the Flemish Government initiated Flanders Impulse Program on Networks for Dementia Research (VIND), the Fund for Scientific Research Vlaanderen (FWO-Vlaanderen), under the frame of E-RARE-2 (PYRAMID) and JPND (STRENGTH and RiMod-FTD), the ALS Liga België and the KU Leuven funds Een Hart voor ALS and Laeversfonds voor ALS Onderzoek. PV holds a senior clinical investigatorship from FWO-Vlaanderen.

REFERENCES

1. Hardiman O, Al-Chalabi A, Chio A, Corr EM, Logroscino G, Robberecht W, et al. Amyotrophic lateral sclerosis. *Nat Rev Dis Primers* (2017) 3:17085. doi: 10.1038/nrdp.2017.85
2. Brooks BR, Miller RG, Swash M, Munsat TL. El Escorial revisited: revised criteria for the diagnosis of amyotrophic lateral sclerosis. *Amyotroph Lateral Scler Other Motor Neuron Disord.* (2000) 1:293–9. doi: 10.1080/146608200300079536
3. de Carvalho M, Dengler R, Eisen A, England JD, Kaji R, Kimura J, et al. Electrodiagnostic criteria for diagnosis of ALS. *Clin Neurophysiol.* (2008) 119:497–503. doi: 10.1016/j.clinph.2007.09.143
4. Schrooten M, Smetcoren C, Robberecht W, Van Damme P. Benefit of the Awaji diagnostic algorithm for amyotrophic lateral sclerosis: a prospective study. *Ann Neurol.* (2011) 70:79–83. doi: 10.1002/ana.22380
5. Paganoni S, Macklin EA, Lee A, Murphy A, Chang J, Zipf A, et al. Diagnostic timelines and delays in diagnosing amyotrophic lateral sclerosis (ALS). *Amyotr Lateral Scler Frontotem Degener.* (2014) 15:453–6. doi: 10.3109/21678421.2014.903974
6. Westeneng HJ, Debray TPA, Visser AE, van Eijk RPA, Rooney JPK, Calvo A, et al. Prognosis for patients with amyotrophic lateral sclerosis: development and validation of a personalised prediction model. *Lancet Neurol.* (2018) 17:423–33. doi: 10.1016/S1474-4422(18)30089-9
7. Turner MR, Kiernan MC, Leigh PN, Talbot K. Biomarkers in amyotrophic lateral sclerosis. *Lancet Neurol.* (2009) 8:94–109. doi: 10.1016/S1474-4422(08)70293-X
8. Bacioglu M, Maia LF, Preische O, Schelle J, Apel A, Kaeser SA, et al. Neurofilament light chain in blood and CSF as marker of disease progression in mouse models and in neurodegenerative diseases. *Neuron* (2016) 91:56–66. doi: 10.1016/j.neuron.2016.05.018
9. Lee MK, Cleveland DW. Neuronal intermediate filaments. *Ann Rev Neurosci.* (1996) 19:187–217. doi: 10.1146/annurev.ne.19.030196.001155
10. Yuan A, Rao MV, Veeranna, Nixon RA. Neurofilaments and neurofilament proteins in health and disease. *Cold Spring Harbor Perspect Biol.* (2017) 9:4. doi: 10.1101/cshperspect.a018309
11. Hoyle JC, Isfort MC, Roggenbuck J, Arnold WD. The genetics of Charcot-Marie-Tooth disease: current trends and future implications for diagnosis and management. *Appl Clin Genet.* (2015) 8:235–43. doi: 10.2147/TACG.S69969
12. Figlewicz DA, Krizus A, Martinoli MG, Meininger V, Dib M, Rouleau GA, et al. Variants of the heavy neurofilament subunit are associated with the development of amyotrophic lateral sclerosis. *Hum Mol Genet.* (1994) 3:1757–61. doi: 10.1093/hmg/3.10.1757
13. Julien JP. Amyotrophic lateral sclerosis. unfolding the toxicity of the misfolded. *Cell* (2001) 104:581–91. doi: 10.1016/S0092-8674(01)00244-6
14. Hirano A, Nakano I, Kurland LT, Mulder DW, Holley PW, Saccomanno G. Fine structural study of neurofibrillary changes in a family with amyotrophic lateral sclerosis. *J Neuropathol Exp Neurol.* (1984) 43:471–80. doi: 10.1097/00005072-198409000-00002
15. Wong NK, He BP, Strong MJ. Characterization of neuronal intermediate filament protein expression in cervical spinal motor neurons in sporadic amyotrophic lateral sclerosis (ALS). *J Neuropathol Exp Neurol.* (2000) 59:972–82. doi: 10.1093/jnen/59.11.972
16. Meier J, Couillard-Despres S, Jacomy H, Gravel C, Julien JP. Extra neurofilament NF-L subunits rescue motor neuron disease caused by overexpression of the human NF-H gene in mice. *J Neuropathol Exp Neurol.* (1999) 58:1099–110. doi: 10.1097/00005072-199910000-00009
17. Williamson TL, Bruijn LI, Zhu Q, Anderson KL, Anderson SD, Julien JP, et al. Absence of neurofilaments reduces the selective vulnerability of motor neurons and slows disease caused by a familial amyotrophic lateral sclerosis-linked superoxide dismutase 1 mutant. *Proc Natl Acad Sci USA.* (1998) 95:9631–6. doi: 10.1073/pnas.95.16.9631
18. Couillard-Despres S, Zhu Q, Wong PC, Price DL, Cleveland DW, Julien JP. Protective effect of neurofilament heavy gene overexpression in motor neuron disease induced by mutant superoxide dismutase. *Proc Natl Acad Sci USA.* (1998) 95:9626–30. doi: 10.1073/pnas.95.16.9626
19. Lu CH, Petzold A, Kalmar B, Dick J, Malaspina A, Greensmith L. Plasma neurofilament heavy chain levels correlate to markers of late stage disease progression and treatment response in SOD1(G93A) mice that model ALS. *PLoS ONE* (2012) 7:e40998. doi: 10.1371/journal.pone.0040998
20. Boylan K, Yang C, Crook J, Overstreet K, Heckman M, Wang Y, et al. Immunoreactivity of the phosphorylated axonal neurofilament H subunit (pNF-H) in blood of ALS model rodents and ALS patients: evaluation of blood pNF-H as a potential ALS biomarker. *J Neurochem.* (2009) 111:1182–91. doi: 10.1111/j.1471-4159.2009.06386.x
21. Gaetani L, Hoglund K, Parnetti L, Pujol-Calderon F, Becker B, Eusebi P, et al. A new enzyme-linked immunosorbent assay for neurofilament light in cerebrospinal fluid: analytical validation and clinical evaluation. *Alzheimers Res Ther.* (2018) 10:8. doi: 10.1186/s13195-018-0339-1
22. Koel-Simmelink MJ, Vennegoor A, Killestein J, Blankenstein MA, Norgren N, Korth C, et al. The impact of pre-analytical variables on the stability of neurofilament proteins in CSF, determined by a novel validated

SinglePlex Luminex assay and ELISA. *J Immunol Methods* (2014) 402:43–9. doi: 10.1016/j.jim.2013.11.008

23. Poesen K, De Schaepdryver M, Stubendorff B, Gille B, Muckova P, Wendler S, et al. Neurofilament markers for ALS correlate with extent of upper and lower motor neuron disease. *Neurology* (2017) 88:2302–9. doi: 10.1212/WNL.0000000000004029
24. Ganesalingam J, An J, Shaw CE, Shaw G, Lacomis D, Bowser R. Combination of neurofilament heavy chain and complement C3 as CSF biomarkers for ALS. *J Neurochem* (2011) 117:528–37. doi: 10.1111/j.1471-4159.2011.07224.x
25. Petzold A, Keir G, Green AJ, Giovannoni G, Thompson EJ. A specific ELISA for measuring neurofilament heavy chain phosphoforms. *J Immunol Methods* (2003) 278:179–90. doi: 10.1016/S0022-1759(03)00189-3
26. Petzold A, Shaw G. Comparison of two ELISA methods for measuring levels of the phosphorylated neurofilament heavy chain. *J Immunol Methods* (2007) 319:34–40. doi: 10.1016/j.jim.2006.09.021
27. Shaw G, Yang C, Ellis R, Anderson K, Parker Mickle J, Scheff S, et al. Hyperphosphorylated neurofilament NF-H is a serum biomarker of axonal injury. *Biochem Biophys Res Commun.* (2005) 336:1268–77. doi: 10.1016/j.bbrc.2005.08.252
28. Norgren N, Karlsson JE, Rosengren L, Stigbrand T. Monoclonal antibodies selective for low molecular weight neurofilaments. *Hybridoma Hybridom.* (2002) 21:53–9. doi: 10.1089/15368590252917647
29. Kuhle J, Barro C, Andreasson U, Derfuss T, Lindberg R, Sandelius A, et al. Comparison of three analytical platforms for quantification of the neurofilament light chain in blood samples: ELISA, electrochemiluminescence immunoassay and Simoa. *Clin Chem Lab Med.* (2016) 54:1655–61. doi: 10.1515/cclm-2015-1195
30. Steinacker P, Feneberg E, Weishaupt J, Brettschneider J, Tumani H, Andersen PM, et al. Neurofilaments in the diagnosis of motoneuron diseases: a prospective study on 455 patients. *J Neurol Neurosurg Psychiatry* (2016) 87:12–20. doi: 10.1136/jnnp-2015-311387
31. Feneberg E, Oeckl P, Steinacker P, Verde F, Barro C, Van Damme P, et al. Multicenter evaluation of neurofilaments in early symptom onset amyotrophic lateral sclerosis. *Neurology* (2018) 90:e22–e30. doi: 10.1212/WNL.0000000000004761
32. Li DW, Ren H, Jeromin A, Liu M, Shen D, Tai H, et al. Diagnostic performance of neurofilaments in chinese patients with amyotrophic lateral sclerosis: a prospective study. *Front Neurol.* (2018) 9:726. doi: 10.3389/fneur.2018.00726
33. Verde F, Steinacker P, Weishaupt JH, Kassubek J, Oeckl P, Halbgebauer S, et al. Neurofilament light chain in serum for the diagnosis of amyotrophic lateral sclerosis. *J Neurol Neurosurg Psychiatry* (2018). doi: 10.1136/jnnp-2018-318704. [Epub ahead of print].
34. Gille B, De Schaepdryver M, Goossens J, Dedeene L, De Vocht J, Oldoni E, et al. Serum neurofilament light chain levels as a marker of upper motor neuron degeneration in patients with amyotrophic lateral sclerosis. *Neuropathol Appl Neurobiol.* (2018). doi: 10.1111/nan.12511. [Epub ahead of print].
35. Reijn TS, Abdo WF, Schelhaas HJ, Verbeek MM. CSF neurofilament protein analysis in the differential diagnosis of ALS. *J Neurol.* (2009) 256:615–9. doi: 10.1007/s00415-009-0131-z
36. Goldstein ME, Sternberger LA, Sternberger NH. Varying degrees of phosphorylation determine microheterogeneity of the heavy neurofilament polypeptide (Nf-H). *J Neuroimmunol.* (1987) 14:135–48. doi: 10.1016/0165-5728(87)90048-8
37. Brettschneider J, Petzold A, Sussmuth SD, Ludolph AC, Tumani H. Axonal damage markers in cerebrospinal fluid are increased in ALS. *Neurology* (2006) 66:852–6. doi: 10.1212/01.wnl.0000203120.85850.54
38. Kuhle J, Regeniter A, Leppert D, Mehling M, Kappos L, Lindberg RL, et al. A highly sensitive electrochemiluminescence immunoassay for the neurofilament heavy chain protein. *J Neuroimmunol.* (2010) 220:114–9. doi: 10.1016/j.jneuroim.2010.01.004
39. De Schaepdryver M, Jeromin A, Gille B, Claeys KG, Herbst V, Brix B, et al. Comparison of elevated phosphorylated neurofilament heavy chains in serum and cerebrospinal fluid of patients with amyotrophic lateral sclerosis. *J Neurol Neurosurg Psychiatry* (2017). 89:367–73. doi: 10.1136/jnnp-2017-316605
40. Weydt P, Oeckl P, Huss A, Muller K, Volk AE, Kuhle J, et al. Neurofilament levels as biomarkers in asymptomatic and symptomatic familial amyotrophic lateral sclerosis. *Ann Neurol.* (2016) 79:152–8. doi: 10.1002/ana.24552
41. Rosengren LE, Karlsson JE, Karlsson JO, Persson LI, Wikkelso C. Patients with amyotrophic lateral sclerosis and other neurodegenerative diseases have increased levels of neurofilament protein in CSF. *J Neurochem.* (1996) 67:2013–8. doi: 10.1046/j.1471-4159.1996.67052013.x
42. Xu Z, Henderson RD, David M, McCombe PA. Neurofilaments as biomarkers for amyotrophic lateral sclerosis: a systematic review and meta-analysis. *PLoS ONE* (2016) 11:e0164625. doi: 10.1371/journal.pone.0164625
43. Zetterberg H, Jacobsson J, Rosengren L, Blennow K, Andersen PM. Cerebrospinal fluid neurofilament light levels in amyotrophic lateral sclerosis: impact of SOD1 genotype. *Eur J Neurol.* (2007) 14:1329–33. doi: 10.1111/j.1468-1331.2007.01972.x
44. Gaiottino J, Norgren N, Dobson R, Topping J, Nissim A, Malaspina A, et al. Increased neurofilament light chain blood levels in neurodegenerative neurological diseases. *PLoS ONE* (2013) 8:e75091. doi: 10.1371/journal.pone.0075091
45. Lu CH, Macdonald-Wallis C, Gray E, Pearce N, Petzold A, Norgren N, et al. Neurofilament light chain: a prognostic biomarker in amyotrophic lateral sclerosis. *Neurology* (2015) 84:2247–57. doi: 10.1212/WNL.0000000000001642
46. Tortelli R, Ruggieri M, Cortese R, D'Errico E, Capozzo R, Leo A, et al. Elevated cerebrospinal fluid neurofilament light levels in patients with amyotrophic lateral sclerosis: a possible marker of disease severity and progression. *Eur J Neurol.* (2012) 19:1561–7. doi: 10.1111/j.1468-1331.2012.03777.x
47. Tortelli R, Copetti M, Ruggieri M, Cortese R, Capozzo R, Leo A, et al. Cerebrospinal fluid neurofilament light chain levels: marker of progression to generalized amyotrophic lateral sclerosis. *Eur J Neurol.* (2015) 22:215–8. doi: 10.1111/ene.12421
48. Menke RA, Gray E, Lu CH, Kuhle J, Talbot K, Malaspina A, et al. CSF neurofilament light chain reflects corticospinal tract degeneration in ALS. *Ann Clin Trans Neurol.* (2015) 2:748–55. doi: 10.1002/acn3.212
49. Oeckl P, Jardel C, Salachas F, Lamari F, Andersen PM, Bowser R, et al. Multicenter validation of CSF neurofilaments as diagnostic biomarkers for ALS. *Amyotr Later Scler Frontotemp Degen.* (2016) 17:404–13. doi: 10.3109/21678421.2016.1167913
50. Boylan KB, Glass JD, Crook JE, Yang C, Thomas CS, Desaro P, et al. Phosphorylated neurofilament heavy subunit (pNF-H) in peripheral blood and CSF as a potential prognostic biomarker in amyotrophic lateral sclerosis. *J Neurol Neurosurg Psychiatry* (2013) 84:467–72. doi: 10.1136/jnnp-2012-303768
51. Gendron TF, Group CONS, Daughrity LM, Heckman MG, Diehl NN, Wuu J, et al. Phosphorylated neurofilament heavy chain: A biomarker of survival for C9ORF72-associated amyotrophic lateral sclerosis. *Ann Neurol.* (2017) 82:139–46. doi: 10.1002/ana.24980
52. Lehnert S, Costa J, de Carvalho M, Kirby J, Kuzma-Kozakiewicz M, Morelli C, et al. Multicentre quality control evaluation of different biomarker candidates for amyotrophic lateral sclerosis. *Amyotr Later Scler Frontotemp Degen.* (2014) 15:344–50. doi: 10.3109/21678421.2014.884592
53. McCombe PA, Pfluger C, Singh P, Lim CY, Airey C, Henderson RD. Serial measurements of phosphorylated neurofilament-heavy in the serum of subjects with amyotrophic lateral sclerosis. *J Neurol Sci.* (2015) 353:122–9. doi: 10.1016/j.jns.2015.04.032
54. Li S, Ren Y, Zhu W, Yang F, Zhang X, Huang X. Phosphorylated neurofilament heavy chain levels in paired plasma and CSF of amyotrophic lateral sclerosis. *J Neurol Sci.* (2016) 367:269–74. doi: 10.1016/j.jns.2016.05.062
55. Chen X, Chen Y, Wei Q, Ou R, Cao B, Zhao B, et al. Assessment of a multiple biomarker panel for diagnosis of amyotrophic lateral sclerosis. *BMC Neurol.* (2016) 16:173. doi: 10.1186/s12883-016-0689-x
56. Oeckl P, Steinacker P, Otto M. Comparison of internal standard approaches for SRM analysis of alpha-synuclein in cerebrospinal fluid. *J Proteome Res.* (2018) 17:516–23. doi: 10.1021/acs.jproteome.7b00660
57. Leinenbach A, Pannee J, Dulffer T, Huber A, Bittner T, Andreasson U, et al. Mass spectrometry-based candidate reference measurement procedure for quantification of amyloid-beta in cerebrospinal fluid. *Clin Chem.* (2014) 60:987–94. doi: 10.1373/clinchem.2013.220392

58. Andreasson U, Kuhlmann J, Pannee J, Umek RM, Stoops E, Vanderstichele H, et al. Commutability of the certified reference materials for the standardization of beta-amyloid 1–42 assay in human cerebrospinal fluid: lessons for tau and beta-amyloid 1–40 measurements. *Clin Chem Lab Med.* (2018). 56:2058–66. doi: 10.1515/cclm-2018-0147
59. Gille B, Dedeene L, Stoops E, Demeyer L, Francois C, Lefever S, et al. Automation on an Open-Access Platform of Alzheimer's Disease Biomarker Immunoassays. *SLAS Technol.* (2018) 23:188–97. doi: 10.1177/2472630317750378
60. Benatar M, Wuu J, Andersen PM, Lombardi V, Malaspina A. Neurofilament light: a candidate biomarker of presymptomatic amyotrophic lateral sclerosis and phenoconversion. *Ann Neurol.* (2018) 84:130–9. doi: 10.1002/ana.25276
61. Gaiani A, Martinelli I, Bello L, Querin G, Puthenparampil M, Ruggero S, et al. Diagnostic and prognostic biomarkers in amyotrophic lateral sclerosis: neurofilament light chain levels in definite subtypes of disease. *JAMA Neurol.* (2017) 74:525–32. doi: 10.1001/jamaneurol.2016.5398
62. Chio A, Ilardi A, Cammarosano S, Moglia C, Montuschi A, Calvo A. Neurobehavioral dysfunction in ALS has a negative effect on outcome and use of PEG and NIV. *Neurology* (2012) 78:1085–9. doi: 10.1212/WNL.0b013e31824e8f53
63. Elamin M, Bede P, Byrne S, Jordan N, Gallagher L, Wynne B, et al. Cognitive changes predict functional decline in ALS: a population-based longitudinal study. *Neurology* (2013) 80:1590–7. doi: 10.1212/WNL.0b013e31828f18ac
64. Illan-Gala I, Alcolea D, Montal V, Dols-Icardo O, Munoz L, de Luna N, et al. CSF sAPPbeta, YKL-40, and NfL along the ALS-FTD spectrum. *Neurology* (2018) 91:e1619–e28. doi: 10.1212/WNL.0000000000006383
65. McCampbell A, Cole T, Wegener AJ, Tomassy GS, Setnicka A, Farley BJ, et al. Antisense oligonucleotides extend survival and reverse decrement in muscle response in ALS models. *J Clin Invest.* (2018) 128:3558–67. doi: 10.1172/JCI99081
66. Disanto G, Barro C, Benkert P, Naegelin Y, Schadelin S, Giardiello A, et al. Serum neurofilament light: a biomarker of neuronal damage in multiple sclerosis. *Ann Neurol.* (2017) 81:857–70. doi: 10.1002/ana.24954
67. Lu CH, Petzold A, Topping J, Allen K, Macdonald-Wallis C, Clarke J, et al. Plasma neurofilament heavy chain levels and disease progression in amyotrophic lateral sclerosis: insights from a longitudinal study. *J Neurol Neurosurg Psychiatry* (2015) 86:565–73. doi: 10.1136/jnnp-2014-307672

10

Increased Interleukin-6 Levels in the Astrocyte-Derived Exosomes of Sporadic Amyotrophic Lateral Sclerosis Patients

*Yong Chen[1], Kailin Xia[1], Lu Chen[1] and Dongsheng Fan[1,2]**

[1] Department of Neurology, Peking University Third Hospital, Beijing, China,

[2] Key Laboratory for Neuroscience, Ministry of Education/National Health Commission, Peking University, Beijing, China

***Correspondence:**
Dongsheng Fan
dsfan2010@aliyun.com

Neuroinflammation plays an important role in amyotrophic lateral sclerosis (ALS) pathogenesis. However, it is difficult to evaluate inflammation of the central nervous system (CNS) or the relationship between neuroinflammation and disease progression in ALS patients. Recent advances in the field of exosomes and CNS-derived exosomes extraction technology provide the possibility of measuring the inflammatory status in the CNS without brain biopsy. In this pilot study, we extracted astrocyte-derived exosomes from the plasma of sporadic ALS patients and age-, sex-matched healthy controls and determined Interleukin-6 (IL-6) levels by an enzyme-linked immunosorbent assay (ELISA). The IL-6 levels in astrocyte-derived exosomes were increased in sALS patients and positively associated with the rate of disease progression. However, the association between IL-6 levels and disease progression rate was limited to patients whose disease duration were less than 12 months. These data suggest an increased inflammatory cascade in the CNS of sALS patients. Our pilot study demonstrates that CNS-derived exosomes could be useful to reveal neuroinflammation of the CNS in ALS patients.

Keywords: amyotrophic lateral sclerosis, astrocytes, exosomes, disease progress, interleukin-6

INTRODUCTION

Amyotrophic lateral sclerosis (ALS) is a rare, progressive neurodegenerative disease that affects upper and lower motor neurons and leads to fatal paralysis (Brown and Al-Chalabi, 2017). Ultimately, most ALS patients die within 3–5 years after disease onset due to respiratory failure. Approximately 90–95% of ALS cases are the sporadic type (sALS), and the remaining cases are the familial type (fALS). To date, more than 20 genes that cause fALS and sALS have been identified (Brown and Al-Chalabi, 2017). Scientific advances in genetic studies in the ALS field have improved our understanding of ALS pathogenesis. However, the exact etiology and pathogenesis of ALS are still unknown. As a result, there is no effective treatment for the disease. Riluzole and edaravone are the only two approved drugs for the treatment of ALS, and they solely delay disease progression for several months (Kumar et al., 2016; Rothstein, 2017).

Numerous intrinsic and extrinsic factors are involved in ALS motor neuron degeneration. One possible factor involved in motor neuron degeneration in ALS is neuroinflammation. Accumulating evidence indicates that ALS patients have chronic inflammation, as demonstrated by activated microglia and astrocytes, as well as infiltration of peripheral monocytes and lymphocytes into the CNS (Zhao et al., 2013; Liu and Wang, 2017). Increased serum/plasma and CSF levels of some cytokines, such as tumor necrosis factor-alpha (TNF-α), interleukin-6 (IL-6), IL-8, and interferon-beta (IFN-β), have been detected in ALS patients when compared to controls (Ono et al., 2001; Mitchell et al., 2009; Fiala et al., 2010; Mitchell et al., 2010; Italiani et al., 2014; Ehrhart et al., 2015; Liu et al., 2015; Hu et al., 2017). Beyond demonstrating ongoing inflammatory processes in ALS patients, these inflammatory biomarkers could also be used as diagnostic and prognostic biomarkers for clinical use because they have been reported to distinguish ALS from healthy or disease controls (Vu and Bowser, 2017; Gonzalez-Garza et al., 2018) and to predict the disease prognosis (Su et al., 2013; Liu et al., 2015). Activated microglia and astrocytes in the CNS play a vital role in the neuroinflammation process in ALS patients; however, the determination of the inflammatory biomarkers in serum/plasma and CSF only indirectly reflects the status of the CNS. Recently, scientific advances in the field of exosomes and CNS-derived exosome extraction technology have provided the possibility of measuring the inflammatory status in the CNS without brain biopsy.

Exosomes are approximately 30–100 nm extracellular vesicles with lipid bilayer membranes that are secreted by almost all types of cells, including neurons, microglia and astrocytes (Raposo and Stoorvogel, 2013; Yanez-Mo et al., 2015). Exosomes contain proteins, lipids and RNA and transfer them between cells. Therefore, exosomes play an important role in intercellular communication. Moreover, different cell types can secrete exosomes with different biomarkers, which could help to identify the exosome source (Beninson and Fleshner, 2014). Due to their specific characteristics, exosomes have attracted large amounts of attention in various studies ranging from mechanistic analyses to clinical research (Jarmalaviciute and Pivoriunas, 2016; Goh et al., 2017). In addition, exosomes can cross the blood-brain barrier (BBB) from both directions. As a result, CNS-derived exosomes can be detected in the blood and may help to reveal the pathophysiology of brain diseases without the use of brain biopsy and CSF analysis (Mustapic et al., 2017). In recent studies, several strategies to extract CNS-derived exosomes from peripheral blood have been reported (Mustapic et al., 2017; Kuwano et al., 2018). However, CNS-derived exosome-based studies focusing on ALS have not been previously reported.

Based on the above information, we hypothesized that inflammatory biomarkers in astrocyte-derived exosomes (ADEs) may increase and may be associated with clinical features in ALS patients. In this pilot study, we extracted ADEs from the plasma of sporadic ALS patients and age-, sex-matched healthy controls to determine the IL-6 levels in ADEs and, ultimately, we detected increased IL-6 levels in ADEs of sALS patients, which were positively associated with the rate of disease progression.

PARTICIPANTS AND METHODS

Participants

This study was approved by the Ethics Committee of the Perking University Third Hospital, Beijing, China. All ALS patients and age-, sex-matched healthy control individuals signed the informed consent before peripheral blood samples were drawn. Patients and controls were recruited from the Department of Neurology of Perking University Third Hospital. Clinically definite and probable sALS patients were diagnosed based on the El Escorial revised criteria (Brooks et al., 2000) and further evaluated by the revised ALS functional rating scale (ALSFRS-R) (Cedarbaum et al., 1999). The rate of disease progression (ΔFS) was calculated as follows: ΔFS = (48 -ALSFRS-R at "time of diagnosis")/duration from onset to diagnosis (month) (Kimura et al., 2006).

Plasma Sampling in ALS Patients and Controls

Samples containing two milliliters of peripheral blood from ALS patients and healthy control individuals were collected into EDTA tubes. To extract plasma, blood samples were centrifuged at 1500 *g* for 10 min to remove blood cells. Then, the supernatant was subjected to another centrifugation at 2500 *g* for 20 min to remove the platelets and cell debris. Finally, the plasma was stored at −80°C until use.

Extraction of ADEs From Plasma

The method to extract the ADEs from plasma was modified from a previously published article (Mustapic et al., 2017). Briefly, 0.25 ml plasma was incubated with 0.2 μl thromboplastin (System Biosciences, Mountain View, CA, United States) for 5 min. Then, 298 μl calcium- and magnesium-free Dulbecco's Balanced Salt Solution (DBS^{-2}) was added with protease inhibitor cocktail (Roche, Indianapolis, IN) and phosphatase inhibitor cocktail (Thermo Fisher Scientific), followed by centrifugation at 10,000 rpm for 5 min at 4°C. The supernatants were harvested, followed by addition of 126 μl per tube of ExoQuick (System Biosciences, Mountain View, CA, United States). After a second centrifugation at 1500 g for 30 min at 4°C, total exosomes were harvested by removing the supernatant. To enrich ADEs, total exosomes were resuspended in 250 μl of ddH_2O with protease inhibitor cocktail and phosphatase inhibitor cocktail and incubated for at least 120 min at 4°C. Then, 1.5 μg biotinylated mouse anti-human glutamine aspartate transporter (ACSA-1) antibody (Miltenyi Biotec, Auburn, CA, United States) in 50 ml of 3% bovine serum albumin (BSA; 1:3.33 dilution of Blocker BSA 10% solution in DBS^{-2}; Thermo Fisher Scientific) was added per tube and mixed for 60 min at room temperature, followed by the addition of 10 μl streptavidin-agarose Ultralink resin (Thermo Fisher Scientific) in 40 ml 3% BSA and incubation with mixing for another 20 min at room temperature. After centrifugation at 400 *g* for 10 min at 4°C, the supernatant was removed, and each pellet was suspended in 200 μl cold 0.1 M glycine-HCl (pH = 3.0) by gentle mixing for 10 s and centrifugation at 4,500 *g* for 5 min. The supernatants were then harvested, and 25 μl of 3% BSA and 15 μl of 1 M Tris-HCl (pH = 8.0) were added. Finally, 260 μl mammalian protein extraction reagent (M-PER, Thermo Fisher Scientific) was added, and the solution was mixed. The resultant 0.5 ml lysates of ADEs were stored at −80°C. Evidence for enrichment of exosomes from neural sources in plasma has been demonstrated previously (Mustapic et al., 2017).

Measurement of IL-6 Levels in ADEs and Plasma

Astrocyte-derived exosome proteins were quantified using a single-plex high-sensitivity and high-dynamic-range ELISA for IL-6 (Rockville, MD, United States Cat# K151AKC) (Chaturvedi et al., 2015) and by using enzyme-linked immunosorbent assay (ELISA) kits for the tetra-spanning exosome marker CD81 (Cusabio Technology, Wuhan, China), according to the suppliers' directions. The mean value for all determinations of CD81 in each assay group was set at 1.00, and the relative values for each sample were used to normalize their recovery. The plasma IL-6 levels in both groups were also measured. The protein levels were measured by board-certified laboratory technicians who were blinded to the clinical information.

To ensure the specificity of the tests, negative control groups were set up in this study. In the negative control group one, the biotinylated anti-ACSA-1 antibody was replaced with 3% BSA. In the negative control group two, the total exosomes solution resuspended from ExoQuick pellet was replaced by ddH2O.

Statistical Analyses

Data are presented as numbers, means and standard deviations, or medians (interquartile range, IQR) as appropriate. Normal distributions of datasets were assessed by the Shapiro–Wilks test. Unpaired Student *t*-tests, χ^2 test or one-way ANOVA, followed by Tukey analysis, were used to examine differences between groups. Pearson's correlation was used for statistical correlation analysis. The differences between groups were considered significant if the *p*-value was less than 0.05 (two-tailed). All statistical analyses and graphs were performed using GraphPad Prism 6 (GraphPad Software Inc., San Diego, United States).

RESULTS

In this pilot study, 40 ALS patients and 39 healthy controls were recruited. The detailed clinical information for these two groups are summarized in **Table 1**. The ALS patients and controls were comparable, as there was no difference in age or sex ratio between the two groups. Of the 40 ALS patients, 12 were bulbar onset and 28 were limber onset; 10 ALS cases were diagnosed as definite, and the remainder were probable. The median delay of diagnosis for all patients was 9.23 months. The mean ALSFRS-R score for the patients was 39.83 ± 1.08, and the median disease progression rate was 0.56. The extracted ADEs were validated by western blot. The result showed that the ADEs were positive for CD63, but negative for calnexin (**Supplementary Figure S1**). The ADEs were also verified by transmission electron microscope (**Supplementary Figure S2**). In the CD81 and IL-6 test, the negative control group one and two were all at background levels. The CD81-normalized levels of IL-6 in ADEs were significantly higher in ALS patients (40.40 ± 2.11 pg/ml) than in controls (22.45 ± 1.90 pg/ml) (**Figure 1A**). However, among 40 ALS patients and 39 healthy controls, the IL-6 was detectable only in 12 controls and 15 ALS patients. There was no difference in detection rate between the two groups. The plasma IL-6 levels ranged from 0.13 to 4.58 pg/mL in controls and 0.39 to 15.69 pg/ml in ALS patients (**Supplementary Figure S3A**). There was no difference in plasma IL-6 levels between controls and ALS patients ($p = 0.3614$) and there was no correlation between IL-6 levels in plasma and ADEs ($r = 0.3384$, $p = 0.2173$ for ALS group; $r = -0.2657$, $p = 0.4038$ for control group; **Supplementary Figures S3B,C**).

The ALS patients were further divided into subgroups according to the following: onset site: bulbar onset (ALS-B) or limber onset (ALS-L); diagnosis level: definite (ALS-D) or probable (ALS-P); and disease duration: less than 12 months (ALS < 12) or greater than or equal to 12 months (ALS ≥ 12). As shown in **Figures 1B–D**, compared with the control group, the levels of IL-6 in ADEs were increased in all ALS subgroups. However, there was no difference between the ALS subgroups.

The correlations of the levels of IL-6 in ADEs with clinical parameters are shown in **Figure 2**. The IL-6 levels correlated positively with the disease progression rate ($r = 0.4696$, $p = 0.002$). However, IL-6 levels in the ADEs of ALS patients did not correlate with total ALSFRS-R scores ($r = -0.2021$, $p = 0.2110$), diagnosis delay ($r = -0.1735$, $p = 0.2845$) or patient age ($r = -0.1087$, $p = 0.5560$). In controls, IL-6 levels also did not correlate with age (data not shown). When the patients were separated into two groups according disease duration (ALS < 12 m or ALS ≥ 12 m), a positive correlation between IL-6 levels and disease progression was only verified in the ALS < 12 m group ($r = 0.6605$, $p = 0.015$) (**Figure 3A**) but not in the ALS ≥ 12 m group ($r = 0.3510$, $p = 0.1291$) (**Figure 3B**).

DISCUSSION

The present study demonstrated that the levels of IL-6 in ADEs of sALS patients were increased and positively associated with the rate of disease progression, especially in patients at an earlier disease stage. These data suggest that the inflammatory cascade is augmented in the CNS of sALS patients. Analysis of CNS-derived exosomes in peripheral blood has recently attracted immense attention. Numerous studies have demonstrated that CNS-derived exosomes could be helpful to understand the

TABLE 1 | Characteristics of ALS patients and healthy controls.

	Control	ALS	*p*
Cases (male/female)	39 (25/14)	40 (26/14)	1
Age (mean ± SE)	55.74 ± 1.32	54.35 ± 2.02	0.57
Onset site: bulbar/limb	NA	12/28	NA
Diagnosis delay (months)	NA	9.23 (9.68)	NA
Definite/probable	NA	10/30	NA
ALSFRS-R	NA	39.83 ± 1.08	NA
ΔFS	NA	0.56 (0.71)	NA
IL-6 (pg/ml)	22.45 ± 1.90	40.40 ± 2.11	<0.001

Diagnosis delay, interval from the initial symptoms to diagnosis; ALSFRS-R, revised amyotrophic lateral sclerosis functional rating scale; ΔFS, disease progression rate.

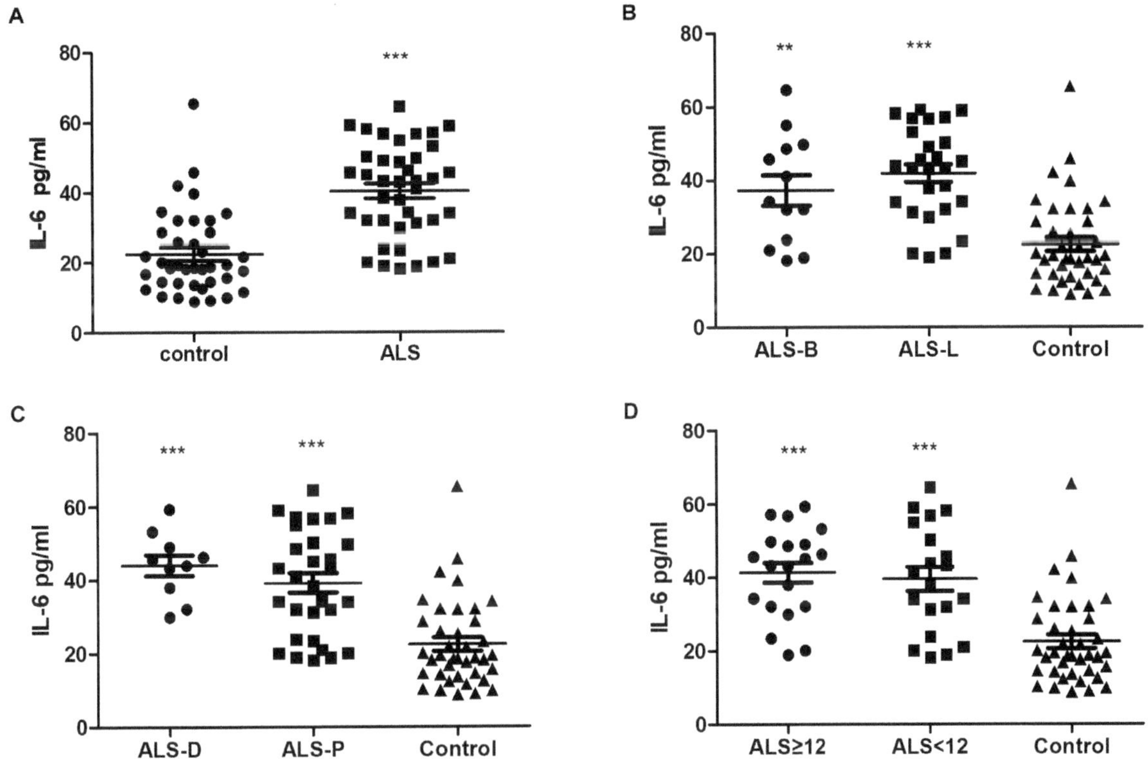

FIGURE 1 | Comparison IL-6 levels in ADEs from plasma of ALS and healthy subjects. Panels **(A–D)** show the levels of IL-6 in ADEs of **(A)** ALS patients and controls; **(B)** ALS patients with bulbar (ALS-B) or limb onset (ALS-L) and controls; **(C)** definite ALS (ALS-D) or probable ALS (ALS-P) and controls; **(D)** ALS duration ≥ 12 months (ALS ≥ 12) or <12 months (ALS < 12) and controls. **, *** indicate $p < 0.01$ and $p < 0.001$, respectively, compared with controls.

pathophysiology of brain disease and the identification of biomarkers (Abner et al., 2016; Winston et al., 2016; Goetzl et al., 2018; Ohmichi et al., 2018). However, to our knowledge, no studies have been reported on CNS-derived exosomes in ALS patients. Therefore, our pilot study is the first to demonstrate that CNS-derived exosomes could be useful to reveal the pathophysiology of CNS in ALS patients.

Several inflammatory biomarkers have been found to be linked to ALS. As a well-known cytokine, IL-6 has been extensively investigated in neurodegenerative disorders and associated with ALS in numerous studies (Sekizawa et al., 1998; Ehrhart et al., 2015; Lu et al., 2016; Blasco et al., 2017; Hu et al., 2017). However, the results are not consistent across all studies (Moreau et al., 2005; Tanaka et al., 2006). In addition, one study reported an increase in IL-6 levels at the late stage of disease (Lu et al., 2016), whereas another study reported that the levels of IL-6 were high at disease onset followed by a subsequent decline (Ehrhart et al., 2015). The plasma IL-6 levels were also measured in this study. However, the IL-6 was detectable in only 12 controls and 15 ALS patients and undetectable in most of the samples. Among the 12 controls and 15 ALS patients, the IL-6 levels were highly variable and no difference has been found between the two groups. The highly variable plasma IL-6 levels in our study and the contradictory results from previous studies indicate that the peripheral IL-6 levels may be influenced by complex factors. A recent study showed that the levels of IL-6 in blood could be influenced by aging and respiratory dysfunction in ALS (Pronto-Laborinho et al., 2019). Thus, determining the IL-6 levels in blood may not be a good way. CNS-derived exosomes could directly reflect the situation in the CNS, and peripheral factors might have little effect on cytokines in CNS-derived exosomes. Therefore, the measurement of IL-6 levels in CNS-derived exosomes, compared with blood or CSF, may be better to illuminate the actual role of IL-6 in ALS. Astrocytes have been reported play an important role in the pathogenesis of ALS, and the predominant CNS source of IL-6 is the activated astrocyte (Van Wagoner and Benveniste, 1999). Hence, in this pilot study, we chose to measure IL-6 levels in ADEs. Compared with the plasma IL-6 levels, the IL-6 levels in ADEs were relatively high and stable and the IL-6 levels in the ADEs didn't correlate with age. Moreover, it was supposed that there may be connection between IL-6 levels in plasma and ADEs. However, no correlation had been found between two groups. All these results indicate that CNS-derived exosomes may be a promising object to help find biomarkers for ALS.

The important findings of our study were that IL-6 levels in ADEs increased in sALS patients and were positively associated with the rate of disease progression. These data suggest that the IL-6 in ADEs may be a candidate biomarker for ALS. However, neuroinflammation is a common phenomenon in almost all neurological disease. Therefore, it is believed that the IL-6 levels in ADEs probably increase in other neurological conditions. Actually, it has been reported that the IL-6 levels in ADEs

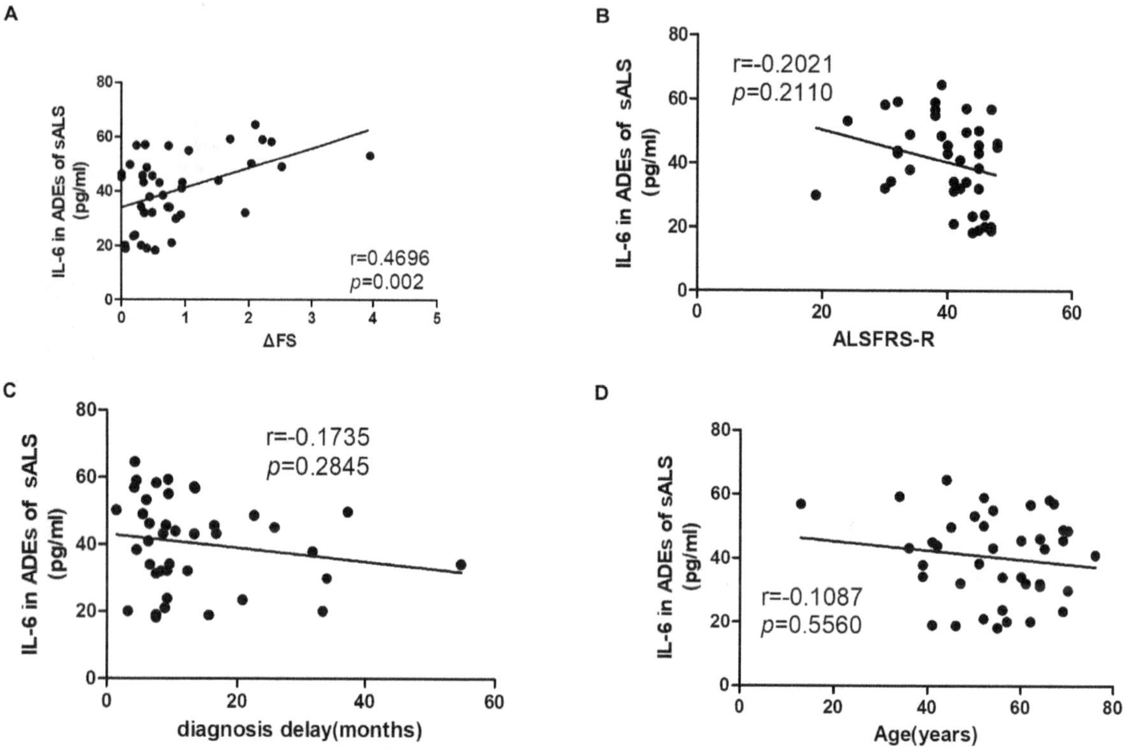

FIGURE 2 | Correlations between IL-6 levels in ADEs of ALS patients with the disease progression rate, ALSFRS-R score, diagnosis delay and patient age. **(A)** shows that the IL-6 levels in ADEs of ALS patients positively correlate with the disease progression rate. However, the IL-6 levels in ADEs of ALS patients do not correlate with the ALSFRS-R score **(B)**, diagnosis delay **(C)**, and patient age **(D)**.

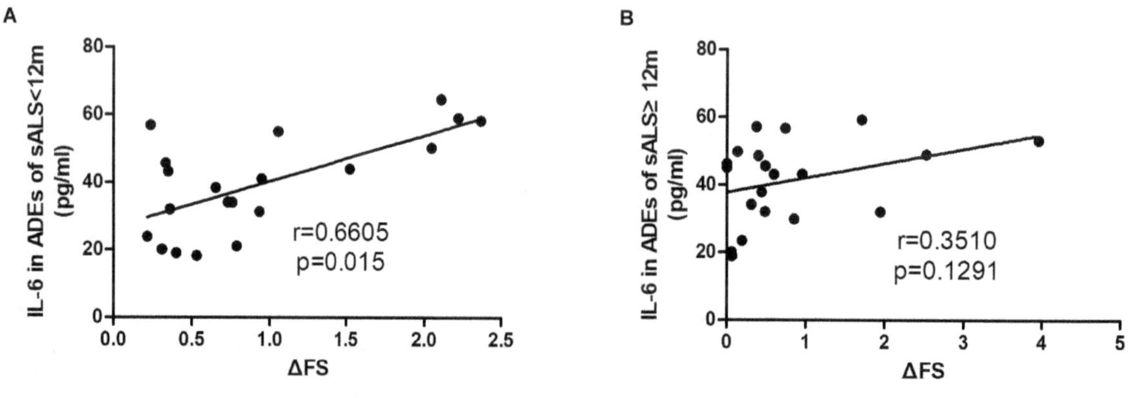

FIGURE 3 | Correlations between IL-6 levels in ADEs of ALS subgroups with the disease progression rate. ALS patients were divided into two groups according to the disease duration. **(A)** The IL-6 levels in ADEs of the ALS < 12 group positively correlate with the disease progression rate. However, the Il-6 levels in ADEs of the ALS12 group do not correlate with the disease progression rate **(B)**.

increased in AD patients (Goetzl et al., 2018). Thus, the IL-6 levels in ADEs may not be suitable to help discriminate ALS from other neurological diseases. According to our study, measuring the IL-6 levels in ADEs may be helpful to reflect the neuroinflammation status and predict disease progression.

We could not determine the precise role of IL-6 in ALS patients because of its complex physiological functions. Increased IL-6 secretion could be a neuroprotective reaction against CNS damage or a pro-inflammatory agent (Spooren et al., 2011). However, most views consider IL-6 as a pro-inflammatory cytokine in ALS patients. The anti-IL-6 antibody, tocilizumab, has been proposed as a therapeutic drug for ALS (Fiala et al., 2013). Therefore, we speculate that the increase in IL-6 observed in this study was harmful to ALS patients. Our further analyses revealed that the levels of IL-6 did not differ between ALS subgroups, and the correlation between IL-6 and the rate of disease progression was only observed during the initial 12 months. These results indicated that IL-6 produced by astrocytes might be more important during the early stage of disease. However, our sample size was limited, and the results should therefore be confirmed in further studies.

CONCLUSION

The present study demonstrated that the levels of IL-6 in ADEs of ALS patients were increased and positively associated with the rate of disease progression, especially in patients at an earlier disease stage. Our pilot study is the first to demonstrate that CNS-derived exosomes could be useful to reveal the pathophysiology of CNS in ALS patients.

AUTHOR CONTRIBUTIONS

DF conceived the study, provided the financial support, and responsible for the project management. DF and YC designed the study, responsible for preparing and revising the manuscript, and had key roles in the study. KX and LC took part in the design of the study and in sample collection, and undertook data checking.

FUNDING

This study was supported by the National Natural Sciences Foundation of China (81873784).

REFERENCES

1. Abner, E. L., Jicha, G. A., Shaw, L. M., Trojanowski, J. Q., and Goetzl, E. J. (2016). Plasma neuronal exosomal levels of Alzheimer's disease biomarkers in normal aging. *Ann. Clin. Transl. Neurol.* 3, 399–403. doi: 10.1002/acn3.309
2. Beninson, L. A., and Fleshner, M. (2014). Exosomes: an emerging factor in stress- induced immunomodulation. *Semin. Immunol.* 26, 394–401. doi: 10.1016/j. smim.2013.12.001
3. Blasco, H., Garcon, G., Patin, F., Veyrat-Durebex, C., Boyer, J., Devos, D., et al. (2017). Panel of oxidative stress and inflammatory biomarkers in ALS: a pilot study. *Can. J. Neurol. Sci.* 44, 90–95. doi: 10.1017/cjn.2016.284
4. Brooks, B. R., Miller, R. G., Swash, M., Munsat, T. L., and World Federation of Neurology Research Group on Motor Neuron Diseases. (2000). El Escorial revisited: revised criteria for the diagnosis of amyotrophic lateral sclerosis, amyotroph lateral scler other motor. *Neuron Disord.* 1, 293–299. doi: 10.1080/ 146608200300079536
5. Brown, R. H., and Al-Chalabi, A. (2017). Amyotrophic lateral sclerosis. *N. Engl. J. Med.* 377, 162–172.
6. Cedarbaum, J. M., Stambler, N., Malta, E., Fuller, C., Hilt, D., Thurmond, B., et al. (1999). The ALSFRS-R: a revised ALS functional rating scale that incorporates assessments of respiratory function. BDNF ALS study group (Phase III). *J. Neurol. Sci.* 169, 13–21. doi: 10.1016/s0022-510x(99)00210-5
7. Chaturvedi, S., Siegel, D., Wagner, C. L., Park, J., van de Velde, H., Vermeulen, J., et al. (2015). Development and validation of panoptic Meso scale discovery assay to quantify total systemic interleukin-6. *Br. J. Clin. Pharmacol.* 80, 687–697. doi: 10.1111/bcp.12652
8. Ehrhart, J., Smith, A. J., Kuzmin-Nichols, N., Zesiewicz, T. A., Jahan, I., Shytle, R. D., et al. (2015). Humoral factors in ALS patients during disease progression. *J. Neuroinflammation* 12:127. doi: 10.1186/s12974-015-0350-4
9. Fiala, M., Chattopadhay, M., La Cava, A., Tse, E., Liu, G., and Lourenco, E. (2010). IL-17A is increased in the serum and in spinal cord CD8 and mast cells of ALS patients. *J. Neuroinflammation* 7:76. doi: 10.1186/1742-2094-7-76
10. Fiala, M., Mizwicki, M. T., Weitzman, R., Magpantay, L., and Nishimoto, N. (2013). Tocilizumab infusion therapy normalizes inflammation in sporadic ALS patients. *Am. J. Neurodegener. Dis.* 2, 129–139.
11. Goetzl, E. J., Schwartz, J. B., Abner, E. L., Jicha, G. A., and Kapogiannis, D. (2018). High complement levels in astrocyte-derived exosomes of Alzheimer disease. *Ann. Neurol.* 83, 544–552. doi: 10.1002/ana.25172
12. Goh, W. J., Zou, S., Ong, W. Y., Torta, F., Alexandra, A. F., Schiffelers, R. M., et al. (2017). Bioinspired cell-derived nanovesicles versus exosomes as drug delivery systems: a cost-effective alternative. *Sci. Rep.* 7:14322. doi: 10.1038/ s41598-017- 14725-x
13. Gonzalez-Garza, M. T., Martinez, H. R., Cruz-Vega, D. E., Hernandez-Torre, M., and Moreno-Cuevas, J. E. (2018). Adipsin. MIP-1b, and IL-8 as CSF biomarker panels for ALS diagnosis. *Dis. Markers* 2018:3023826. doi: 10.1155/ 2018/3023826
14. Hu, Y., Cao, C., Qin, X. Y., Yu, Y., Yuan, J., Zhao, Y., et al. (2017). Increased peripheral blood inflammatory cytokine levels in amyotrophic lateral sclerosis: a meta-analysis study. *Sci. Rep.* 7:9094. doi: 10.1038/ s41598-017-09097-1
15. Italiani, P., Carlesi, C., Giungato, P., Puxeddu, I., Borroni, B., Bossu, P., et al. (2014). Evaluating the levels of interleukin-1 family cytokines in sporadic amyotrophic lateral sclerosis. *J. Neuroinflammation* 11:94. doi: 10.1186/1742-2094- 11-94
16. Jarmalaviciute, A., and Pivoriunas, A. (2016). Exosomes as a potential novel therapeutic tools against neurodegenerative diseases. *Pharmacol. Res.* 113(Pt B), 816–822. doi: 10.1016/j.phrs.2016.02.002
17. Kimura, F., Fujimura, C., Ishida, S., Nakajima, H., Furutama, D., Uehara, H., et al. (2006). Progression rate of ALSFRS-R at time of diagnosis predicts survival time in ALS. *Neurology* 66, 265–267. doi: 10.1212/01.wnl.0000194316.91908.8a
18. Kumar, V., Islam, A., Hassan, M. I., and Ahmad, F. (2016). Therapeutic progress in amyotrophic lateral sclerosis-beginning to learning. *Eur. J. Med. Chem.* 121, 903–917. doi: 10.1016/j.ejmech.2016.06.017
19. Kuwano, N., Kato, T. A., Mitsuhashi, M., Sato-Kasai, M., Shimokawa, N., Hayakawa, K., et al. (2018). Neuron-related blood inflammatory markers as an objective evaluation tool for major depres sive disorder: an exploratory pilot case-control study. *J. Affect Disord.* 240, 88–98. doi: 10.1016/j.jad.2018.0 7.040
20. Liu, J., Gao, L., and Zang, D. (2015). Elevated levels of IFN-gamma in CSF and serum of patients with amyotrophic lateral sclerosis. *PLoS One* 10:e0136937. doi: 10.1371/journal.pone.0136937
21. Liu, J., and Wang, F. (2017). Role of neuroinflammation in amyotrophic lateral sclerosis: cellular mechanisms and therapeutic implications. *Front. Immunol.* 8:1005. doi: 10.3389/fimmu.2017.01005
22. Lu, C. H., Allen, K., Oei, F., Leoni, E., Kuhle, J., and Tree, T. (2016). Systemic inflammatory response and neuromuscular involvement in amyotrophic lateral sclerosis. *Neurol. Neuroimmunol. Neuroinflamm.* 3:e244. doi: 10.1212/NXI. 0000000000000244
23. Mitchell, R. M., Freeman, W. M., Randazzo, W. T., Stephens, H. E., Beard, J. L., Simmons, Z., et al. (2009). A CSF biomarker panel for identification of patients with amyotrophic lateral sclerosis. *Neurology* 72, 14–19. doi: 10.1212/01.wnl. 0000333251.36681.a5
24. Mitchell, R. M., Simmons, Z., Beard, J. L., Stephens, H. E., and Connor, J. R. (2010). Plasma biomarkers associated with ALS and their relationship to iron homeostasis. *Mus. Nerve* 42, 95–103. doi: 10.1002/mus.21625
25. Moreau, C., Devos, D., Brunaud-Danel, V., Defebvre, L., Perez, T., Destee, A., et al. (2005). Elevated IL-6 and TNF-alpha levels in patients with ALS: inflammation or hypoxia? *Neurology* 65, 1958 1960. doi: 10.1212/01. wnl.0000188907.973 39.76
26. Mustapic, M., Eitan, E., Werner, J. K. Jr., Berkowitz, S. T., Lazaropoulos, M. P., Tran, J., et al. (2017). Plasma extracellular vesicles enriched for neuronal origin: a potential window into brain pathologic processes. *Front. Neurosci.* 11:278. doi: 10.3389/fnins.2017.00278
27. Ohmichi, T., Mitsuhashi, M., Tatebe, H., Kasai, T., Ali El-Agnaf, O. M., and Tokud a, T. (2018). Quantification of brain-derived extracellular vesicles in plasma as a biomarker to diagnose Parkinson's and related diseases. *Parkin. Relat. Disord.* 61, 82–87. doi: 10.1016/j.parkreldis.2018.11.021
28. Ono, S., Hu, J., Shimizu, N., Imai, T., and Nakagawa, H. (2001). Increased interleukin-6 of skin and serum in amyotrophic lateral sclerosis. *J. Neurol. Sci.* 187, 27–34. doi: 10.1016/s0022-510x(01)00514-7
29. Pronto-Laborinho, A., Pinto, S., Gromicho, M., Pereira, M., Swash, M., and de Carvalho, M. (2019). Interleukin-6 and amyotrophic lateral sclerosis. *J. Neurol. Sci.* 398, 50–53. doi: 10.1016/j.jns.2019.01.026

30. Raposo, G., and Stoorvogel, W. (2013). Extracellular vesicles: exosomes, microvesicles, and friends. *J. Cell. Biol.* 200, 373–383. doi: 10.1083/jcb. 201211138
31. Rothstein, J. D. (2017). Edaravone: a new drug approved for ALS. *Cell* 171:725. doi: 10.1016/j.cell.2017.10.011
32. Sekizawa, T., Openshaw, H., Ohbo, K., Sugamura, K., Itoyama, Y., and Niland, J. C. (1998). Cerebrospinal fluid interleukin 6 in amyotrophic lateral sclerosis: immunological parameter and comparison with inflammatory and non-inflammatory central nervous system diseases. *J. Neurol. Sci.* 154, 194–199. doi: 10.1016/s0022-510x(97)00 228-1
33. Spooren, A., Kolmus, K., Laureys, G., Clinckers, R., De Keyser, J., Haegeman, G., et al. (2011). Interleukin-6, a mental cytokine. *Brain Res. Rev.* 67, 157–183. doi: 10.1016/j.brainresrev.2011.01.002
34. Su, X. W., Simmons, Z., Mitchell, R. M., Kong, L., Stephens, H. E., and Connor, J. R. (2013). Biomarker-based predictive models for prognosis in amyotrophic lateral sclerosis. *JAMA Neurol.* 70, 1505–1511. doi: 10.1001/jamaneurol.2013.4646
35. Tanaka, M., Kikuchi, H., Ishizu, T., Minohara, M., Osoegawa, M., and Motomura, K. (2006). Intrathecal upregulation of granulocyte colony stimulating factor and its neuroprotective actions on motor neurons in amyotrophic lateral sclerosis. *J. Neuropathol. Exp. Neurol.* 65, 816–825. doi: 10.1097/01.jnen.0000232025. 84238.e1
36. Van Wagoner, N. J., and Benveniste, E. N. (1999). Interleukin-6 expression and regulation in astrocytes. *J. Neuroimmunol.* 100, 124–139. doi: 10.1016/ s0165- 5728(99)00187-3
37. Vu, L. T., and Bowser, R. (2017). Fluid-Based biomarkers for amyotrophic lateral sclerosis. *Neurotherapeutics* 14, 119–134. doi: 10.1007/s13311-016-0503-x
38. Winston, C. N., Goetzl, E. J., Akers, J. C., Carter, B. S., Rockenstein, E. M., Galasko, D., et al. (2016). Prediction of conversion from mild cognitive impairment to dementia with neuronally derived blood exosome protein profile. *Alzheimers Dement* 3, 63–72. doi: 10.1016/j.dadm.2016.04.001
39. Yanez-Mo, M., Siljander, P. R., Andreu, Z., Zavec, A. B., Borras, F. E., and Buzas, E. I. (2015). Biological properties of extracellular vesicles and their physiological functions. *J. Extracell. Vesicles* 4:27066. doi: 10.3402/jev.v4.27066
40. Zhao, W., Beers, D. R., and Appel, S. H. (2013). Immune-mediated mechanisms in the pathoprogression of amyotrophic lateral sclerosis. *J. Neuroimmune. Pharmacol.* 8, 888–899. doi: 10.1007/s11481-013-9489-x

11

Clinical and Radiological Markers of Extra-Motor Deficits in Amyotrophic Lateral Sclerosis

Foteini Christidi[1], Efstratios Karavasilis[2], Michail Rentzos[1], Nikolaos Kelekis[2], Ioannis Evdokimidis[1] and Peter Bede[3]*

[1] First Department of Neurology, Aeginition Hospital, National and Kapodistrian University of Athens, Athens, Greece, [2] Second Department of Radiology, University General Hospital Attikon, National and Kapodistrian University of Athens, Athens, Greece, [3] Computational Neuroimaging Group, Academic Unit of Neurology, Trinity College Dublin, Dublin, Ireland

***Correspondence:**
Foteini Christidi
christidi.f.a@gmail.com

Amyotrophic lateral sclerosis (ALS) is now universally recognized as a complex multisystem disorder with considerable extra-motor involvement. The neuropsychological manifestations of frontotemporal, parietal, and basal ganglia involvement in ALS have important implications for compliance with assistive devices, survival, participation in clinical trials, caregiver burden, and the management of individual care needs. Recent advances in neuroimaging have been instrumental in characterizing the biological substrate of heterogeneous cognitive and behavioral deficits in ALS. In this review we discuss the clinical and radiological aspects of cognitive and behavioral impairment in ALS focusing on the recognition, assessment, and monitoring of these symptoms.

Keywords: amyotrophic lateral sclerosis, extra-motor involvement, cognition, behavior, neuropsychological deficits, neuroimaging

INTRODUCTION

Amyotrophic lateral sclerosis (ALS) is the most common form of motor neuron disease (MND), a progressive neurodegenerative condition defined by concomitant lower and upper motor neuron degeneration (1). Motor symptoms include muscle weakness, fasciculations, cramps, as well as spasticity and brisk reflexes that accrue to considerable limb and bulbar disability over time, and eventually respiratory failure (1). The identification of TAR DNA-binding protein 43 (TDP-43) positive ubiquitinated cytoplasmic inclusions in almost all patients with ALS and more than half of patients with frontotemporal dementia (FTD) has placed ALS on the so-called "ALS-FTD continuum," highlighting the considerable clinical, pathophysiological, and neuroimaging overlap between the two neurodegenerative conditions (2).

Although mentioned in early descriptions of ALS (3, 4), cognitive and behavioral deficits and frank dementia were previously considered atypical of ALS. It is not until the end of the twentieth century that clinical and research interest shifted to the extra-motor features of ALS and it has been gradually recognized as a genuine multisystem disease (5–8).

Neuropsychological deficits in ALS range from mild impairment to full-blown FTD. Up to 65% of ALS patients exhibit some cognitive or behavioral impairment (9–12) and 6–15% of sporadic ALS patients meet diagnostic criteria for FTD (10–13). While hexanucleotide repeat expansions in *C9ORF72* are often associated with ALS-FTD (14), extra-motor symptoms are not unique to this mutation and extra-motor neuroimaging findings can also be readily identified in a significant proportion of C9 negative patients (15, 16). The early recognition of extra-motor involvement in

ALS is crucial due to its impact on functional decline (17), survival (18), compliance with assistive devices (19), decision-making, and engagement in end-of-life and legal decisions (20).

COGNITIVE DYSFUNCTION

Much attention has been initially focused on executive dysfunction (21, 22) in ALS which has been gradually complemented by the characterization of language (23, 24), memory (25, 26), praxis (27), and theory of mind deficits (28) (**Table 1**). Population-based studies have confirmed distinct cognitive phenotypes without executive impairment (10, 11, 29).

Executive Dysfunction

Executive dysfunction is the most commonly cited facet of cognitive impairment in ALS. Executive function however is an umbrella term encompassing several relatively distinct higher-order processes, such as planning, organization, goal-directed activity, working memory, initiation, behavioral regulation, and inhibitory control, as well as situation-appropriate decision-making on the basis of projected positive and negative outcomes in novel, complex or ambiguous situations (30). In addition, tests of verbal (i.e., phonemic and semantic/category) and figural/design fluency are also often conceptualized as proxies of executive performance (31).

Verbal fluency impairment has been consistently reported in ALS (11, 22, 24, 27, 32–46). Coexisting phonemic and semantic fluency dysfunction or phonemic fluency deficits alone are often linked to executive dysfunction, while isolated semantic fluency deficits are associated with impaired semantic memory processing. Semantic (24, 34, 40, 44, 46, 47) and figural (34, 46) fluency are not typically impaired in ALS. A verbal fluency index has been proposed and is now widely utilized to account for patients' motor disability (32, 48). Other executive processes are also affected in ALS, such as concept formation and mental flexibility (24, 27, 33, 35, 36, 41, 49–53) which is typically examined by the Wisconsin Card Sorting Test or the Dellis-Kaplan Executive Function System Card Sorting Test (31). However, not all neuropsychology studies corroborate these findings (34, 38, 39, 45, 46, 54–56). Several studies have specifically evaluated mental set shifting ability in ALS using the Trail Making Test; most of them identifying considerable dysfunction (37, 42, 47, 55, 57), while others have not captured such deficits (58, 59). Response inhibition and attentional control are typically examined by the Stroop test, and are often impaired in ALS (11, 27, 35–37, 51, 53, 57, 60), but unaffected cohorts have also been reported (39, 40, 44, 49). ALS patients also often exhibit difficulties in maintaining, manipulating and retrieving information relying on working memory (27, 32, 34, 37, 43, 46, 61), but preserved working memory has also been observed (39, 44, 51, 54, 55, 58, 62). Subtle deficits in reasoning and coordinating rules have been found using ecologically valid measures of executive functions (44, 63).

Memory Deficits

Following inconsistent initial reports, memory dysfunction in ALS has received increasing attention recently (7, 64). While autobiographic memory seems to be preserved in ALS (65), semantic memory is often affected (66). Episodic memory is the most commonly evaluated memory domain in ALS, typically tested by list-learning tests, associate-learning tests, prose memory, as well as visual memory tests (7). Several studies have reported mild to moderate episodic memory impairments which are often interpreted as the corollary of underlying executive deficits (27, 35, 37, 39, 41, 67–69). Memory impairment in ALS is rarely identified in isolation (11), but using data-driven taxonomy approaches a subgroup of patients may show non-executive memory dysfunction (29). Several studies have found impaired encoding (37, 60, 68), retrieval (12, 17, 37, 60, 70) consolidation and recognition (26, 60), although recognition deficits in ALS are not universally recognized (11, 37, 41). Visual memory dysfunction has also been noted in ALS (12), although visual recall is typically less affected than delayed verbal recall (7). Neuroimaging studies have contributed to the characterization of ALS-associated memory impairment highlighting mesial temporal lobe involvement irrespective of frontal lobe pathology (64).

Language Deficits

Language deficits in ALS have traditionally attracted less attention compared to other cognitive domains and have been mostly appraised in association with ALS-FTD (7, 23, 71, 72). However, language dysfunction is increasingly recognized as a core feature of ALS and has been consistently detected in patients without executive dysfunction (24, 29, 73). Patients with ALS show impaired syntactic processing (74), deficits in verb naming and action verb processing (75, 76). Selective impairment in action knowledge (77) has been directly associated with motor cortex degeneration (78) suggesting a link between action execution and action conceptualization (79). Grammatical errors such as incomplete utterances (73, 74) and omission of determiners (73) have been reported in ALS and seem to be dissociable from the patients' motor and executive deficits (73). Phonemic and semantic paraphasias have also been reported (74, 80). Patients with ALS may find narrative discourse particularly challenging due to difficulties to establish (81) and adhere to the main topic of conversation (73, 81). Frequent pauses are another key characteristic of narrative speech in ALS in both demented and non-demented ALS cohorts (82). Syntactic comprehension deficits have also been detected in up to 72% of patients with ALS (83, 84).

Visuo-Perceptive and Visuo-Constructive Deficits

Visuo-perceptive and visuo-constructive functions are seldom specifically examined in ALS. Existing studies tend to focus on visuospatial memory measures and often fail to reach definite conclusions (37, 41, 46, 47, 85). Based on large meta-analyses, these domains are not significantly affected in ALS (7). The relative absence of visuo-perceptual deficits is further supported by the lack of reports on Balint's syndrome in ALS and is consistent with limited occipital involvement on neuroimaging (86) and pathology (87). While praxis deficits are also rarely

TABLE 1 | Most characteristic neuropsychological deficits in ALS categorised per cognitive domain.

Main cognitive domains	Target processes/main deficits	Representative studies (First author, year, sample size ALS/Control)
Executive functions	Verbal fluency	Ludolph, 1992 (21/12); Kew, 1993 (16/16); Abrahams, 1995 (12/6); Massman, 1996 (146/–); Abrahams, 1996 (12/6); Abrahams, 1997 (52/28); Frank, 1997 (74/56); Rakowicz, 1998 (18/24); Abrahams, 2000 (21/25); Lomen- Hanagasi, 2002 (20/13); Hoerth, 2003 (44/–); Abrahams, 2004 (28/18); Abrahams, 2005 (20/18); Pinkhardt, 2008 (20/20); Wicks, 2009 (41/35); Witgert, 2010 (225/–); Stukovnik, 2010 (22/21); Phukan, 2012 (160/110); Taylor, 2013 (51/35)
	Concept formation and mental flexibility	Abrahams, 1996 (12/6); Massman, 1996 (146/-); Abrahams, 1997 (52/28); Frank, 1997 (74/56); Evdokimidis, 2002 (51/28); Moretti, 2002 (14/15); Lomen-Hoerth, 2003 (44/-); Schreiber, 2005 (52/-); Libon, 2012 (41/25); Zalonis, 2012 (48/47); Taylor, 2013 (51/35)
	Mental set shifting	Hartikainen, 1993 (24/26); Hanagasi, 2002 (20/13); Kilani, 2004 (18/19); Witgert, 2010 (225/–)
	Response inhibition and attentional control	Abrahams, 1997 (52/28); Frank, 1997 (74/56); Hanagasi, 2002 (20/13); Moretti, 2002 (14/15); Lomen-Hoerth, 2003 (44/-); Sterling, 2010 (355/-); Christidi, 2012 (22/22); Phukan, 2012 (160/110); Zalonis, 2012 (48/47)
	Working memory	Abrahams, 1997 (52/28); Rakowicz, 1998 (18/24); Abrahams, 2000 (21/25); Hanagasi, 2002 (20/13); Abrahams, 2004 (28/18); Abrahams, 2005 (20/18); Lillo, 2012 (20/18)
	Reasoning and coordinating rules using ecologically valid measures	Meier, 2010 (18/18); Stukovnik, 2010 (22/21)
Memory	Episodic memory encoding	Hanagasi, 2002 (20/13); Mantovan, 2003 (20/20); Christidi, 2012 (22/22)
	Episodic memory retrieval	Hanagasi, 2002 (20/13); Ringholz, 2005 (279/129); Christidi, 2012 (22/22); Elamin, 2013 (186/120); Raaphorst, 2015 (26/21)
	Episodic memory consolidation/recognition	Machts, 2014 (40/40); Christidi, 2012 (22/22)
	Visual delayed recall	Ringholz, 2005 (279/129)
	Semantic memory	Hervieu-Begue, 2016 (15/-)
Language	Verb naming and action verb processing	Bak, 2001 (6/20); Grossman, 2008 (34/25); York, 2014 (36/13); Papeo, 2015 (21/14)
	Grammatical errors	Ash, 2015 (26/19); Tsermentseli, 2015 (26/26)
	Phonemic and semantic paraphasias	Roberts-South, 2012 (16/12); Tsermentseli, 2015 (26/26)
	Establishing and adhering to the main topic of conversations	Ash, 2015 (26/19); Bambini, 2016 (33/33)
	Narrative speech pauses	Yunusova, 2016 (85/33)
	Syntactic processing/comprehension	Yoshizawa, 2014 (25/–); Tsermentseli, 2015 (26/26); Kamminga, 2016 (35/23)
Praxis	Constructive apraxia	Abrahams, 1997 (52/28)
	Orofacial apraxia	Lobo, 2013 (1/–)
	Speech apraxia	Duffy, 2007 (7/–)
	Respiratory apraxia	Pinto, 2007 (1/–)
Social cognition	Theory of mind	Meier, 2010 (18/18); Girardi, 2011 (19/20); Burke, 2016 (59/59)
	Emotional processing and ability to recognize emotional facial expressions	Palmieri, 2010 (9/10); Girardi, 2011 (19/20); Crespi, 2014 (22/55); Savage, 2014 (29/30); Andrews, 2017 (33/22)
	Ability to describe intentions and feelings of others	Gibbons, 2007 (16/16); Staios, 2013 (35/30); Cerami, 2014 (20/56)
	Empathy	Girardi, 2011 (19/20); Cerami, 2014 (20/56)
	Social inferences	Staios, 2013 (35/30); Savage, 2014 (29/30)
Behavior	Apathy	Grossman, 2007 (45/–); Chio, 2010 (70/–); Witgert, 2010 (225/–); Girardi, 2011 (19/20); Radakovic, 2016 (83/83)
	Disinhibition	Grossman, 2007 (45/–); Terada, 2011 (24/–)
	Pathological crying and laughing	McCullagh, 1999 (18/10); Palmieri, 2009 (32/39); Olney, 2011 (35/–); Brooks, 2013 (9/–); Floeter, 2014 (22/28); Christidi, 2018 (56/25)

ALS, amyotrophic lateral sclerosis.

reported in ALS (27), orofacial (88), speech (89), and respiratory (90) apraxia have been sporadically reported.

Social Cognition Deficits

Social cognition refers to a diverse set of cognitive skills that allow humans to understand themselves, interact with and understand others and are crucial to adopt situation-appropriate, goal-directed behaviors in everyday social interactions (91). Despite considerable variations, deficits in theory of mind, empathy, social perception, social behavior are now recognized as key elements of the ALS-associated cognitive profile (7, 28, 92). It is however still unclear if these deficits are linked to executive dysfunction (29, 93–98) or may be related to non-executive domains, such as episodic memory function and visuospatial abilities (99). Patients with ALS may also exhibit impaired emotional processing and ability to interpret emotional facial expressions, especially with comorbid FTD (96, 100–102). Impairments in complex facial affect recognition, affective prosody recognition and cross-modal integration have also been found in non-demented ALS cohorts (103). Multiple subcomponents of theory of mind seem to be affected in ALS, including the ability to describe the intentions and feelings of others (95, 98, 104), to recognize and provide explanations for social "faux pas" (63) and evaluate object preferences based on the interpretation of eye gaze direction (96, 105). Loss of empathy (96), impaired emotional empathy attribution (95), and erroneous social inferences (98, 100) have also been reported in non-demented ALS cohorts.

Behavioral Deficits

The clinical link between ALS and FTD is exemplified by overlapping behavioral changes which are similar to those observed in behavioral variant of FTD (106). These deficits are typically identified through a structured clinical interview with the caregivers or through validated questionnaires. Perseveration, apathy and disinhibition are the most commonly reported behavioral alterations, followed by loss of disease insight, indifference, loss of interest, aggression, irritability, and lability (107).

Apathy is the most commonly reported behavioral symptom in non-demented ALS (42, 45, 96, 108, 109), which used to be assessed by generic behavioral instruments, such as the Frontal Systems Behavior Scale (110) and the Frontal Behavioral Inventory (111), until the development of ALS-specific scales, such as the Dimensional Apathy Scale (112) which appraises initiation, executive and emotional apathy. Initiation apathy is thought to be particularly prevalent in ALS (113). ALS patients with apathy may require prompts to initiate or follow through with a task, including self-care, feeding, and taking medications. They may appear poorly motivated, aloof or uninterested. Apathy may impact of rehabilitation, hamper gait initiation, and curb communication efforts especially in the presence of bulbar impairment. It can be mistaken for low mood, depression and withdrawal by inexperienced observers. Disinhibition is more readily identified and reported by caregivers, and can precede (108) or follow (114) motor disability. Disinhibited behavior can manifest in rude, offensive, flirtatious comments, puns, "Witzelsucht" often violating social norms, personal space and may result in careless or impulsive decisions. Purchasing expensive items on a whim, hoarding, compulsive behavior, overeating, and developing a preference for sweets have also been reported (115).

Hallucinations have been reported by several groups (116–119) and are sometimes associated with the C9orf72 genotype. Symptomatic treatment includes the judicious use of small dose atypical antipsychotics, if necessary.

Patients with pseudobulbar affect or pathological crying and laughing exhibit sudden situation-inappropriate emotional responses (120–122) which may have a negative impact on their quality of life (123) and lead to social isolation or social stigma. It is most commonly associated with UMN-type bulbar dysfunction (124), but frontal abnormalities, executive dysfunction, basal ganglia pathology and impaired cerebellar gating mechanisms have also been linked this symptom (27, 122, 125–128).

INSIGHTS FROM NEUROIMAGING

Neuroimaging techniques provide optimal non-invasive tools to characterize extra-motor pathology in ALS underpinning cognitive and behavioral deficits and also permit exploratory correlations with clinical measures (129, 130).

Structural Imaging

Voxel based morphometry (VBM) and surface-based morphometry (SBM) are reproducible, validated and widely-used pipelines that use high resolution 3D T1-weighted MR images to identify focal GM alterations. Beyond the consensus on motor cortex atrophy (131), many studies also detect multifocal frontotemporal and parietal GM changes (132). GM abnormalities have also been identified in subcortical structures (133), such as the hippocampus (134–136), amygdala (137, 138), thalamus (134, 135, 139, 140), and insula (141, 142). Reduced GM density in occipital (139, 143–145) and cerebellar (139, 146) regions is less commonly reported. GM alterations in extra-motor areas have been linked to structure-specific cognitive and behavioral deficits in ALS (147, 148). Recent studies have highlighted extra-motor cortical changes in ALS patients without overt cognitive impairment (134, 135, 146, 149, 150). The anatomical patterns of extra-motor gray matter involvement in ALS further support the notion of the ALS-FTD continuum (72).

White matter integrity in ALS is most commonly evaluated by diffusion tensor imaging (DTI). Reduced fractional anisotropy and increased axial and radial diffusivity in the corticospinal tracts and corpus callosum are hallmark features of ALS (151, 152). Extra-motor white matter pathology has been consistently detected in frontal (139, 153–160), temporal (53, 154, 161), cingular (162), parahippocampal (25, 157, 160), insular (160), thalamic (141, 159, 163), and cerebellar regions (86, 146, 164). Similarly to gray matter analyses, extra-motor white matter involvement has also been identified in ALS patients without overt cognitive impairment (146).

Metabolic Imaging

MR spectroscopy in ALS has consistently revealed decreased N-acetyl aspartate (NAA)/choline and NAA/creatine ratios in motor regions (165–167), but whole brain spectroscopy also detected extra-motor NAA reductions in frontal, parietal, thalamic and occipital areas (168, 169).

Most positron emission tomography (PET) studies in ALS use 18F-FDG PET, but TSPO, $GABA_A$ (11C-flumazenil) and 5-HT1A receptor (11C-WAY100635) radioligands have also been utilized (170). Hypometabolism in motor regions is a characteristic FDG-PET finding in ALS (171–174), but extra-motor changes in dorsolateral prefrontal, orbitofrontal, anterior frontal, anterior temporal, fusiform, and occipital regions have also been reported (171–174). Frontotemporal hypometabolism has been linked to cognitive performance (22, 39, 172), is thought to precede atrophy (175) and has been linked to shorter survival (176). There is also evidence of hypermetabolism in the hippocampus, amygdala midbrain, pons and cerebellum (173, 174, 177). PET imaging has identified microglial activation in frontotemporal, thalamic, midbrain, and pontine regions suggestive of extra-motor inflammation (178–181). Widespread reduction of 11C-Flumazenil binding to $GABA_A$ in sporadic ALS has been interpreted as inhibitory dysfunction (182) and is regarded as a one of cornerstones of ALS pathogenesis (183). Reduced serotonin receptor binding has also been reported in ALS using the 11C-WAY100635 radio-ligand (184).

Functional Imaging

Resting state fMRI enables the assessment of functional connectivity between different brain regions by evaluating synchronized neuronal activity at rest. Reduced (185–189) and increased (183, 190) functional connectivity have both been reported in sensorimotor networks of ALS patients which may be explained by the different sub-regions evaluated (191–193) and also by the inclusion of patients in different disease-stages. Similarly, both reduced and increased functional connectivity alterations have been reported in extra-motor areas which mediate cognitive and behavioral functions (187, 188, 193, 194). The functional connectivity of the default mode network (DMN) has been reported to be both decreased (187, 189, 193) and increased (193, 195). Increased functional connectivity has been detected in the DMN using graph theory-based analyses (196). Increased (193) and decreased (186, 189, 193) fronto-parietal network integrity has been both reported. Reduced "executive control network" (middle frontal cortex) and "salience network" (medial prefrontal cortex, insula) connectivity has been described in ALS cohorts without dementia (189). Increased connectivity in ALS has either been interpreted as evidence of attempted compensation for structural degeneration (197, 198) or proof of inhibitory dysfunction (183, 190, 199).

Task-based fMRI studies in ALS have consistently revealed the recruitment of pre- and supplementary motor regions when executing motor tasks. Additional activation has also been observed in areas associated with motor learning areas, such as the basal ganglia and cerebellum (200, 201). Despite difference in study protocols, an activation shift to premotor (202, 203), temporal and parietal regions (203–205) has been often noted. Cognitive paradigms have been particularly helpful in capturing frontotemporal network alterations. Impaired verbal fluency was linked to reduced frontotemporal, parietal, and cingulate activation in non-demented ALS patients (46). Impaired frontal inhibitory control was confirmed by a number of fMRI paradigms, such as Stroop, negative priming, antisaccade tasks, go/no-go tasks etc. Increased activation during the Stroop paradigm and decreased activation in negative priming conditions has been reported mostly in left hemispheric regions (206). Increased activation in supplementary and frontal eye fields and reduced activation in dorsolateral prefrontal cortex have been noted in antisaccade tasks (207). Furthermore, in go/no-go paradigms, ALS patients show increased inhibition-related activation in frontal and basal ganglia regions and increased execution-related activity in contralateral sensorimotor

TABLE 2 | ALS-specific instruments to screen for cognitive and behavioral changes at baseline and during the course of the disease.

Screening instrument	Duration of administration	Cognitive and behavioral domains examined	Parallel forms for longitudinal assessment	Validation in non-English speaking populations
Edinburgh Cognitive and Behavioral ALS Screen (ECAS)	15–20 min	Executive functions, Social cognition, Language, Visuoconstruction, Memory Behavioral changes (including psychotic symptoms)	Yes	American-English; Belgium; Chinese; Croatian; Czech; Dutch; French; German; Swiss-German; Greek; Hebrew; Italian; Japanese; Norwegian; Polish; Portuguese; Russian; Slovak; Slovenian; Spanish; Swedish; Welsh
ALS Cognitive and Behavioral Screen (ALS-CBS)	<10 min	Executive functions including attention, concentration, mental tracking and monitoring, verbal fluency Behavioral changes	Yes	Brazilian; Spanish; Greek
ALS Brief Cognitive Assessment (ALS-BCA)	5 min	Executive functions (working memory, set-shifting), Frontally-mediated language function, Delayed verbal recall, Behavioral changes	N/A	N/A
Beaumont Behavioral Inventory (BBI)	5–10 min	Frontal Behavioral symptoms; Executive functions; Language; Psychotic symptoms	N/A	N/A
Motor Neuron Disease Behavioral Instrument (MiND-B)	<10 min	Behavioral symptoms	N/A	N/A
ALS Frontotemporal Dementia Questionnaire (ALS-FTD-Q)	5–10 min	Behavioral symptoms (it also includes 3 items for memory, concentration and orientation in time)	N/A	N/A

regions (208). Few studies have specifically examined the functional correlates of social cognition to date. Patients with ALS tend to show increased activation compared to healthy participants in the right supramarginal, anterior cingulate and bilateral dorsolateral prefrontal cortex in response to socio-emotional stimuli (56, 209). The combined use of motor and memory tasks on fMRI enables the longitudinal characterization of divergent motor and extra-motor functional changes. Increased motor activation was found in ALS compared to controls at baseline, which has decreased on the follow-up assessment, suggestive of failing compensation. Contrary to the functional motor changes, hippocampal activation increased on follow-up when novel stimuli was presented (210).

RELEVANCE TO CLINICAL CARE

The detection (48), expert evaluation (11), categorization (211), and follow-up (17) of extra-motor deficits in ALS is crucially important for individualized patient care. While screening tests (**Table 2**) are useful for the detection of gross deficits, expert review by neuropsychologists is indicated for accurate patient classification. Adherence to treatment, compliance with assistive devices, participation in clinical trials, making informed financial and end-of-life decisions, choices in participating in non-licensed treatments are just some of the aspects of a patient journey which may be significantly affected by cognitive or behavioral deficits (19, 212). Cognitive impairment in ALS is widely regarded as a negative prognostic indicator and linked to reduced survival (17, 18, 213). Neuropsychological deficits in ALS are thought to be associated with increased caregiver burden (214, 215) and reduced quality of life (216). The recognition of the far-reaching effects of neuropsychological deficits on nearly all aspects of ALS care, caregiver support, resource allocation, and prognosis, led to the inclusion of specialist neuropsychologists as core members of ALS multidisciplinary teams worldwide (217, 218). The careful evaluation of motor deficits which are not directly linked to the corticospinal axis and are not reflected in the ALSFRS-R score, such as extra-pyramidal deficits are also crucial (219). Extra-pyramidal deficits may contribute to falls and gait impairment and are increasingly investigated in neuroimaging studies (220, 221). These symptoms may present early in the course of the disease, and contribute the clinical heterogeneity of the condition (220, 222). Postural instability and rigidity may be associated with other extra-motor deficits, and potentially linked to poor survival (205, 223). There is some controversy about the chronology of motor and extra-motor involvement in ALS. Extra-motor manifestations, such as dementia (224, 225), psychiatric features (226), and extra-pyramidal symptoms (227) have been reported to precede motor symptoms in some cases, and there is also compelling evidence of early extra-motor pathology in cognitively normal ALS patients (134, 135, 146).

RESEARCH OPPORTUNITIES AND FUTURE DIRECTIONS

Even though the high incidence of cognitive impairment and its impact on individualized patient care are now universally recognized, the neuropsychological aspects of ALS are seldom considered for patient stratification in clinical trials (228). Several ALS-specific cognitive screening tests have now been validated, but generic tests, such as MOCA and MMSE are still in use in some clinics. While neuropsychological scores are often adjusted for motor-disability and depression, medication-effects, fatigue, and hypoxia are seldom considered when interpreting cognitive performance on various instruments. Despite sporadic reports, the full spectrum of psychiatric manifestations and the precise incidence of psychosis remain to be established in ALS (119, 229, 230). Certain cognitive domains, such as memory and praxis have not been exhaustively characterized in ALS to date. Relatively little is known of the neuropsychological profile of ALS-causing mutation carriers before they develop motor symptoms (231–233). The gaps in our current understanding of extra-motor pathology in ALS shape future study designs. Novel technologies such as online assessments, internet-based data collection, mobile phone apps, and wearable devices are emerging research resources. Irrespective of specific neuropsychological instruments, the early detection, and careful of monitoring of cognitive deficits in ALS is pivotal for optimized patient and caregiver support and tailoring precision management strategies to individual patient needs.

AUTHOR CONTRIBUTIONS

The paper was drafted by FC, EK, and PB and has been reviewed for intellectual content by MR, NK, and IE.

ACKNOWLEDGMENTS

FC is supported by the State Scholarships Foundation (I.K.Y.; Postdoctoral Support; EP ANADEDBM/ESPA 2014–2020). Peter Bede's group is supported by the Health Research Board (HRB–Ireland; HRB EIA-2017-019), the Andrew Lydon scholarship, the Irish Institute of Clinical Neuroscience IICN–Novartis Ireland Research Grant, the Iris O'Brien Foundation, the Perrigo Clinician-Scientist Research Fellowship, and the Research Motor Neuron (RMN–Ireland) Foundation.

REFERENCES

1. Kiernan MC, Vucic S, Cheah BC, Turner MR, Eisen A, Hardiman O, et al. Amyotrophic lateral sclerosis. *Lancet* (2011) 377:942–55. doi: 10.1016/S0140-6736(10)61156-7
2. Neumann M, Sampathu DM, Kwong LK, Truax AC, Micsenyi MC, Chou TT, et al. Ubiquitinated TDP–43 in frontotemporal lobar degeneration and amyotrophic lateral sclerosis. *Science* (2006) 314:130–3. doi: 10.1126/science.1134108
3. Gallassi R, Montagna P, Ciardulli C, Lorusso S, Mussuto V, Stracciari A. Cognitive impairment in motor neuron disease. *Acta Neurol Scand.* (1985) 71:480–4. doi: 10.1111/j.1600-0404.1985.tb03231.x
4. David AS, Gillham RA. Neuropsychological study of motor neuron disease. *Psychosomatics* (1986) 27:441–5. doi: 10.1016/S0033-3182(86)72673-X

5. Silani V, Ludolph A, Fornai F. The emerging picture of ALS: a multisystem, not only a "motor neuron disease. *Arch Ital Biol.* (2017) 155:99–109.
6. Hudson AJ. Amyotrophic lateral sclerosis and its association with dementia, parkinsonism and other neurological disorders: a review. *Brain* (1981) 104:217–47. doi: 10.1093/brain/104.2.217
7. Beeldman E, Raaphorst J, Klein Twennaar M, de Visser M, Schmand BA, de Haan RJ. The cognitive profile of ALS: a systematic review and meta-analysis update. *J Neurol Neurosurg Psychiatry* (2016) 87:611–9. doi: 10.1136/jnnp-2015-310734
8. Beeldman E, Raaphorst J, Klein Twennaar M, Govaarts R, Pijnenburg YAL, de Haan RJ, et al. The cognitive profile of behavioural variant FTD and its similarities with ALS: a systematic review and meta-analysis. *J Neurol Neurosurg Psychiatry* (2018) 89:995–1002. doi: 10.1136/jnnp-2017-317459
9. Goldstein LH, Abrahams S. Changes in cognition and behaviour in amyotrophic lateral sclerosis: nature of impairment and implications for assessment. *Lancet Neurol.* (2013) 12:368–80. doi: 10.1016/S1474-4422(13)70026-7
10. Montuschi A, Iazzolino B, Calvo A, Moglia C, Lopiano L, Restagno G, et al. Cognitive correlates in amyotrophic lateral sclerosis: a population-based study in Italy. *J Neurol Neurosurg Psychiatry* (2015) 86:168–73. doi: 10.1136/jnnp-2013-307223
11. Phukan J, Elamin M, Bede P, Jordan N, Gallagher L, Byrne S, et al. The syndrome of cognitive impairment in amyotrophic lateral sclerosis: a population-based study. *J Neurol Neurosurg Psychiatry* (2012) 83:102–8. doi: 10.1136/jnnp-2011-300188
12. Ringholz GM, Appel SH, Bradshaw M, Cooke NA, Mosnik DM, Schulz PE. Prevalence and patterns of cognitive impairment in sporadic ALS. *Neurology* (2005) 65:586–90. doi: 10.1212/01.wnl.0000172911.39167.b6
13. Trojsi F, Siciliano M, Femiano C, Santangelo G, Lunetta C, Calvo A, et al. Comorbidity of dementia with amyotrophic lateral sclerosis (ALS): insights from a large multicenter Italian cohort. *J Neurol.* (2017) 264:2224–31. doi: 10.1007/s00415-017-8619-4
14. Renton AE, Majounie E, Waite A, Simon-Sanchez J, Rollinson S, Gibbs JR, et al. A hexanucleotide repeat expansion in C9ORF72 is the cause of chromosome 9p21-linked ALS-FTD. *Neuron* (2011) 72:257–68. doi: 10.1016/j.neuron.2011.09.010
15. Crockford C, Newton J, Lonergan K, Chiwera T, Booth T, Chandran S, et al. ALS-specific cognitive and behavior changes associated with advancing disease stage in ALS. *Neurology* (2018) 91:e1370–80. doi: 10.1212/WNL.0000000000006317
16. Byrne S, Elamin M, Bede P, Shatunov A, Walsh C, Corr B, et al. Cognitive and clinical characteristics of patients with amyotrophic lateral sclerosis carrying a C9orf72 repeat expansion: a population-based cohort study. *Lancet Neurol.* (2012) 11:232–40. doi: 10.1016/S1474-4422(12)70014-5
17. Elamin M, Bede P, Byrne S, Jordan N, Gallagher L, Wynne B, et al. Cognitive changes predict functional decline in ALS: a population-based longitudinal study. *Neurology* (2013) 80:1590–7. doi: 10.1212/WNL.0b013e31828f18ac
18. Elamin M, Phukan J, Bede P, Jordan N, Byrne S, Pender N, et al. Executive dysfunction is a negative prognostic indicator in patients with ALS without dementia. *Neurology* (2011) 76:1263–9. doi: 10.1212/WNL.0b013e318214359f
19. Olney RK, Murphy J, Forshew D, Garwood E, Miller BL, Langmore S, et al. The effects of executive and behavioral dysfunction on the course of ALS. *Neurology* (2005) 65:1774–7. doi: 10.1212/01.wnl.0000188759.87240.8b
20. Merrilees J, Klapper J, Murphy J, Lomen-Hoerth C, Miller BL. Cognitive and behavioral challenges in caring for patients with frontotemporal dementia and amyotrophic lateral sclerosis. *Amyotroph Lateral Scler.* (2010) 11:298–302. doi: 10.3109/17482961003605788
21. Abrahams S, Goldstein LH, Lloyd CM, Brooks DJ, Leigh PN. Cognitive deficits in non-demented amyotrophic lateral sclerosis patients: a neuropsychological investigation. *J Neurol Sci.* (1995) 129(Suppl.):54–5. doi: 10.1016/0022-510X(95)00063-8
22. Abrahams S, Leigh PN, Kew JJ, Goldstein LH, Lloyd CM, Brooks DJ. A positron emission tomography study of frontal lobe function (verbal fluency) in amyotrophic lateral sclerosis. *J Neurol Sci.* (1995) 129(Suppl.):44–6. doi: 10.1016/0022-510X(95)00060-F
23. Pinto-Grau M, Hardiman O, Pender N. The study of language in the amyotrophic lateral sclerosis - frontotemporal spectrum disorder: a systematic review of findings and new perspectives. *Neuropsychol Rev.* (2018) 28:251–68. doi: 10.1007/s11065-018-9375-7
24. Taylor LJ, Brown RG, Tsermentseli S, Al-Chalabi A, Shaw CE, Ellis CM, et al. Is language impairment more common than executive dysfunction in amyotrophic lateral sclerosis? *J Neurol Neurosurg Psychiatry* (2013) 84:494–8. doi: 10.1136/jnnp-2012-303526
25. Christidi F, Karavasilis E, Zalonis I, Ferentinos P, Giavri Z, Wilde EA, et al. Memory-related white matter tract integrity in amyotrophic lateral sclerosis: an advanced neuroimaging and neuropsychological study. *Neurobiol Aging* (2017) 49:69–78. doi: 10.1016/j.neurobiolaging.2016.09.014
26. Machts J, Bittner V, Kasper E, Schuster C, Prudlo J, Abdulla S, et al. Memory deficits in amyotrophic lateral sclerosis are not exclusively caused by executive dysfunction: a comparative neuropsychological study of amnestic mild cognitive impairment. *BMC Neurosci.* (2014) 15:83. doi: 10.1186/1471-2202-15-83
27. Abrahams S, Goldstein LH, Al-Chalabi A, Pickering A, Morris RG, Passingham RE, et al. Relation between cognitive dysfunction and pseudobulbar palsy in amyotrophic lateral sclerosis. *J Neurol Neurosurg Psychiatry* (1997) 62:464–72. doi: 10.1136/jnnp.62.5.464
28. Bora E. Meta-analysis of social cognition in amyotrophic lateral sclerosis. *Cortex* (2017) 88:1–7. doi: 10.1016/j.cortex.2016.11.012
29. Consonni M, Catricala E, Dalla Bella E, Gessa VC, Lauria G, Cappa SF. Beyond the consensus criteria: multiple cognitive profiles in amyotrophic lateral sclerosis? *Cortex* (2016) 81:162–7. doi: 10.1016/j.cortex.2016.04.014
30. Goldstein S. *Handbook of Executive Functioning.* New York, NY: Springer (2014).
31. Lezak MD. *Neuropsychological Assessment.* 5th ed. ed Oxford New York, NY: Oxford University Press (2012) p. 1161.
32. Abrahams S, Leigh PN, Harvey A, Vythelingum GN, Grise D, Goldstein LH. Verbal fluency and executive dysfunction in amyotrophic lateral sclerosis (ALS). *Neuropsychologia* (2000) 38:734–47. doi: 10.1016/S0028-3932(99)00146-3
33. Abrahams S, Goldstein LH, Kew JJ, Brooks DJ, Lloyd CM, Frith CD, et al. Frontal lobe dysfunction in amyotrophic lateral sclerosis. A PET study. *Brain* (1996) 119(Pt. 6):2105–20.
34. Abrahams S, Leigh PN, Goldstein LH. Cognitive change in ALS: a prospective study. *Neurology* (2005) 64:1222–6. doi: 10.1212/01.WNL.0000156519.41681.27
35. Frank B, Haas J, Heinze HJ, Stark E, Munte TF. Relation of neuropsychological and magnetic resonance findings in amyotrophic lateral sclerosis: evidence for subgroups. *Clin Neurol Neurosurg.* (1997) 99:79–86. doi: 10.1016/S0303-8467(97)80001-7
36. Lomen-Hoerth C, Murphy J, Langmore S, Kramer JH, Olney RK, Miller B. Are amyotrophic lateral sclerosis patients cognitively normal? *Neurology* (2003) 60:1094–7. doi: 10.1212/01.WNL.0000055861.95202.8D
37. Hanagasi HA, Gurvit IH, Ermutlu N, Kaptanoglu G, Karamursel S, Idrisoglu HA, et al. Cognitive impairment in amyotrophic lateral sclerosis: evidence from neuropsychological investigation and event-related potentials. *Brain Res Cogn Brain Res.* (2002) 14:234–44. doi: 10.1016/S0926-6410(02)00110-6
38. Kew JJ, Goldstein LH, Leigh PN, Abrahams S, Cosgrave N, Passingham RE, et al. The relationship between abnormalities of cognitive function and cerebral activation in amyotrophic lateral sclerosis. A neuropsychological and positron emission tomography study. *Brain* (1993) 116(Pt 6):1399–423.
39. Ludolph AC, Langen KJ, Regard M, Herzog H, Kemper B, Kuwert T, et al. Frontal lobe function in amyotrophic lateral sclerosis: a neuropsychologic and positron emission tomography study. *Acta Neurol Scand.* (1992) 85:81–9. doi: 10.1111/j.1600-0404.1992.tb04003.x
40. Pinkhardt EH, Jurgens R, Becker W, Molle M, Born J, Ludolph AC, et al. Signs of impaired selective attention in patients with amyotrophic lateral sclerosis. *J Neurol.* (2008) 255:532–8. doi: 10.1007/s00415-008-0734-9
41. Massman PJ, Sims J, Cooke N, Haverkamp LJ, Appel V, Appel SH. Prevalence and correlates of neuropsychological deficits in amyotrophic lateral sclerosis. *J Neurol Neurosurg Psychiatry* (1996) 61:450–5. doi: 10.1136/jnnp.61.5.450
42. Witgert M, Salamone AR, Strutt AM, Jawaid A, Massman PJ, Bradshaw M, et al. Frontal-lobe mediated behavioral dysfunction in amyotrophic lateral sclerosis. *Eur J Neurol.* (2010) 17:103–10. doi: 10.1111/j.1468-1331.2009.02801.x

43. Rakowicz WP, Hodges JR. Dementia and aphasia in motor neuron disease: an underrecognised association? *J Neurol Neurosurg Psychiatry* (1998) 65:881–9. doi: 10.1136/jnnp.65.6.881
44. Stukovnik V, Zidar J, Podnar S, Repovs G. Amyotrophic lateral sclerosis patients show executive impairments on standard neuropsychological measures and an ecologically valid motor-free test of executive functions. *J Clin Exp Neuropsychol.* (2010) 32:1095–109. doi: 10.1080/13803391003749236
45. Wicks P, Abrahams S, Papps B, Al-Chalabi A, Shaw CE, Leigh PN, et al. SOD1 and cognitive dysfunction in familial amyotrophic lateral sclerosis. *J Neurol.* (2009) 256:234–41. doi: 10.1007/s00415-009-0078-0
46. Abrahams S, Goldstein LH, Simmons A, Brammer M, Williams SC, Giampietro V, et al. Word retrieval in amyotrophic lateral sclerosis: a functional magnetic resonance imaging study. *Brain* (2004) 127(Pt 7):1507–17. doi: 10.1093/brain/awh170
47. Hartikainen P, Helkala EL, Soininen H, Riekkinen P, Sr. Cognitive and memory deficits in untreated Parkinson's disease and amyotrophic lateral sclerosis patients: a comparative study. *J Neural Transm Park Dis Dement Sect.* (1993) 6:127–37. doi: 10.1007/BF02261006
48. Abrahams S, Newton J, Niven E, Foley J, Bak TH. Screening for cognition and behaviour changes in ALS. *Amyotroph Lateral Scler Frontotemporal Degener.* (2014) 15:9–14. doi: 10.3109/21678421.2013.805784
49. Evdokimidis I, Constantinidis TS, Gourtzelidis P, Smyrnis N, Zalonis I, Zis PV, et al. Frontal lobe dysfunction in amyotrophic lateral sclerosis. *J Neurol Sci.* (2002) 195:25–33. doi: 10.1016/S0022-510X(01)00683-9
50. Libon DJ, McMillan C, Avants B, Boller A, Morgan B, Burkholder L, et al. Deficits in concept formation in amyotrophic lateral sclerosis. *Neuropsychology* (2012) 26:422–9. doi: 10.1037/a0028668
51. Moretti R, Torre P, Antonello RM, Carraro N, Cazzato G, Bava A. Complex cognitive disruption in motor neuron disease. *Dement Geriatr Cogn Disord.* (2002) 14:141–50. doi: 10.1159/000063600
52. Schreiber H, Gaigalat T, Wiedemuth-Catrinescu U, Graf M, Uttner I, Muche R, et al. Cognitive function in bulbar- and spinal-onset amyotrophic lateral sclerosis. A longitudinal study in 52 patients. *J Neurol. (*2005) 252:772–81. doi: 10.1007/s00415-005-0739-6
53. Zalonis I, Christidi F, Paraskevas G, Zabelis T, Evdokimidis I, Kararizou E. Can executive cognitive measures differentiate between patients with spinal- and bulbar-onset amyotrophic lateral sclerosis? *Arch Clin Neuropsychol.* (2012) 27:348–54. doi: 10.1093/arclin/acs031
54. Hammer A, Vielhaber S, Rodriguez-Fornells A, Mohammadi B, Munte TF. A neurophysiological analysis of working memory in amyotrophic lateral sclerosis. *Brain Res.* (2011) 1421:90–9. doi: 10.1016/j.brainres.2011.09.010
55. Kilani M, Micallef J, Soubrouillard C, Rey-Lardiller D, Demattei C, Dib M, et al. A longitudinal study of the evolution of cognitive function and affective state in patients with amyotrophic lateral sclerosis. *Amyotroph Lateral Scler Other Motor Neuron Disord.* (2004) 5:46–54. doi: 10.1080/14660820310017560
56. Lule D, Diekmann V, Anders S, Kassubek J, Kubler A, Ludolph AC, et al. Brain responses to emotional stimuli in patients with amyotrophic lateral sclerosis (ALS). *J Neurol.* (2007) 254:519–27. doi: 10.1007/s00415-006-0409-3
57. Sterling LE, Jawaid A, Salamone AR, Murthy SB, Mosnik DM, McDowell E, et al. Association between dysarthria and cognitive impairment in ALS: a prospective study. *Amyotroph Lateral Scler.* (2010) 11:46–51. doi: 10.3109/17482960903207997
58. Jelsone-Swain L, Persad C, Votruba KL, Weisenbach SL, Johnson T, Gruis KL, et al. The relationship between depressive symptoms, disease state, and cognition in amyotrophic lateral sclerosis. *Front Psychol.* (2012) 3:542. doi: 10.3389/fpsyg.2012.00542
59. Mioshi E, Lillo P, Yew B, Hsieh S, Savage S, Hodges JR, et al. Cortical atrophy in ALS is critically associated with neuropsychiatric and cognitive changes. *Neurology* (2013) 80:1117–23. doi: 10.1212/WNL.0b013e31828869da
60. Christidi F, Zalonis I, Smyrnis N, Evdokimidis I. Selective attention and the three-process memory model for the interpretation of verbal free recall in amyotrophic lateral sclerosis. *J Int Neuropsychol Soc.* (2012) 18:809–18. doi: 10.1017/S1355617712000562
61. Lillo P, Mioshi E, Burrell JR, Kiernan MC, Hodges JR, Hornberger M. Grey and white matter changes across the amyotrophic lateral sclerosis-frontotemporal dementia continuum. *PLoS ONE* (2012) 7:e43993. doi: 10.1371/journal.pone.0043993
62. Newsom-Davis IC, Lyall RA, Leigh PN, Moxham J, Goldstein LH. The effect of non-invasive positive pressure ventilation (NIPPV) on cognitive function in amyotrophic lateral sclerosis (ALS): a prospective study. *J Neurol Neurosurg Psychiatry* (2001) 71:482–7. doi: 10.1136/jnnp.71.4.482
63. Meier SL, Charleston AJ, Tippett LJ. Cognitive and behavioural deficits associated with the orbitomedial prefrontal cortex in amyotrophic lateral sclerosis. *Brain* (2010) 133:3444–57. doi: 10.1093/brain/awq254
64. Christidi F, Karavasilis E, Velonakis G, Ferentinos P, Rentzos M, Kelekis N, et al. The clinical and radiological spectrum of hippocampal pathology in amyotrophic lateral sclerosis. *Front Neurol.* (2018) 9:523. doi: 10.3389/fneur.2018.00523
65. Hsieh S, Irish M, Foxe D, Caga J, Devenney E, Ahmed R, et al. My memories are important to me: changes in autobiographical memory in amyotrophic lateral sclerosis. *Neuropsychology* (2016) 30:920–30. doi: 10.1037/neu0000291
66. Hervieu-Begue M, Rouaud O, Graule Petot A, Catteau A, Giroud M. Semantic memory assessment in 15 patients with amyotrophic lateral sclerosis. *Revue Neurol.* (2016) 172:307–12. doi: 10.1016/j.neurol.2015.10.009
67. Iwasaki Y, Kinoshita M, Ikeda K, Takamiya K, Shiojima T. Cognitive impairment in amyotrophic lateral sclerosis and its relation to motor disabilities. *Acta Neurol Scand.* (1990) 81:141–3. doi: 10.1111/j.1600-0404.1990.tb00950.x
68. Mantovan MC, Baggio L, Dalla Barba G, Smith P, Pegoraro E, Soraru G, et al. Memory deficits and retrieval processes in ALS. *Eur J Neurol.* (2003) 10:221–7. doi: 10.1046/j.1468-1331.2003.00607.x
69. Abe K, Fujimura H, Toyooka K, Sakoda S, Yorifuji S, Yanagihara T. Cognitive function in amyotrophic lateral sclerosis. *J Neurol Sci.* (1997) 148:95–100. doi: 10.1016/S0022-510X(96)05338-5
70. Raaphorst J, van Tol MJ, de Visser M, van der Kooi AJ, Majoie CB, van den Berg LH, et al. Prose memory impairment in amyotrophic lateral sclerosis patients is related to hippocampus volume. *Eur J Neurol.* (2015) 22:547–54. doi: 10.1111/ene.12615
71. Bede P, Omer T, Finegan E, Chipika RH, Iyer PM, Doherty MA, et al. Connectivity-based characterisation of subcortical grey matter pathology in frontotemporal dementia and ALS: a multimodal neuroimaging study. *Brain Imag Behav.* (2018). doi: 10.1007/s11682-018-9837-9. [Epub ahead of print].
72. Omer T, Finegan E, Hutchinson S, Doherty M, Vajda A, McLaughlin RL, et al. Neuroimaging patterns along the ALS-FTD spectrum: a multiparametric imaging study. *Amyotroph Lateral Scler Frontotemporal Degener.* (2017) 18:611–23. doi: 10.1080/21678421.2017.1332077
73. Ash S, Olm C, McMillan CT, Boller A, Irwin DJ, McCluskey L, et al. Deficits in sentence expression in amyotrophic lateral sclerosis. *Amyotroph Lateral Scler Frontotemporal Degener.* (2015) 16:31–9. doi: 10.3109/21678421.2014.974617
74. Tsermentseli S, Leigh PN, Taylor LJ, Radunovic A, Catani M, Goldstein LH. Syntactic processing as a marker for cognitive impairment in amyotrophic lateral sclerosis. *Amyotroph Lateral Scler Frontotemporal Degener.* (2015) 17:69–76. doi: 10.3109/21678421.2015.1071397
75. Bak TH, O'Donovan DG, Xuereb JH, Boniface S, Hodges JR. Selective impairment of verb processing associated with pathological changes in Brodmann areas 44 and 45 in the motor neurone disease-dementia-aphasia syndrome. *Brain* (2001) 124(Pt 1):103–20. doi: 10.1093/brain/124.1.103
76. Papeo L, Cecchetto C, Mazzon G, Granello G, Cattaruzza T, Verriello L, et al. The processing of actions and action-words in amyotrophic lateral sclerosis patients. *Cortex* (2015) 64:136–47. doi: 10.1016/j.cortex.2014.10.007
77. Grossman M, Anderson C, Khan A, Avants B, Elman L, McCluskey L. Impaired action knowledge in amyotrophic lateral sclerosis. *Neurology* (2008) 71:1396–401. doi: 10.1212/01.wnl.0000319701.50168.8c
78. York C, Olm C, Boller A, McCluskey L, Elman L, Haley J, et al. Action verb comprehension in amyotrophic lateral sclerosis and Parkinson's disease. *J Neurol.* (2014) 261:1073–9. doi: 10.1007/s00415-014-7314-y
79. Bak TH, Chandran S. What wires together dies together: verbs, actions and neurodegeneration in motor neuron disease. *Cortex* (2012) 48:936–44. doi: 10.1016/j.cortex.2011.07.008
80. Roberts-South A, Findlater K, Strong MJ, Orange JB. Longitudinal changes in discourse production in amyotrophic lateral sclerosis.

Semin Speech Language (2012) 33:79–94. doi: 10.1055/s-0031-1301165
81. Bambini V, Arcara G, Martinelli I, Bernini S, Alvisi E, Moro A, et al. Communication and pragmatic breakdowns in amyotrophic lateral sclerosis patients. *Brain Language* (2016) 153–154:1–12. doi: 10.1016/j.bandl.2015.12.002
82. Yunusova Y, Graham NL, Shellikeri S, Phuong K, Kulkarni M, Rochon E, et al. Profiling speech and pausing in amyotrophic lateral sclerosis (ALS) and frontotemporal dementia (FTD). *PLoS ONE* (2016) 11:e0147573. doi: 10.1371/journal.pone.0147573
83. Kamminga J, Leslie FVC, Hsieh S, Caga J, Mioshi E, Hornberger M, et al. Syntactic comprehension deficits across the FTD-ALS continuum. *Neurobiol Aging* (2016) 41:11–8. doi: 10.1016/j.neurobiolaging.2016.02.002
84. Yoshizawa K, Yasuda N, Fukuda M, Yukimoto Y, Ogino M, Hata W, et al. Syntactic comprehension in patients with amyotrophic lateral sclerosis. *Behav Neurol.* (2014) 2014:230578. doi: 10.1155/2014/230578
85. Strong MJ, Grace GM, Orange JB, Leeper HA, Menon RS, Aere C. A prospective study of cognitive impairment in ALS. *Neurology* (1999) 53:1665–70. doi: 10.1212/WNL.53.8.1665
86. Bede P, Iyer PM, Schuster C, Elamin M, McLaughlin RL, Kenna K, et al. The selective anatomical vulnerability of ALS: 'disease-defining' and 'disease-defying' brain regions. *Amyotroph Lateral Scler Frontotemporal Degener.* (2016) 17:561–70. doi: 10.3109/21678421.2016.1173702
87. Geser F, Brandmeir NJ, Kwong LK, Martinez-Lage M, Elman L, McCluskey L, et al. Evidence of multisystem disorder in whole-brain map of pathological TDP—43 in amyotrophic lateral sclerosis. *Arch Neurol.* (2008) 65:636–41. doi: 10.1001/archneur.65.5.636
88. Lobo PP, Pinto S, Rocha L, Reimao S, de Carvalho M. Orofacial apraxia in motor neuron disease. *Case Rep Neurol.* (2013) 5:47–51. doi: 10.1159/000349895
89. Duffy JR, Peach RK, Strand EA. Progressive apraxia of speech as a sign of motor neuron disease. *Am J Speech Language Pathol.* (2007) 16:198–208. doi: 10.1044/1058-0360(2007/025)
90. Pinto S, Pinto A, Atalaia A, Peralta R, de Carvalho M. Respiratory apraxia in amyotrophic lateral sclerosis. *Amyotr Lateral Scler.* (2007) 8:180–4. doi: 10.1080/17482960701249340
91. Adolphs R. The social brain: neural basis of social knowledge. *Ann Rev Psychol.* (2009) 60:693–716. doi: 10.1146/annurev.psych.60.110707.163514
92. Christidi F, Migliaccio R, Santamaria-Garcia H, Santangelo G, Trojsi F. Social cognition dysfunctions in neurodegenerative diseases: neuroanatomical correlates and clinical implications. *Behav Neurol.* (2018) 2018:1849794. doi: 10.1155/2018/1849794
93. Carluer L, Mondou A, Buhour MS, Laisney M, Pelerin A, Eustache F, et al. Neural substrate of cognitive theory of mind impairment in amyotrophic lateral sclerosis. *Cortex* (2015) 65:19–30. doi: 10.1016/j.cortex.2014.12.010
94. Cavallo M, Adenzato M, Macpherson SE, Karwig G, Enrici I, Abrahams S. Evidence of social understanding impairment in patients with amyotrophic lateral sclerosis. *PLoS ONE* (2011) 6:e25948. doi: 10.1371/journal.pone.0025948
95. Cerami C, Dodich A, Canessa N, Crespi C, Iannaccone S, Corbo M, et al. Emotional empathy in amyotrophic lateral sclerosis: a behavioural and voxel-based morphometry study. *Amyotroph Lateral Scler Frontotemporal Degener.* (2014) 15:21–9. doi: 10.3109/21678421.2013.785568
96. Girardi A, MacPherson SE, Abrahams S. Deficits in emotional and social cognition in amyotrophic lateral sclerosis. *Neuropsychology* (2011) 25:53–65. doi: 10.1037/a0020357
97. Watermeyer TJ, Brown RG, Sidle KC, Oliver DJ, Allen C, Karlsson J, et al. Executive dysfunction predicts social cognition impairment in amyotrophic lateral sclerosis. *J Neurol.* (2015) 262:1681–90. doi: 10.1007/s00415-015-7761-0
98. Staios M, Fisher F, Lindell AK, Ong B, Howe J, Reardon K. Exploring sarcasm detection in amyotrophic lateral sclerosis using ecologically valid measures. *Front Hum Neurosci.* (2013) 7:178. doi: 10.3389/fnhum.2013.00178
99. Trojsi F, Siciliano M, Russo A, Passaniti C, Femiano C, Ferrantino T, et al. Theory of mind and its neuropsychological and quality of life correlates in the early stages of amyotrophic lateral sclerosis. *Front Psychol.* (2016) 7:1934. doi: 10.3389/fpsyg.2016.01934
100. Savage SA, Lillo P, Kumfor F, Kiernan MC, Piguet O, Hodges JR. Emotion processing deficits distinguish pure amyotrophic lateral sclerosis from frontotemporal dementia. *Amyotroph Lateral Scler Frontotemporal Degener.* (2014) 15:39–46. doi: 10.3109/21678421.2013.809763
101. Palmieri A, Naccarato M, Abrahams S, Bonato M, D'Ascenzo C, Balestreri S, et al. Right hemisphere dysfunction and emotional processing in ALS: an fMRI study. *J Neurol.* (2010) 257:1970–8. doi: 10.1007/s00415-010-5640-2
102. Crespi C, Cerami C, Dodich A, Canessa N, Arpone M, Iannaccone S, et al. Microstructural white matter correlates of emotion recognition impairment in Amyotrophic Lateral Sclerosis. *Cortex* (2014) 53:1–8. doi: 10.1016/j.cortex.2014.01.002
103. Andrews SC, Staios M, Howe J, Reardon K, Fisher F. Multimodal emotion processing deficits are present in amyotrophic lateral sclerosis. *Neuropsychology* (2017) 31:304–10. doi: 10.1037/neu0000323
104. Gibbons ZC, Snowden JS, Thompson JC, Happe F, Richardson A, Neary D. Inferring thought and action in motor neurone disease. *Neuropsychologia* (2007) 45:1196–207. doi: 10.1016/j.neuropsychologia.2006.10.008
105. Burke T, Elamin M, Bede P, Pinto-Grau M, Lonergan K, Hardiman O, et al. Discordant performance on the 'Reading the Mind in the Eyes' Test, based on disease onset in amyotrophic lateral sclerosis. *Amyotroph Lateral Scler Frontotemporal Degener.* (2016) 17:467–72. doi: 10.1080/21678421.2016.1177088
106. Elamin M, Pinto-Grau M, Burke T, Bede P, Rooney J, O'Sullivan M, et al. Identifying behavioural changes in ALS: validation of the Beaumont Behavioural Inventory (BBI). *Amyotroph Lateral Scler Frontotemporal Degener.* (2017) 18:68–73. doi: 10.1080/21678421.2016.1248976.
107. Raaphorst J, Beeldman E, De Visser M, De Haan RJ, Schmand B. A systematic review of behavioural changes in motor neuron disease. *Amyotroph Lateral Scler.* (2012) 13:493–501. doi: 10.3109/17482968.2012.656652
108. Grossman AB, Woolley-Levine S, Bradley WG, Miller RG. Detecting neurobehavioral changes in amyotrophic lateral sclerosis. *Amyotroph Lateral Scler.* (2007) 8:56–61. doi: 10.1080/17482960601044106
109. Chio A, Vignola A, Mastro E, Giudici AD, Iazzolino B, Calvo A, et al. Neurobehavioral symptoms in ALS are negatively related to caregivers' burden and quality of life. *Eur J Neurol.* (2010) 17:1298–303. doi: 10.1111/j.1468-1331.2010.03016.x
110. Grace J, Mallow, P.F. *Frontal Systems Behavior Scale.* Lutz, FL: Psychological Assessment Resources (2001).
111. Kertesz A, Davidson W, Fox H. Frontal behavioral inventory: diagnostic criteria for frontal lobe dementia. *Can J Neurol Sci.* (1997) 24:29–36.
112. Radakovic R, Abrahams S. Developing a new apathy measurement scale: dimensional apathy scale. *Psychiatry Res.* (2014) 219:658–63. doi: 10.1016/j.psychres.2014.06.010
113. Radakovic R, Stephenson L, Colville S, Swingler R, Chandran S, Abrahams S. Multidimensional apathy in ALS: validation of the Dimensional Apathy Scale. *J Neurol Neurosurg Psychiatry* (2016) 87:663–9. doi: 10.1136/jnnp-2015-310772
114. Terada T, Obi T, Yoshizumi M, Murai T, Miyajima H, Mizoguchi K. Frontal lobe-mediated behavioral changes in amyotrophic lateral sclerosis: are they independent of physical disabilities? *J Neurol Sci.* (2011) 309:136–40. doi: 10.1016/j.jns.2011.06.049
115. Turner MR, Talbot K. Sweet food preference in amyotrophic lateral sclerosis. *Pract Neurol.* (2017) 17:128–9. doi: 10.1136/practneurol-2016-001554
116. Snowden JS, Rollinson S, Thompson JC, Harris JM, Stopford CL, Richardson AM, et al. Distinct clinical and pathological characteristics of frontotemporal dementia associated with C9ORF72 mutations. *Brain* (2012) 135(Pt 3):693–708. doi: 10.1093/brain/awr355
117. Kertesz A, Ang LC, Jesso S, MacKinley J, Baker M, Brown P, et al. Psychosis and hallucinations in frontotemporal dementia with the C9ORF72 mutation: a detailed clinical cohort. *Cogn Behav Neurol.* (2013) 26:146–54. doi: 10.1097/WNN.0000000000000008
118. Nitrini R, Rosemberg S. Psychotic symptoms in dementia associated with motor neuron disease: a pathophysiological hypothesis. *J Neuropsychiatry Clin Neurosci.* (1998) 10:456–8. doi: 10.1176/jnp.10.4.456
119. Lillo P, Garcin B, Hornberger M, Bak TH, Hodges JR. Neurobehavioral features in frontotemporal dementia with amyotrophic lateral sclerosis. *Arch Neurol.* (2010) 67:826–30. doi: 10.1001/archneurol.2010.146

120. Noh SM, Chung SJ, Kim KK, Kang DW, Lim YM, Kwon SU, et al. Emotional disturbance in CADASIL: its impact on quality of life and caregiver burden. *Cerebrovasc Dis.* (2014) 37:188–94. doi: 10.1159/000357798
121. Lauterbach EC, Cummings JL, Kuppuswamy PS. Toward a more precise, clinically-informed pathophysiology of pathological laughing and crying. *Neurosci Biobehav Rev.* (2013) 37:1893–916. doi: 10.1016/j.neubiorev.2013.03.002
122. Bede P, Finegan E. Revisiting the pathoanatomy of pseudobulbar affect: mechanisms beyond corticobulbar dysfunction. *Amyotroph Lateral Scler Frontotemporal Degener.* (2018) 19:4–6. doi: 10.1080/21678421.2017.1392578
123. Brooks BR, Crumpacker D, Fellus J, Kantor D, Kaye RE. PRISM: a novel research tool to assess the prevalence of pseudobulbar affect symptoms across neurological conditions. *PLoS ONE* (2013) 8:e72232. doi: 10.1371/journal.pone.0072232
124. Palmieri A, Abrahams S, Soraru G, Mattiuzzi L, D'Ascenzo C, Pegoraro E, et al. Emotional Lability in MND: Relationship to cognition and psychopathology and impact on caregivers. *J Neurol Sci.* (2009) 278:16–20. doi: 10.1016/j.jns.2008.10.025
125. McCullagh S, Moore M, Gawel M, Feinstein A. Pathological laughing and crying in amyotrophic lateral sclerosis: an association with prefrontal cognitive dysfunction. *J Neurol Sci.* (1999) 169:43–8. doi: 10.1016/S0022-510X(99)00214-2
126. Olney NT, Goodkind MS, Lomen-Hoerth C, Whalen PK, Williamson CA, Holley DE, et al. Behaviour, physiology and experience of pathological laughing and crying in amyotrophic lateral sclerosis. *Brain* (2011) 134(Pt 12):3458–69. doi: 10.1093/brain/awr297
127. Floeter MK, Katipally R, Kim MP, Schanz O, Stephen M, Danielian L, et al. Impaired corticopontocerebellar tracts underlie pseudobulbar affect in motor neuron disorders. *Neurology* (2014) 83:620–7. doi: 10.1212/WNL.0000000000000693
128. Christidi F, Karavasilis E, Ferentinos P, Xirou S, Velonakis G, Rentzos M, et al. Investigating the neuroanatomical substrate of pathological laughing and crying in amyotrophic lateral sclerosis with multimodal neuroimaging techniques. *Amyotroph Lateral Scler Frontotemporal Degener.* (2018) 19(1–2):12–20. doi: 10.1080/21678421.2017.1386689
129. Verstraete E, Turner MR, Grosskreutz J, Filippi M, Benatar M. Mind the gap: The mismatch between clinical and imaging metrics in ALS. *Amyotroph Lateral Scler Frontotemporal Degener.* (2015) 16:524–9. doi: 10.3109/21678421.2015.1051989
130. Bede P, Querin G, Pradat PF. The changing landscape of motor neuron disease imaging: the transition from descriptive studies to precision clinical tools. *Curr Opin Neurol.* (2018) 31:431–8. doi: 10.1097/WCO.0000000000000569
131. Shen D, Cui L, Fang J, Cui B, Li D, Tai H. Voxel-wise meta-analysis of gray matter changes in amyotrophic lateral sclerosis. *Front Aging Neurosci.* (2016) 8:64. doi: 10.3389/fnagi.2016.00064
132. Bede P, Hardiman O. Lessons of ALS imaging: Pitfalls and future directions - A critical review. *NeuroImage Clin.* (2014) 4:436–43. doi: 10.1016/j.nicl.2014.02.011
133. Bede P, Elamin M, Byrne S, McLaughlin RL, Kenna K, Vajda A, et al. Basal ganglia involvement in amyotrophic lateral sclerosis. *Neurology* (2013) 81:2107–15. doi: 10.1212/01.wnl.0000437313.80913.2c
134. Bede P, Bokde A, Elamin M, Byrne S, McLaughlin RL, Jordan N, et al. Grey matter correlates of clinical variables in amyotrophic lateral sclerosis (ALS): a neuroimaging study of ALS motor phenotype heterogeneity and cortical focality. *J Neurol Neurosurg Psychiatry* (2013) 84:766–73. doi: 10.1136/jnnp-2012-302674
135. Bede P, Bokde AL, Byrne S, Elamin M, McLaughlin RL, Kenna K, et al. Multiparametric MRI study of ALS stratified for the C9orf72 genotype. *Neurology* (2013) 81:361–9. doi: 10.1212/WNL.0b013e31829c5eee
136. Westeneng HJ, Verstraete E, Walhout R, Schmidt R, Hendrikse J, Veldink JH, et al. Subcortical structures in amyotrophic lateral sclerosis. *Neurobiol Aging* (2015) 36:1075–82. doi: 10.1016/j.neurobiolaging.2014.09.002
137. Pinkhardt EH, van Elst LT, Ludolph AC, Kassubek J. Amygdala size in amyotrophic lateral sclerosis without dementia: an *in vivo* study using MRI volumetry. *BMC Neurol.* (2006) 6:48. doi: 10.1186/1471-2377-6-48
138. Machts J, Loewe K, Kaufmann J, Jakubiczka S, Abdulla S, Petri S, et al. Basal ganglia pathology in ALS is associated with neuropsychological deficits. *Neurology* (2015) 85:1301–9. doi: 10.1212/WNL.0000000000002017
139. Thivard L, Pradat PF, Lehericy S, Lacomblez L, Dormont D, Chiras J, et al. Diffusion tensor imaging and voxel based morphometry study in amyotrophic lateral sclerosis: relationships with motor disability. *J Neurol Neurosurg Psychiatry* (2007) 78:889–92. doi: 10.1136/jnnp.2006.101758
140. Chang JL, Lomen-Hoerth C, Murphy J, Henry RG, Kramer JH, Miller BL, et al. A voxel-based morphometry study of patterns of brain atrophy in ALS and ALS/FTLD. *Neurology* (2005) 65:75–80. doi: 10.1212/01.wnl.0000167602.38643.29
141. Schuster C, Kasper E, Machts J, Bittner D, Kaufmann J, Benecke R, et al. Focal thinning of the motor cortex mirrors clinical features of amyotrophic lateral sclerosis and their phenotypes: a neuroimaging study. *J Neurol.* (2013) 260:2856–64. doi: 10.1007/s00415-013-7083-z
142. Bede P, Hardiman O. Longitudinal structural changes in ALS: a three time-point imaging study of white and gray matter degeneration. *Amyotroph Lateral Scler Frontotemporal Degener.* (2018) 19:232–41. doi: 10.1080/21678421.2017.1407795
143. Agosta F, Valsasina P, Riva N, Copetti M, Messina MJ, Prelle A, et al. The cortical signature of amyotrophic lateral sclerosis. *PLoS ONE* (2012) 7:e42816. doi: 10.1371/journal.pone.0042816
144. Mezzapesa DM, Ceccarelli A, Dicuonzo F, Carella A, De Caro MF, Lopez M, et al. Whole-brain and regional brain atrophy in amyotrophic lateral sclerosis. *AJNR Am J Neuroradiol.* (2007) 28:255–9.
145. Mezzapesa DM, D'Errico E, Tortelli R, Distaso E, Cortese R, Tursi M, et al. Cortical thinning and clinical heterogeneity in amyotrophic lateral sclerosis. *PLoS ONE* (2013) 8:e80748. doi: 10.1371/journal.pone.0080748
146. Christidi F, Karavasilis E, Riederer F, Zalonis I, Ferentinos P, Velonakis G, et al. Gray matter and white matter changes in non-demented amyotrophic lateral sclerosis patients with or without cognitive impairment: a combined voxel-based morphometry and tract-based spatial statistics whole-brain analysis. *Brain Imaging Behav.* (2018) 12:547–63. doi: 10.1007/s11682-017-9722-y
147. Alruwaili AR, Pannek K, Coulthard A, Henderson R, Kurniawan ND, McCombe P. A combined tract-based spatial statistics and voxel-based morphometry study of the first MRI scan after diagnosis of amyotrophic lateral sclerosis with subgroup analysis. *J Neuroradiol.* (2018) 45:41–8. doi: 10.1016/j.neurad.2017.03.007
148. Murphy JM, Henry RG, Langmore S, Kramer JH, Miller BL, Lomen-Hoerth C. Continuum of frontal lobe impairment in amyotrophic lateral sclerosis. *Arch Neurol.* (2007) 64:530–4. doi: 10.1001/archneur.64.4.530
149. Agosta F, Ferraro PM, Riva N, Spinelli EG, Chio A, Canu E, et al. Structural brain correlates of cognitive and behavioral impairment in MND. *Hum Brain Map.* (2016) 37:1614–26. doi: 10.1002/hbm.23124
150. Masuda M, Senda J, Watanabe H, Epifanio B, Tanaka Y, Imai K, et al. Involvement of the caudate nucleus head and its networks in sporadic amyotrophic lateral sclerosis-frontotemporal dementia continuum. *Amyotroph Lateral Scler Frontotemporal Degener.* (2016) 17:571–9. doi: 10.1080/21678421.2016.1211151
151. Zhang F, Chen G, He M, Dai J, Shang H, Gong Q, et al. Altered white matter microarchitecture in amyotrophic lateral sclerosis: A voxel-based meta-analysis of diffusion tensor imaging. *NeuroImage Clin.* (2018) 19:122–9. doi: 10.1016/j.nicl.2018.04.005
152. Foerster BR, Dwamena BA, Petrou M, Carlos RC, Callaghan BC, Churchill CL, et al. Diagnostic accuracy of diffusion tensor imaging in amyotrophic lateral sclerosis: a systematic review and individual patient data meta-analysis. *Acad Radiol.* (2013) 20:1099–106. doi: 10.1016/j.acra.2013.03.017
153. Abe O, Yamada H, Masutani Y, Aoki S, Kunimatsu A, Yamasue H, et al. Amyotrophic lateral sclerosis: diffusion tensor tractography and voxel-based analysis. *NMR Biomed.* (2004) 17:411–6. doi: 10.1002/nbm.907
154. Agosta F, Pagani E, Rocca MA, Caputo D, Perini M, Salvi F, et al. Voxel-based morphometry study of brain volumetry and diffusivity in amyotrophic lateral sclerosis patients with mild disability. *Hum Brain Map.* (2007) 28:1430–8. doi: 10.1002/hbm.20364
155. Ciccarelli O, Behrens TE, Johansen-Berg H, Talbot K, Orrell RW, Howard RS, et al. Investigation of white matter pathology in ALS and PLS

using tract-based spatial statistics. *Hum Brain Map.* (2009) 30:615–24. doi: 10.1002/hbm.20527

156. Filippini N, Douaud G, Mackay CE, Knight S, Talbot K, Turner MR. Corpus callosum involvement is a consistent feature of amyotrophic lateral sclerosis. *Neurology* (2010) 75:1645–52. doi: 10.1212/WNL.0b013e3181fb84d1
157. Keil C, Prell T, Peschel T, Hartung V, Dengler R, Grosskreutz J. Longitudinal diffusion tensor imaging in amyotrophic lateral sclerosis. *BMC Neurosci.* (2012) 13:141. doi: 10.1186/1471-2202-13-141
158. Rosskopf J, Muller HP, Dreyhaupt J, Gorges M, Ludolph AC, Kassubek J. Ex post facto assessment of diffusion tensor imaging metrics from different MRI protocols: preparing for multicentre studies in ALS. *Amyotroph Lateral Scler Frontotemporal Degener.* (2015) 16:92–101. doi: 10.3109/21678421.2014.977297
159. Sach M, Winkler G, Glauche V, Liepert J, Heimbach B, Koch MA, et al. Diffusion tensor MRI of early upper motor neuron involvement in amyotrophic lateral sclerosis. *Brain* (2004) 127(Pt 2):340–50. doi: 10.1093/brain/awh041
160. Sage CA, Van Hecke W, Peeters R, Sijbers J, Robberecht W, Parizel P, et al. Quantitative diffusion tensor imaging in amyotrophic lateral sclerosis: revisited. *Hum Brain Map.* (2009) 30:3657–75. doi: 10.1002/hbm.20794
161. Sato K, Aoki S, Iwata NK, Masutani Y, Watadani T, Nakata Y, et al. Diffusion tensor tract-specific analysis of the uncinate fasciculus in patients with amyotrophic lateral sclerosis. *Neuroradiology* (2010) 52:729–33. doi: 10.1007/s00234-010-0653-1
162. Prell T, Peschel T, Hartung V, Kaufmann J, Klauschies R, Bodammer N, et al. Diffusion tensor imaging patterns differ in bulbar and limb onset amyotrophic lateral sclerosis. *Clin Neurol Neurosurg.* (2013) 115:1281–7. doi: 10.1016/j.clineuro.2012.11.031
163. Sarica A, Cerasa A, Vasta R, Perrotta P, Valentino P, Mangone G, et al. Tractography in amyotrophic lateral sclerosis using a novel probabilistic tool: a study with tract-based reconstruction compared to voxel-based approach. *J Neurosci Methods* (2014) 224:79–87. doi: 10.1016/j.jneumeth.2013.12.014
164. Bede P, Elamin M, Byrne S, McLaughlin RL, Kenna K, Vajda A, et al. Patterns of cerebral and cerebellar white matter degeneration in ALS. *J Neurol Neurosur Psychiatry* (2015) 86:468–70. doi: 10.1136/jnnp-2014-308172
165. Foerster BR, Carlos RC, Dwamena BA, Callaghan BC, Petrou M, Edden RA, et al. Multimodal MRI as a diagnostic biomarker for amyotrophic lateral sclerosis. *Ann Clin Transl Neurol.* (2014) 1:107–14. doi: 10.1002/acn3.30
166. Sivak S, Bittsansky M, Kurca E, Turcanova-Koprusakova M, Grofik M, Nosal V, et al. Proton magnetic resonance spectroscopy in patients with early stages of amyotrophic lateral sclerosis. *Neuroradiology* (2010) 52:1079–85. doi: 10.1007/s00234-010-0685-6
167. Pyra T, Hui B, Hanstock C, Concha L, Wong JC, Beaulieu C, et al. Combined structural and neurochemical evaluation of the corticospinal tract in amyotrophic lateral sclerosis. *Amyotroph Lateral Scler.* (2010) 11:157–65. doi: 10.3109/17482960902756473
168. Verma G, Woo JH, Chawla S, Wang S, Sheriff S, Elman LB, et al. Whole-brain analysis of amyotrophic lateral sclerosis by using echo-planar spectroscopic imaging. *Radiology* (2013) 267:851–7. doi: 10.1148/radiol.13121148
169. Usman U, Choi C, Camicioli R, Seres P, Lynch M, Sekhon R, et al. Mesial prefrontal cortex degeneration in amyotrophic lateral sclerosis: a high-field proton MR spectroscopy study. *AJNR Am J Neuroradiol.* (2011) 32:1677–80. doi: 10.3174/ajnr.A2590
170. Cistaro A, Cuccurullo V, Quartuccio N, Pagani M, Valentini MC, Mansi L. Role of PET and SPECT in the study of amyotrophic lateral sclerosis. *BioMed Res Int.* (2014) 2014:237437. doi: 10.1155/2014/237437
171. Pagani M, Chio A, Valentini MC, Oberg J, Nobili F, Calvo A, et al. Functional pattern of brain FDG-PET in amyotrophic lateral sclerosis. *Neurology* (2014) 83:1067–74. doi: 10.1212/WNL.0000000000000792
172. Renard D, Collombier L, Castelnovo G, Fourcade G, Kotzki PO, LaBauge P. Brain FDG-PET changes in ALS and ALS-FTD. *Acta Neurologica Belgica.* (2011) 111:306–9.
173. Van Laere K, Vanhee A, Verschueren J, De Coster L, Driesen A, Dupont P, et al. Value of 18fluorodeoxyglucose-positron-emission tomography in amyotrophic lateral sclerosis: a prospective study. *JAMA Neurol.* (2014) 71:553–61. doi: 10.1001/jamaneurol.2014.62
174. Cistaro A, Valentini MC, Chio A, Nobili F, Calvo A, Moglia C, et al. Brain hypermetabolism in amyotrophic lateral sclerosis: a FDG PET study in ALS of spinal and bulbar onset. *Eur J Nuclear Med Mol Imag.* (2012) 39:251–9. doi: 10.1007/s00259-011-1979-6
175. Rajagopalan V, Pioro EP. Comparing brain structural MRI and metabolic FDG-PET changes in patients with ALS-FTD: 'the chicken or the egg?' question. *J Neurol Neurosurg Psychiatry* (2015) 86:952–8. doi: 10.1136/jnnp-2014-308239
176. Van Weehaeghe D, Ceccarini J, Delva A, Robberecht W, Van Damme P, Van Laere K. Prospective validation of 18F-FDG brain PET discriminant analysis methods in the diagnosis of amyotrophic lateral sclerosis. *J Nuclear Med.* (2016) 57:1238–43. doi: 10.2967/jnumed.115.166272
177. Cistaro A, Pagani M, Montuschi A, Calvo A, Moglia C, Canosa A, et al. The metabolic signature of C9ORF72-related ALS: FDG PET comparison with nonmutated patients. *Eur J Nuclear Med Mol Imag.* (2014) 41:844–52. doi: 10.1007/s00259-013-2667-5
178. Turner MR, Cagnin A, Turkheimer FE, Miller CC, Shaw CE, Brooks DJ, et al. Evidence of widespread cerebral microglial activation in amyotrophic lateral sclerosis: an [11C](R)-PK11195 positron emission tomography study. *Neurobiol Dis.* (2004) 15:601–9. doi: 10.1016/j.nbd.2003.12.012
179. Corcia P, Tauber C, Vercoullie J, Arlicot N, Prunier C, Praline J, et al. Molecular imaging of microglial activation in amyotrophic lateral sclerosis. *PLoS ONE* (2012) 7:e52941. doi: 10.1371/journal.pone.0052941
180. Zurcher NR, Loggia ML, Lawson R, Chonde DB, Izquierdo-Garcia D, Yasek JE, et al. Increased *in vivo* glial activation in patients with amyotrophic lateral sclerosis: assessed with [(11)C]-PBR28. *NeuroImage Clin.* (2015) 7:409–14. doi: 10.1016/j.nicl.2015.01.009
181. Johansson A, Engler H, Blomquist G, Scott B, Wall A, Aquilonius SM, et al. Evidence for astrocytosis in ALS demonstrated by [11C](L)-deprenyl-D2 PET. *J Neurol Sci.* (2007) 255:17–22. doi: 10.1016/j.jns.2007.01.057
182. Lloyd CM, Richardson MP, Brooks DJ, Al-Chalabi A, Leigh PN. Extramotor involvement in ALS: PET studies with the GABA(A) ligand [(11)C]flumazenil. *Brain* (2000) 123(Pt 11):2289–96. doi: 10.1093/brain/123.11.2289
183. Douaud G, Filippini N, Knight S, Talbot K, Turner MR. Integration of structural and functional magnetic resonance imaging in amyotrophic lateral sclerosis. *Brain* (2011) 134(Pt 12):3470–9. doi: 10.1093/brain/awr279
184. Turner MR, Rabiner EA, Hammers A, Al-Chalabi A, Grasby PM, Shaw CE, et al. [11C]-WAY100635 PET demonstrates marked 5-HT1A receptor changes in sporadic ALS. *Brain* (2005) 128(Pt 4):896–905. doi: 10.1093/brain/awh428
185. Jelsone-Swain LM, Fling BW, Seidler RD, Hovatter R, Gruis K, Welsh RC. Reduced interhemispheric functional connectivity in the motor cortex during rest in limb-onset amyotrophic lateral sclerosis. *Front Syst Neurosci.* (2010) 4:158. doi: 10.3389/fnsys.2010.00158
186. Tedeschi G, Trojsi F, Tessitore A, Corbo D, Sagnelli A, Paccone A, et al. Interaction between aging and neurodegeneration in amyotrophic lateral sclerosis. *Neurobiol Aging* (2012) 33:886–98. doi: 10.1016/j.neurobiolaging.2010.07.011
187. Mohammadi B, Kollewe K, Samii A, Krampfl K, Dengler R, Munte TF. Changes of resting state brain networks in amyotrophic lateral sclerosis. *Exp Neurol.* (2009) 217:147–53. doi: 10.1016/j.expneurol.2009.01.025
188. Fekete T, Zach N, Mujica-Parodi LR, Turner MR. Multiple kernel learning captures a systems-level functional connectivity biomarker signature in amyotrophic lateral sclerosis. *PLoS ONE* (2013) 8:e85190. doi: 10.1371/journal.pone.0085190
189. Trojsi F, Esposito F, de Stefano M, Buonanno D, Conforti FL, Corbo D, et al. Functional overlap and divergence between ALS and bvFTD. *Neurobiol Aging* (2015) 36:413–23. doi: 10.1016/j.neurobiolaging.2014.06.025
190. Agosta F, Canu E, Inuggi A, Chio A, Riva N, Silani V, et al. Resting state functional connectivity alterations in primary lateral sclerosis. *Neurobiol Aging* (2014) 35:916–25. doi: 10.1016/j.neurobiolaging.2013.09.041
191. Agosta F, Valsasina P, Absinta M, Riva N, Sala S, Prelle A, et al. Sensorimotor functional connectivity changes in amyotrophic lateral sclerosis. *Cerebr Cortex* (2011) 21:2291–8. doi: 10.1093/cercor/bhr002
192. Zhou F, Xu R, Dowd E, Zang Y, Gong H, Wang Z. Alterations in regional functional coherence within the sensory-motor network in amyotrophic lateral sclerosis. *Neurosci Lett.* (2014) 558:192–6. doi: 10.1016/j.neulet.2013.11.022

193. Agosta F, Canu E, Valsasina P, Riva N, Prelle A, Comi G, et al. Divergent brain network connectivity in amyotrophic lateral sclerosis. *Neurobiol Aging* (2013) 34:419–27. doi: 10.1016/j.neurobiolaging.2012.04.015
194. Luo C, Chen Q, Huang R, Chen X, Chen K, Huang X, et al. Patterns of spontaneous brain activity in amyotrophic lateral sclerosis: a resting-state FMRI study. *PLoS ONE* (2012) 7:e45470. doi: 10.1371/journal.pone.0045470
195. Tietz F HV, Prell T, Penzlin S, Ilse B, Bokemeyer M, et al. The resting state default mode network (DMN) is pathologically hyperactive in amyotrophic lateral sclerosis. *Amyotroph Lateral Scler Frontotemporal Degener.* (2012) 13:171. doi: 10.3389/fnins.2016.00204
196. Heimrath J, Gorges M, Kassubek J, Muller HP, Birbaumer N, Ludolph AC, et al. Additional resources and the default mode network: Evidence of increased connectivity and decreased white matter integrity in amyotrophic lateral sclerosis. *Amyotroph Lateral Scler Frontotemporal Degener.* (2014) 15:537–45. doi: 10.3109/21678421.2014.911914
197. Chiò A, Pagani M, Agosta F, Calvo A, Cistaro A, Filippi M. Neuroimaging in amyotrophic lateral sclerosis: insights into structural and functional changes. *Lancet Neurol.* (2014) 13:1228–40. doi: 10.1016/S1474-4422(14)70167-X
198. Bede P. Deciphering neurodegeneration: A paradigm shift from focality to connectivity. *Neurology* (2017) 89:1758–9. doi: 10.1212/WNL.0000000000004582
199. Turner MR, Kiernan MC. Does interneuronal dysfunction contribute to neurodegeneration in amyotrophic lateral sclerosis? *Amyotroph Lateral Scler.* (2012) 13:245–50. doi: 10.3109/17482968.2011.636050
200. Schoenfeld MA, Tempelmann C, Gaul C, Kuhnel GR, Duzel E, Hopf JM, et al. Functional motor compensation in amyotrophic lateral sclerosis. *J Neurol.* (2005) 252:944–52. doi: 10.1007/s00415-005-0787-y
201. Konrad C, Jansen A, Henningsen H, Sommer J, Turski PA, Brooks BR, et al. Subcortical reorganization in amyotrophic lateral sclerosis. *Exp Brain Res.* (2006) 172:361–9. doi: 10.1007/s00221-006-0352-7
202. Konrad C, Henningsen H, Bremer J, Mock B, Deppe M, Buchinger C, et al. Pattern of cortical reorganization in amyotrophic lateral sclerosis: a functional magnetic resonance imaging study. *Exp Brain Res.* (2002) 143:51–6. doi: 10.1007/s00221-001-0981-9
203. Cosottini M, Pesaresi I, Piazza S, Diciotti S, Cecchi P, Fabbri S, et al. Structural and functional evaluation of cortical motor areas in Amyotrophic Lateral Sclerosis. *Exp Neurol.* (2012) 234:169–80. doi: 10.1016/j.expneurol.2011.12.024
204. Stanton BR, Williams VC, Leigh PN, Williams SC, Blain CR, Jarosz JM, et al. Altered cortical activation during a motor task in ALS. Evidence for involvement of central pathways. *J Neurol.* (2007) 254:1260–7. doi: 10.1007/s00415-006-0513-4
205. Poujois A, Schneider FC, Faillenot I, Camdessanche JP, Vandenberghe N, Thomas-Anterion C, et al. Brain plasticity in the motor network is correlated with disease progression in amyotrophic lateral sclerosis. *Hum Brain Map.* (2013) 34:2391–401. doi: 10.1002/hbm.22070
206. Goldstein LH, Newsom-Davis IC, Bryant V, Brammer M, Leigh PN, Simmons A. Altered patterns of cortical activation in ALS patients during attention and cognitive response inhibition tasks. *J Neurol.* (2011) 258:2186–98. doi: 10.1007/s00415-011-6088-8
207. Witiuk K, Fernandez-Ruiz J, McKee R, Alahyane N, Coe BC, Melanson M, et al. Cognitive deterioration and functional compensation in ALS measured with fMRI using an inhibitory task. *J Neurosci.* (2014) 34:14260–71. doi: 10.1523/JNEUROSCI.1111-14.2014
208. Mohammadi B, Kollewe K, Cole DM, Fellbrich A, Heldmann M, Samii A, et al. Amyotrophic lateral sclerosis affects cortical and subcortical activity underlying motor inhibition and action monitoring. *Hum Brain Mapp.* (2015) 36:2878–89. doi: 10.1002/hbm.22814
209. Passamonti L, Fera F, Tessitore A, Russo A, Cerasa A, Gioia CM, et al. Dysfunctions within limbic-motor networks in amyotrophic lateral sclerosis. *Neurobiol Aging* (2013) 34:2499–509. doi: 10.1016/j.neurobiolaging.2013.05.016
210. Stoppel CM, Vielhaber S, Eckart C, Machts J, Kaufmann J, Heinze HJ, et al. Structural and functional hallmarks of amyotrophic lateral sclerosis progression in motor- and memory-related brain regions. *NeuroImage Clin.* (2014) 5:277–90. doi: 10.1016/j.nicl.2014.07.007
211. Strong MJ, Grace GM, Freedman M, Lomen-Hoerth C, Woolley S, Goldstein LH, et al. Consensus criteria for the diagnosis of frontotemporal cognitive and behavioural syndromes in amyotrophic lateral sclerosis. *Amyotroph Lateral Scler.* (2009) 10:131–46. doi: 10.1080/17482960802654364
212. Bede P, Oliver D, Stodart J, van den Berg L, Simmons Z, D OB, et al. Palliative care in amyotrophic lateral sclerosis: a review of current international guidelines and initiatives. *J Neurol Neurosurg Psychiatry* (2011) 82:413–8. doi: 10.1136/jnnp.2010.232637
213. Elamin M, Bede P, Montuschi A, Pender N, Chio A, Hardiman O. Predicting prognosis in amyotrophic lateral sclerosis: a simple algorithm. *J Neurol.* (2015) 262:1447–54. doi: 10.1007/s00415-015-7731-6
214. Burke T, Elamin M, Galvin M, Hardiman O, Pender N. Caregiver burden in amyotrophic lateral sclerosis: a cross-sectional investigation of predictors. *J Neurol.* (2015) 262:1526–32. doi: 10.1007/s00415-015-7746-z
215. Andrews SC, Pavlis A, Staios M, Fisher F. Which behaviours? Identifying the most common and burdensome behaviour changes in amyotrophic lateral sclerosis. *Psychol Health Med.* (2017) 22:483–92. doi: 10.1080/13548506.2016.1164871
216. Bock M, Duong YN, Kim A, Allen I, Murphy J, Lomen-Hoerth C. Progression and effect of cognitive-behavioral changes in patients with amyotrophic lateral sclerosis. *Neurol Clin Pract.* (2017) 7:488–98. doi: 10.1212/CPJ.0000000000000397
217. Van den Berg JP, Kalmijn S, Lindeman E, Veldink JH, de Visser M, Van der Graaff MM, et al. Multidisciplinary ALS care improves quality of life in patients with ALS. *Neurology* (2005) 65:1264–7. doi: 10.1212/01.wnl.0000180717.29273.12
218. Hardiman O. Multidisciplinary care in ALS: expanding the team. *Amyotroph Lateral Scler.* (2012) 13:165. doi: 10.3109/17482968.2012.657006
219. Desai J, Swash M. Extrapyramidal involvement in amyotrophic lateral sclerosis: backward falls and retropulsion. *J Neurol Neurosurg Psychiatry* (1999) 67:214–6. doi: 10.1136/jnnp.67.2.214
220. Feron M, Couillandre A, Mseddi E, Termoz N, Abidi M, Bardinet E, et al. Extrapyramidal deficits in ALS: a combined biomechanical and neuroimaging study. *J Neurol.* (2018). doi: 10.1007/s00415-018-8964-y. [Epub ahead of print].
221. Chio A, Calvo A, Cammarosano S, Dematteis F, Artusi CA, Pagani M, et al. Extrapyramidal involvement in ALS: a prospective population-based study (P4.314). *Neurology* (2017) 79:1983–9. doi: 10.1212/WNL.0b013e3182735d36.
222. Pupillo E, Bianchi E, Messina P, Chiveri L, Lunetta C, Corbo M, et al. Extrapyramidal and cognitive signs in amyotrophic lateral sclerosis: a population based cross-sectional study. *Amyotroph Lateral Scler Frontotemporal Degener.* (2015) 16:324–30. doi: 10.3109/21678421.2015.1040028
223. McCluskey L, Vandriel S, Elman L, Van Deerlin VM, Powers J, Boller A, et al. ALS-Plus syndrome: non-pyramidal features in a large ALS cohort. Journal of the neurological *Sciences* (2014) 345:118–24. doi: 10.1016/j.jns.2014.07.022
224. Giordana MT, Ferrero P, Grifoni S, Pellerino A, Naldi A, Montuschi A. Dementia and cognitive impairment in amyotrophic lateral sclerosis: a review. *Neurol Sci.* (2011) 32:9–16. doi: 10.1007/s10072-010-0439-6
225. Khan AM. Rare presentation of amyotrophic lateral sclerosis as frontotemporal dementia: a case report. *Open Access J Toxicol.* (2017) 1:555566. doi: 10.19080/OAJT.2017.01.555566
226. Turner MR, Goldacre R, Talbot K, Goldacre MJ. Psychiatric disorders prior to amyotrophic lateral sclerosis. *Ann Neurol.* (2016) 80:935–8. doi: 10.1002/ana.24801
227. Qureshi AI, Wilmot G, Dihenia B, Schneider JA, Krendel DA. Motor neuron disease with parkinsonism. *Arch Neurol.* (1996) 53:987–91. doi: 10.1001/archneur.1996.00550100061015
228. Mitsumoto H, Brooks BR, Silani V. Clinical trials in amyotrophic lateral sclerosis: why so many negative trials and how can trials be improved? *Lancet Neurol.* (2014) 13:1127–38. doi: 10.1016/S1474-4422(14)70129-2
229. Cui B, Cui L, Liu M, Ma J, Fang J. Amyotrophic lateral sclerosis with frontotemporal dementia presented with prominent psychosis. *Chin Med J.* (2014) 127:3996–8.
230. Snowden JS, Adams J, Harris J, Thompson JC, Rollinson S, Richardson A, et al. Distinct clinical and pathological phenotypes in frontotemporal dementia associated with MAPT, PGRN and C9orf72 mutations.

Amyotroph Lateral Scler Frontotemporal Degener. (2015) 16:497–505. doi: 10.3109/21678421.2015.1074700

231. Benatar M, Wuu J. Presymptomatic studies in ALS: rationale, challenges, and approach. *Neurology* (2012) 79:1732–9. doi: 10.1212/WNL.0b013e31826e9b1d
232. Bertrand A, Wen J, Rinaldi D, Houot M, Sayah S, Camuzat A, et al. Early cognitive, structural, and microstructural changes in presymptomatic C9orf72 carriers younger than 40 years. *JAMA Neurol.* (2018) 75:236–45. doi: 10.1001/jamaneurol.2017.4266
233. Eisen A, Kiernan M, Mitsumoto H, Swash M. Amyotrophic lateral sclerosis: a long preclinical period? *J Neurol Neurosurg Psychiatry* (2014) 85:1232–8. doi: 10.1136/jnnp-2013-307135

12

Kynurenine Pathway Metabolites as Biomarkers for Amyotrophic Lateral Sclerosis

*Vanessa X. Tan and Gilles J. Guillemin**

Macquarie University Centre for MND Research, Department of Biological Sciences, Faculty of Medicine and Health Sciences, Macquarie University, Sydney, NSW, Australia

***Correspondence:**
Gilles J. Guillemin
gilles.guillemin@mq.edu.au

Amyotrophic Lateral Sclerosis (ALS) currently lacks a robust and well-defined biomarker that can 1) assess the progression of the disease, 2) predict and/or delineate the various clinical subtypes, and 3) evaluate or predict a patient's response to treatments. The kynurenine Pathway (KP) of tryptophan degradation represent a promising candidate as it is involved with several neuropathological features present in ALS including neuroinflammation, excitotoxicity, oxidative stress, immune system activation and dysregulation of energy metabolism. Some of the KP metabolites (KPMs) can cross the blood brain barrier, and many studies have shown their levels are dysregulated in major neurodegenerative diseases including ALS. The KPMs can be easily analyzed in body fluids and tissue and as they are small molecules, and are stable. KPMs have a Janus face action, they can be either or both neurotoxic and/or neuroprotective depending of their levels. This mini review examines and presents evidence supporting the use of KPMs as a relevant set of biomarkers for ALS, and highlights the criteria required to achieve a valid biomarker set for ALS.

Keywords: kynurenine pathway, amyotrophic lateral sclerosis, biomarker development, neurodegeneration, motor neuron disease, neuroinflammation and neurodegeneration, tryptophan

AMYOTROPHIC LATERAL SCLEROSIS

The diagnosis of amyotrophic lateral sclerosis (ALS) can only be fully confirmed by the post mortem detection of ALS-associated protein inclusions such as TDP-43 and SOD1 (Turner et al., 2013). Coupled with the spectrum of symptoms seen in the clinical presentation of ALS, the diagnosis of ALS relies on presentation to a neurologist and the elimination of other neurological and/or muscular diseases such as Kennedy's disease or myasthenia gravis, based on the El Escorial criteria that requires the assessment of disease progression (Brooks et al., 2000; Lambrechts et al., 2007; Al-Chalabi et al., 2016; Hardiman et al., 2017). This results in the average time from onset of symptoms after diagnosis of ALS being 10 months, in a disease with survival of 24–48 months (Chiò et al., 2009; Hardiman et al., 2017).

Abbreviations: 3HAA, 3-hydroxyanthranilic acid; 3HK, 3-hydroxykynurenine; 5-HT, serotonin; AA, anthranilic acid; ALS, amyotrophic lateral sclerosis; BBB, blood brain barrier; BH4, tetrahydrobiopterin; ChAT, choline acetyltransferase; CNS, central nervous system; CSF, cerebrospinal fluid; GCMS, gas chromatography mass spectrometry; HPLC, high performance liquid chromatography; IHC, immunohistochemistry; KP, kynurenine pathway; KPM, KP metabolites; KTR, kynurenine: tryptophan Ratio; KYN, kynurenine; KYNA, kynurenic acid; LC-MS/MS, liquid chromatography tandem mass spectrometry; MS, multiple sclerosis; NAD+, nicotinamide adenine dinucleotide; NMDA, *N*-methyl-D-aspartate; PIC, picolinic acid; QUIN, quinolinic acid; QUINA, quinaldic acid; SOD1, Cu/Zn superoxide dismutase; TRP, tryptophan; XA, xanthurenic acid.

Defined as characteristic that is objectively measured and evaluated as an indicator of normal biological process, pathogenic process, or a pharmacogenomic process to therapeutic intervention, biomarkers include genomics, proteomics, metabolomics, neurophysiology, and neuroimaging (Ganesalingam and Bowser, 2010; Turner et al., 2011). The lack of a reliable biomarker for ALS hampers a rapid, definitive diagnosis of disease, determination of ALS subtypes, monitoring of disease progression in patients, and limits the ability of clinicians and scientists to achieve an unbiased assessment of the efficiency of new treatments (Turner et al., 2009; Ganesalingam and Bowser, 2010). For patients and their families, a sensitive and specific biomarkers could allow detection of ALS at early stages, and allow the prognosis of the clinical subtype of ALS to predict disease aggressivity and subtype (Ganesalingam and Bowser, 2010; Al-Chalabi et al., 2016). This research gap in biomarker discovery and development for ALS comes not only as an impediment for patients and their families, but also at a cost to the pharmaceutical industries, through the monitoring of drug effects and disease progression in clinical trials. In particular, the repeated failure of drugs demonstrating clinical efficacy, and the inability to detect improvements, or non-improvements rapidly (Aggarwal and Cudkowicz, 2008; Ganesalingam and Bowser, 2010; Petrov et al., 2017).

THE KYNURENINE PATHWAY

One of the hallmarks of ALS is the presence of neuroinflammation and the kynurenine pathway (KP) is known to be strongly induced by inflammatory cytokines such as IFN-γ (McGeer and McGeer, 2002; Moffett and Namboodiri, 2003; Chen et al., 2010; Oxenkrug, 2011). The KP is the major route of tryptophan (TRP) catabolism, and feeds into the serotonin pathway, immune related tetrahydrobiopterin (BH4) pathway, glycolysis, and *de novo* nicotinamide adenine dinucleotide (NAD+) pathway (**Figure 1**) (Stone, 1993; Grant et al., 2010; Oxenkrug, 2013; Sasaki, 2019); linking it to fatigue, depression, inflammation, and decrease in energy metabolism (Sandyk, 2006; Grant et al., 2010; Oxenkrug, 2013).

The essential amino acid tryptophan originates from the diet, if which up to 85% is bound to albumin in blood circulation, and 99% metabolized in the liver (Quagliariello et al., 1964; Yuwiler et al., 1977; Badawy, 2017). Activation of the KP is achieved by the triggering of the first enzyme of the pathway, indoleamine 2,3 dioxygenase (IDO1) (Guillemin et al., 2005c; Badawy, 2017). This results in the production of several neuroactive metabolites such as the excitotoxins quinolinic acid (QUIN), and 3-hydroxykynurenine (3HK) by activated monocytic cells (Guillemin et al., 2003b); and the neuroprotective kynurenic acid (KA) and picolinic acid (PIC) by astrocytes and neurons, respectively (Heyes et al., 1988; Beninger et al., 1994; Guillemin et al., 2001, 2007; Badawy, 2017). The KP is active in most cell types, particularly in the liver (Takikawa et al., 1986; Heyes et al., 1997), and is highly activated in monocytic cells during inflammation (Jones et al., 2015). Only a limited number of KP can cross the blood brain barrier (BBB). TRP, Kynurenine (KYN), 3HK, anthranilic acid (AA) are actively transported by the large neutral amino acid carrier system; and others via passive diffusion (Fukui et al., 1991; Ruddick et al., 2006). This indicates that peripheral activation of the KP by inflammation can be translocated to the central nervous system (CNS), altering immune regulation and increasing neurotoxicity (Owe-Young et al., 2008). In the CNS, most cells contain the complete set of KP enzymes, and are capable of degrading TRP (Guillemin et al., 2005c; Lee et al., 2017). However, neurons, astrocytes and oligodendrocytes are incapable of synthesizing QUIN, only activated microglia and infiltrating macrophages produce QUIN (Guillemin et al., 2000; Lim et al., 2007).

The concept of using kynurenine pathway metabolites (KPMs) as markers for diseases dates back to the 1950s (Musajo et al., 1955; Tompsett, 1959), where excretion of KPMs were observed in the urine of patients diagnosed with cancer, rheumatoid arthritis, cardiovascular events and fevers (Musajo et al., 1955; Takahashi et al., 1956; Tompsett, 1959; McMillan, 1960; McManus and Jackson, 1968; Mawatari et al., 1995). More recently, the KP is investigated mostly in other liquid biopsies such as serum and plasma (Lewitt et al., 2013). The levels of the KPMs has been shown to be well correlated between the cerebrospinal fluid (CSF) and blood (Curzon, 1979; Chen et al., 2010; Myint, 2012; Jacobs et al., 2019), however, they are not always identical; and only few studies (Curzon, 1979; Widner et al., 2002; Chen et al., 2010; Zuo et al., 2016; Havelund et al., 2017; Lim et al., 2017; Jacobs et al., 2019) correlate the KP levels in different biofluids from the same patients at the same time. KPMs have been historically measured using thin layer chromatography, and detected under UV light, or via radioactive metabolites (Musajo et al., 1955, 1956; McMillan, 1960; McManus and Jackson, 1968; Shibata, 1988). Today, KPMs are more often measured using more sensitive methods and equipment such as high performance liquid chromatography (HPLC), Gas chromatography mass spectrometry (GCMS), and liquid chromatography tandem mass spectrometry (LC-MS/MS) (Heyes and Markey, 1988; Bizzarri et al., 1990; Smythe et al., 2003; de Jong et al., 2009; Pedersen et al., 2013; Miller et al., 2018). The most commonly measured KPMs are TRP, KYN, and KYNA, and are often presented as ratios. As they are small molecules, the KPMs such as KYN, KYNA, Xanthurenic acid (XA) and AA have been shown to be stable. With the exception of 3-hydroxy anthranilic acid (3HAA), which is known to be particularly unstable over time and sensitive to light (Darlington et al., 2010; Midttun et al., 2014).

Ex vivo, the KPMs have been measured using immunohistochemistry (IHC) in tissue sections (Guillemin et al., 2005a; Steiner et al., 2011; Lim et al., 2013). More recently, techniques such as tissue-based Matrix-assisted laser desorption/ionization (MALDI) Mass spectrometry Imaging (MSI) and tissue microarray has been used to not only detect, but localize the presence of TRP and KYN in tumors *ex vivo* (Puccetti et al., 2015; Ait-Belkacem et al., 2017). This specific localization will allow for focal observation of KPMs changes within tissue, and targeted applications of monitoring and altering of the KP if this can be translated *in vivo*.

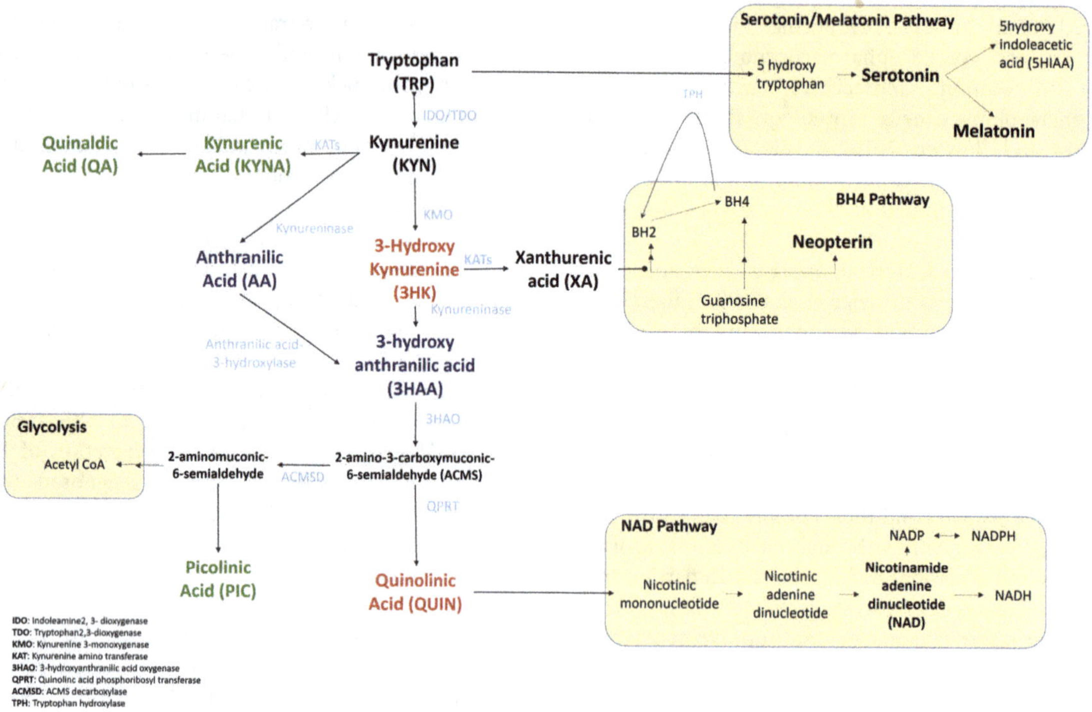

FIGURE 1 | The Kynurenine Pathway and its downstream pathways of Serotonin/Melatonin, BH4, Glycolysis, and NAD+. Tryptophan is converted into serotonin and melatonin, that regulate mood and sleep. The tetrahydrobiopterin (BH4) pathway interacts with the KP in three ways, (1) the sharing of the enzyme TPH that degrades tryptophan, (2) the inhibition of a key BH4 pathway enzyme, sepiapterin reductase, (3) both BH4 and KP are induced by inflammatory cytokines. Tryptophan also feeds into the glycolysis cycle via ACMS, affecting ATP production. Finally, the KP is the *de novo* synthesis pathway of NAD+ which is associated with cellular energy, repair and fatigue. The key KPMs are bolded, neurotoxic metabolites represented in red, neuroprotective metabolites in green, and dual functioning in blue.

Using the levels of KPMs, the activity of their associated enzymes can be derived as a proxy of the concentrations of direct derivatives of the metabolites as a ratio (Darlington et al., 2007; Sathyasaikumar et al., 2011; Lim et al., 2013) – most commonly measuring IDO1 via the Kynurenine: Tryptophan ratio (K/T ratio; KTR); or via direct enzymatic assays (Sathyasaikumar et al., 2011). Although few studies have looked at the direct correlation between metabolite ratio and enzymatic concentrations (Baran et al., 1999).

In vitro, neurotoxic KPMs such as QUIN and 3HK, have been shown to induce neurodegeneration and neuronal cell death through excitotoxicity, *N*-methyl-D-aspartate (NMDA) receptor antagonism, increased glutamate release, and the production of reactive oxygen species (Kim and Choi, 1987; Koh and Choi, 1988; Khaspekov et al., 1989; Nakagami et al., 1996; Shoki et al., 1998; Guidetti and Schwarcz, 1999; Leipnitz et al., 2007; Guillemin, 2012b; Kalonia et al., 2012; Pierozan et al., 2015). The neurotoxic mechanisms of QUIN is well established, and overlaps with mechanisms of neurodegeneration in ALS such as excitotoxicity, hyperphosphorylation, and protein dysfunction (Pierozan et al., 2010; Guillemin, 2012a; Lee et al., 2017). Some of the KPMs such as KYNA, PIC, and 3HAA have neuroprotective and immunomodulatory properties (Foster et al., 1984; Behan and Stone, 2000; Grant et al., 2009; Krause et al., 2011; Lugo-Huitrón et al., 2011). Other KPMs such as 3HAA, have both neurotoxic and neuroprotective functions depending on their relative concentrations (Colín-González et al., 2013; Pérez-González et al., 2017). The KPMs can influence each other levels (Perkins and Stone, 1982; Jhamandas et al., 1990), and the balance of KPMs is crucial for managing the equilibrium between neurotoxicity and neuroprotection. The dysregulation of KPMs, especially excessive QUIN production, has been correlated with variations of other neuroinflammatory markers (Heyes et al., 1992; Guillemin et al., 2003a; Kalonia et al., 2011), making the modulation of KPMs a plausible target for the regulation of the immune response within the CNS (Stone et al., 2012; Bohár et al., 2015; Jacobs and Lovejoy, 2018).

Using these modern techniques, the KP has been investigated as a marker for progression, severity, and prognostic for diseases such as systemic lupus erythematosus (Perl, 2015; Åkesson et al., 2018), cancers (Jin et al., 2015; Zuo et al., 2016; Xie et al., 2017; Huang et al., 2018; Liu et al., 2018; Khan et al., 2019), cardiovascular disease (Sun et al., 2013; Zuo et al., 2016), lung cancer and chronic obstructive pulmonary disease (Chuang et al., 2014; Zinellu et al., 2018), chronic kidney disease and diabetes (Hirayama et al., 2012; Zhao, 2013), acquired immunodeficiency syndrome (AIDS) and HIV-dementia (Fuchs et al., 1990; Heyes et al., 1991; Sardar et al., 2002; Guillemin et al., 2005b; Favre et al., 2010; Lee et al., 2016; Wang et al., 2019), pancreatic cysts (Park et al., 2013), acute myeloid leukemia and lymphomas

(Giusti et al., 1996; Finger et al., 2017), vitamin levels (Midttun et al., 2014), tuberculosis (Weiner et al., 2012; Feng et al., 2015), malaria (Medana et al., 2003), irritable bowel syndrome (IBS) (Clarke et al., 2012; Gupta et al., 2012), rheumatoid arthritis (Spiera and Vallarino, 1969; Schroecksnadel et al., 2003), growth deficits (Kosek et al., 2016), obesity (Mangge et al., 2014), and preeclampsia (Nilsen et al., 2012). In the nervous system, the KP has been shown to associate with pathologies such as stroke (Darlington et al., 2007), schizophrenia (Müller and Schwarz, 2006; Kegel et al., 2014; Oxenkrug et al., 2016), Parkinson's (Ogawa et al., 1992; Widner et al., 2002; Lewitt et al., 2013; Havelund et al., 2017), neuropsychiatric disorders such as depression and stress (Mackay et al., 2009; Gabbay et al., 2010; Olsson et al., 2010; Steiner et al., 2011; Kocki et al., 2012; Erhardt et al., 2013; Comai et al., 2016; Küster et al., 2017; Huang et al., 2018; Kuwano et al., 2018), suicide (Erhardt et al., 2013; Bay-Richter et al., 2015; Brundin et al., 2016), multiple sclerosis (Rejdak et al., 2002; Lim et al., 2017), Alzheimer's disease (Guillemin et al., 2005a; Hartai et al., 2007), Huntington's disease (Schwarcz et al., 1988; Beal et al., 1990; Stoy et al., 2005; Byrne and Wild, 2016), brain tumors (Adams et al., 2012, 2014), Autism Spectrum Disorders, and Attention Deficit Hyperactivity Disorder (ADHD) (Aarsland et al., 2015; Bryn et al., 2017). More recently, studies have demonstrated that the KPMs could be used for the prognosis of MS, and also to differentiate between disease subtypes (Aeinehband et al., 2015; Lim et al., 2017).

AMYOTROPHIC LATERAL SCLEROSIS AND KYNURENINE-ASSOCIATED PATHWAYS

The levels of KPMs are known to be dysregulated in the serum, CSF, and tissue of ALS patients (Ilzecka et al., 2003; Chen et al., 2010) (**Table 1**). The first study by Ilzecka et al. (2003) investigated the presence of KYNA in ALS patients and matching healthy controls. Broadly, the results did not show any significant differences in the levels of KYNA between patients and controls in either serum or CSF. However, CSF KYNA was higher in (1) patients with severe clinical status; and (2) in patients with bulbar onset, compared to patients with limb onset. The authors concluded that this increase likely associated with the neuroprotective role of KYNA. The authors also showed that the concentrations of KYNA in CSF and in serum were not correlated, indicating that KYNA in the CNS is mostly produced in the brain by astrocytes (Guillemin et al., 2001), and this confirms that KYNA is able to cross the BBB and may be imported from the PNS. This is supported by the presence of astrogliosis as part of the neuroinflammatory features found in ALS brain. In 2010, our team reported increased levels of TRP, KYN, and QUIN in both CSF and serum. This study did not investigate KYNA or astrogliosis as Ilzecka et al. did, however, does confirm the neuroinflammatory status in ALS patients, with presence of activated microglia and activation of the KP in the motor cortex.

Other studies have indirectly reported associations between ALS and the KPMs. Jhamandas et al. (1990) showed that injections of the excitotoxin QUIN and 3HAA, directly into the rat brain, triggers a decrease in choline acetyltransferase (ChAT) activity, and that KYNA, PIC, quinaldic acid (QUINA), and AA co-injections could antagonize the QUIN-induced neurotoxicity. In addition, QUIN injections were associated with neuronal loss, but also glial proliferation, highlighting the important roles played by KPMs in neuroinflammation and glial activation in ALS.

Aside from the KP, tryptophan is also metabolized by pinealocytes into serotonin (5-HT), and then melatonin, a serotonin downstream metabolite. Pinealocytes are external to the BBB, and thus directly affected by the KP in the periphery, but not directly by the KP in the CNS (Ruddick et al., 2006). Within the brain, serotonin is modulated by tryptophan levels. A decrease in serotonin levels has been linked to depression through tryptophan depletion (Owens and Nemeroff, 1994; Ruddick et al., 2006; Maes et al., 2011), and with the decrease of melatonin, and sleep disturbances, which are both symptoms in ALS patients (Sandyk, 2006). Furthermore, motoneurons affected in ALS are heavily innervated by serotoninergic neurons; whereas those resistant to ALS-associated degeneration are less innervated by serotonin neurons, possibly linking serotonin with induction of neuronal excitability and neurodegeneration. The roles of serotonin in ALS has been reviewed (Sandyk, 2006). Melatonin has been shown to confer neuroprotection in ALS patients and Cu/Zn superoxide dismutase (SOD1) mice models, likely by decreasing systemic oxidative stress, caspase activation, and by increasing ATP availability to increase cell repair mechanisms to limit neuronal death (Weishaupt et al., 2006; Zhang et al., 2013).

The metabolic pathway of tryptophan degradation also feeds into the cell's energy metabolism through the production of NAD+ and glycolysis. Its dysregulation increases the risk for the development of neurodegenerative diseases as many repair and neuroprotective systems perform at a suboptimal level. NAD+ depletion can lead to fatigue (Procaccini et al., 2016; Camandola and Mattson, 2017; Sasaki, 2019). Altered energy metabolism has also been investigated in ALS (Dupuis et al., 2004; Ngo and Steyn, 2015), and has been shown to be altered by QUIN via the respiratory chain and Krebs cycle (Ribeiro et al., 2006; Colín-González et al., 2015). The NAD+ pathway represents an important therapeutic avenue, and is being targeted using precursors such as nicotinamide phosphoribosyl transferase, or nicotinamide ribosyl directed at ageing, neurodegeneration, and in particular, axonal degeneration (Sasaki et al., 2006; Imai and Yoshino, 2013; Verdin, 2015; Pehar et al., 2018).

A pathway that has been understudied in ALS is the tetrahydrobiopterin (BH4) pathway (**Figure 1**). Interconnected to the KP via the modulatory effect of XA, and as a co-substrate for tryptophan hydroxylase (Zhang et al., 2006; Cronin et al., 2018), studies on BH4 have largely focused on inflammation, pain and neuroprotection (Oxenkrug, 2007; Ghisoni et al., 2015; Cronin et al., 2018). BH4 is strongly associated with neuroinflammation, and is also an essential co-factor in nitric oxide synthases in oxidative stress (Sakai et al., 1995; Guix et al., 2005; Cronin et al., 2018) - both pathological features present in ALS. Several reports have associated BH4 with neurodegeneration, such as the differential methylation of BH4

TABLE 1 | Summary of Kynurenine Pathway metabolite levels in controls and ALS patients collated from Ilzecka and Chen.

References	KPM	Population	Serum	CSF	Trend observed	
					Serum	**CSF**
Ilzecka	Kyna pmol/ml	Control (*n* = 14)	59.6 ± 20.5	2.41 ± 1.7		
		ALS (*n* = 16)	57.8 ± 35.0	1.59 ± 0.9	Mild > Severe	Control < Bulbar
		Bulbar (*n* = 6)	59.5 ± 39.3	3.61 ± 2.0	Control > Severe	Bulbar > Limb
		Limb (*n* = 10)	59.6 ± 31.2	1.70 ± 1.0	clinical status	Control < Severe
		Mild clinical status (*n* = 6)	81.6 ± 41.2	1.75 ± 09		clinical status
		Severe clinical status (*n* = 8)	39.9 ± 14.7	3.26 ± 2.1		
Chen	TRP (μM)	Control (*n* = 17)	75.0 ± 10.5	2.58 ± 0.16	Control < ALS**	Control < ALS**
		ALS(140)	143.3 + 5.6	5.0 ± 0.2		
		sALS (*n* = 133)	133.3 ± 6.0	4.67 ± 0.19		
		fALS (*n* = 7)	166.4 ± 20.7	5.20 ± 0.87		
		Bulbar (*n* = 31)	128.2 ± 10.6	4.58 ± 0.33		
		Limb (*n* = 109)	137.3 ± 6.9	4.73 ± 0.22		
	KYN (μM)	Control (*n* = 17)	2.52 ± 0.19	0.027 ± 0.00	Control < ALS**	Control < ALS**
		ALS(140)	4.0 + 0.2	0.23 + 0.02		
		sALS (*n* = 133)	4.05 ± 0.21	0.22 ± 0.01		
		fALS (*n* = 7)	3.24 ± 0.36	0.26 ± 0.05		
		Bulbar (*n* = 31)	3.99 ± 0.29	0.22 ± 0.02		
		Limb (*n* = 109)	4.00 ± 0.24	0.21 ± 0.03		
	PIC (μM)	Control (*n* = 35)	2.4 ± 0.4	0.51 ± 0.11	Control > ALS*	Control > ALS (*p* = 0.09)
		ALS(140)	1.4 + 0.1	0.36 + 0.03		
		sALS (*n* = 133)	1.46 ± 0.13	0.35 ± 0.07		
		fALS (*n* = 7)	1.80 ± 0.51	0.60 ± 0.21		
		Bulbar (*n* = 31)	1.45 ± 0.16	0.30 ± 0.06		
		Limb (*n* = 109)	1.49 ± 0.10	0.35 ± 0.07		
	QUIN (μM)	Control (*n* = 35)	0.30 ± 0.03	0.038 ± 0.004	Control < ALS*	Control < ALS*
		ALS(140)	0.37 + 0.02	0.053 + 0.005		
		sALS (*n* = 133)	0.38 ± 0.02	0.05 ± 0.01		
		fALS (*n* = 7)	0.36 ± 0.04	0.04 ± 0.01		
		Bulbar (*n* = 31)	0.43 ± 0.04	0.04 ± 0.01		
		Limb (*n* = 109)	0.36 ± 0.02	0.05 ± 0.01		
	IDO Activity (K/T ratio)	Control (*n* = 17)	0.039 ± 0.004	0.011 ± 0.001		Control < ALS
		ALS (*n* = 40)	0.037 ± 0.0025	0.044 + 0.002		
		sALS (*n* = 133)	0.04 ± 0.00	0.04 ± 0.00		
		fALS (*n* = 7)	0.02 ± 0.00	0.04 ± 0.01		
		Bulbar (*n* = 31)	0.04 ± 0.00	0.04 ± 0.00		
		Limb (*n* = 109)	0.04 ± 0.00	0.04 ± 0.00		

Mild clinical status defined as mild to moderate according to Munsat, Severe clinical status defined as severe to terminal according to Munsat. KMP, KP metabolites; Kyna, kynurenic acid; TRP, tryptophan; KYN, kynurenine; PIC, picolinic acid; QUIN, quinolinic acid; IDO, indoleamine dioxygenase; K/T ratio, kynurenine/tryptophan ratio; sALS, sporadic ALS; fALS, familial ALS. $^{*}p < 0.05$; $^{**}p < 0.0001$.

in monozygotic twins discordant for ALS (Young et al., 2017); and particularly in Parkinson's Disease (Choi et al., 2004; Foxton et al., 2007; Yoon et al., 2010).

With all these evidences associating the KP in ALS, especially the unbalance between neuroprotective and neurotoxic metabolites, the KPMs represent a relevant set of biomarkers to characterize disease subtypes and to assess disease progression. As mentioned previously, such biomarkers are lacking especially for the response to treatments and for testing new drugs in clinical trials. One of the main reasons supporting the role of KPMs as a biomarker for ALS is its association with neuroinflammation. The KTR (indication of IDO activity, and thus KP activation) is a very sensitive and specific marker for inflammation. This KTR ratio is well suited as a surrogate progressive, or end-point marker for neuroinflammation. Apart from CSF, body fluids such as blood and urine are easiest to collect. Measurement of KPMs levels in blood present a rapid and reliable set of markers as there are validated quantification methods, and they are stable. However, there are still some limitations using the KPMs as a biomarker for diseases.

Firstly, a potential pitfall using the KPMs as a biomarker for neurological diseases and psychological disorders is that KP activation is not specific of one disease as it is present in all neuroinflammatory diseases. Thus, the KP cannot be used a diagnostic marker, but is relevant as a prognostic/progression marker, and to identify disease subtypes. Diagnostically, the KPMs still have a great potential as a confirmatory biomarker in conjunction with a shortlisted clinical diagnosis, or subtype. For example in MS, we were able to differentiate MS subtypes from patients diagnosed with MS (Lim et al., 2017). Similarly, when a patient is suspected to have ALS, or has been diagnosed with ALS by a neurologist, the KPMs can be used to differentiate between disease subtypes (e.g., bulbar or lower motor neuron symptoms) and be able to differentiate between patients predicted to be fast or slow progressors. The addition of other inflammatory markers such as cytokines, chemokines, C Protein Reactive, etc, in combination with KPMs would increase the sensitivity and specificity of the biomarker set.

Secondly, the biological functions of all the KPMs are not fully understood – it is a very complex system that is intertwined other regulatory pathways such as BH4 (Cronin et al., 2018), and ultimately regulate the immune system. Further, there is only a limited direct correlation between enzymatic activities and the metabolite formation and their ratios. This is not a key issue in using the KP as surrogate biomarkers, as the crux is that the KPM ratios (ratios of the bioactive metabolites) are what confer biological activity and biomarker association; rather than the function of measuring the enzyme activity. The levels of KPMs in the general population has been directly investigated by Zuo et al. (2016) (n = 7015) and Gostner et al. (2015) (n = 100), which showed that some KPMs are influenced by both age (KTR, KYN, HAA), and gender (TRP) (de Bie et al., 2016a,b). Further, tryptophan has been shown to increase through to adolescence (Lepage et al., 1997) and in adulthood (Mangge et al., 2014). An earlier study by Medana et al. (2003) investigated the KPMs in Malawian children and Vietnamese adults who were affected by Malaria, showing that increases in QA and PIC in both populations could predict a fatal outcome. On the contrary, differences in KA levels in Malawian children as compared to Vietnamese adults (Medana et al., 2003), although it is unclear if this difference was attribute to age, disease, or ethnicity. Further, the correlation of the KPMs in different biofluids need to be better established for correlation and pathway studies. Urine represents the ideal biofluid as it is non-invasive. However, it is not homeostatic, and apart from early studies when the KP was discovered in urine (Musajo et al., 1955, 1956; Tompsett, 1959; McMillan, 1960; Mawatari et al., 1995), only few recent studies have analyzed the KPMs in urine (Fukuwatari et al., 2004; Pedersen et al., 2013; Dolina et al., 2014). Recent research mostly use serum or plasma to assess the KPMs (Darlington et al., 2007; Favre et al., 2010; Hirayama et al., 2012; Aarsland et al., 2015; Comai et al., 2016; Oxenkrug et al., 2016; Lim et al., 2017), and some when available, CSF (Erhardt et al., 2013; Havelund et al., 2017; Sühs et al., 2019). Further, the KP has been proposed as therapeutic intervention for neurodegenerative diseases such as ALS, and has been well reviewed (Füvesi et al., 2012).

As for other potential candidate biomarkers for ALS, the need for defined classifications of ALS subtypes or stages of disease progression (Gil et al., 2017) is critical. Standardized operation procedures for a defined analysis of progression rate, imaging, biopsy retrieval and storage, and biomarker analysis techniques need to be implemented to ensure consistency across centers to achieve an objective assessment. Biobanks storing clinical and biopsies of patient and control samples will be crucial to achieving the aim of a clinically applicable biomarker for ALS.

CONCLUSION

Overall, the KPMs have potential to be used as a sensitive and specific biomarker for patients diagnosed with ALS. Such markers would also have the ability to be used for surrogate clinical and prognostic biomarkers as we previously demonstrated for MS (Lim et al., 2017) and Alzheimer's disease (Chatterjee et al., 2018; Jacobs et al., 2019). The strong correlation of the KP with neuroinflammation, depression, and immune regulation makes it a valid candidate as a surrogate biomarker for ALS, for disease progression (fast/slow progressors) and possibly disease subtyping. Combining the KPM levels together with (1) other markers of inflammation or neurodegeneration, (2) clinical information, and (3) imaging would strongly increase both sensitivity and specificity of the biomarker set.

AUTHOR CONTRIBUTIONS

VT wrote the first draft of the manuscript. Both authors contributed to manuscript revision and read and approved the submitted version.

FUNDING

This research was supported by the MND Research Institute of Australia, FightMND, CreAte ALS Association, and Macquarie University.

REFERENCES

1. Aarsland, T. I. M., Landaas, E. T., Hegvik, T.-A., Ulvik, A., Halmøy, A., Ueland, P. M., et al. (2015). Serum concentrations of kynurenines in adult patients with attention-deficit hyperactivity disorder (ADHD): a case-control study. *Behav. Brain Funct.* 11:36. doi: 10.1186/s12993-015-0080-x
2. Adams, S., Braidy, N., Bessesde, A., Brew, B. J., Grant, R., Teo, C., et al. (2012). The Kynurenine pathway in brain tumor pathogenesis. *Cancer Res.* 72, 5649–5657. doi: 10.1158/0008-5472.CAN-12-0549
3. Adams, S., Teo, C., McDonald, K. L., Zinger, A., Bustamante, S., Lim, C. K., et al. (2014). Involvement of the Kynurenine pathway in human glioma pathophysiology. *PLoS One* 9:e112945. doi: 10.1371/journal.pone.0112945
4. Aeinehband, S., Brenner, P., Ståhl, S., Bhat, M., Fidock, M. D., Khademi, M., et al. (2015). Cerebrospinal fluid kynurenines in multiple sclerosis; relation to disease course and neurocognitive symptoms. *Brain Behav. Immun.* 51, 47–55. doi: 10.1016/j.bbi.2015. 07.016
5. Aggarwal, S., and Cudkowicz, M. (2008). ALS drug development: reflections from the past and a way forward. *Neurotherapeutics* 5, 516–527. doi: 10.1016/j.nurt. 2008.08.002
6. Ait-Belkacem, R., Bol, V., Hamm, G., Schramme, F., Van Den Eynde, B., Poncelet, L., et al. (2017). Microenvironment tumor metabolic interactions highlighted

by qMSI: application to the Tryptophan-Kynurenine pathway in immuno-oncology. *SLAS Discov.* 22, 1182–1192. doi: 10.1177/2472555217712659

7. Åkesson, K., Pettersson, S., Ståhl, S., Surowiec, I., Hedenström, M., Eketjäll, S., et al. (2018). Kynurenine pathway is altered in patients with SLE and associated with severe fatigue. *Lupus Sci. Med.* 5:e000254. doi: 10.1136/lupus-2017-000254
8. Al-Chalabi, A., Hardiman, O., Kiernan, M. C., Chiò, A., Rix-Brooks, B., and van den Berg, L. H. (2016). Amyotrophic lateral sclerosis: moving towards a new classification system. *Lancet Neurol.* 15, 1182–1194. doi: 10.1016/S1474-4422(16)30199-5
9. Badawy, A. A. (2017). Kynurenine pathway of tryptophan metabolism: regulatory and functional aspects. *Int. J. Tryptophan. Res.* 10:1178646917691938. doi: 10. 1177/1178646917691938
10. Baran, H., Jellinger, K., and Deecke, L. (1999). Kynurenine metabolism in Alzheimer's disease. *J. Neural Transm.* 106, 165–181.
11. Bay-Richter, C., Linderholm, K. R., Lim, C. K., Samuelsson, M., Träskman-Bendz, L., Guillemin, G. J., et al. (2015). A role for inflammatory metabolites as modulators of the glutamate N-methyl-d-aspartate receptor in depression and suicidality. *Brain Behav. Immun.* 43, 110–117. doi: 10.1016/J.BBI.2014.07.012
12. Beal, M. F., Matson, W. R., Swartz, K. J., Gamache, P. H., and Bird, E. D. (1990). Kynurenine pathway measurements in Huntington's disease striatum: evidence for reduced formation of Kynurenic Acid. *J. Neurochem.* 55, 1327–1339. doi: 10.1111/j.1471-4159.1990.tb03143.x
13. Behan, W. M. H., and Stone, T. W. (2000). Role of kynurenines in the neurotoxic actions of kainic acid. *Br. J. Pharmacol.* 129, 1764–1770. doi: 10.1038/sj.bjp.0703250
14. Beninger, R. J., Colton, A. M., Ingles, J. L., Jhamandas, K., and Boegman, R. J. (1994). Picolinic acid blocks the neurotoxic but not the neuroexcitant properties of quinolinic acid in the rat brain: evidence from turning behaviour and tyrosine hydroxylase immunohistochemistry. *Neuroscience* 61, 603–612. doi: 10.1016/ 0306-4522(94)90438-3
15. Bizzarri, M., Catizone, A., Pompei, M., Chiappini, L., Curini, L., and Lagana, A. (1990). Determination of urinary tryptophan and its metabolites along the nicotinic acid pathway by high performance liquid chromatography with ultraviolet detection. *Biomed. Chromatogr.* 4, 24–27. doi: 10.1002/bmc.1130040104
16. Bohár, Z., Toldi, J., Fülöp, F., Vécsei, L., Bohár, Z., Toldi, J., et al. (2015). Changing the face of Kynurenines and neurotoxicity: therapeutic considerations. *Int. J. Mol. Sci.* 16, 9772–9793. doi: 10.3390/ijms16059772
17. Brooks, B. R., Miller, R. G., Swash, M., and Munsat, T. L. (2000). El Escorial revisited: revised criteria for the diagnosis of amyotrophic lateral sclerosis. *Amyotroph. Lateral Scler.* 1, 293–299. doi: 10.1080/146608200300079536
18. Brundin, L., Sellgren, C. M., Lim, C. K., Grit, J., Pålsson, E., Landén, M., et al. (2016). An enzyme in the kynurenine pathway that governs vulnerability to suicidal behavior by regulating excitotoxicity and neuroinflammation. *Transl. Psychiatry* 6:e865. doi: 10.1038/tp.2016.133
19. Bryn, V., Verkerk, R., Skjeldal, O. H., Saugstad, O. D., and Ormstad, H. (2017). Kynurenine pathway in autism spectrum disorders in children. *Neuropsychobiology* 76, 82–88. doi: 10.1159/000488157
20. Byrne, L. M., and Wild, E. J. (2016). Cerebrospinal fluid biomarkers for Huntington's disease. *J. Huntingtons Dis.* 5, 1–13. doi: 10.3233/JHD-160196 Camandola, S., and Mattson, M. P. (2017). Brain metabolism in health, aging, and neurodegeneration. *EMBO J.* 36, 1474–1492. doi: 10.15252/embj.201695810 Chatterjee, P., Goozee, K., Lim, C. K., James, I., Shen, K., Jacobs, K. R., et al. (2018).
21. Alterations in serum kynurenine pathway metabolites in individuals with high neocortical amyloid-β load: a pilot study. *Sci. Rep.* 8:8008. doi: 10.1038/s41598-018-25968-7
22. Chen, Y., Stankovic, R., Cullen, K. M., Meininger, V., Garner, B., Coggan, S., et al. (2010). The Kynurenine pathway and inflammation in amyotropic lateral sclerosis. *Neurotox. Res.* 18, 132–142. doi: 10.1007/s12640-009-9129-7
23. Chiò, A., Mora, G., Calvo, A., Mazzini, L., Bottacchi, E., and Mutani, R. (2009). Epidemiology of ALS in Italy: a 10-year prospective population-based study. *Neurology* 72, 725–731. doi: 10.1212/01.wnl.0000343008.26874.d1
24. Choi, H. J., Kim, S. W., Lee, S. Y., and Hwang, O. (2004). Dopamine- dependent cytotoxicity of tetrahydrobiopterin: a possible mechanism for selective neurodegeneration in Parkinson's disease. *J. Neurochem.* 86, 143–152. doi: 10.1046/j.1471-4159.2003.01808.x
25. Chuang, S.-C., Fanidi, A., Magne Ueland, P., Relton, C., Midttun, O., Vollset, E., et al. (2014). Circulating biomarkers of tryptophan and the Kynurenine pathway and lung cancer risk. *Cancer Epidemiol Biomarkers Prev.* 23, 461–468. doi: 10.1158/1055-9965.EPI-13-0770
26. Clarke, G., McKernan, D. P., Gaszner, G., Quigley, E. M., Cryan, J. F., and Dinan, T. G. (2012). A distinct profile of tryptophan metabolism along the Kynurenine pathway downstream of toll-like receptor activation in irritable Bowel Syndrome. *Front. Pharmacol.* 3:90. doi: 10.3389/fphar.2012.00090
27. Colín-González, A. L., Maldonado, P. D., and Santamaría, A. (2013). 3- Hydroxykynurenine: an intriguing molecule exerting dual actions in the central nervous system. *Neurotoxicology* 34, 189–204. doi: 10.1016/j.neuro.2012.11.007 Colín-González, A. L., Paz-Loyola, A. L., Serratos, I., Seminotti, B., Ribeiro, C. A. J., Leipnitz, G., et al. (2015). Toxic synergism between quinolinic acid and organic acids accumulating in glutaric acidemia type I and in disorders of propionate metabolism in rat brain synaptosomes: relevance for metabolic acidemias. *Neuroscience* 308, 64–74. doi: 10.1016/J.NEUROSCIENCE.2015.09.002.
28. Comai, S., Bertazzo, A., Vachon, J., Daigle, M., Toupin, J., Côté, G., et al. (2016). Tryptophan via serotonin/kynurenine pathways abnormalities in a large cohort of aggressive inmates: markers for aggression. *Prog. Neuropsychopharmacol. Biol. Psychiatry* 70, 8–16. doi: 10.1016/j.pnpbp.2016.04.012
29. Cronin, S. J. F., Seehus, C., Weidinger, A., Talbot, S., Reissig, S., Seifert, M., et al. (2018). The metabolite BH4 controls T cell proliferation in autoimmunity and cancer. *Nature* 563, 564–568. doi: 10.1038/s41586-018-0701-2
30. Curzon, G. (1979). "Relationships between plasma, CSF and brain tryptophan," in *Transport Mechanisms of Tryptophan in Blood Cells, Nerve Cells, and at the Blood-Brain Barrier*, ed. P. Baumann (Vienna: Springer), 81–92. doi: 10.1007/978-3-7091-2243-3_7
31. Darlington, L. G., Forrest, C. M., Mackay, G. M., Smith, R. A., Smith, A. J., Stoy, N., et al. (2010). On the biological importance of the 3-hydroxyanthranilic acid: anthranilic acid ratio. *Int. J. Tryptophan Res.* 3, 51–59. doi: 10.4137/IJTR.S4282 Darlington, L. G., Mackay, G. M., Forrest, C. M., Stoy, N., George, C., and Stone, W. (2007). Altered kynurenine metabolism correlates with infarct volume in stroke. *Eur. J. Neurosci.* 26, 2211–2221. doi: 10.1111/j.1460-9568.2007.05838.x
32. de Bie, J., Lim, C. K., and Guillemin, G. J. (2016a). Kynurenines, gender and neuroinflammation; showcase Schizophrenia. *Neurotox. Res.* 30, 285–294. doi: 10.1007/s12640-016-9641-5
33. de Bie, J., Lim, C. K., and Guillemin, G. J. (2016b). Progesterone alters kynurenine pathway activation in IFN-γ-activated macrophages - relevance for neuroinflammatory diseases. *Int. J. Tryptophan Res.* 9, 89–93. doi: 10.4137/IJTR. S40332
34. de Jong, W. H. A., Smit, R., Bakker, S. J. L., de Vries, E. G. E., and Kema, I. P. (2009). Plasma tryptophan, kynurenine and 3-hydroxykynurenine measurement using automated on-line solid-phase extraction HPLC–tandem mass spectrometry. *J. Chromatogr.* B 877, 603–609. doi: 10.1016/j.jchromb.2009.01.015
35. Dolina, S., Margalit, D., Malitsky, S., and Rabinkov, A. (2014). Attention-deficit hyperactivity disorder (ADHD) as a pyridoxine-dependent condition: urinary diagnostic biomarkers. *Med. Hypotheses* 82, 111–116. doi: 10.1016/J.MEHY.2013.11.018
36. Dupuis, L., Oudart, H., René, F., Gonzalez de Aguilar, J.-L., and Loeffler, J.-P. (2004). Evidence for defective energy homeostasis in amyotrophic lateral sclerosis: benefit of a high-energy diet in a transgenic mouse model. *Proc. Natl. Acad. Sci. U.S.A.* 101, 11159–11164. doi: 10.1073/pnas.0402026101
37. Erhardt, S., Lim, C. K., Linderholm, K. R., Janelidze, S., Lindqvist, D., Samuelsson, M., et al. (2013). Connecting inflammation with glutamate agonism in suicidality. *Neuropsychopharmacology* 38, 743–752. doi: 10.1038/npp. 2012.248
38. Favre, D., Mold, J., Hunt, P. W., Kanwar, B., Loke, P., Seu, L., et al. (2010). Tryptophan catabolism by indoleamine 2,3-dioxygenase 1 alters the balance of TH17 to regulatory T cells in HIV disease. *Sci. Transl. Med.* 2:32ra36. doi: 10.1126/scitranslmed.3000632
39. Feng, S., Du, Y.-Q., Zhang, L. L., Zhang, L. L., Feng, R.-R., and Liu, S.-
40. Y. (2015). Analysis of serum metabolic profile by ultra-performance liquid chromatography-mass spectrometry for biomarkers discovery: application in a pilot study to discriminate patients with tuberculosis. *Chin. Med. J.* 128, 159–168. doi: 10.4103/0366-6999.149188
41. Finger, E., Wong, J., Gray, J., Rock, D., Loberg, R., Fitzpatrick, D., et al. (2017). Utilization of metabolomics to identify biomarkers in hematological malignancies: role of IDO and the Tryptophan pathway. *Blood* 130:5100.
42. Foster, A. C., Vezzani, I., and French, E. D. (1984). Kynurenic acid blocks neurotoxicity and seizures induc- Ed in rats by the related brain metabolite quinolinic acid. *Neurosci. Lett.* 48, 273–278. doi: 10.1016/0304-3940(84) 90050-8
43. Foxton, R. H., Land, J. M., and Heales, S. J. R. (2007). Tetrahydrobiopterin availability in Parkinson's and Alzheimer's disease; potential pathogenic mechanisms. *Neurochem. Res.* 32, 751–756. doi: 10.1007/s11064-006-9201-0
44. Fuchs, D., Forsman, A., Hagberg, L., Larsson, M., Norkrans, G., Reibnegger, G., et al. (1990). Immune activation and decreased tryptophan in patients with HIV-1 infection. *J. Interferon Res.* 10, 599–603. doi: 10.1089/jir.1990.10.599

45. Fukui, S., Schwarcz, R., Rapoport, S. I., Takada, Y., and Smith, Q. R. (1991). Blood? brain barrier transport of Kynurenines: implications for brain synthesis and metabolism. *J. Neurochem.* 56, 2007–2017. doi: 10.1111/j.1471-4159.1991.tb03460.x
46. Fukuwatari, T., Wada, H., Sasaki, R., and Shibata, K. (2004). Effects of excess nicotinamide administration on the urinary excretion of nicotinamide N - Oxide and nicotinuric acid by rats. *Biosci. Biotechnol. Biochem.* 68, 44–50. doi: 10.1271/bbb.68.44
47. Füvesi, J., Rajda, C., Bencsik, K., Toldi, J., and Vécsei, L. (2012). The role of kynurenines in the pathomechanism of amyotrophic lateral sclerosis and multiple sclerosis: therapeutic implications. *J. Neural Transm.* 119, 225–234. doi: 10.1007/s00702-012-0765-3
48. Gabbay, V., Klein, R. G., Katz, Y., Mendoza, S., Guttman, L. E., Alonso, C. M., et al. (2010). The possible role of the kynurenine pathway in adolescent depression with melancholic features. *J. Child Psychol. Psychiatry* 51, 935–943. doi: 10.1111/ j.1469-7610.2010.02245.x
49. Ganesalingam, J., and Bowser, R. (2010). The application of biomarkers in clinical trials for motor neuron disease. *Biomark. Med.* 4, 281–297. doi: 10.2217/bmm. 09.71
50. Ghisoni, K., Martins Rde, P., Barbeito, L., and Latini, A. (2015). Neopterin as a potential cytoprotective brain molecule. *J. Psychiatr. Res.* 71, 134–139. doi: 10.1016/j.jpsychires.2015.10.003
51. Gil, J., Preux, P., Alioum, A., Ketzoian, C., Desport, J., Druet-cabanac, M., et al. (2017). Disease progression and survival in ALS: first multi-state model approach Disease progression and survival in ALS: first multi-state model approach. *Amyotroph. Lateral Scler.* 8, 224–229. doi: 10.1080/17482960701278562
52. Giusti, R. M., Maloney, E. M., Hanchard, B., Morgan, O. S., Steinberg, S. M., Wachter, H., et al. (1996). Differential patterns of serum biomarkers of immune activation in human T-cell lymphotropic virus type I-associated myelopathy/ tropical spastic paraparesis, and adult T-cell leukemia/lymphoma. *Cancer Epidemiol. Biomark. Prev.* 5, 699–704.
53. Gostner, J. M., Geisler, S., Becker, K., Fuchs, D., Mayersbach, P., Schennach, H., et al. (2015). Serum tryptophan, kynurenine, phenylalanine, tyrosine and neopterin concentrations in 100 healthy blood donors. *Pteridines* 26, 31–36. doi: 10.1515/pterid-2014-0015
54. Grant, R., Nguyen, S., and Guillemin, G. (2010). Kynurenine pathway metabolism is involved in the maintenance of the intracellular NAD concentration in human primary astrocytes. *Int. J. Tryptophan Res.* 3, 151–156.
55. Grant, R. S., Coggan, S. E., and Smythe, G. A. (2009). The physiological action of picolinic acid in the human brain. *Int. J. Tryptophan Res.* 2, 71–79.
56. Guidetti, P., and Schwarcz, R. (1999). 3-Hydroxykynurenine potentiates quinolinate but not NMDA toxicity in the rat striatum. *Eur. J. Neurosci.* 11, 3857–3863. doi: 10.1046/j.1460-9568.1999.00806.x
57. Guillemin, G. J. (2012a). Quinolinic acid, the inescapable neurotoxin. *FEBS J.* 279, 1356–1365. doi: 10.1111/j.1742-4658.2012.08485.x
58. Guillemin, G. J. (2012b). Quinolinic acid: neurotoxicity. *FEBS J.* 279:1355. doi: 10.1111/j.1742-4658.2012.08493.x
59. Guillemin, G. J., Brew, B. J., Noonan, C. E., Takikawa, O., and Cullen, K. M. (2005a). Indoleamine 2,3 dioxygenase and quinolinic acid immunoreactivity in Alzheimer's disease hippocampus. *Neuropathol. Appl. Neurobiol.* 31, 395–404. doi: 10.1111/j.1365-2990.2005.00655.x
60. Guillemin, G. J., Kerr, S. J., and Brew, B. J. (2005b). Involvement of quinolinic acid in AIDS dementia complex. *Neurotox. Res.* 7, 103–123. doi: 10.1007/bf03033781
61. Guillemin, G. J., Smythe, G., Takikawa, O., and Brew, B. J. (2005c). Expression of indoleamine 2,3-dioxygenase and production of quinolinic acid by human microglia, astrocytes, and neurons. *Glia* 49, 15–23. doi: 10.1002/glia.20090
62. Guillemin, G. J., Croitoru-Lamoury, J., Dormont, D., Armati, P. J., and Brew, B. J. (2003a). Quinolinic acid upregulates chemokine production and chemokine receptor expression in astrocytes. *Glia* 41, 371–381. doi: 10.1002/glia.10175
63. Guillemin, G. J., Smith, D. G., Smythe, G. A., Armati, P. J., and Brew, B. J. (2003b). Expression of the kynurenine pathway enzymes in human microglia and macrophages. *Adv. Exp. Med. Biol.* 527, 105–112. doi: 10.1007/978-1-4615-0135-0_12
64. Guillemin, G. J., Cullen, K. M., Lim, C. K., Smythe, G. A., Garner, B., Kapoor, V., et al. (2007). Characterization of the kynurenine pathway in human neurons. *J. Neurosci.* 27, 12884–12892. doi: 10.1523/JNEUROSCI.4101-07.2007
65. Guillemin, G. J., Kerr, S. J., Smythe, G. A., Smith, D. G., Kapoor, V., Armati, P. J., et al. (2001). Kynurenine pathway metabolism in human astrocytes: a paradox for neuronal protection. *J. Neurochem.* 78, 842–853. doi: 10.1046/j.1471-4159.2001.00498.x
66. Guillemin, G. J. J., Smith, D. G. G., Kerr, S. J. J., Smythe, G. A. A., Kapoor, V., Armati, P. J. J., et al. (2000). Characterisation of kynurenine pathway metabolism in human astrocytes and implications in neuropathogenesis. *Redox Rep.* 5, 108–111. doi: 10.1179/135100000101535375
67. Guix, F. X., Uribesalgo, I., Coma, M., and Muñoz, F. J. (2005). The physiology and pathophysiology of nitric oxide in the brain. *Prog. Neurobiol.* 76, 126–152. doi: 10.1016/j.pneurobio.2005.06.001
68. Gupta, N. K., Thaker, A. I., Kanuri, N., Riehl, T. E., Rowley, C. W., Stenson, W. F., et al. (2012). Serum analysis of tryptophan catabolism pathway: correlation with Crohn's disease activity. *Inflamm. Bowel Dis.* 18, 1214–1220. doi: 10.1002/ibd. 21849
69. Hardiman, O., Al Chalabi, A., Chio, A., Corr, E. M., Logroscino, G., Robberecht, W., et al. (2017). Amyotrophic lateral sclerosis. *Nat. Rev. Dis. Prim.* 3:17071. Hartai, Z., Juhász, A., Rimanóczy, Á, Janáky, T., Donkó, T., Dux, L., et al. (2007).
70. Decreased serum and red blood cell kynurenic acid levels in Alzheimer's disease. *Neurochem. Int.* 50, 308–313. doi: 10.1016/j.neuint.2006.08.012
71. Havelund, J. F., Andersen, A. D., Binzer, M., Blaabjerg, M., Heegaard, N. H. H., Stenager, E., et al. (2017). Changes in kynurenine pathway metabolism in Parkinson patients with L-DOPA-induced dyskinesia. *J. Neurochem.* 142, 756–766. doi: 10.1111/jnc.14104
72. Heyes, M. P., Brew, B., Martin, A., Markey, S. P., Price, R. W., Bhalla, R. B., et al. (1991). Cerebrospinal fluid quinolinic acid concentrations are increased in acquired immune deficiency syndrome. *Adv. Exp. Med. Biol.* 294, 687–690. doi: 10.1007/978-1-4684-5952-4_94
73. Heyes, M. P., Brew, B. J., Saito, K., Quearry, B. J., Price, R. W., Lee, K., et al. (1992). Inter-relationships between quinolinic acid, neuroactive kynurenines, neopterin and β2-microglobulin in cerebrospinal fluid and serum of HIV-1-infected patients. *J. Neuroimmunol.* 40, 71–80. doi: 10.1016/0165-5728(92) 90214-6
74. Heyes, M. P., Chen, C. Y., Major, E. O., and Saito, K. (1997). Different kynurenine pathway enzymes limit quinolinic acid formation by various human cell types. *Biochem. J.* 326(Pt 2), 351–356. doi: 10.1042/bj3260351
75. Heyes, M. P., Hutto, B., and Markey, S. P. (1988). 4-chloro-3-hydroxyanthranilate inhibits brain 3-hydroxyanthranate oxidase. *Neurochem. Int.* 13, 405–408. doi: 10.1016/0197-0186(88)90015-0
76. Heyes, M. P., and Markey, S. P. (1988). Quantification of quinolinic acid in rat brain, whole blood, and plasma by gas chromatography and negative chemical ionization mass spectrometry: effects of systemic l-tryptophan administration on brain and blood quinolinic acid concentrations. *Anal. Biochem.* 174, 349–359. doi: 10.1016/0003-2697(88)90556-8
77. Hirayama, A., Nakashima, E., Sugimoto, M., Akiyama, S., Sato, W., Maruyama, S., et al. (2012). Metabolic profiling reveals new serum biomarkers for differentiating diabetic nephropathy. *Anal. Bioanal. Chem.* 404, 3101–3109. doi: 10.1007/s00216-012-6412-x
78. Huang, J. Y., Butler, L. M., Midttun, Ø., Ulvik, A., Wang, R., Jin, A., et al. (2018). A prospective evaluation of serum kynurenine metabolites and risk of pancreatic cancer. *PLoS One* 13:e0196465. doi: 10.1371/journal.pone.019 6465
79. Ilzecka, J., Kocki, T., Stelmasiak, Z., and Turski, W. A. (2003). Endogenous protectant kynurenic acid in amyotrophic lateral sclerosis. *Acta Neurol. Scand.* 107, 412–418. doi: 10.1034/j.1600-0404.2003.00076.x
80. Imai, S., and Yoshino, J. (2013). The importance of NAMPT/NAD/SIRT1 in the systemic regulation of metabolism and ageing. *Diabetes Obes. Metab.* 15, 26–33. doi: 10.1111/dom.12171
81. Jacobs, K. R., Lim, C. K., Blennow, K., Zetterberg, H., Chatterjee, P., Martins, R. N., et al. (2019). Correlation between plasma and CSF concentrations of kynurenine pathway metabolites in Alzheimer's disease and relationship to amyloid-β and tau. *Neurobiol. Aging* 80, 11–20. doi: 10.1016/j.neurobiolaging.2019.03.015
82. Jacobs, K. R., and Lovejoy, D. B. (2018). Inhibiting the kynurenine pathway in spinal cord injury: multiple therapeutic potentials? *Neural Regen. Res.* 13, 2073–2076. doi: 10.4103/1673-5374.241446
83. Jhamandas, K., Boegman, R. J. J., Beninger, R. J. J., and Bialik, M. (1990). Quinolinate-induced cortical cholinergic damage: modulation by tryptophan metabolites. *Brain Res.* 529, 185–191. doi: 10.1016/0006-8993(90)90826-W
84. Jin, H., Zhang, Y., You, H., Tao, X., Wang, C., Jin, G., et al. (2015). Prognostic significance of kynurenine 3-monooxygenase and effects on proliferation, migration and invasion of human hepatocellular carcinoma. *Sci. Rep.* 5:10466. doi: 10.1038/srep10466
85. Jones, S. P., Franco, N. F., Varney, B., Sundaram, G., Brown, D. A., de Bie, J., et al. (2015). Expression of the Kynurenine pathway in human peripheral blood mononuclear cells: implications for inflammatory and neurodegenerative disease. *PLoS One* 10:e0131389. doi: 10.1371/journal.pone.0131389
86. Kalonia, H., Kumar, P., and Kumar, A. (2011). Attenuation of proinflammatory

cytokines and apoptotic process by verapamil and diltiazem against quinolinic acid induced Huntington like alterations in rats. *Brain Res.* 1372, 115–126. doi: 10.1016/j.brainres.2010.11.060

87. Kalonia, H., Mishra, J., and Kumar, A. (2012). Targeting neuro-inflammatory cytokines and oxidative stress by minocycline attenuates quinolinic-acid-induced Huntington's disease-like symptoms in rats. *Neurotox. Res.* 22, 310–320. doi: 10.1007/s12640-012-9315-x
88. Kegel, M. E., Bhat, M., Skogh, E., Samuelsson, M., Lundberg, K., Dahl, M.-L., et al. (2014). Imbalanced kynurenine pathway in schizophrenia. *Int. J. Tryptophan Res.* 7, 15–22. doi: 10.4137/IJTR.S16800
89. Khan, A., Choi, S. A., Na, J., Pamungkas, A. D., Jung, K. J., Jee, S. H., et al. (2019). Noninvasive serum metabolomic profiling reveals elevated Kynurenine pathway's metabolites in humans with prostate cancer. *J. Proteome Res.* 18, 1532–1541. doi: 10.1021/acs.jproteome.8b00803
90. Khaspekov, L., Kida, E., Victorov, I., and Mossakowski, M. J. (1989). Neurotoxic effect induced by quinolinic acid in dissociated cell culture of mouse hippocampus. *J. Neurosci. Res.* 22, 150–157. doi: 10.1002/jnr.4902 20207
91. Kim, J. P., and Choi, D. W. (1987). Quinolinate neurotoxicity in cortical cell culture. *Neuroscience* 23, 423–432. doi: 10.1016/0306-4522(87)90066-2
92. Kocki, T., Wnuk, S., Kloc, R., Kocki, J., Owe-Larsson, B., and Urbanska, E. M. (2012). New insight into the antidepressants action: modulation of kynurenine pathway by increasing the kynurenic acid/3-hydroxykynurenine ratio. *J. Neural Transm.* 119, 235–243. doi: 10.1007/s00702-011-0668-8
93. Koh, J. Y., and Choi, D. W. (1988). Vulnerability of cultured cortical neurons to damage by excitotoxins: differential susceptibility of neurons containing NADPH-diaphorase. *J. Neurosci.* 8, 2153–2163. doi: 10.1523/jneurosci.08-06-02153.1988
94. Kosek, M. N., Mduma, E., Kosek, P. S., Lee, G. O., Svensen, E., Pan, W. K. Y., et al. (2016). Plasma tryptophan and the Kynurenine–tryptophan ratio are associated with the acquisition of statural growth deficits and oral vaccine underperformance in populations with environmental enteropathy. *Am. J. Trop. Med. Hyg.* 95, 928–937. doi: 10.4269/ajtmh.16-0037
95. Krause, D., Suh, H.-S., Tarassishin, L., Cui, Q. L., Durafourt, B. A., Choi, N., et al. (2011). The tryptophan metabolite 3-hydroxyanthranilic acid plays anti-inflammatory and neuroprotective roles during inflammation. *Am. J. Pathol.* 179, 1360–1372. doi: 10.1016/j.ajpath.2011.05.048
96. Küster, O. C., Laptinskaya, D., Fissler, P., Schnack, C., Zügel, M., Nold, V., et al. (2017). Novel blood-based biomarkers of cognition, stress, and physical or cognitive training in older adults at risk of Dementia: preliminary evidence for a role of BDNF, Irisin, and the Kynurenine pathway. *J. Alzheimer's Dis.* 59, 1097–1111. doi: 10.3233/JAD-170447
97. Kuwano, N., Kato, T. A., Setoyama, D., Sato-Kasai, M., Shimokawa, N., Hayakawa, K., et al. (2018). Tryptophan-kynurenine and lipid related metabolites as blood biomarkers for first-episode drug-naïve patients with major depressive disorder: an exploratory pilot case-control study. *J. Affect. Disord.* 231, 74–82. doi: 10.1016/J.JAD.2018.01.014
98. Lambrechts, D., Robberecht, W., and Carmeliet, P. (2007). Heterogeneity in motoneuron disease. *Trends Neurosci.* 30, 536–544. doi: 10.1016/j.tins.2007. 07.002
99. Lee, J.-M. M., Tan, V., Lovejoy, D., Braidy, N., Rowe, D. B., Brew, B. J., et al. (2017). Involvement of quinolinic acid in the neuropathogenesis of amyotrophic lateral sclerosis. *Neuropharmacology* 112, 346–364. doi: 10.1016/j.neuropharm.2016.05.011
100. Lee, S. A., Mefford, J. A., Huang, Y., Witte, J. S., Martin, J. N., Haas, D. W., et al. (2016). Host genetic predictors of the kynurenine pathway of tryptophan catabolism among treated HIV-infected Ugandans. *AIDS* 30, 1807–1815. doi: 10.1097/QAD.0000000000001124
101. Leipnitz, G., Schumacher, C., Dalcin, K. B., Scussiato, K., Solano, A., Funchal, C., et al. (2007). In vitro evidence for an antioxidant role of 3-hydroxykynurenine and 3-hydroxyanthranilic acid in the brain. *Neurochem. Int.* 50, 83–94. doi: 10.1016/j.neuint.2006.04.017
102. Lepage, N., Mcdonald, N., Dallaire, L., and Lambert, M. (1997). Diet-related reference values for plasma amino acids in newborns measured by reversed-phase HPLC. *Clin. Chem.* 43, 2397–2402.
103. Lewitt, P. A., Li, J., Lu, M., Beach, T. G., Adler, C. H., and Guo, L. (2013). 3-hydroxykynurenine and other Parkinson's disease biomarkers discovered by metabolomic analysis. *Mov. Disord.* 28, 1653–1660. doi: 10.1002/mds.25555
104. Lim, C. K., Bilgin, A., Lovejoy, D. B., Tan, V., Bustamante, S., Taylor, B. V., et al. (2017). Kynurenine pathway metabolomics predicts and provides mechanistic insight into multiple sclerosis progression. *Sci. Rep.* 7:41473. doi: 10.1038/srep41473
105. Lim, C. K., Smythe, G. A., Stocker, R., Brew, B. J., and Guillemin, G. J. (2007). Characterization of the kynurenine pathway in human oligodendrocytes. *Int. Congr. Ser.* 1304, 213–217. doi: 10.1016/J.ICS.2007.07.011
106. Lim, C. K., Yap, M. M. C., Kent, S. J., Gras, G., Samah, B., Batten, J. C., et al. (2013). Characterization of the kynurenine pathway and quinolinic Acid production in macaque macrophages. *Int. J. Tryptophan Res.* 6, 7–19. doi: 10.4137/IJTR. S11789
107. Liu, H., Ding, L., Zhang, H., Mellor, D., Wu, H., Zhao, D., et al. (2018). The metabolic factor Kynurenic acid of Kynurenine pathway predicts major depressive disorder. *Front. Psychiatry* 9:552. doi: 10.3389/fpsyt.2018.00552
108. Lugo-Huitrón, R., Blanco-Ayala, T., Ugalde-Muñiz, P., Carrillo-Mora, P., Pedraza- Chaverrí, J., Silva-Adaya, D., et al. (2011). On the antioxidant properties of kynurenic acid: free radical scavenging activity and inhibition of oxidative stress. *Neurotoxicol. Teratol.* 33, 538–547. doi: 10.1016/J.NTT.2011.07.002
109. Mackay, G. M., Forrest, C. M., Christofides, J., Bridel, M. A., Mitchell, S., Cowlard, R., et al. (2009). Kynurenine metabolites and inflammation markers in depressed patients treated with fluoxetine or counselling. *Clin. Exp. Pharmacol. Physiol.* 36, 425–435. doi: 10.1111/j.1440-1681.2008.05077.x
110. Maes, M., Leonard, B. E., Myint, A. M., Kubera, M., and Verkerk, R. (2011). The new "5-HT" hypothesis of depression: cell-mediated immune activation induces indoleamine 2,3-dioxygenase, which leads to lower plasma tryptophan and an increased synthesis of detrimental tryptophan catabolites (TRYCATs), both of which contribute to th. *Prog. Neuro Psychopharmacol. Biol. Psychiatry* 35, 702–721. doi: 10.1016/j.pnpbp.2010.12.017
111. Mangge, H., Summers, K. L., Meinitzer, A., Zelzer, S., Almer, G., Prassl, R., et al. (2014). Obesity-related dysregulation of the Tryptophan-Kynurenine metabolism: role of age and parameters of the metabolic syndrome. *Obesity* 22, 195–201. doi: 10.1002/oby.20491
112. Mawatari, K., Oshida, K., Iinuma, F., and Watanabe, M. (1995). Determination of quinolinic acid in human urine by liquid chromatography with fluorimetric detection. *Anal. Chim. Acta* 302, 179–183. doi: 10.1016/0003-2670(94)00493-6 McGeer, P. L., and McGeer, E. G. (2002). Inflammatory processes in amyotrophic lateral sclerosis. *Muscle Nerve* 26, 459–470. doi: 10.1002/mus.10191 McManus, I. R., and Jackson, M. (1968). Isolation and assay of radioactive urinary kynurenic and xanthurenic acids. *Anal. Biochem.* 23, 163–172. doi: 10.1016/ 0003-2697(68)90022-5
113. McMillan, M. (1960). The identification of a fluorescent reducing substance in the urine of patients with rheumatoid arthritis: the excretion of 3-hydroxyanthranilic acid in this and other conditions. *J. Clin. Pathol.* 13, 140–148. doi: 10.1136/JCP.13.2.140
114. Medana, I. M., Day, N. P. J., Salahifar-Sabet, H., Stocker, R., Smythe, G., Bwanaisa, L., et al. (2003). Metabolites of the Kynurenine pathway of tryptophan metabolism in the cerebrospinal fluid of Malawian Children with Malaria. *J. Infect. Dis.* 188, 844–849. doi: 10.1086/377583
115. Midttun, Ø, Townsend, M. K., Nygård, O., Tworoger, S. S., Brennan, P., Johansson, M., et al. (2014). Most blood biomarkers related to vitamin status, one- carbon metabolism, and the Kynurenine pathway show adequate preanalytical stability and within-person reproducibility to allow assessment of exposure or nutritional status in healthy women and cardiovascular patients. *J. Nutr.* 144, 784–790. doi: 10.3945/jn.113.189738
116. Miller, D., Tan, L., Dorshorst, D., Morrissey, K., Mahrus, S., Milanowski, D., et al. (2018). A validated surrogate analyte LC–MS/MS assay for quantitation of endogenous kynurenine and tryptophan in human plasma. *Bioanalysis* 10, 1307–1317. doi: 10.4155/bio-2018-0044
117. Moffett, J. R., and Namboodiri, M. A. (2003). Tryptophan and the immune response. *Immunol. Cell Biol.* 81, 247–265. doi: 10.1046/j.1440-1711.2003.t01-1-01177.x
118. Müller, N., and Schwarz, M. (2006). Schizophrenia as an inflammation-mediated dysbalance of glutamatergic neurotransmission. *Neurotox. Res.* 10, 131–148. doi: 10.1007/BF03033242
119. Musajo, L., Benassi, C. A., and Parpajola, A. (1955). Isolation of Kynurenine and 3-Hydroxykynurenine from human pathological urine. *Nature* 175, 855–856. doi: 10.1038/175855a0
120. Musajo, L., Benassi, C. A., and Parpajola, A. (1956). Excretion and isolation of kynurenine and 3-hydroxykynurenine from human pathological urine. *Clin. Chim. Acta* 1, 229–235. doi: 10.1016/0009-8981(56)90069-9
121. Myint, A. M. (2012). Kynurenines: from the perspective of major psychiatric disorders. *FEBS J.* 279, 1375–1385. doi: 10.1111/j.1742-4658.2012.08551.x
122. Nakagami, Y., Saito, H., and Katsuki, H. (1996). 3-Hydroxykynurenine toxicity on the rat striatum in vivo. *Jpn. J. Pharmacol.* 71, 183–186. doi: 10.1254/jjp.71.183 Ngo, S. T., and Steyn, F. J. (2015). The interplay between metabolic homeostasis and neurodegeneration: insights into the neurometabolic nature of amyotrophic lateral sclerosis. *Cell Regen.* 4:5. doi: 10.1186/s13619-015-0019-6

123. Nilsen, R. M., Bjørke-Monsen, A.-L., Midttun, O., Nygård, O., Pedersen, E. R., Ulvik, A., et al. (2012). Maternal tryptophan and kynurenine pathway metabolites and risk of preeclampsia. *Obstet. Gynecol.* 119, 1243–1250. doi: 10.1097/AOG.0b013e318255004e
124. Ogawa, T., Matson, W. R., Beal, M. F., Myers, R. H., Bird, E. D., Milbury, P., et al. (1992). Kynurenine pathway abnormalities in Parkinson's disease. *Neurology* 42, 1702–1706. doi: 10.1212/WNL.42.9.1702
125. Olsson, S. K., Samuelsson, M., Saetre, P., Lindström, L., Jönsson, E. G., Nordin, C., et al. (2010). Elevated levels of kynurenic acid in the cerebrospinal fluid of patients with bipolar disorder. *J. Psychiatry Neurosci.* 35, 195–199. doi: 10.1503/jpn.090180
126. Owens, M. J., and Nemeroff, C. B. (1994). Role of serotoninin the pathophysiology of depression:focus on the serotonintransporter. *Clin. Chem.* 40, 288–295.
127. Owe-Young, R., Webster, N. L., Mukhtar, M., Pomerantz, R. J., Smythe, G., Walker, D., et al. (2008). Kynurenine pathway metabolism in human blood-brain-barrier cells: implications for immune tolerance and neurotoxicity. *J. Neurochem.* 105, 1346–1357. doi: 10.1111/j.1471-4159.2008.05241.x
128. Oxenkrug, G. (2013). Insulin resistance and dysregulation of tryptophan-kynurenine and kynurenine-nicotinamide adenine dinucleotide metabolic pathways. *Mol. Neurobiol.* 48, 294–301. doi: 10.1007/s12035-013-8497-4
129. Oxenkrug, G., van der Hart, M., Roeser, J., and Summergrad, P. (2016). Anthranilic acid: a potential biomarker and treatment target for Schizophrenia. *Ann. psychiatry Ment. Heal.* 4:1059.
130. Oxenkrug, G. F. (2007). Genetic and hormonal regulation of Tryptophan-Kynurenine metabolism. *Ann. N. Y. Acad. Sci.* 1122, 35–49. doi: 10.1196/annals. 1403.003
131. Oxenkrug, G. F. (2011). Interferon-gamma-inducible kynurenines/pteridines inflammation cascade: implications for aging and aging-associated psychiatric and medical disorders NIH public access. *J. Neural Transm.* 118, 75–85. doi: 10.1007/s00702-010-0475-7
132. Park, W. G., Wu, M., Bowen, R., Zheng, M., Fitch, W. L., Pai, R. K., et al. (2013). Metabolomic-derived novel cyst fluid biomarkers for pancreatic cysts: glucose and kynurenine. *Gastrointest. Endosc.* 78, 295.e2–302.e2. doi: 10.1016/j.gie. 2013.02.037
133. Pedersen, E. R., Svingen, G. F. T., Schartum-Hansen, H., Ueland, P. M., Ebbing, M., Nordrehaug, J. E., et al. (2013). Urinary excretion of kynurenine and tryptophan, cardiovascular events, and mortality after elective coronary angiography. *Eur. Heart J.* 34, 2689–2696. doi: 10.1093/eurheartj/eht264
134. Pehar, M., Harlan, B. A., Killoy, K. M., and Vargas, M. R. (2018). Nicotinamide adenine dinucleotide metabolism and neurodegeneration. *Antioxid. Redox Signal.* 28, 1652–1668. doi: 10.1089/ars.2017.7145
135. Pérez-González, A., Raú Alvarez-Idaboy, J., and Galano, A. (2017). Dual antioxidant/pro-oxidant behavior of the tryptophan metabolite 3-hydroxyanthranilic acid: a theoretical investigation of reaction mechanisms and kinetics. *New J. Chem.* 41, 3829–3845. doi: 10.1039/c6nj03980d
136. Perkins, M. N. N., and Stone, T. W. W. (1982). An iontophoretic investigation of the actions of convulsant kynurenines and their interaction with the endogenous excitant quinolinic acid. *Brain Res.* 247, 184–187. doi: 10.1016/0006-8993(82)91048-4
137. Perl, A. (2015). mTOR activation is a biomarker and a central pathway to autoimmune disorders, cancer, obesity, and aging. *Ann. N. Y. Acad. Sci.* 1346, 33–44. doi: 10.1111/nyas.12756
138. Petrov, D., Mansfield, C., Moussy, A., and Hermine, O. (2017). ALS clinical trials review: 20 years of failure. Are we any closer to registering a new treatment?. *Front. Aging Neurosci.* 9:68. doi: 10.3389/fnagi.2017.00068
139. Pierozan, P., Ferreira, F., de Lima, B. O., and Pessoa-Pureur, R. (2015). Quinolinic acid induces disrupts cytoskeletal homeostasis in striatal neurons. Protective role of astrocyte-neuron interaction. *J. Neurosci. Res.* 93, 268–284. doi: 10.1002/ jnr.23494
140. Pierozan, P., Zamoner, A., Krombauer Soska, Â, Bristot Silvestrin, R., Oliveira Loureiro, S., Heimfarth, L., et al. (2010). Acute intrastriatal administration of quinolinic acid provokes hyperphosphorylation of cytoskeletal intermediate filament proteins in astrocytes and neurons of rats. *Exp. Neurol.* 224, 188–196. doi: 10.1016/j.expneurol.2010.03.009
141. Procaccini, C., Santopaolo, M., Faicchia, D., Colamatteo, A., Formisano, L., de Candia, P., et al. (2016). Role of metabolism in neurodegenerative disorders. *Metabolism* 65, 1376–1390. doi: 10.1016/J.METABOL.2016.05.018
142. Puccetti, P., Fallarino, F., Italiano, A., Soubeyran, I., MacGrogan, G., Debled, M., et al. (2015). Accumulation of an endogenous tryptophan-derived metabolite in colorectal and breast cancers. *PLoS One* 10:e0122046. doi: 10.1371/journal. pone.0122046
143. Quagliariello, E., Papa, S., Saccone, C., and Alifano, A. (1964). Effect of 3-Hydroxyanthranilic acid on the mitochondrial respiratory system. *Biochem J.* 91, 137–146. doi: 10.1042/bj0910137
144. Rejdak, K., Bartosik-Psujek, H., Dobosz, B., Kocki, T., Grieb, P., Giovannoni, G., et al. (2002). Decreased level of kynurenic acid in cerebrospinal fluid of relapsing-onset multiple sclerosis patients. *Neurosci. Lett.* 331, 63–65. doi: 10. 1016/S0304-3940(02)00710-3
145. Ribeiro, C. A. J., Grando, V., Dutra Filho, C. S., Wannmacher, C. M. D., and Wajner, M. (2006). Evidence that quinolinic acid severely impairs energy metabolism through activation of NMDA receptors in striatum from developing rats. *J. Neurochem.* 99, 1531–1542. doi: 10.1111/j.1471-4159.2006. 04199.x
146. Ruddick, J. P., Evans, A. K., Nutt, D. J., Lightman, S. L., Rook, G. A. W., and Lowry, C. A. (2006). Tryptophan metabolism in the central nervous system: medical implications. *Expert Rev. Mol. Med.* 8, 1–27. doi: 10.1017/s1462399406000068
147. Sakai, N., Kaufman, S., and Milstien, S. (1995). Parallel induction of nitric oxide and tetrahydrobiopterin synthesis by cytokines in rat glial cells. *J. Neurochem.* 65, 895–902. doi: 10.1046/j.1471-4159.1995.65020895.x
148. Sandyk, R. (2006). Serotonergic mechanisms in amyotrophic lateral sclerosis. *Int. J. Neurosci.* 116, 775–826. doi: 10.1080/00207450600754087
149. Sardar, A. M., Bell, J. E., and Reynolds, G. P. (2002). Increased concentrations of the Neurotoxin 3-Hydroxykynurenine in the frontal cortex of HIV-1-positive patients. *J. Neurochem.* 64, 932–935. doi: 10.1046/j.1471-4159.1995.64020932.x
Sasaki, Y. (2019). Metabolic aspects of neuronal degeneration: from a NAD+ point of view. *Neurosci. Res.* 139, 9–20. doi: 10.1016/j.neures.2018.07.001
150. Sasaki, Y., Araki, T., and Milbrandt, J. (2006). Stimulation of nicotinamide adenine dinucleotide biosynthetic pathways delays axonal degeneration after axotomy. *J. Neurosci.* 26, 8484–8491. doi: 10.1523/JNEUROSCI.2320-06.2006
151. Sathyasaikumar, K. V., Stachowski, E. K., Wonodi, I., Roberts, R. C., Rassoulpour, A., McMahon, R. P., et al. (2011). Impaired kynurenine pathway metabolism in the prefrontal cortex of individuals with schizophrenia. *Schizophr. Bull.* 37, 1147–1156. doi: 10.1093/schbul/sbq112
152. Schroecksnadel, K., Kaser, S., Ledochowski, M., Neurauter, G., Mur, E., Herold, M., et al. (2003). Increased degradation of tryptophan in blood of patients with rheumatoid arthritis. *J. Rheumatol.* 30, 1935–1939.
153. Schwarcz, R., Okuno, E., White, R. J., Birdt, E. D., and Whetsell, W. O. (1988). 3-Hydroxyanthranilate oxygenase activity is increased in the brains of Huntington disease victims (kynurenines/quinolinic acid/excitotoins/ neurodegenerative disorders). *Neurobiology* 85, 4079–4081. doi: 10.1073/pnas.85.11.4079
154. Shibata, K. (1988). Fluorimetric micro-determination of kynurenic acid, an endogenous blocker of neurotoxicity, by high-performance liquid chromatography. *J. Chromatogr. B Biomed. Sci. Appl.* 430, 376–380. doi: 10. 1016/S0378-4347(00)83173-4
155. Shoki, O., Nobuyoshi, N., Hiroshi, S., Hiroshi, K., Okuda, S., Nishiyama, N., et al. (1998). 3-Hydroxykynurenine, an endogenous oxidative stress generator, causes neuronal cell death with apoptotic features and region selectivity. *J. Neurochem.* 70, 299–307. doi: 10.1046/j.1471-4159.1998.70010299.x
156. Smythe, G. A., Poljak, A., Bustamante, S., Braga, O., Maxwell, A., Grant, R., et al. (2003). ECNI GC-MS analysis of picolinic and quinolinic acids and their amides in human plasma, CSF, and brain tissue. *Adv. Exp. Med. Biol.* 527, 705–712. doi: 10.1007/978-1-4615-0135-0_83
157. Spiera, H., and Vallarino, R. (1969). Serum kynurenine in rheumatoid arthritis. *J. Clin. Invest.* 48, 856–859. doi: 10.1172/JCI106043
158. Steiner, J., Walter, M., Gos, T., Guillemin, G. J., Bernstein, H.-G., Sarnyai, Z., et al. (2011). Severe depression is associated with increased microglial quinolinic acid in subregions of the anterior cingulate gyrus: evidence for an immune-modulated glutamatergic neurotransmission? *J. Neuroinflamm.* 8:94. doi: 10. 1186/1742-2094-8-94
159. Stone, T. (1993). Neuropharmacology of quinolinic and kynurenic acids. *Pharmacol. Rev.* 45, 309–379.
160. Stone, T. W., Forrest, C. M., and Darlington, L. G. (2012). Kynurenine pathway inhibition as a therapeutic strategy for neuroprotection. *FEBS J.* 279, 1386–1397. doi: 10.1111/j.1742-4658.2012.08487.x
161. Stoy, N., Mackay, G. M., Forrest, C. M., Christofides, J., Egerton, M., Stone, T. W., et al. (2005). Tryptophan metabolism and oxidative stress in patients with Huntington's disease. *J. Neurochem.* 93, 611–623. doi: 10.1111/j.1471-4159. 2005.03070.x
162. Sühs, K.-W., Novoselova, N., Kuhn, M., Seegers, L., Kaever, V., Müller-Vahl, K., et al. (2019). Kynurenine is a cerebrospinal fluid biomarker for bacterial and viral central nervous system infections. *J. Infect. Dis.* 220, 127–138. doi: 10.1093/ infdis/jiz048
163. Sun, M., Gao, X., Zhang, D., Ke, C., Hou, Y., Fan, L., et al. (2013). Identification

of biomarkers for unstable angina by plasma metabolomic profiling. *Mol. Biosyst.* 9:3059. doi: 10.1039/c3mb70216b

164. Takahashi, H., Kaihara, M., and Pricet, J. M. (1956). The conversion of kynurenic acid to quinaldic acid by humans and rats. *J. Biol. Chem.* 223, 705–708.

165. Takikawa, O., Yoshida, R., Kido, R., and Hayaishi, O. (1986). Tryptophan degradation in mice initiated by indoleamine 2,3-dioxygenase. *J. Biol. Chem.* 261, 3648–3653.

166. Tompsett, S. L. (1959). The determination in urine of some metabolites of tryptophan-kynurenine, anthranilic acid and 3-hydroxyanthranilic acid-and reference to the presence of o-aminophenol in urine. *Clin. Chim. Acta* 4, 411–419. doi: 10.1016/0009-8981(59)90112-3

167. Turner, M. R., Bowser, R., Bruijn, L., Dupuis, L., Ludolph, A., McGrath, M., et al. (2013). Mechanisms, models and biomarkers in amyotrophic lateral sclerosis. *Amyotroph. Lateral Scler. Frontotemporal Degener.* 14(Suppl. 1), 19–32. doi: 10.3109/21678421.2013.778554

168. Turner, M. R., Grosskreutz, J., Kassubek, J., Abrahams, S., Agosta, F., Benatar, M., et al. (2011). Towards a neuroimaging biomarker for amyotrophic lateral sclerosis. *Lancet Neurol.* 10, 400–403. doi: 10.1016/S1474-4422(11)70049-7

169. Turner, M. R., Kiernan, M. C., Leigh, P. N., and Talbot, K. (2009). Biomarkers in amyotrophic lateral sclerosis. *Lancet Neurol.* 8, 94–109. doi: 10.1016/S1474- 4422(08)70293-X

170. Verdin, E. (2015). NAD+ in aging, metabolism, and neurodegeneration. *Science* 350, 1208–1213. doi: 10.1126/science.aac4854

171. Wang, M., Dong, X., Huang, Y., Su, J., Dai, X., Guo, Y., et al. (2019). Activation of the kynurenine pathway is associated with poor outcome in Pneumocystis pneumonia patients infected with HIV: results of 2?months cohort study. *BMC Infect. Dis.* 19:223. doi: 10.1186/s12879-019-3851-4

172. Weiner, J., Parida, S. K., Maertzdorf, J., Black, G. F., Repsilber, D., Telaar, A., et al. (2012). Biomarkers of inflammation, immunosuppression and stress are revealed by metabolomic profiling of tuberculosis patients. *PLoS One* 7:e40221. doi: 10.1371/journal.pone.0040221

173. Weishaupt, J. H., Bartels, C., Pölking, E., Dietrich, J., Rohde, G., Poeggeler, B., et al. (2006). Reduced oxidative damage in ALS by high-dose enteral melatonin treatment. *J. Pineal Res.* 41, 313–323. doi: 10.1111/j.1600-079X.2006.00377.x

174. Widner, B., Leblhuber, F., and Fuchs, D. (2002). Increased neopterin production and tryptophan degradation in advanced Parkinson's disease. *J. Neural Transm.* 109, 181–189. doi: 10.1007/s007020200014

175. Xie, H., Hou, Y., Cheng, J., Openkova, M. S., Xia, B., Wang, W., et al. (2017). Metabolic profiling and novel plasma biomarkers for predicting survival in epithelial ovarian cancer. *Oncotarget* 8, 32134–32146. doi: 10.18632/oncotarget.16739

176. Yoon, N. S., Cho, Y., Lee, S. Y., Choi, H. J., and Hwang, O. (2010). Inactivation of aconitase by Tetrahydrobiopterin in DArgic Cells: relevance to PD. *Exp. Neurobiol.* 19, 23–29. doi: 10.5607/en.2010.19.1.23

177. Young, P. E., Jew, S. K., Buckland, M. E., Pamphlett, R., and Suter, C. M. (2017). Epigenetic differences between monozygotic twins discordant for amyotrophic lateral sclerosis (ALS) provide clues to disease pathogenesis. *PLoS One* 12:e0182638. doi: 10.1371/journal.pone.0182638

178. Yuwiler, A., Oldendorf, W. H., Geller, E., and Braun, L. (1977). Effect of albumin binding and amino acid competition on tryptophan uptake into brain. *J. Neurochem.* 28, 1015–1023. doi: 10.1111/j.1471-4159.1977.tb10664.x

179. Zhang, X., Beaulieu, J.-M., Gainetdinov, R. R., and Caron, M. G. (2006). Functional polymorphisms of the brain serotonin synthesizing enzyme tryptophan hydroxylase-2. *Cell. Mol. Life Sci.* 63, 6–11. doi: 10.1007/s00018-005-5417-4

180. Zhang, Y., Cook, A., Kim, J., Baranov, S. V., Jiang, J., Smith, K., et al. (2013). Melatonin inhibits the caspase-1/cytochrome c/caspase-3 cell death pathway, inhibits MT1 receptor loss and delays disease progression in a mouse model of amyotrophic lateral sclerosis. *Neurobiol. Dis.* 55, 26–35. doi: 10.1016/J.NBD.2013.03.008

181. Zhao, J. (2013). Plasma Kynurenic Acid/Tryptophan Ratio: a sensitive and reliable biomarker for the assessment of renal function. *Ren. Fail.* 35, 648–653. doi: 10.3109/0886022X.2013.790301

182. Zinellu, A., Fois, A. G., Zinellu, E., Sotgiu, E., Sotgia, S., Arru, D., et al. (2018). Increased kynurenine plasma concentrations and kynurenine-tryptophan ratio in mild-to-moderate chronic obstructive pulmonary disease patients. *Biomark. Med.* 12, 229–237. doi: 10.2217/bmm-2017-0280

183. Zuo, H., Ueland, P. M., Ulvik, A., Eussen, S. J. P. M., Vollset, S. E., Nygård, O., et al. (2016). Plasma biomarkers of inflammation, the kynurenine pathway, and risks of all-cause, cancer, and cardiovascular disease mortality. *Am. J. Epidemiol.* 183, 249–258. doi: 10.1093/aje/kwv242

13

White Matter Microstructure Breakdown in the Motor Neuron Disease Spectrum: Recent Advances Using Diffusion Magnetic Resonance Imaging

Silvia Basaia[1], Massimo Filippi[1,2], Edoardo G. Spinelli[1] and Federica Agosta[1]*

[1] Neuroimaging Research Unit, Institute of Experimental Neurology, Division of Neuroscience, Vita-Salute San Raffaele University, Milan, Italy, [2] Department of Neurology, Institute of Experimental Neurology, Division of Neuroscience, San Raffaele Scientific Institute, Vita-Salute San Raffaele University, Milan, Italy

***Correspondence:**
Federica Agosta
agosta.federica@hsr.it

Motor neuron disease (MND) is a fatal progressive neurodegenerative disorder characterized by the breakdown of the motor system. The clinical spectrum of MND encompasses different phenotypes classified according to the relative involvement of the upper or lower motor neurons (LMN) and the presence of genetic or cognitive alterations, with clear prognostic implications. However, the pathophysiological differences of these phenotypes remain largely unknown. Recently, magnetic resonance imaging (MRI) has been recognized as a helpful *in-vivo* MND biomarker. An increasing number of studies is applying advanced neuroimaging techniques in order to elucidate the pathophysiological processes and to identify quantitative outcomes to be used in clinical trials. Diffusion tensor imaging (DTI) is a non-invasive method to detect white matter alterations involving the upper motor neuron and extra-motor white matter tracts. According to this background, the aim of this review is to highlight the key role of MRI and especially DTI, summarizing cross-sectional and longitudinal results of different approaches applied in MND. Current literature suggests that DTI is a promising tool in order to define anatomical "signatures" of the different phenotypes of MND and to track *in vivo* the progressive spread of pathological proteins aggregates.

Keywords: amyotrophic lateral sclerosis, motor neuron disease, diffusion tensor imaging, fractional anisotropy, network analysis, magnetic resonance imaging, structural connectomics

INTRODUCTION

Motor neuron disease (MND) is a group of fatal neurodegenerative diseases characterized by progressive damage of the upper motor neurons (UMN) in the cortex and/or lower motor neurons (LMN) in the brainstem and spinal cord. Depending on the relative involvement of UMN and LMN, MND can be classified in a wide range of clinical phenotypes (including amyotrophic lateral sclerosis [ALS], primary lateral sclerosis [PLS], and progressive muscular atrophy [PMA]), characterized by different clinical presentation and progression rate. Advanced brain imaging techniques, such as magnetic resonance imaging (MRI), have been developed over the last decades in order to detect *in vivo* structural and functional brain abnormalities and to monitor neurodegeneration in the central nervous system of MND patients. Although neurodegeneration primarily affects the gray matter (GM), pathological alterations in the white matter (WM) have also been reported (1), involving not only the corticospinal tract (CST), but also non-motor regions (2).

The present review aims to discuss the current state of the art of MRI within different phenotypes of MND, focusing on WM microstructural alterations, underlining the role of MRI as a tool to understand disease pathophysiology and to provide potential biomarkers for diagnosis and prognostic stratification. Moreover, we also highlight emerging techniques, such as graph analysis, that will likely provide further insights in disease pathogenesis and might help in monitoring disease progression.

DIFFUSION TENSOR IMAGING

Basic Principles

Diffusion tensor imaging (DTI) is the most common MRI technique that allows to investigate WM microstructural changes. DTI is based on the random diffusion of water molecules in the fiber bundles, also known as Brownian motion (3). DTI analysis relies on the concept that, in a spherical volume, the diffusion of water has no preferential direction and spreads equally in three different directions (λ1, λ2, and λ3). Nevertheless, the movement of water molecules within the WM is approximately elliptical, having the greatest movement along axons (axial diffusivity [λ1]) caused by the restriction in the minor axes (radial diffusivity [λ2 and λ3]) imposed by myelin. In order to analyze the diffusion of water molecules, it is possible to define four parameters: (1) fractional anisotropy (FA), which describes how strongly directional is the movement of water molecules within the tissue; (2) radial diffusivity (RD, which is the average of λ2 and λ3); (3) axial diffusivity (AD, or λ1); (4) mean diffusivity (MD, obtained by the average of diffusion in the λ1, λ2, and λ3 axes). While the first three parameters (FA, RD, and AD) describe the spatial variation of water movement, MD reflects the average displacement of water molecules within the volume of interest. Axonal integrity will preserve diffusion parallel to the main fiber direction, resulting in higher FA and lower MD, while damage to the WM will lead to lower FA and higher MD (4). To date, there are several approaches to analyze DTI metrics: regions of interest (ROI) approach, whole-brain voxel-wise methods or tract-based spatial statistics (TBSS). These techniques provide complementary information and are characterized by relative strengths and limitations. The ROI approach is based on the delineation of defined areas or the reconstruction of WM tracts of interest in each subject's native space, in order to extract average DTI metrics to be compared among subjects; although this procedure allows a precise anatomical definition of WM structures and does not involve the coregistration of multiple scan images, it masks local alterations by averaging all voxels within the ROI, usually needs an *a priori* hypothesis and might be influenced by inter-subject anatomical variability (5). The most straightforward approach to assess local DTI alterations is to coregister all subjects' scans and perform statistical tests among groups within each voxel of the whole-brain WM mask; however, whole-brain voxel-wise approaches are sensitive to registration errors (6). To reduce the effects of local misregistrations, TBSS projects all voxels of the DTI image onto the nearest location on a "skeleton" delineating the main WM tracts (7). In addition to these methods, graph theory is one of the most recent approaches to investigate WM changes, building models of structural connectivity in brain disorders based on nodes and edges (8). Current evidence provided by each of these techniques for the study of MND is summarized in the following paragraphs.

The weakness of DTI is the lack of specificity in voxels presenting multiple fiber populations (termed "crossing fibers") (9). In order to overcome this problem, novel data acquisition approaches have been proposed such as high angular resolution diffusion imaging (HARDI), neurite orientation dispersion and density imaging (NODDI) and diffusion spectrum imaging. Although these approaches hold the promise to provide further insights on the pathogenic mechanisms underlying WM degeneration and are likely sensitive to even subtle alterations in several neurodegenerative conditions (10), current evidence in the context of MND is scarce and should be considered preliminary (11, 12).

DTI Signatures in ALS

Several studies have consistently demonstrated decreased FA and increased MD, RD, and AD along the entire CST in ALS patients relative to healthy controls (13–18). Several studies showed specific alterations of DTI metrics only in some parts of the CST: subcortical WM of the precentral gyrus, corona radiata, posterior limb of the internal capsule, cerebral peduncles and pons (19–21). DTI studies have also detected altered metrics in the middle and posterior part of the corpus callosum in ALS patients relative to healthy controls (22, 23). Cervical cord studies also consistently showed DTI alterations in the lateral columns of ALS patients (24–27), which were more severe at more distal cervical segments (25).

Many neuroimaging studies characterized the structural "signatures" in ALS patients with specific underlying genetic mutations. In particular, diffuse WM abnormalities were observed in *C9orf72* repeat expansion carriers (the most common genetic mutation) (28, 29). Particularly, *C9orf72* patients showed an involvement of the CST, whole corpus callosum and superior longitudinal fasciculus compared with healthy controls, in terms of decreased FA and increased MD (29). Only few structural MRI studies were performed in carriers of pathogenic mutations in *SOD1*, showing a relative preservation of brain motor networks compared to sporadic ALS patients (30, 31).

Cross-sectional DTI studies shed light on the pathophysiological processes associated with the development of ALS. However, the definition of biomarkers that could track progressive changes over time has crucial importance. To date, relatively few longitudinal studies focused on DTI changes over time in these patients, due to the difficulties in enrolling enough cases with a rapidly evolving disease who could undergo an appropriate number of follow-up scans. Most of the studies, using a ROI approach or TBSS, showed decreasing values of FA over time in CST, corpus callosum, frontal areas and cerebellum (21, 32–35). One study demonstrated also that diffusivity increased both in the external and internal capsule (21). Nevertheless, there are also studies showing inconsistent results, probably due to different sample sizes, follow-up intervals and, most importantly, the heterogeneity of MND patients (36–38). The same limitations apply to the few longitudinal studies assessing the evolution of cervical cord DTI alterations (27, 36) that showed diverging results about the entity of cord FA decrease over time. One recent study was performed in ALS patients carrying *C9orf72* mutation, demonstrating the spreading of diffusivity alterations from anterior to posterior WM regions over a 6-month period (39).

Phenotyping the MND Spectrum

DTI measures might also be crucial to distinguish different MND phenotypes. Indeed, DTI metrics were widely used for the identification of "signatures" in PLS. In particular, one study demonstrated that PLS patients showed lower CST FA values relative to healthy controls and ALS patients (40). Degeneration in extra-motor areas has also been found to be similar (41) or even more severe (40) in PLS patients compared to ALS patients. Furthermore, widespread DTI alterations were found to correlate with the severity of cognitive deficits in PLS patients (42). On the other hand, the least extensive microstructural changes were observed in patients with predominant LMN involvement, with diverging results in literature concerning the extent and significance of such damage (43–45). Particularly, a recent two-center study suggested that WM integrity was disrupted along the CST and in frontal and prefrontal regions in patients with predominant LMN disease relative to healthy controls (46). Only patients with predominant LMN involvement and a higher rate of disease progression showed significant WM alterations in the specific ALS-related tract systems (46).

Clinical and Neuropsychological Correlations

Many DTI studies aimed to test the relationship between WM changes and clinical and neuropsychological measures in MND. Decreased FA in the CST related with disease severity and rate of disease progression in ALS, identifying an association between worsening disability and degeneration of WM tracts, both in the brain (21) and the cervical cord (24, 27). These findings support the potential use of connectivity measures as markers of disease progression in ALS. Inconsistencies among different studies have been reported as for the relationship between DTI measures and disease duration in ALS patients, as longer disease duration has been paradoxically associated with both increased FA (47) and increased MD values of the CST (48). These discrepancies may be explained by the different progression rates of the two samples. DTI changes in the CST and corpus callosum, as well as in the cingulum, inferior longitudinal, inferior fronto-occipital, and uncinate fasciculi have been found to correlate with performance at cognitive tests assessing attention and executive functions (49). Additional extensive WM damage to extra-motor frontotemporal tracts has also been shown, underlying variable degree of behavioral and cognitive disturbances in ALS patients (45, 50, 51). Particularly, one study demonstrated that WM abnormalities of the corpus callosum and frontotemporal tracts, including uncinate, cingulum, and superior longitudinal fasciculi, are the best predictor of executive and non-executive deficits and behavioral changes within the MND spectrum (51).

Network-Based Analyses

Network-based analysis of structural connections is a new powerful technique that allows studying the brain of healthy subjects or patients with neurodegenerative disorders. The techniques mentioned so far allow to map WM tracts individually using DTI. Recently, neuroimaging research has moved to the study of the human connectome, which aims to map all the possible pathways of the human brain (52). With such new approach, it is possible to provide information about how networks are embedded and interact in the brain. Using graph analysis and connectomics, brain regions can be depicted as a set of nodes, linked by edges representing structural connections. Maps of structural connectivity are created following the following steps: (1) network nodes are identified applying a selected atlas of GM structures to the brain; (2) following definition of the brain regions, WM tracts are reconstructed using DTI; (3) streamlines of the whole brain touching each couple *i* and *j* of the segmented GM nodes are selected; (4) the number of streamlines is calculated for each tract and inserted into a matrix; (5) for each structural connection, the level of microstructural integrity is measured extracting the mean FA, MD, RD, and AD values; (6) finally, all the values are inserted into four different matrices. From the analysis of these matrices, it is possible to provide information concerning the topological organization of network architecture (53). Many studies have examined the global and local graph metrics such as: (1) nodal strength and degree, which provide information regarding the effect of a node in the network; (2) clustering coefficient and local efficiency, which reflect the level of local organization of a network; (3) path length, that is the number of steps needed to connect each pair of nodes; (4) global efficiency, calculated as the inverse of path length, which represents the efficacy of a network to communicate between each pair of nodes; (5) modularity, which gives information regarding segregation of a network, reflecting the level of modular organization (54, 55). To date, modifications of brain topological organization and disruption of structural connectivity have been associated with several neurodegenerative disorders (56–58), including MND.

In a first cross-sectional study, structural brain networks were compared between ALS patients and healthy controls applying network-based statistics (59). ALS patients showed regions with reduced WM connectivity, centered around the primary but also included secondary motor regions (frontal cortex and pallidum). In addition, overall efficiency and clustering coefficient were found to be decreased in ALS patients. A second study studied WM alterations using network analysis, comparing results with those obtained using TBSS (60). The results, consistent with the previous study, showed an impaired motor-frontal-subcortical subnetwork in the ALS patients compared with controls (60). The study also revealed that the results obtained with the network analysis have a strong correspondence with voxel-based approaches (60).

To date, only a few longitudinal studies aimed to investigate the effect of ALS on the brain network over-time. Particularly, one study showed an expanding sub-network of impaired brain connections after six months, with a central role of the primary motor regions (61). The loss of structural connectivity was found to propagate to frontal and parietal regions, supporting the idea that disease spreads along WM connections following a pattern classified into sequential stages (62).

DTI as a Non-invasive *in-vivo* Biomarker of Disease Spreading

Neuropathological studies identified the cytoplasmic inclusions of TDP-43 as the molecular hallmark in up to 98% of ALS cases (63). In the last few years, several studies have speculated that the progressive regional accumulation of TDP-43 aggregates in the brain might be reflected by the consecutive deterioration of WM fiber tracts (61). In light of this, DTI-based approaches have been used to study propagation patterns in the brain of MND patients. A DTI study, using a tract of interest-based staging approach, confirmed the neuropathological progression of ALS in the following order: CST (stage 1); corticorubral and corticopontine tracts (stage 2); corticostriatal pathway (stage 3) and proximal portion of the perforant path (stage 4) (64). Furthermore, the extracted tracts of interest were used to categorize ALS patients into the predefined stages according with their WM damage. Staging categorization at baseline was able to classify 72% of the ALS patients into the different stages. After 6 months, there was an increase in ALS stage in 27% of ALS patients (64). Recent studies applied the *in-vivo* staging approach also to phenotypic variants of ALS. One study aimed to figure out if PLS might be a separate disease or just a slowly progressive variant of ALS (41). Microstructural changes were analyzed using the same approach as "classical" ALS, demonstrating that ALS and PLS patients showed identical alterations in the ALS-related tract systems, considering consequently PLS as phenotypical variant of ALS (41) (**Figure 1**).

The previously considered studies investigated pathology spreading in ALS-related tracts that were selected *a priori*, according with *post-mortem* neuropathological stages. In order to overcome this *a-priori* selection, one study applied network analysis to investigate the underlying pathogenic mechanism of ALS (65). The results showed that regions involved by TDP-43 pathology in early disease stages are highly structurally interconnected in the brain (65). Furthermore, brain regions of subsequent neuropathological stages were found more closely interconnected than regions of more distant stages (65), suggesting that spread of TDP-43 in ALS occurs along axonal pathways (**Figure 2**). The DTI-based *in-vivo* staging of MND patients needs to be confirmed in future longitudinal studies with *post-mortem* confirmation.

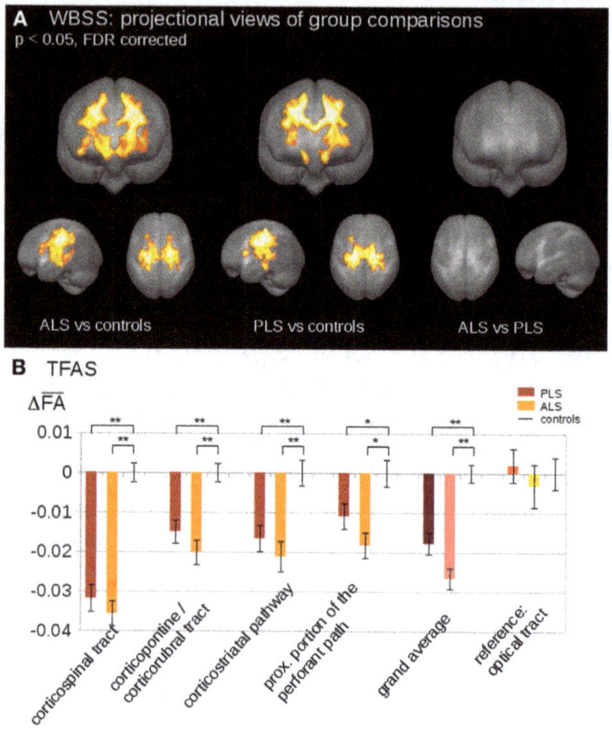

FIGURE 1 | (A) Whole brain-based spatial statistics (WBSS) of fractional anisotropy (FA) maps at the group level for amyotrophic lateral sclerosis (ALS) patients, primary lateral sclerosis (PLS) patients, and controls. WBSS of FA maps demonstrated multiple clusters of regional FA reductions at $p < 0.05$ (corrected for multiple comparisons), projectional views. **(B)** Tractwise fractional anisotropy statistics (TFAS) of FA maps at the group level for ALS patients, PLS patients, and controls. TFAS demonstrated significant regional FA reductions in ALS-related tract systems and in the grand average between ALS patients and controls as well as between PLS patients and controls. No alterations between groups were observed in the reference tract. $^*p < 0.05$, $^{**}p < 0.001$. Reproduced with permission from Müller et al. NeuroImage Clinical 2018 (41) (published open-access under a CC BY-NC-ND 4.0 license).

DISCUSSION AND FUTURE DIRECTIONS

In the context of therapeutic trials, it is essential to identify a useful biomarker that might help for diagnosis, stratification and tracking the disease progression within the MND spectrum. In order to provide new drugs that could aid the early treatment of the disease, the identification of such biomarker is a crucial point to be addressed. Within such a framework, MRI has been long recognized as *in-vivo* biomarker and, in the last few years, an increasing number of studies applied advanced neuroimaging techniques in order to understand the underlying mechanisms in MND. Particularly, we highlighted the important role of DTI, as a very useful tool in order to characterize microstructural changes during the progression of the disease, to find "signatures" of the different phenotype of MND and to track *in vivo* the progressive spread of TDP-43 aggregates. In order to detect WM changes of different phenotypes of MND, cross-sectional studies were performed highlighting alterations within specific tracts, especially in the CST as well as in the corpus callosum. In light of the fact that decreased FA and increased MD describe the microstructural damage in MND patients, we support the idea that the most potential promising DTI biomarkers are FA or MD changes in the CST and corpus callosum. Additionally, connectivity

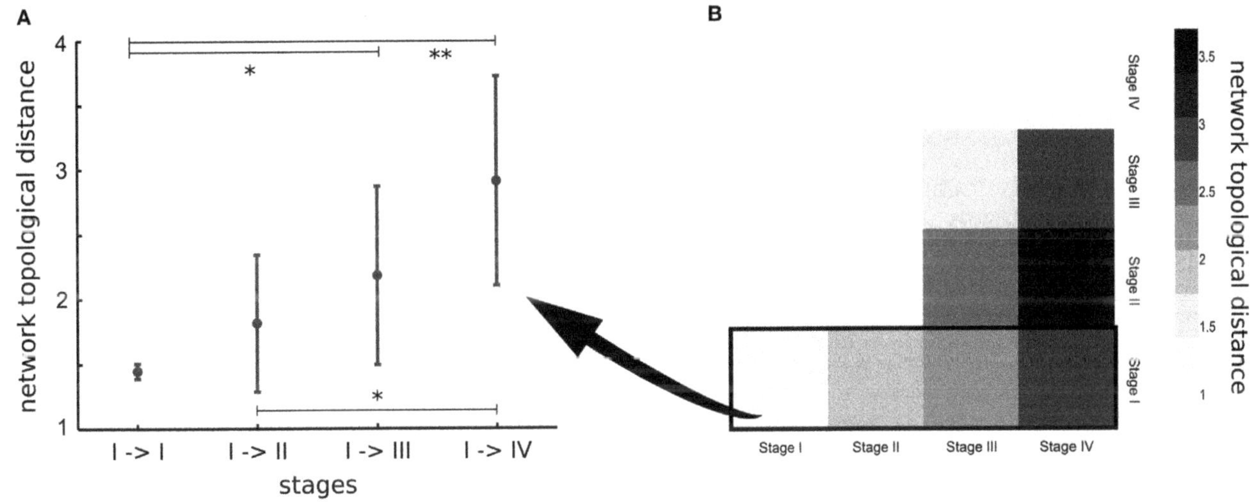

FIGURE 2 | (A) Network topological distance between nodes of stage I, stage I and stage II, stages I, and III and between stages I and IV show a strong ordering effect ($p = 0.002$). Significance of differences in network topological distances between stages is marked as follows: $^*p < 0.05$, $^{**}p < 0.005$. **(B)** Matrix of mean network topological distances between all four stages. Reproduced with permission from Schmidt et al. NeuroImage 2016 (65) (published open-access under a CC BY-NC-ND 4.0 license).

measures might potentially be considered as a marker of disease progression. This is because decreased FA and disease severity and rate of disease progression are highly correlated. In the last few years, the focus has shifted towards the analysis of disease progression. Particularly, several longitudinal neuroimaging studies are confirming the recently proposed neuropathological staging model (62), demonstrating an expanding subnetwork of impaired brain connections from the primary motor cortex to frontal and parietal regions. All these findings support the idea that WM tract involvement might be a valid biomarker to assess *in vivo* the spreading of pathological proteins and to track the neurodegeneration process.

In conclusion, DTI analysis has the potential to be a valid technique for use at the individual patient level in the future. However, there is urgent need for more longitudinal studies. The combination of the *in vivo* staging using longitudinal DTI scans with the *post-mortem* classification might be very useful to understand deeply the pathophysiology of the disease and to provide as soon as possible disease-modifying therapies.

AUTHOR CONTRIBUTIONS

SB drafted the first version of the manuscript. All the authors discussed/edited the draft producing the final version of the manuscript.

FUNDING

The study was partially supported by the European Research Council (grant number 714388 NeuroTRACK).

REFERENCES

1. Rafalowska J, Dziewulska D. White matter injury in amyotrophic lateral sclerosis (ALS). *Folia Neuropathol.* (1996) 34:87–91
2. Smith MC. Nerve fibre degeneration in the brain in amyotrophic lateral sclerosis. *J Neurol Neurosurg Psychiatry.* (1960) 23:269–82. doi: 10.1136/jnnp.23.4.269
3. Le Bihan D, Breton E, Lallemand D, Grenier P, Cabanis E, Laval-Jeantet M. MR imaging of intravoxel incoherent motions: application to diffusion and perfusion in neurologic disorders. *Radiology.* (1986) 161:401–7. doi: 10.1148/radiology.161.2.3763909
4. Basser PJ, Mattiello J, LeBihan D. Estimation of the effective self-diffusion tensor from the NMR spin echo. *J Magn Reson B.* (1994) 103:247–54. doi: 10.1006/jmrb.1994.1037
5. Snook L, Plewes C, Beaulieu C. Voxel based versus region of interest analysis in diffusion tensor imaging of neurodevelopment. *Neuroimage.* (2007) 34:243–52. doi: 10.1016/j.neuroimage.2006.07.021
6. Bookstein FL. "Voxel-based morphometry" should not be used with imperfectly registered images. *Neuroimage.* (2001) 14:1454–62. doi: 10.1006/nimg.2001.0770
7. Smith SM, Jenkinson M, Johansen-Berg H, Rueckert D, Nichols TE, Mackay CE, et al. Tract-based spatial statistics: voxelwise analysis of multi-subject diffusion data. *Neuroimage.* (2006) 31:1487–505. doi: 10.1016/j.neuroimage.2006.02.024
8. Iturria-Medina Y, Canales-Rodriguez EJ, Melie-Garcia L, Valdes-Hernandez PA, Martinez-Montes E, Aleman-Gomez Y, et al. Characterizing brain anatomical connections using diffusion weighted MRI and graph theory. *Neuroimage.* (2007) 36:645–60. doi: 10.1016/j.neuroimage.2007.02.012
9. Douaud G, Jbabdi S, Behrens TE, Menke RA, Gass A, Monsch AU, et al. DTI measures in crossing-fibre areas: increased diffusion anisotropy reveals early white matter alteration in MCI and mild Alzheimer's disease. *Neuroimage.* (2011) 55:880–90. doi: 10.1016/j.neuroimage.2010.12.008
10. Barritt AW, Gabel MC, Cercignani M, Leigh PN. Emerging magnetic resonance imaging techniques and analysis methods in amyotrophic lateral sclerosis. *Front Neurol.* (2018) 9:1065. doi: 10.3389/fneur.2018.01065

11. Trojsi F, Caiazzo G, Di Nardo F, Fratello M, Santangelo G, Siciliano M, et al. High angular resolution diffusion imaging abnormalities in the early stages of amyotrophic lateral sclerosis. *J Neurol Sci.* (2017) 380:215–22. doi: 10.1016/j.jns.2017.07.039
12. Broad RJ, Gabel MC, Dowell NG, Schwartzman DJ, Seth AK, Zhang H, et al. Neurite orientation and dispersion density imaging (NODDI) detects cortical and corticospinal tract degeneration in ALS. *J Neurol Neurosurg Psychiatry.* (2018) doi: 10.1136/jnnp-2018-318830. [Epub ahead of print].
13. Iwata NK, Aoki S, Okabe S, Arai N, Terao Y, Kwak S, et al. Evaluation of corticospinal tracts in ALS with diffusion tensor MRI and brainstem stimulation. *Neurology.* (2008) 70:528–32. doi: 10.1212/01.wnl.0000299186.72374.19
14. Yin H, Cheng SH, Zhang J, Ma L, Gao Y, Li D, et al. Corticospinal tract degeneration in amyotrophic lateral sclerosis: a diffusion tensor imaging and fibre tractography study. *Ann Acad Med Singapore.* (2008) 37:411–5.
15. Metwalli NS, Benatar M, Nair G, Usher S, Hu X, Carew JD. Utility of axial and radial diffusivity from diffusion tensor MRI as markers of neurodegeneration in amyotrophic lateral sclerosis. *Brain Res.* (2010) 1348:156–64. doi: 10.1016/j.brainres.2010.05.067
16. Stagg CJ, Knight S, Talbot K, Jenkinson M, Maudsley AA, Turner MR. Whole-brain magnetic resonance spectroscopic imaging measures are related to disability in ALS. *Neurology.* (2013) 80:610–5. doi: 10.1212/WNL.0b013e318281ccec
17. Sarica A, Cerasa A, Vasta R, Perrotta P, Valentino P, Mangone G, et al. Tractography in amyotrophic lateral sclerosis using a novel probabilistic tool: a study with tract-based reconstruction compared to voxel-based approach. *J Neurosci Methods.* (2014) 224:79–87. doi: 10.1016/j.jneumeth.2013.12.014
18. Müller HP, Turner MR, Grosskreutz J, Abrahams S, Bede P, Govind V, et al. A large-scale multicentre cerebral diffusion tensor imaging study in amyotrophic lateral sclerosis. *J Neurol Neurosurg Psychiatry.* (2016) 87:570–9. doi: 10.1136/jnnp-2015-311952
19. Thivard L, Pradat PF, Lehericy S, Lacomblez L, Dormont D, Chiras J, et al. Diffusion tensor imaging and voxel based morphometry study in amyotrophic lateral sclerosis: relationships with motor disability. *J Neurol Neurosurg Psychiatry.* (2007) 78:889–92. doi: 10.1136/jnnp.2006.101758
20. Canu E, Agosta F, Riva N, Sala S, Prelle A, Caputo D, et al. The topography of brain microstructural damage in amyotrophic lateral sclerosis assessed using diffusion tensor MR imaging. *AJNR Am J Neuroradiol.* (2011) 32:1307–14. doi: 10.3174/ajnr.A2469
21. Keil C, Prell T, Peschel T, Hartung V, Dengler R, Grosskreutz J. Longitudinal diffusion tensor imaging in amyotrophic lateral sclerosis. *BMC Neurosci.* (2012) 13:141. doi: 10.1186/1471-2202-13-141
22. Sach M, Winkler G, Glauche V, Liepert J, Heimbach B, Koch MA, et al. Diffusion tensor MRI of early upper motor neuron involvement in amyotrophic lateral sclerosis. *Brain.* (2004) *127*:340–50. doi: 10.1093/brain/awh041
23. Agosta F, Pagani E, Rocca MA, Caputo D, Perini M, Salvi F, et al. Voxel-based morphometry study of brain volumetry and diffusivity in amyotrophic lateral sclerosis patients with mild disability. *Hum Brain Mapp.* (2007) 28:1430–8. doi: 10.1002/hbm.20364
24. Valsasina P, Agosta F, Benedetti B, Caputo D, Perini M, Salvi F, et al. Diffusion anisotropy of the cervical cord is strictly associated with disability in amyotrophic lateral sclerosis. *J Neurol Neurosurg Psychiatry.* (2007) 78:480–4. doi: 10.1136/jnnp.2006.100032
25. Nair G, Carew JD, Usher S, Lu D, Hu XP, Benatar M. Diffusion tensor imaging reveals regional differences in the cervical spinal cord in amyotrophic lateral sclerosis. *Neuroimage.* (2010) 53:576–83. doi: 10.1016/j.neuroimage.2010.06.060
26. Cohen-Adad J, Zhao W, Keil B, Ratai EM, Triantafyllou C, Lawson R, et al. 7-T MRI of the spinal cord can detect lateral corticospinal tract abnormality in amyotrophic lateral sclerosis. *Muscle Nerve.* (2013) 47:760–2. doi: 10.1002/mus.23720
27. El Mendili MM, Cohen-Adad J, Pelegrini-Issac M, Rossignol S, Morizot-Koutlidis R, Marchand-Pauvert V, et al. Multi-parametric spinal cord MRI as potential progression marker in amyotrophic lateral sclerosis. *PLoS ONE.* (2014) 9:e95516. doi: 10.1371/journal.pone.0095516
28. Bede P, Bokde AL, Byrne S, Elamin M, McLaughlin RL, Kenna K, et al. Multiparametric MRI study of ALS stratified for the C9orf72 genotype. *Neurology.* (2013) 81:361–9. doi: 10.1212/WNL.0b013e31829c5eee
29. Agosta F, Ferraro PM, Riva N, Spinelli EG, Domi T, Carrera P, et al. Structural and functional brain signatures of C9orf72 in motor neuron disease. *Neurobiol Aging.* (2017) 57:206–19. doi: 10.1016/j.neurobiolaging.2017.05.024
30. Stanton BR, Shinhmar D, Turner MR, Williams VC, Williams SC, Blain CR, et al. Diffusion tensor imaging in sporadic and familial (D90A SOD1) forms of amyotrophic lateral sclerosis. *Arch Neurol.* (2009) 66:109–15. doi: 10.1001/archneurol.2008.527
31. Agosta F, Spinelli EG, Marjanovic IV, Stevic Z, Pagani E, Valsasina P, et al. Unraveling ALS due to SOD1 mutation through the combination of brain and cervical cord MRI. *Neurology.* (2018) 90:e707–16. doi: 10.1212/WNL.0000000000005002
32. van der Graaff MM, Sage CA, Caan MW, Akkerman EM, Lavini C, Majoie CB, et al. Upper and extra-motoneuron involvement in early motoneuron disease: a diffusion tensor imaging study. *Brain.* (2011) 134:1211–28. doi: 10.1093/brain/awr016
33. Menke RA, Korner S, Filippini N, Douaud G, Knight S, Talbot K, et al. Widespread grey matter pathology dominates the longitudinal cerebral MRI and clinical landscape of amyotrophic lateral sclerosis. *Brain.* (2014) 137:2546–55. doi: 10.1093/brain/awu162
34. Bede P, Elamin M, Byrne S, McLaughlin RL, Kenna K, Vajda A, et al. Patterns of cerebral and cerebellar white matter degeneration in ALS. *J Neurol Neurosurg Psychiatry.* (2015) 86:468–70. doi: 10.1136/jnnp-2014-308172
35. Cardenas-Blanco A, Machts J, Acosta-Cabronero J, Kaufmann J, Abdulla S, Kollewe K, et al. Structural and diffusion imaging versus clinical assessment to monitor amyotrophic lateral sclerosis. *Neuroimage Clin.* (2016) 11:408–14. doi: 10.1016/j.nicl.2016.03.011
36. Agosta F, Rocca MA, Valsasina P, Sala S, Caputo D, Perini M, et al. A longitudinal diffusion tensor MRI study of the cervical cord and brain in amyotrophic lateral sclerosis patients. *J Neurol Neurosurg Psychiatry.* (2009) 80:53–5. doi: 10.1136/jnnp.2008.154252
37. Kwan JY, Meoded A, Danielian LE, Wu T, Floeter MK. Structural imaging differences and longitudinal changes in primary lateral sclerosis and amyotrophic lateral sclerosis. *Neuroimage Clin.* (2012) 2:151–60. doi: 10.1016/j.nicl.2012.12.003
38. Menke RA, Agosta F, Grosskreutz J, Filippi M, Turner MR. Neuroimaging endpoints in amyotrophic lateral sclerosis. *Neurotherapeutics.* (2017) 14:11–23. doi: 10.1007/s13311-016-0484-9
39. Floeter MK, Danielian LE, Braun LE, Wu T. Longitudinal diffusion imaging across the C9orf72 clinical spectrum. *J Neurol Neurosurg Psychiatry.* (2018) 89:53–60. doi: 10.1136/jnnp-2017-316799
40. Agosta F, Galantucci S, Riva N, Chio A, Messina S, Iannaccone S, et al. Intrahemispheric and interhemispheric structural network abnormalities in PLS and ALS. *Hum Brain Mapp.* (2014) 35:1710–22. doi: 10.1002/hbm.22286
41. Müller HP, Agosta F, Gorges M, Kassubek R, Spinelli EG, Riva N, et al. Cortico-efferent tract involvement in primary lateral sclerosis and amyotrophic lateral sclerosis: a two-centre tract of interest-based DTI analysis. *Neuroimage Clin.* (2018) 20:1062–9. doi: 10.1016/j.nicl.2018.10.005
42. Canu E, Agosta F, Galantucci S, Chio A, Riva N, Silani V, et al. Extramotor damage is associated with cognition in primary lateral sclerosis patients. *PLoS ONE.* (2013) 8:e82017. doi: 10.1371/journal.pone.0082017
43. Prudlo J, Bissbort C, Glass A, Grossmann A, Hauenstein K, Benecke R, et al. White matter pathology in ALS and lower motor neuron ALS variants: a diffusion tensor imaging study using tract-based spatial statistics. *J Neurol.* (2012) 259:1848–59. doi: 10.1007/s00415-012-6420-y
44. Rosenbohm A, Müller HP, Hubers A, Ludolph AC, Kassubek J. Corticoefferent pathways in pure lower motor neuron disease: a diffusion tensor imaging study. *J Neurol.* (2016) 263:2430–7. doi: 10.1007/s00415-016-8281-2
45. Spinelli EG, Agosta F, Ferraro PM, Riva N, Lunetta C, Falzone YM, et al. Brain MR imaging in patients with lower motor neuron-predominant disease. *Radiology.* (2016) 280:545–56. doi: 10.1148/radiol.2016151846
46. Müller HP, Agosta F, Riva N, Spinelli EG, Comi G, Ludolph AC, et al. Fast progressive lower motor neuron disease is an ALS variant: a two-centre

tract of interest-based MRI data analysis. *Neuroimage Clin.* (2018) 17:145–52. doi: 10.1016/j.nicl.2017.10.008

47. Iwata NK, Kwan JY, Danielian LE, Butman JA, Tovar-Moll F, Bayat E, et al. White matter alterations differ in primary lateral sclerosis and amyotrophic lateral sclerosis. *Brain.* (2011) 134:2642–55. doi: 10.1093/brain/awr178
48. Ellis CM, Simmons A, Jones DK, Bland J, Dawson JM, Horsfield MA, et al. Diffusion tensor MRI assesses corticospinal tract damage in ALS. *Neurology.* (1999) 53:1051–8. doi: 10.1212/WNL.53.5.1051
49. Sarro L, Agosta F, Canu E, Riva N, Prelle A, Copetti M, et al. Cognitive functions and white matter tract damage in amyotrophic lateral sclerosis: a diffusion tensor tractography study. *AJNR Am J Neuroradiol.* (2011) 32:1866–72. doi: 10.3174/ajnr.A2658
50. Lillo P, Mioshi E, Burrell JR, Kiernan MC, Hodges JR, Hornberger M. Grey and white matter changes across the amyotrophic lateral sclerosis-frontotemporal dementia continuum. *PLoS ONE.* (2012) 7:e43993. doi: 10.1371/journal.pone.0043993
51. Agosta F, Ferraro PM, Riva N, Spinelli EG, Chio A, Canu E, et al. Structural brain correlates of cognitive and behavioral impairment in MND. *Hum Brain Mapp.* (2016) 37:1614–26. doi: 10.1002/hbm.23124
52. Bullmore E, Sporns O. Complex brain networks: graph theoretical analysis of structural and functional systems. *Nat Rev Neurosci.* (2009) 10:186–98. doi: 10.1038/nrn2575
53. Stam CJ, van Straaten EC. The organization of physiological brain networks. *Clin Neurophysiol.* (2012) 123:1067–87. doi: 10.1016/j.clinph.2012.01.011
54. Watts DJ, Strogatz SH. Collective dynamics of 'small-world' networks. *Nature.* (1998) 393:440–2. doi: 10.1038/30918
55. Sporns O, Chialvo DR, Kaiser M, Hilgetag CC. Organization, development and function of complex brain networks. *Trends Cogn Sci.* (2004) 8:418–25. doi: 10.1016/j.tics.2004.07.008
56. Filippi M, Basaia S, Canu E, Imperiale F, Meani A, Caso F, et al. Brain network connectivity differs in early-onset neurodegenerative dementia. *Neurology.* (2017) 89:1764–72. doi: 10.1212/WNL.0000000000004577
57. Galantucci S, Agosta F, Stefanova E, Basaia S, van den Heuvel MP, Stojkovic T, et al. Structural brain connectome and cognitive impairment in parkinson disease. *Radiology.* (2017) 283:515–25. doi: 10.1148/radiol.2016160274
58. Filippi M, Basaia S, Canu E, Imperiale F, Magnani G, Falautano M, et al. Changes in functional and structural brain connectome along the Alzheimer's disease continuum. *Mol Psychiatry.* (2018) doi: 10.1038/s41380-018-0067-8. [Epub ahead of print].
59. Verstraete E, Veldink JH, Mandl RC, van den Berg LH, van den Heuvel MP. Impaired structural motor connectome in amyotrophic lateral sclerosis. *PLoS ONE.* (2011) 6:e24239. doi: 10.1371/journal.pone.0024239
60. Buchanan CR, Pettit LD, Storkey AJ, Abrahams S, Bastin ME. Reduced structural connectivity within a prefrontal-motor-subcortical network in amyotrophic lateral sclerosis. *J Magn Reson Imaging.* (2015) 41:1342–52. doi: 10.1002/jmri.24695
61. Verstraete E, Veldink JH, van den Berg LH, van den Heuvel MP. Structural brain network imaging shows expanding disconnection of the motor system in amyotrophic lateral sclerosis. *Hum Brain Mapp.* (2014) 35:1351–61. doi: 10.1002/hbm.22258
62. Brettschneider J, Del Tredici K, Toledo JB, Robinson JL, Irwin DJ, Grossman M, et al. Stages of pTDP-43 pathology in amyotrophic lateral sclerosis. *Ann Neurol.* (2013) 74:20–38. doi: 10.1002/ana.23937
63. Neumann M, Sampathu DM, Kwong LK, Truax AC, Micsenyi MC, Chou TT, et al. Ubiquitinated TDP-43 in frontotemporal lobar degeneration and amyotrophic lateral sclerosis. *Science.* (2006) 314:130–3. doi: 10.1126/science.1134108
64. Kassubek J, Müller HP, Del Tredici K, Brettschneider J, Pinkhardt EH, Lule D, et al. Diffusion tensor imaging analysis of sequential spreading of disease in amyotrophic lateral sclerosis confirms patterns of TDP-43 pathology. *Brain.* (2014) *137*:1733–40. doi: 10.1093/brain/awu090
65. Schmidt R, de Reus MA, Scholtens LH, van den Berg LH, van den Heuvel MP. Simulating disease propagation across white matter connectome reveals anatomical substrate for neuropathology staging in amyotrophic lateral sclerosis. *Neuroimage.* (2016) 124:762–9. doi: 10.1016/j.neuroimage.2015.04.005

14

Biomarkers of Metabolism in Amyotrophic Lateral Sclerosis

*Siobhan E. Kirk[1], Timothy J. Tracey[1], Frederik J. Steyn[1,2] and Shyuan T. Ngo[1,2,3]**

[1] The Australian Institute for Bioengineering and Nanotechnology, The University of Queensland, Brisbane, QLD, Australia, [2] Centre for Clinical Research, The University of Queensland, Brisbane, QLD, Australia, [3] Queensland Brain Institute, The University of Queensland, Brisbane, QLD, Australia

***Correspondence:**
Shyuan T. Ngo
s.ngo@uq.edu.au

Amyotrophic lateral sclerosis (ALS) is a neurodegenerative disorder characterized by the deterioration of motor neurons. However, this complex disease extends beyond the boundaries of the central nervous system, with metabolic alterations being observed at the systemic and cellular level. While the number of studies that assess the role and impact of metabolic perturbations in ALS is rapidly increasing, the use of metabolism biomarkers in ALS remains largely underinvestigated. In this review, we discuss current and potential metabolism biomarkers in the context of ALS. Of those for which data does exist, there is limited insight provided by individual markers, with specificity for disease, and lack of reproducibility and efficacy in informing prognosis being the largest drawbacks. However, given the array of metabolic markers available, the potential exists for a panel of metabolism biomarkers, which may complement other current biomarkers (including neurophysiology, imaging, as well as CSF, blood and urine markers) to overturn these limitations and give rise to new diagnostic and prognostic indicators.

Keywords: amyotrophic lateral sclerosis, ALS, metabolism, biomarker, motor neurone disease

OVERVIEW

Amyotrophic lateral sclerosis (ALS) is a progressive neurodegenerative disease caused by the death of motor neurons in the brain and spinal cord. The loss of neuronal input leads to progressive paralysis and patient mortality within 2–5 years from diagnosis (1). ALS likely arises from a combination of genetic susceptibility and environmental exposures (2, 3), although it is recognized that ALS is a complex, multi-system disease (4, 5).

Given the complex and heterogeneous nature of ALS, diagnosis and tracking of prognosis remains difficult. Current diagnostic criteria typically follow tests to rule out other pathological causes of symptoms and include: indicators of upper and lower motor neuron involvement, nerve conduction tests, electromyography and "watchful waiting" (4). As a result, researchers have attempted to utilize a wide range of biomarkers—observable biological measurements that confirm the presence or progression of a change in body status, as a means of diagnosing and following disease progression. While the current range of biomarkers in ALS offer some diagnostic and prognostic benefit, there is a need to identify a biomarker that satisfies the following six attributes: specificity to disease; reproducibility; appearance early in the disease; stability across the diurnal period; independence of dietary status and behavior; and a notable change during disease progression. By meeting these criteria, a biomarker can be used to reliably identify and track disease progression, in a manner that can easily be reproduced in a clinical setting.

Metabolic perturbations occur in ALS patients and in mouse models of the disease; both at the systemic and cellular level (6, 7). Clinically, an increase in resting energy expenditure (REE) and decline in body mass index (BMI) is linked to worse outcome (8–10), suggesting prognostic potential in metabolic biomarkers. Given that changes in metabolic status are generally reflected in overall body weight, body composition, and tissue/cellular metabolic function, metabolic changes at the anthropometric, tissue and cellular levels may represent appreciable metabolism biomarkers of ALS onset, progression, and/or severity (**Figure 1**). A list of the potential biomarkers of metabolism in ALS, and their quality relative to the aforementioned identifying attributes are summarized in **Table 1**.

ANTHROPOMETRIC BODY MEASURES

Lower premorbid BMI is associated with increased risk for ALS (11–13), and the degree of decline in premorbid BMI predicts ALS risk and survival (14, 15). Lower BMI, or a decline in BMI following diagnosis correlates with worse survival (16, 17), although this association is not always observed (18, 19, 23, 24). Rather, the mortality risk for ALS relative to BMI exists as a U-shaped curve, in which mortality decreases with increasing BMI, until BMI levels indicate premorbid obesity. Thereafter, mortality risk increases again (8, 20). This seemingly complex association could be explained by changes in body composition throughout disease progression.

BMI is often used as an indirect measure of fatness. However, conventional anthropometric measures of BMI and body adiposity index (BAI) do not always accurately reflect changes in fat and/or fat free mass (FFM) in ALS (69). In this regard, fat mass (FM) and FFM at diagnosis are not associated with survival risk (14), yet redistribution of adipose tissue does occur in ALS (29), and visceral fat is correlated with functional status and survival (28). Moreover, serial assessment of body FM indicates that increases in FM are associated with longer survival (14). While a decrease in FFM serves as an independent prognostic factor for shorter survival in ALS (23), we did not identify any studies that document progressive changes in muscle mass as a potential marker of disease progression in ALS. As a hallmark of ALS, however, there is potential to use the loss of FFM as a marker of disease progression. Such measures must consider the technical difficulties associated with assessing FFM in patients who experience significant and progressive disability, while also accounting for whole body and regional changes in FFM, which differ greatly between patients.

Despite BMI and BAI being poor predictors of body composition in ALS, changes in BMI may offer reliable measures for progressive changes in the overall nutritional status of the patient, and by proxy, disease progression. As documented by Kasarskis et al. a progressive decline in body weight is commonly observed in ALS patients in the months prior to death, and this reduction in body weight or BMI likely reflects a state of undernutrition (25). In recent years, lower BMI has been found to be associated with lower ALSFRS-R scores (70), and a loss of body weight (14, 21, 23, 24, 26, 27, 71) and BMI (14, 17, 22, 24) throughout disease course is consistently associated with shorter survival. Not surprisingly, these observations, while serving as markers for disease progression, have resulted in the adoption of interventions aimed at slowing weight loss in ALS (72).

SKELETAL MUSCLE PATHOLOGY

With findings suggesting that FFM is a prognostic factor in ALS (23), analysis of skeletal muscle, the primary component of FFM, may offer insights into tissue-specific metabolism biomarkers. Assessment of cellular metabolic changes in skeletal muscle can be challenging, especially when weighing the clinical benefit against that of an invasive procedure on a patient undergoing significant muscle wasting. Furthermore, heterogeneity in site of disease onset leads to variable muscle pathophysiology between patients (73).

Despite these limitations, creatine kinase, an enzyme that is linked with muscle damage and deterioration, has been studied intensely in ALS. While not strictly a metabolic marker, creatine kinase can be considered as an important modulator of body composition (74). As such, it may indirectly influence systemic metabolic processes. Numerous reports of increased creatine kinase in ALS (36–43), and particularly in limb-onset patients (38, 43), highlight the potential for its use as a marker of disease. However, contradictory observations of associations between creatine kinase and clinical parameters of disease, and disease progression and survival attest to the need for further investigations into determining the utility of creatine kinase as a biomarker in ALS.

MITOCHONDRIAL DYSFUNCTION

In human ALS muscle, mitochondrial defects including dysregulation of respiratory complex I (44), decreased respiratory complex I and IV activity (45, 75), decreased muscle mitochondrial protein expression (75) and upregulation of muscular mitochondrial uncoupling protein 3 (76) indicate that impairments in mitochondrial function could serve as a metabolic marker of ALS. It should be noted, however, that these studies were unable to correlate mitochondrial defects with functional parameters of disease progression, despite studies in animal models reporting a strong relationship between the two (77–79). Therefore, while there is clear evidence of mitochondrial defects in ALS, mitochondrial defects *per se* cannot currently be used as a biomarker due to the difficulty in both easily observing these defects in a clinical setting, and linking such defects to a marker of disease progression and/or survival. Instead, emphasis could be placed on the assessment of the more easily detectable metabolites that drive mitochondrial function.

GLUCOSE METABOLISM

Glucose use in the brain of ALS patients has been evaluated using fluorodeoxyglucose F18 positron emission tomography (F18-PET) (30–33). These studies have identified decreased glucose use in the primary motor cortex of ALS patients, suggesting that this brain region is hypometabolic (32). Other studies have reported a decrease in the use of glucose across other brain regions

TABLE 1 | Classification of potential biomarkers of metabolism in amyotrophic lateral sclerosis (ALS).

Marker	Observation	Utility as a biomarker in ALS						Biomarker Score	References
		Specific to ALS	Reproducible	Pre-diagnostic	Diurnal stability	Independence	Change with progression		
ANTHROPOMETRIC MARKERS									
Body mass index (BMI)	Lower BMI is an indicator of poor prognosis. U-shaped association; lower BMI is associated with increased risk and faster progression whereas BMI in the range of morbid obesity is associated with shorter survival. Degree of premorbid loss of BMI predicts risk of ALS	N	N	Y	Y	N	*Variable*	**2.5**	(8, 11–22)
Body weight	Weight loss correlates with faster disease progression; weight loss suggested as a risk factor for ALS	N	N	N	Y	N	*Variable*	**1.5**	(14, 21, 23–27)
Fat mass	Fat mass at diagnosis is not a determinant of survival. Increased fat mass is correlated with longer survival	N	N	*Insufficient data*	Y	N	Y	**2**	(14, 28)
Fat free mass	Fat free mass at diagnosis is not a determinant of survival. Loss of fat free mass is associated with shorter survival	N	Y	*Insufficient data*	Y	N	Y	**3**	(14, 23)
Fat distribution	Redistribution and increased deposition of fat in muscle	N	*Insufficient data*	*Insufficient data*	Y	N	*Insufficient data*	**1**	(29)
IMAGING MARKERS									
Brain glucose use	Hypometabolism specific to select brain regions; varies between studies	N	*Insufficient data*	*Insufficient data*	*Likely*	*Likely*	Y	**2**	(30–33)
Spinal cord glucose use	Hypermetabolism; changes in glucose metabolism correlates with disease progression	N	*Insufficient data*	*Insufficient data*	*Likely*	*Likely*	*Variable*	**1.5**	(34, 35)
MUSCLE MARKERS									
Creatine kinase	Increased in blood; variability in correlation with disease progression/survival. Greater increase observed in male subjects and limb-onset ALS	N	Y	Y	*Likely*	*Likely*	*Variable*	**3.5**	(36–43)
Mitochondrial function	Decreased activity of complex I and IV. Activity also declines over course of disease	N	*Insufficient data*	*Insufficient data*	Y	Y	*Variable*	**2.5**	(44, 45)
PDK4 levels	Increase in pyruvate dehydrogenase kinase 4 (PDK4) correlated with increased denervation and fuel switch	N	*Insufficient data*	*Insufficient data*	Y	Y	*Likely*	**2.5**	(46)
Glucose	Increased	N	N	*Insufficient data*	N	N	N	**0**	(47)
Sphingolipids	Increased	N	*Insufficient data*	*Insufficient data*	N	N	Y	**1**	(48)
Phosphatidylcholine	Increased	N	*Insufficient data*	*Insufficient data*	N	N	N	**0**	(48)

(Continued)

TABLE 1 | Continued

Marker	Observation	Utility as a biomarker in ALS						Biomarker Score	References
		Specific to ALS	Reproducible	Pre-diagnostic	Diurnal stability	Independence	Change with progression		
Cholesterol + Carriers	Increased	N	*Insufficient data*	*Insufficient data*	N	N	N	**0**	(49)
Lactate	Increased	N	*Insufficient data*	*Insufficient data*	N	N	*Insufficient data*	**0**	(47, 50)
CEREBROSPINAL FLUID (CSF) MARKERS									
Pyruvate	Increased	N	*Insufficient data*	*Insufficient data*	N	N	*Insufficient data*	**0**	(51)
Insulin	Decreased	N	*Insufficient data*	*Insufficient data*	N	N	N	**0**	(52)
Growth hormone	Decreased	N	*Insufficient data*	*Insufficient data*	N	N	N	**0**	(52)
CIRCULATING MARKERS (BLOOD, PLASMA AND SERUM)									
Glucose	Increased (33% of patients achieve World Health Organization (WHO) criteria for impaired glucose tolerance)	N	N	*Insufficient data*	N	N	N	**0**	(53)
Mannose	Increased	N	N	*Insufficient data*	N	N	*Insufficient data*	**0**	(54)
Free fatty acids	Increased	N	N	*Insufficient data*	N	N	N	**0**	(53)
Sphingolipids	Increased	N	N	*Insufficient data*	N	N	N	**0**	(54)
Cholesterol + Carriers	Major variations and contradictory reports mask any specific trend	N	N	*Insufficient data*	N	N	*Variable*	**0.5**	(53, 55–62)
β-hydroxy-butyrate	Increased	N	N	*Insufficient data*	N	N	*Insufficient data*	**0**	(63)
2-hydroxy-butyrate	Increased	N	N	*Insufficient data*	N	N	*Insufficient data*	**0**	(54)
α-ketoglutarate	Increased	N	N	*Insufficient data*	N	N	*Insufficient data*	**0**	(54)
Acetate	Increased	N	N	*Insufficient data*	N	N	*Insufficient data*	**0**	(63)
Adiponectin	Increased	N	N	*Insufficient data*	N	N	N	**0**	(64)

(Continued)

TABLE 1 | Continued

Marker	Observation	Utility as a Biomarker in ALS						Biomarker Score	References
		Specific to ALS	Reproducible	Pre-diagnostic	Diurnal stability	Independence	Change with progression		
Cortisol	Increased	N	N	*Insufficient data*	N	N	N	**0**	(65)
Cortisol (morning peak)	Decreased	N	N	*Insufficient data*	N	N	N	**0**	(65)
Insulin	Decreased	N	N	*Insufficient data*	N	N	N	**0**	(52, 64)
Gastric inhibitory peptide	Decreased	N	N	*Insufficient data*	N	N	N	**0**	(64)
Ghrelin	Decreased	N	N	*Insufficient data*	N	N	N	**0**	(64, 66)
SALIVA MARKERS									
Cortisol (night-time)	Increased	N	*Insufficient data*	*Insufficient data*	N	*Likely*	*Insufficient data*	**0.5**	(67)
Cortisol (Stress-induced)	Decreased	N	*Insufficient data*	*Insufficient data*	N	*Likely*	*Insufficient data*	**0.5**	(67)
Cortisol (circadian rhythm)	Decreased	N	*Insufficient data*	*Insufficient data*	N	*Likely*	*Insufficient data*	**0.5**	(67)
URINE MARKERS									
p75 neurotrophin receptor extracellular domain	Increased	N	*Likely*	*Insufficient data*	Y	Y	Y	**3.5**	(68)

The strength of proposed biomarkers are scored relative to their potential to serve as markers that are specific to ALS, and that conform to the requirements as detailed in text.
Specific to ALS refers to uniqueness of the marker to ALS over other diseases, reproducible refers to whether the indicated change is reproducible across patient cohorts, pre-diagnostic indicates where changes are apparent prior to symptom onset, diurnal stability refers to the consistency of the marker throughout the day, independence indicates the ability of the marker to remain stable regardless of changes in food intake or behavior, change with progression identifies whether the marker changes as disease progresses. For each potential biomarker, a score out of 6 was determined (biomarker score, indicated in bold), where Y (Yes) = 1 point, N (No) = 0 points, Variable = 0.5 points, Likely (supported by animal or statistical modeling studies) = 0.5 points, and Insufficient data = 0 points.

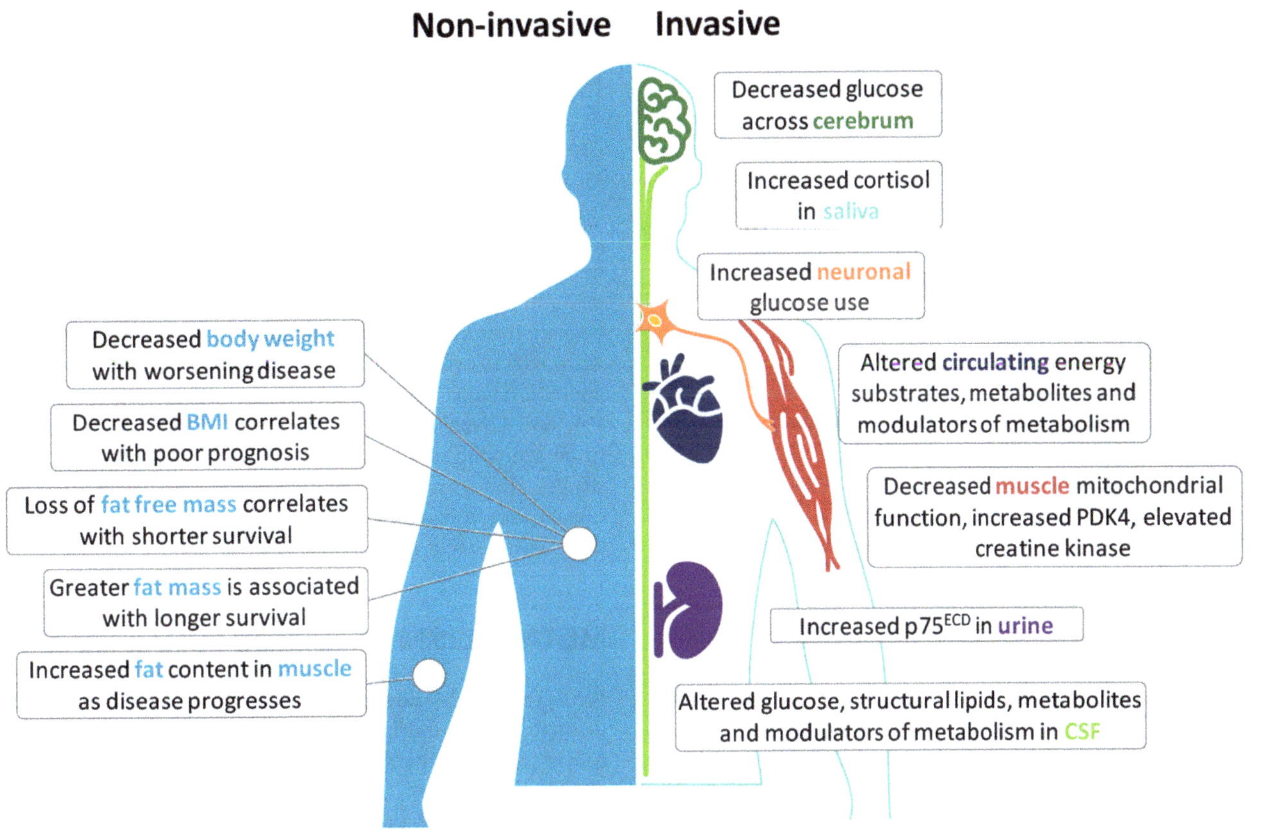

FIGURE 1 | Potential metabolism biomarkers in amyotrophic lateral sclerosis (ALS). Metabolic alterations in ALS offer opportunities to use metabolism biomarkers for the diagnosis, categorization, and tracking of disease. Non-invasive anthropometric measures include body weight, body mass index (BMI), fat free mass, fat mass, and fat distribution. Invasive measures include the use of F18-PET to assess glucose metabolism in the central nervous system, or require the sampling of saliva, blood, cerebrospinal fluid (CSF), muscle tissue, and urine. Although few independent markers are specific, reproducible or able to track disease in ALS, used together with complementary biomarkers (including neurophysiology and imaging), these markers may provide deeper insights into metabolic perturbations that are potentially involved in the onset and progression of disease.

(31, 33); although this may reflect the differences in experimental cohorts. In this regard, Claassen et al. investigated a cohort of patients with primary lateral sclerosis, while the study by Ludolph et al. evaluated ALS patients with both upper and lower motor symptoms. Given that the degree of cerebral hypometabolism in ALS is correlated with the duration of clinically-identified symptoms (30), the ability of the motor cortex to utilize glucose may allow for monitoring of disease progression. However, since brain glucose hypometabolism is not specific to ALS (80), its use as a diagnostic/prognostic marker is limited.

F18-PET has also been used to assess the uptake and utilization of glucose in the cervical spinal cords of ALS patients (34, 35, 81). Overall, observations of spinal cord glucose hypermetabolism (34, 35, 81) is congruent with increased levels of glucose in the CSF of ALS patients (47). In a study by Yamashita et al. glucose hypermetabolism on the ipsilateral side to the patient's symptoms was found to be positively correlated with ALSFRS-R, suggesting that changes in spinal cord glucose metabolism are specific to the affected corticospinal tract and the degree of disease severity (35). By contrast, the study by Marini et al. reported spinal cord glucose hypermetabolism independent of disease duration and functional impairment (34). As such, the degree of glucose use in the spinal cord may present some use for diagnostic testing, but provides limited insights for evaluation of disease progression and prognosis. Indeed, glucose hypermetabolism in the spinal cord extends to other neurological conditions (82, 83), thereby limiting its use as a specific biomarker for ALS. Finally, as the reproducibility of F18-PET in both the brain and spinal cord is low (84), more rigorous testing is required to determine if results are consistent across a heterogeneous ALS population.

Alterations in glucose metabolism in ALS extend beyond the central nervous system (CNS). Glucose tolerance tests conducted by Pradat et al. indicate that ALS patients have a significant increase in blood glucose levels following the provision of a glucose load when compared to age- and sex-matched controls. Within ALS patients, a degree of heterogeneity was observed, with 33% of participants meeting World Health Organization criteria for impaired glucose tolerance (53). Impaired glucose tolerance is in line with reports of insulin resistance in ALS

(85), and could explain observations of increased expression of pyruvate dehydrogenase kinase 4 (PDK4) in skeletal muscle of ALS patients (46). Similarly, mannose, an epimer of glucose that has recently been shown to be a predictor of insulin resistance (86), has been reported to be significantly increased in the plasma of ALS patients (54). While the assessment of glucose tolerance and insulin resistance is relatively straightforward, these tests lack reproducibility and specificity to ALS (87–89). Therefore, although glucose metabolism is altered in ALS, it cannot be used as an independent biomarker for ALS diagnosis and prognosis.

FATTY ACIDS AND KETONES

In patients with ALS, the resting level of circulating free fatty acids (FFAs) is significantly increased (53). While higher levels of FFAs has been linked to impaired glucose tolerance in ALS, it has not been shown to be correlated with any markers of disease progression or severity. Ketones, including β-hydroxy-butyrate (63) and 2-hydroxy-butyrate and α-ketoglutarate (54), which are produced through fatty acid metabolism under fasting conditions, are also significantly increased in ALS. Similar to FFAs, no correlations have been observed between disease status and the expression of ketones. Thus, FFAs and ketones cannot currently be considered as reliable biomarkers for ALS, and the lack of specificity for ALS-centric pathology indicate that they may not present as particularly valuable diagnostic markers individually.

DOWNSTREAM METABOLITES

Metabolites, the downstream indicators of metabolic function, are also impacted in ALS. While not specific to ALS, altered expression of metabolites may offer a potential avenue for biomarker discovery. In line with disease heterogeneity, reported levels of metabolites in the blood and CSF are variable. Notably, the levels of lactate (47, 50) and pyruvate (51) in the CNS are increased, potentially reflecting an increase in metabolic output, or increased release of metabolites into the CSF following neuronal deterioration. Given that mitochondrial dysfunction is observed in ALS, further evaluation of the ratio between these metabolites may hold significant informative value in ALS due to the diagnostic value of this test for mitochondrial disorders (90).

Blood levels of acetate are increased in ALS (63), although this is not readily observed in the CSF (47, 51). Acetate is a key metabolite in the oxidation of fatty acids. As acetate synthesis precedes the formation of citric acid in the Krebs cycle, changes in circulating acetate may occur due to excess production via an increase in fatty acid oxidation, increased release from deteriorating muscle cells, or other disruptions to mitochondrial membrane integrity (e.g., due to the presence of free radicals). Such potential mechanisms align with ALS pathology. As a whole, downstream metabolites hold promise as potential biomarkers, and further work that can interrogate relationships between metabolites and clinical parameters of disease would add merit to their use as metabolic biomarkers of disease.

ENDOCRINE MODULATORS OF METABOLISM

Insulin is an anabolic hormone that has been reported to be decreased in the blood (64) and CSF (52) of ALS patients. By contrast, other studies have reported no significant differences in plasma insulin levels in ALS patients (91, 92). Other anabolic hormones that have been found to be decreased in ALS include growth hormone (in CSF and blood) (52, 92–94) and gastric inhibitory peptide in blood (64). Conversely, hormones that promote catabolism, such as cortisol (65, 67), and adiponectin (64) are increased or dysregulated in saliva and blood of patients with ALS. Furthermore, ghrelin, an important modulator of appetite, is also reduced in the plasma/blood of ALS patients (64, 66). Given that alterations in these hormones are likely to be symbolic of a change in metabolic function/homeostasis, studies that confirm a link between endocrine markers of metabolism and clinical markers of disease offer potential for their development as prognostic biomarkers.

METABOLISM OF STRUCTURAL LIPIDS

While fatty acids and their derivatives serve as energy substrates through mitochondrial respiration, they also play an essential role in maintaining cellular integrity. Phospholipids, particularly phosphatidylcholine, are significantly increased in the CSF of ALS patients (48). Sphingolipids, such as stearoyl sphingomyelin and ceramide, are also increased in patient blood (48, 54). Interestingly, in the study by Blasco et al. predictions of clinical measurements, such as ALSFRS-R, were found to be correlated to CSF sphingomyelins and triglycerides with long-chain fatty acids (48). Such findings are favorable for the development of biomarker assays, but further tests are required to confirm the reliability of predictive models, before use as a prognostic biomarker.

An increase in cholesterol esters has been observed in ALS patient spinal cord (95). However, cholesterol and its carriers prove to be more difficult to characterize, with variable levels of HDL and LDL cholesterol being reported in ALS. In a population-based longitudinal study, a positive association was found between LDL cholesterol and ALS risk (55), however, there was no indication of the impact of LDL on disease progression or mortality. Nonetheless, this could serve as a diagnostic biomarker for ALS risk. Previously, higher levels of cholesterol, LDL, as well as an elevated LDL/HDL ratio in ALS patient blood have been correlated with increased survival (56–58). Conversely, similar increases in total cholesterol, LDL, and HDL cholesterol in ALS patient blood (59, 60) and CSF (49) have not been found to be correlated with disease progression. Furthermore, a small number of studies contradict these findings, reporting that cholesterol, LDL, and HDL levels do not vary between ALS patients and controls (53, 61, 62), although lower levels of serum lipids may correlate with worse respiratory function (61). Based on these contradictory observations, the validity of cholesterol as a biomarker remains uncertain. Further studies that address these disparate data are required.

NOVEL METABOLISM-ASSOCIATED BIOMARKERS

p75 neurotrophin receptor (NTR) belongs to the tumor necrosis factor family of receptors. It is a transmembrane receptor which binds neurotrophins and pro-neurotrophins (96). p75NTR has been implicated in processes of energy expenditure (97), glucose uptake, and insulin sensitivity (98). In ALS, the secretion of the extracellular domain of p75NTR ($p75^{ECD}$) in urine was recently established as a biomarker for disease progression and prognosis (68, 99). Urinary $p75^{ECD}$ increases as disease progresses, and an elevation of urinary $p75^{ECD}$ is observed alongside a decrease in ALSFRS-R scores (68). While it is not clear if increases in urinary $p75^{ECD}$ in ALS match metabolic derangements that accompany disease progression (such as changes in energy metabolism, glucose uptake and insulin sensitivity), the introduction of $p75^{ECD}$ as a fluid biomarker in ALS provides an opportunity for the evaluation and possible co-development of metabolism-associated biomarkers.

CONCLUSION

The complexity and heterogeneity of disease between patients limits the scope for the use of a single reliable biomarker of ALS. Significant changes in metabolism seen in ALS may represent a potential avenue for biomarker development. As documented in this review, a range of markers might be relevant (**Figure 1**). However, as investigations into the cause for metabolic derangements in ALS are ongoing, and little emphasis has been placed on the development of metabolism biomarkers as diagnostic or prognostic indicators, few reliable metabolism biomarkers exist (**Table 1**). Moreover, because metabolic alterations in ALS likely arise from the dysregulation of a number of processes, the utility of biomarkers for assessing early or progressive changes in the metabolic state of ALS patients would necessitate the development of a panel that captures the spectrum of metabolic changes that occur at the systemic and cellular level.

As there is no single biomarker for ALS that sufficiently meets the six major attributes of a biomarker, it is clear that the assessment of biomarkers that cover multiple dimensions of the disease is needed in order to generate a comprehensive view of the state of disease. The complementary assessment of metabolism markers alongside other biomarkers including neurophysiology, imaging, as well as CSF, blood, and urine markers may form a more convincing and reliable diagnostic/prognostic platform, while providing insights into the multifactorial nature of disease.

AUTHOR CONTRIBUTIONS

SEK, TJT, FJS, and STN conducted the literature search and wrote the manuscript. FJS produced all artwork. STN critically revised the manuscript.

FUNDING

TJT is supported by an Australian Postgraduate Award from the University of Queensland, and a Postgraduate top-up grant from the Motor Neurone Disease Research Institute of Australia. STN is supported by the Scott Sullivan MND Research Fellowship (MND and Me Foundation, The Royal Brisbane and Women's Hospital Foundation, and the Queensland Brain Institute) and the Australian Institute for Bioengineering and Nanotechnology.

REFERENCES

1. Mitchell JD, Borasio GD. Amyotrophic lateral sclerosis. *Lancet.* (2007) 369:2031–41. doi: 10.1016/S0140-6736(07)60944-1
2. Al-Chalabi A, Calvo A, Chio A, Colville S, Ellis CM, Hardiman O, et al. Analysis of amyotrophic lateral sclerosis as a multistep process: a population-based modelling study. *Lancet Neurol.* (2014) 13:1108–13. doi: 10.1016/S1474-4422(14)70219-4
3. Chio A, Mazzini L, D'Alfonso S, Corrado L, Canosa A, Moglia C, et al. The multistep hypothesis of ALS revisited: the role of genetic mutations. *Neurology.* (2018) 91:e635–42. doi: 10.1212/WNL.0000000000005996
4. Kiernan MC, Vucic S, Cheah BC, Turner MR, Eisen A, Hardiman O, et al. Amyotrophic lateral sclerosis. *Lancet.* (2011) 377:942–55. doi: 10.1016/S0140-6736(10)61156-7
5. Brown RH, Al-Chalabi A. Amyotrophic lateral sclerosis. *N Engl J Med.* (2017) 377:162–72. doi: 10.1056/NEJMra1603471
6. Dupuis L, Oudart H, Rene F, Gonzalez de Aguilar JL, Loeffler JP. Evidence for defective energy homeostasis in amyotrophic lateral sclerosis: benefit of a high-energy diet in a transgenic mouse model. *Proc Natl Acad Sci USA.* (2004) 101:11159–64. doi: 10.1073/pnas.0402026101
7. Dupuis L, Pradat PF, Ludolph AC, Loeffler JP. Energy metabolism in amyotrophic lateral sclerosis. *Lancet Neurol.* (2011) 10:75–82. doi: 10.1016/S1474-4422(10)70224-6
8. Paganoni S, Deng J, Jaffa M, Cudkowicz ME, Wills AM. Body mass index, not dyslipidemia, is an independent predictor of survival in amyotrophic lateral sclerosis. *Muscle Nerve.* (2011) 44:20–4. doi: 10.1002/mus.22114
9. Jesus P, Fayemendy P, Nicol M, Lautrette G, Sourisseau H, Preux PM, et al. Hypermetabolism is a deleterious prognostic factor in patients with amyotrophic lateral sclerosis. *Eur J Neurol.* (2018) 25:97–104. doi: 10.1111/ene.13468
10. Steyn FJ, Ioannides ZA, van Eijk RPA, Heggie S, Thorpe KA, Ceslis A, et al. Hypermetabolism in ALS is associated with greater functional decline and shorter survival. *J Neurol Neurosurg Psychiatry.* (2018) 89:1016–23. doi: 10.1136/jnnp-2017-317887
11. Scarmeas N, Shih T, Stern Y, Ottman R, Rowland LP. Premorbid weight, body mass, and varsity athletics in ALS. *Neurology.* (2002) 59:773–5. doi: 10.1212/WNL.59.5.773
12. Doyle P, Brown A, Beral V, Reeves G, Green J. Incidence of and risk factors for Motor Neurone Disease in UK women: a prospective study. *BMC Neurol.* (2012) 12:25. doi: 10.1186/1471-2377-12-25
13. O'Reilly EJ, Wang H, Weisskopf MG, Fitzgerald KC, Falcone G, McCullough ML, et al. Premorbid body mass index and risk of amyotrophic lateral sclerosis. *Amyotroph Lateral Scler Frontotemporal Degener.* (2013) 14:205–11. doi: 10.3109/21678421.2012.735240
14. Marin B, Desport JC, Kajeu P, Jesus P, Nicolaud B, Nicol M, et al. Alteration of nutritional status at diagnosis is a prognostic factor for survival of amyotrophic lateral sclerosis patients. *J Neurol Neurosurg Psychiatry.* (2011) 82:628–34. doi: 10.1136/jnnp.2010.211474
15. Mariosa D, Beard JD, Umbach DM, Bellocco R, Keller J, Peters TL, et al. Body mass index and amyotrophic lateral sclerosis: a study of US military veterans. *Am J Epidemiol.* (2017) 185:362–71. doi: 10.1093/aje/kww140

16. Desport JC, Preux PM, Truong CT, Courat L, Vallat JM, Couratier P. Nutritional assessment and survival in ALS patients. *Amyotroph Lateral Scler Other Motor Neuron Disord.* (2000) 1:91–6. doi: 10.1080/14660820050515386
17. Jawaid A, Murthy SB, Wilson AM, Qureshi SU, Amro MJ, Wheaton M, et al. A decrease in body mass index is associated with faster progression of motor symptoms and shorter survival in ALS. *Amyotroph Lateral Scler.* (2010) 11:542–8. doi: 10.3109/17482968.2010.482592
18. Wolf J, Safer A, Wohrle JC, Palm F, Nix WA, Maschke M, et al. Factors predicting one-year mortality in amyotrophic lateral sclerosis patients—data from a population-based registry. *BMC Neurol.* (2014) 14:197. doi: 10.1186/s12883-014-0197-9
19. Wolf J, Safer A, Wohrle JC, Palm F, Nix WA, Maschke M, et al. Factors predicting survival in ALS patients—data from a population-based registry in Rhineland-Palatinate, Germany. *Neuroepidemiology.* (2015) 44:149–55. doi: 10.1159/000381625
20. Reich-Slotky R, Andrews J, Cheng B, Buchsbaum R, Levy D, Kaufmann P, et al. Body mass index (BMI) as predictor of ALSFRS-R score decline in ALS patients. *Amyotroph Lateral Scler Frontotemporal Degener.* (2013) 14:212–6. doi: 10.3109/21678421.2013.770028
21. Peter RS, Rosenbohm A, Dupuis L, Brehme T, Kassubek J, Rothenbacher D, et al. Life course body mass index and risk and prognosis of amyotrophic lateral sclerosis: results from the ALS registry Swabia. *Eur J Epidemiol.* (2017) 32:901–8. doi: 10.1007/s10654-017-0318-z
22. Shimizu T, Nagaoka U, Nakayama Y, Kawata A, Kugimoto C, Kuroiwa Y, et al. Reduction rate of body mass index predicts prognosis for survival in amyotrophic lateral sclerosis: a multicenter study in Japan. *Amyotroph Lateral Scler.* (2012) 13:363–6. doi: 10.3109/17482968.2012.678366
23. Roubeau V, Blasco H, Maillot F, Corcia P, Praline J. Nutritional assessment of amyotrophic lateral sclerosis in routine practice: value of weighing and bioelectrical impedance analysis. *Muscle Nerve.* (2015) 51:479–84. doi: 10.1002/mus.24419
24. Fasano A, Fini N, Ferraro D, Ferri L, Vinceti M, Errals, et al. Percutaneous endoscopic gastrostomy, body weight loss and survival in amyotrophic lateral sclerosis: a population-based registry study. *Amyotroph Lateral Scler Frontotemporal Degener.* (2017) 18:233–42. doi: 10.1080/21678421.2016.1270325
25. Kasarskis EJ, Berryman S, Vanderleest JG, Schneider AR, McClain CJ. Nutritional status of patients with amyotrophic lateral sclerosis: relation to the proximity of death. *Am J Clin Nutr.* (1996) 63:130–7. doi: 10.1093/ajcn/63.1.130
26. Stambler N, Charatan M, Cedarbaum JM. Prognostic indicators of survival in ALS. *ALS CNTF Treatment Study Group Neurology.* (1998) 50:66–72. doi: 10.1212/WNL.50.1.66
27. Clavelou P, Blanquet M, Peyrol F, Ouchchane L, Gerbaud L. Rates of progression of weight and forced vital capacity as relevant measurement to adapt Amyotrophic Lateral Sclerosis management for patient result of a French multicentre cohort survey. *J Neurol Sci.* (2013) 331:126–31. doi: 10.1016/j.jns.2013.06.002
28. Lindauer E, Dupuis L, Muller HP, Neumann H, Ludolph AC, Kassubek J. Adipose tissue distribution predicts survival in amyotrophic lateral sclerosis. *PLoS ONE.* (2013) 8:e67783. doi: 10.1371/journal.pone.0067783
29. Gerevini S, Agosta F, Riva N, Spinelli EG, Pagani E, Caliendo G, et al. MR imaging of brachial plexus and limb-girdle muscles in patients with amyotrophic lateral sclerosis. *Radiology.* (2016) 279:553–61. doi: 10.1148/radiol.2015150559
30. Dalakas MC, Hatazawa J, Brooks RA, Di Chiro G. Lowered cerebral glucose utilization in amyotrophic lateral sclerosis. *Ann Neurol.* (1987) 22:580–6. doi: 10.1002/ana.410220504
31. Ludolph AC, Langen KJ, Regard M, Herzog H, Kemper B, Kuwert T, et al. Frontal lobe function in amyotrophic lateral sclerosis: a neuropsychologic and positron emission tomography study. *Acta Neurol Scand.* (1992) 85:81–9. doi: 10.1111/j.1600-0404.1992.tb04003.x
32. Claassen DO, Josephs KA, Peller PJ. The stripe of primary lateral sclerosis: focal primary motor cortex hypometabolism seen on fluorodeoxyglucose F18 positron emission tomography. *Arch Neurol.* (2010) 67:122–5. doi: 10.1001/archneurol.2009.298
33. Pagani M, Chio A, Valentini MC, Oberg J, Nobili F, Calvo A, et al. Functional pattern of brain FDG-PET in amyotrophic lateral sclerosis. *Neurology.* (2014) 83:1067–74. doi: 10.1212/WNL.0000000000000792
34. Marini C, Cistaro A, Campi C, Calvo A, Caponnetto C, Nobili FM, et al. A PET/CT approach to spinal cord metabolism in amyotrophic lateral sclerosis. *Eur J Nucl Med Mol Imaging.* (2016) 43:2061–71. doi: 10.1007/s00259-016-3440-3
35. Yamashita T, Hatakeyama T, Sato K, Fukui Y, Hishikawa N, Ohta Y, et al. Flow-metabolism uncoupling in the cervical spinal cord of ALS patients. *Neurol Sci.* (2017) 38:659–65. doi: 10.1007/s10072-017-2823-y
36. Williams ER, Bruford A. Creatine phosphokinase in motor neurone disease. *Clin Chim Acta.* (1970) 27:53–6. doi: 10.1016/0009-8981(70)90373-6
37. Sinaki M, Mulder DW. Amyotrophic-lateral-sclerosis—relationship between serum creatine-kinase level and patient survival. *Arch Phys Med Rehabil.* (1986) 67:169–71. doi: 10.1016/0003-9993(86)90064-X
38. Felice KJ, North WA. Creatine kinase values in amyotrophic lateral sclerosis. *J Neurol Sci.* (1998) 160:S30–2. doi: 10.1016/S0022-510X(98)00195-6
39. Ilzecka J, Stelmasiak Z. Creatine kinase activity in amyotrophic lateral sclerosis patients. *Neurol Sci.* (2003) 24:286–7. doi: 10.1007/s10072-003-0158-3
40. Lima AF, Evangelista T, de Carvalho M. Increased creatine kinase and spontaneous activity on electromyography, in amyotrophic lateral sclerosis. *Electromyogr Clin Neurophysiol.* (2003) 43:189–92.
41. Gibson SB, Kasarskis EJ, Hu N, Pulst SM, Mendiondo MS, Matthews DE, et al. Relationship of creatine kinase to body composition, disease state, and longevity in ALS. *Amyotroph Lateral Scler Frontotemporal Degener.* (2015) 16:473–7. doi: 10.3109/21678421.2015.1062516
42. Rafiq MK, Lee E, Bradburn M, McDermott CJ, Shaw PJ. Creatine kinase enzyme level correlates positively with serum creatinine and lean body mass, and is a prognostic factor for survival in amyotrophic lateral sclerosis. *Eur J Neurol.* (2016) 23:1071–8. doi: 10.1111/ene.12995
43. Tai HF, Cui LY, Guan YZ, Liu MS, Li XG, Shen DC, et al. Correlation of creatine kinase levels with clinical features and survival in amyotrophic lateral sclerosis. *Front Neurol.* (2017) 8:322. doi: 10.3389/fneur.2017.00322
44. Wiedemann FR, Winkler K, Kuznetsov AV, Bartels C, Vielhaber S, Feistner H, et al. Impairment of mitochondrial function in skeletal muscle of patients with amyotrophic lateral sclerosis. *J Neurol Sci.* (1998) 156:65–72. doi: 10.1016/S0022-510X(98)00008-2
45. Echaniz-Laguna A, Zoll J, Ponsot E, N'Guessan B, Tranchant C, Loeffler JP, et al. Muscular mitochondrial function in amyotrophic lateral sclerosis is progressively altered as the disease develops: a temporal study in man. *Exp Neurol.* (2006) 198:25–30. doi: 10.1016/j.expneurol.2005.07.020
46. Palamiuc L, Schlagowski A, Ngo ST, Vernay A, Grosch S, Henriques A, et al. A metabolic switch towards lipid use in glycolytic muscle is an early pathologic event in a mouse model of Amyotrophic Lateral Sclerosis. *EMBO Mol Med.* (2015) 7:526–46. doi: 10.15252/emmm.201404433
47. Toczylowska B, Jamrozik Z, Liebert A, Kwiecinski H. NMR-based metabonomics of cerebrospinal fluid applied to amyotrophic lateral sclerosis. *Biocybernet Biomed Eng.* (2013) 33:21–32. doi: 10.1016/S0208-5216(13)70053-6
48. Blasco H, Veyrat-Durebex C, Bocca C, Patin F, Vourc'h P, Nzoughet JK, et al. Lipidomics reveals cerebrospinal-fluid signatures of ALS. *Sci Rep.* (2017) 7:17652. doi: 10.1038/s41598-017-17389-9
49. Abdel-Khalik J, Yutuc E, Crick PJ, Gustafsson JA, Warner M, Roman G, et al. Defective cholesterol metabolism in amyotrophic lateral sclerosis. *J Lipid Res.* (2017) 58:267–78. doi: 10.1194/jlr.P071639
50. Gray E, Larkin JR, Claridge TDW, Talbot K, Sibson NR, Turner MR. The longitudinal cerebrospinal fluid metabolomic profile of amyotrophic lateral sclerosis. *Amyotroph Lateral Scler Frontotemporal Degener.* (2015) 16:456–63. doi: 10.3109/21678421.2015.1053490
51. Blasco H, Corcia P, Moreau C, Veau S, Fournier C, Vourc'h P, et al. H-1-NMR-based metabolomic profiling of CSF in early amyotrophic lateral sclerosis. *PLoS ONE.* (2010) 5:e13223. doi: 10.1371/journal.pone.0013223
52. Bilic E, Rudan I, Kusec V, Zurak N, Delimar D, Zagar M. Comparison of the growth hormone, IGF-1 and insulin in cerebrospinal fluid and serum between patients with motor neuron disease and healthy controls. *Eur J Neurol.* (2006) 13:1340–5. doi: 10.1111/j.1468-1331.2006.01503.x
53. Pradat PF, Bruneteau G, Gordon PH, Dupuis L, Bonnefont-Rousselot D, Simon D, et al. Impaired glucose tolerance in patients with

amyotrophic lateral sclerosis. *Amyotroph Lateral Scler.* (2010) 11:166–71. doi: 10.3109/17482960902822960

54. Lawton KA, Cudkowicz ME, Brown MV, Alexander D, Caffrey R, Wulff JE, et al. Biochemical alterations associated with ALS. *Amyotroph Lateral Scler.* (2012) 13:110–8. doi: 10.3109/17482968.2011.619197
55. Mariosa D, Hammar N, Malmstrom H, Ingre C, Jungner I, Ye WM, et al. Blood biomarkers of carbohydrate, lipid, and apolipoprotein metabolisms and risk of amyotrophic lateral sclerosis: a more than 20-year follow-up of the Swedish AMORIS cohort. *Ann Neurol.* (2017) 81:718–28. doi: 10.1002/ana.24936
56. Dupuis L, Corcia P, Fergani A, Gonzalez De Aguilar JL, Bonnefont-Rousselot D, Bittar R, et al. Dyslipidemia is a protective factor in amyotrophic lateral sclerosis. *Neurology.* (2008) 70:1004–9. doi: 10.1212/01.wnl.0000285080.70324.27
57. Dorst J, Kuhnlein P, Hendrich C, Kassubek J, Sperfeld AD, Ludolph AC. Patients with elevated triglyceride and cholesterol serum levels have a prolonged survival in amyotrophic lateral sclerosis. *J Neurol.* (2011) 258:613–7. doi: 10.1007/s00415-010-5805-z
58. Ikeda K, Hirayama T, Takazawa T, Kawabe K, Iwasaki Y. Relationships between disease progression and serum levels of lipid, urate, creatinine and ferritin in japanese patients with amyotrophic lateral sclerosis: a cross-sectional study. *Intern Med.* (2012) 51:1501–8. doi: 10.2169/internalmedicine.51.7465
59. Rafiq MK, Lee E, Bradburn M, McDermott CJ, Shaw PJ. Effect of lipid profile on prognosis in the patients with amyotrophic lateral sclerosis: insights from the olesoxime clinical trial. *Amyotroph Lateral Scler Frontotemporal Degener.* (2015) 16:478–84. 10.3109/21678421.2015.1062517
60. Delaye JB, Patin F, Piver E, Bruno C, Vasse M, Vourc'h P, et al. Low IDL-B and high LDL-1 subfraction levels in serum of ALS patients. *J Neurol Sci.* (2017) 380:124–7. doi: 10.1016/j.jns.2017.07.019
61. Chio A, Calvo A, Ilardi A, Cavallo E, Moglia C, Mutani R, et al. Lower serum lipid levels are related to respiratory impairment in patients with ALS. *Neurology.* (2009) 73:1681–5. doi: 10.1212/WNL.0b013e3181c1df1e
62. Huang R, Guo X, Chen X, Zheng Z, Wei Q, Cao B, et al. The serum lipid profiles of amyotrophic lateral sclerosis patients: a study from south-west China and a meta-analysis. *Amyotroph Lateral Scler Frontotemporal Degener.* (2015) 16:359–65. doi: 10.3109/21678421.2015.1047454
63. Kumar A, Bala L, Kalita J, Misra UK, Singh RL, Khetrapal CL, et al. Metabolomic analysis of serum by ^{1}H NMR spectroscopy in amyotrophic lateral sclerosis. *Clin Chim Acta.* (2010) 411:563–7. doi: 10.1016/j.cca.2010.01.016
64. Ngo ST, Steyn FJ, Huang L, Mantovani S, Pfluger CMM, Woodruff TM, et al. Altered expression of metabolic proteins and adipokines in patients with amyotrophic lateral sclerosis. *J Neurol Sci.* (2015) 357:22–7. doi: 10.1016/j.jns.2015.06.053
65. Spataro R, Volanti P, Vitale F, Meli F, Colletti T, Di Natale A, et al. Plasma cortisol level in amyotrophic lateral sclerosis. *J Neurol Sci.* (2015) 358:282–6. doi: 10.1016/j.jns.2015.09.011
66. Czell D, Baldinger R, Schneider U, Neuwirth C, Weber M. The role of the SenseWear device and ghrelin for metabolism in amyotrophic lateral sclerosis. *Amyotroph Lateral Scler Frontotemporal Degener.* (2016) 17:295–6. doi: 10.3109/21678421.2015.1113299
67. Patacchioli FR, Monnazzi P, Scontrini A, Tremante E, Caridi I, Brunetti E, et al. Adrenal dysregulation in amyotrophic lateral sclerosis. *J Endocrinol Invest.* (2003) 26:Rc23–5. doi: 10.1007/BF03349149
68. Shepheard SR, Wuu J, Cardoso M, Wiklendt L, Dinning PG, Chataway T, et al. Urinary p75(ECD) A prognostic, disease progression, and pharmacodynamic biomarker in ALS. *Neurology.* (2017) 88:1137–43. doi: 10.1212/WNL.0000000000003741
69. Ioannides ZA, Steyn FJ, Henderson RD, McCombe PA, Ngo ST. Anthropometric measures are not accurate predictors of fat mass in ALS. *Amyotroph Lateral Scler Frontotemporal Degener.* (2017) 18:486–91. doi: 10.1080/21678421.2017.1317811
70. Park Y, Park J, Kim Y, Baek H, Kim SH. Association between nutritional status and disease severity using the amyotrophic lateral sclerosis (ALS) functional rating scale in ALS patients. *Nutrition.* (2015) 31:1362–7. doi: 10.1016/j.nut.2015.05.025
71. Moglia C, Calvo A, Grassano M, Canosa A, Manera U, D'Ovidio F, et al. Early weight loss in amyotrophic lateral sclerosis: outcome relevance and clinical correlates in a population-based cohort. *J Neurol Neurosurg Psychiatry.* (2019). doi: 10.1136/jnnp-2018-319611. [Epub ahead of print].
72. Ngo ST, Mi JD, Henderson RD, McCombe PA, Steyn FJ. Exploring targets and therapies for amyotrophic lateral sclerosis: current insights into dietary interventions. *Degener Neurol Neuromuscular Dis.* (2017) 7:95–108. doi: 10.2147/DNND.S120607
73. Wijesekera LC, Leigh PN. Amyotrophic lateral sclerosis. *Orphanet J Rare Dis.* (2009) 4:3. doi: 10.1186/1750-1172-4-3
74. Saks VA, Ventura-Clapier R, Aliev MK. Metabolic control and metabolic capacity: two aspects of creatine kinase functioning in the cells. *Biochim Biophys Acta.* (1996) 1274:81–8. doi: 10.1016/0005-2728(96)00011-4
75. Vielhaber S, Kunz D, Winkler K, Wiedemann FR, Kirches E, Feistner H, et al. Mitochondrial DNA abnormalities in skeletal muscle of patients with sporadic amyotrophic lateral sclerosis. *Brain.* (2000) 123:1339–48. doi: 10.1093/brain/123.7.1339
76. Dupuis L, di Scala F, Rene F, de Tapia M, Oudart H, Pradat PF, et al. Up-regulation of mitochondrial uncoupling protein 3 reveals an early muscular metabolic defect in amyotrophic lateral sclerosis. *FASEB J.* (2003) 17:2091–3. doi: 10.1096/fj.02-1182fje
77. Dobrowolny G, Aucello M, Rizzuto E, Beccafico S, Mammucari C, Boncompagni S, et al. Skeletal muscle is a primary target of SOD1G93A-mediated toxicity. *Cell Metab.* (2008) 8:425–36. doi: 10.1016/j.cmet.2008.09.002
78. Dupuis L, Gonzalez de Aguilar JL, Echaniz-Laguna A, Eschbach J, Rene F, Oudart H, et al. Muscle mitochondrial uncoupling dismantles neuromuscular junction and triggers distal degeneration of motor neurons. *PLoS ONE.* (2009) 4:e5390. doi: 10.1371/journal.pone.0005390
79. Wong M, Martin LJ. Skeletal muscle-restricted expression of human SOD1 causes motor neuron degeneration in transgenic mice. *Hum Mol Genet.* (2010) 19:2284–302. doi: 10.1093/hmg/ddq106
80. Zilberter Y, Zilberter M. The vicious circle of hypometabolism in neurodegenerative diseases: ways and mechanisms of metabolic correction. *J Neurosci Res.* (2017) 95:2217–35. doi: 10.1002/jnr.24064
81. Marini C, Morbelli S, Cistaro A, Campi C, Caponnetto C, Bauckneht M, et al. Interplay between spinal cord and cerebral cortex metabolism in amyotrophic lateral sclerosis. *Brain.* (2018) 141:2272–9. doi: 10.1093/brain/awy152
82. Dubey N, Miletich RS, Wasay M, Mechtler LL, Bakshi R. Role of fluorodeoxyglucose positron emission tomography in the diagnosis of neurosarcoidosis. *J Neurol Sci.* (2002) 205:77–81. doi: 10.1016/S0022-510X(02)00225-3
83. Daulatzai MA. Cerebral hypoperfusion and glucose hypometabolism: key pathophysiological modulators promote neurodegeneration, cognitive impairment, and Alzheimer's disease. *J Neurosci Res.* (2017) 95:943–72. doi: 10.1002/jnr.23777
84. Phelps ME, Huang SC, Hoffman EJ, Selin C, Sokoloff L, Kuhl DE. Tomographic measurement of local cerebral glucose metabolic rate in humans with (F-18)2-fluoro-2-deoxy-D-glucose: validation of method. *Ann Neurol.* (1979) 6:371–88. doi: 10.1002/ana.410060502
85. Reyes ET, Perurena OH, Festoff BW, Jorgensen R, Moore WV. Insulin resistance in amyotrophic lateral sclerosis. *J Neurol Sci.* (1984) 63:317–24. doi: 10.1016/0022-510X(84)90154-0
86. Lee S, Zhang C, Kilicarslan M, Piening BD, Bjornson E, Hallstrom BM, et al. Integrated network analysis reveals an association between plasma mannose levels and insulin resistance. *Cell Metab.* (2016) 24:172–84. doi: 10.1016/j.cmet.2016.05.026
87. Norhammar A, Tenerz A, Nilsson G, Hamsten A, Efendic S, Ryden L, et al. Glucose metabolism in patients with acute myocardial infarction and no previous diagnosis of diabetes mellitus: a prospective study. *Lancet.* (2002) 359:2140–4. doi: 10.1016/S0140-6736(02)09089-X
88. Nathan DM, Davidson MB, DeFronzo RA, Heine RJ, Henry RR, Pratley R, et al. Impaired fasting glucose and impaired glucose tolerance: implications for care. *Diabetes Care.* (2007) 30:753–9. doi: 10.2337/dc07-9920
89. de la Monte SM. Insulin resistance and neurodegeneration: progress towards the development of new therapeutics for Alzheimer's disease. *Drugs.* (2017) 77:47–65. doi: 10.1007/s40265-016-0674-0

90. De Pinieux G, Chariot P, Ammi-saïd M, Louarn F, Lejonc JL, Astier A, et al. Lipid-lowering drugs and mitochondrial function: effects of HMG-CoA reductase inhibitors on serum ubiquinone and blood lactate/pyruvate ratio. *Br J Clin Pharmacol.* (1996) 42:333–7. doi: 10.1046/j.1365-125.1996.04178.x
91. Perurena OH, Festoff BW. Reduction in insulin-receptors in amyotrophic-lateral-sclerosis correlates with reduced insulin sensitivity. *Neurology.* (1987) 37:1375–9. doi: 10.1212/WNL.37.8.1375
92. Pellecchia MT, Pivonello R, Monsurro MR, Trojsi F, Longo K, Piccirillo G, et al. The GH-IGF system in amyotrophic lateral sclerosis: correlations between pituitary GH secretion capacity, insulin-like growth factors and clinical features. *Eur J Neurol.* (2010) 17:666–71. doi: 10.1111/j.1468-1331.2009.02896.x
93. Morselli LL, Bongioanni P, Genovesi M, Licitra R, Rossi B, Murri L, et al. Growth hormone secretion is impaired in amyotrophic lateral sclerosis. *Clin Endocrinol.* (2006) 65:385–8. doi: 10.1111/j.1365-2265.2006.02609.x
94. Sacca F, Quarantelli M, Rinaldi C, Tucci T, Piro R, Perrotta G, et al. A randomized controlled clinical trial of growth hormone in amyotrophic lateral sclerosis: clinical, neuroimaging, and hormonal results. *J Neurol.* (2011) 259:132–8. doi: 10.1007/s00415-011-6146-2
95. Cutler RG, Pedersen WA, Camandola S, Rothstein JD, Mattson MP. Evidence that accumulation of ceramides and cholesterol esters mediates oxidative stress-induced death of motor neurons in amyotrophic lateral sclerosis. *Ann Neurol.* (2002) 52:448–57. doi: 10.1002/ana.10312
96. Chao MV. The p75 neurotrophin receptor. *J Neurobiol.* (1994) 25:1373–85. doi: 10.1002/neu.480251106
97. Baeza-Raja B, Sachs BD, Li PP, Christian F, Vagena E, Davalos D, et al. p75 Neurotrophin receptor regulates energy balance in obesity. *Cell Rep.* (2016) 14:255–68. doi: 10.1016/j.celrep.2015.12.028
98. Baeza-Raja B, Li P, Le Moan N, Sachs BD, Schachtrup C, Davalos D, et al. p75 neurotrophin receptor regulates glucose homeostasis and insulin sensitivity. *Proc Natl Acad Sci USA.* (2012) 109:5838–43. doi: 10.1073/pnas.1103638109
99. Shepheard SR, Chataway T, Schultz DW, Rush RA, Rogers ML. The extracellular domain of neurotrophin receptor p75 as a candidate biomarker for amyotrophic lateral sclerosis. *PLoS ONE.* (2014) 9:e87398. doi: 10.1371/journal.pone.0087398

15

Body Mass Index in Mild Cognitive Impairment According to Age, Sex, Cognitive Intervention and Hypertension and Risk of Progression to Alzheimer's Disease

*Soo Hyun Joo[1], Se Hee Yun[2], Dong Woo Kang[1], Chang Tae Hahn[3], Hyun Kook Lim[4] and Chang Uk Lee[1]**

[1] Department of Psychiatry, Seoul St. Mary's Hospital, College of Medicine, The Catholic University of Korea, Seoul, South Korea, [2] Seocho Center for Dementia, Seoul, South Korea, [3] Department of Psychiatry, Daejeon St. Mary's Hospital, College of Medicine, The Catholic University of Korea, Seoul, South Korea, [4] Department of Psychiatry, Yeouido St. Mary's Hospital, College of Medicine, The Catholic University of Korea, Seoul, South Korea

***Correspondence:**
Chang Uk Lee
jihan@catholic.ac.kr

Introduction: Mild cognitive impairment (MCI) is a prodromal stage of dementia. The association of body mass index (BMI) and progression to Alzheimer's disease (AD) in MCI subjects according to age, sex, and cognitive intervention remains unknown. We investigated the relationship between BMI and the risk of progression to AD in subjects with MCI, as well as the effect of BMI on progression to AD depending on age, sex, cognitive intervention, and chronic diseases.

Methods: Three hundred and eighty-eight MCI subjects were followed for 36.3 ± 18.4 months, prospectively. They underwent neuropsychological testing more than twice during the follow-up period. The MCI subjects were categorized into underweight, normal weight, overweight, and obese subgroups. The associations between baseline BMI and progression to AD over the follow-up period were estimated using Cox proportional hazard regression models. Data were analyzed after stratification by age, sex, cognitive intervention, and chronic diseases.

Results: After adjustment for the covariates, the underweight MCI group had a higher risk of progression to AD [hazard ratio (HR): 2.38, 95% confidence interval (CI): 1.17–4.82] relative to the normal weight group. After stratifying by age, sex, cognitive intervention, and chronic diseases, this effect remained significant among females (HR: 3.15, 95% CI: 1.40–7.10), the older elderly ≥75 years old (HR: 3.52, 95% CI: 1.42–8.72), the non-intervention group (HR: 3.06, 95%CI: 1.18–7.91), and the hypertensive group (HR: 4.71, 95% CI: 1.17–18.99).

Conclusion: These data indicate that underweight could be a useful marker for identifying individuals at increased risk for AD in MCI subjects. This association is even stronger in females, older elderly subjects, the non-cognitive intervention group, and the hypertensive group.

Keywords: body mass index, mild cognitive impairment, Alzheimer's disease, intervention, CERAD

INTRODUCTION

Mild cognitive impairment (MCI) is a prodromal stage of dementia. According to epidemiological studies, approximately 5–15% of individuals with MCI will progress to dementia each year [1, 2]. Furthermore, there is no disease-modifying treatment for AD. Therefore, identifying risk factors at the MCI stage is critical because correcting modifiable risk factors can lower the incidence of dementia and the identification of non-modifiable risk factors can predict the progression of MCI to Alzheimer disease (AD).

Recently, there has been increasing evidence of the relationship between the body mass index (BMI) of normal cognitive individuals and risk of dementia. There are differences in the association between midlife BMI and dementia compared to late-life BMI and dementia. Being overweight or obese in mid-life is a risk factor for dementia [3–5], but in late-life being underweight is a risk factor [5–7]. However, there are few studies on the relationship between BMI and AD in MCI subjects. A recent study of 228 MCI subjects reported that the overweight or obese group had a reduced risk of both dementia and AD, while the underweight group had a higher risk of dementia but not AD, compared to the normal weight group [8]. Other study has investigated this relationship in MCI subjects, suggesting that, the underweight group had a higher risk while the obese group had a lower risk of AD compared to the normal weight group [9]. However, these two studies did not consider the heterogeneity of MCI subjects. The MCI group is composed of individuals with various demographics characteristics and life-styles. We suspected that BMI might have a different impact depending on individual's age, sex, cognitive intervention status, or chronic diseases, unlike finding from the two recent studies described above. In particular, cognitive intervention may improve cognitive reserve and prevent progression to dementia [10]. Therefore, the impact of BMI on the onset of AD may be different in individuals who have received cognitive intervention compared to a non-intervention group.

We hypothesized that BMI in MCI subjects can predict the progression to AD, and BMI may have a different effect depending on age, sex, cognitive intervention status, and chronic diseases. Therefore, we followed a cohort of MCI subjects prospectively to investigate the relationship between baseline BMI status and the risk of progression to AD in MCI subjects, as well as the effect of BMI on progression to AD depending on age, sex, cognitive intervention status, and chronic diseases.

MATERIALS AND METHODS

Study Population

We recruited MCI subjects at the Seocho Center for Dementia, which is one of the 25 regional dementia support centers in Seoul, South Korea. Each participant underwent a detailed clinical interview and standardized neuropsychological battery, namely the Korean version of the Consortium to Establish a Registry for Alzheimer's disease (CERAD-K). Then, the psychiatrist employed a common standardized diagnostic assessment protocol that included measures for the diagnoses of normal cognition, MCI, and dementia. Participants diagnosed with MCI were eligible to take the CERAD-K test at least once every 6 months. Participants diagnosed with dementia were sent to the hospital for further evaluation. After diagnosis, participants could choose to attend cognitive intervention programs according to their particular cognitive level.

Enrollment started in September 2008 and ended in February 2015. The calculation of the follow-up period for each subject of the cohort was equal to the interval between enrollment and the diagnosis of dementia or end of follow-up. We screened 1,905 participants. We excluded 833 participants who were initially diagnosed with normal cognition or dementia. 684 participants were excluded because they did not follow-up. The final cohort consisted of 388 MCI participants who underwent neuropsychological testing more than twice. All participants were over 60 years old.

Diagnostic Assessments

A diagnosis of MCI was made by criteria recommended by the international working group [11]. Objective cognitive impairment of MCI was defined as a performance score of 1.5 *SD* below the respective age-, education-, and gender-specific normative means in at least one of the cognitive test included in the CERAD-K neuropsychological battery. This battery consisted of verbal fluency (VF), the 15-item Boston Naming Test (BNT), the Mini Mental Status Examination (MMSE), word list memory (WLM), constructional praxis (CP), word list recall (WLR), word list recognition (WLRc), and constructional recall (CR) [12]. All MCI subjects had an overall Clinical Dementia Rating of 0.5.

Dementia was defined as by the criteria of the fourth edition of the Diagnostic and Statistical Manual of Mental Disorders (DSM-IV) and required objective evidence of cognitive deficits (confirmed by neuropsychological testing) and social and/or occupational dysfunction (confirmed by impairments in ADL). We used the criteria of the National Institute of Neurological and Communicative Disorders and Stroke (NINCDS) and the Alzheimer's Disease and Related Disorders Association (ADRDA) for a diagnosis of AD [13].

BMI Categories

The weights and heights of all MCI subjects were measured using standard scales while the subjects were dressed in indoor clothing without shoes; using these data, BMI (kilograms/meters squared) was calculated at baseline. MCI subjects were categorized into four BMI subgroups based on the World Health Organization's (WHO) recommendations for Asian populations: underweight (BMI: <18.5 kg/m2), normal weight (18.5–22.9 kg/m2), overweight (23.0–24.9 kg/m2), and obese (BMI $\geq$ 25 kg/m2) [14–16].

Cognitive Intervention

Cognitive intervention is defined as engagement in a range of activities aimed at general enhancement of cognitive and social functioning in a nonspecific manner [10]. This term is a concept that includes cognitive training, cognitive rehabilitation, and cognitive stimulation. Our cognitive intervention includes group programs consisting of memory training, recreational activities

TABLE 1 | Baseline clinical characteristics of MCI subjects according to BMI category (line No. 191).

	All subjects	Underweight	Normal	Overweight	Obese	*p*-value
Number	388	24	160	120	84	
Female, *n* (%)	257 (66.2)	18 (75.0)	112 (70.0)	69 (57.5)	58 (69.1)	0.101
Baseline age, years	74.5 ± 7.6	77.1 ± 7.0	75.2 ± 8.3	74.4 ± 6.9	72.7 ± 6.9	0.029
<75, *n* (%)	200 (51.6)	7 (29.2)	76 (47.5)	66 (55.0)	51 (60.7)	0.026
≥75, *n* (%)	188 (48.5)	17 (70.8)	84 (52.5)	54 (45.0)	33 (39.3)	
Education, years	9.3 ± 5.0	10.4 ± 5.4	9.0 ± 4.8	9.4 ± 5.1	9.3 ± 5.1	0.445
Hypertension, *n* (%)	199 (51.7)	8 (33.3)	69 (44.0)	71 (59.2)	51 (60.7)	0.006
Diabetes mellitus, *n* (%)	70 (18.2)	1 (4.2)	29 (18.5)	26 (21.7)	14 (16.7)	0.232
Hyperlipidemia, *n* (%)	80 (20.8)	6 (25.0)	32 (20.4)	27 (22.5)	15 (17.9)	0.819
Heart disease, *n* (%)	46 (12.0)	3 (12.5)	13 (8.3)	14 (11.8)	16 (19.1)	0.110
Cerebrovascular disease, *n* (%)	28 (7.3)	1 (4.2)	10 (6.4)	8 (6.7)	9 (10.7)	0.557
Follow-up duration, months	36.3 ± 18.4	36.5 ± 22.1	37.1 ± 18.5	35.5 ± 18.7	36.0 ± 16.7	0.905
MMSE score	21.1 ± 4.1	20.4 ± 3.0	20.4 ± 4.4	21.8 ± 3.9	21.6 ± 3.8	0.007
CERAD-K total score	51.0 ± 14.1	48.0 ± 12.0	48.7 ± 15.3	52.6 ± 12.4	54.0 ± 13.8	0.014
Cognitive intervention						
Absent	236 (60.8)	19 (79.2)	106 (66.3)	58 (48.3)	53 (63.1)	0.004
Attended	152 (39.2)	5 (20.8)	54 (33.8)	62 (51.7)	31 (36.9)	

Data are presented as the mean ± standard deviation or frequency (percentage). P-values were calculated by the Kruskal-Wallis test or chi square test. MCI, mild cognitive impairment; BMI, body mass index; MMSE, Mini-Mental Status Examination; CERAD-K, Korean version of the Consortium to Establish a Registry for Alzheimer's Disease.

TABLE 2 | Cox proportional hazard regression for risk of AD in MCI subjects according to baseline BMI (line No. 206).

	Unadjusted		Model 1		Model 2	
	Crude HR (95% CI)	*p*-value	Adjusted HR (95% CI)	*p*-value	Adjusted HR (95% CI)	*p*-value
BMI						
Underweight	**2.09 (1.11–3.92)**	**0.023**	**2.00 (1.03–3.86)**	**0.039**	**2.38 (1.17–4.82)**	**0.017**
Normal weight	Reference		Reference		Reference	
Overweight	0.62 (0.35–1.10)	0.099	0.66 (0.37–1.17)	0.150	0.78 (0.42–1.45)	0.434
Obese	0.51 (0.25–1.06)	0.069	0.59 (0.28–1.23)	0.160	0.71 (0.33–1.53)	0.380

Model 1: Adjusted for age, sex, and education; Model 2: Adjusted for Model 1 plus CERAD-K total score, cognitive intervention, hypertension, diabetes mellitus, hyperlipidemia, heart disease, and cerebrovascular disease. AD, Alzheimer's disease; MCI, mild cognitive impairment; BMI, body mass index; HR, hazard ratio; CI, confidence interval. Statistically significant values are shown in bold.

(games, crafts, and learning to play musical instruments), and physical training implemented by the Seocho Center for Dementia. Each intervention was performed 2–3 times per week for 1 h. The presence of cognitive intervention was defined as attending one of these programs during the follow-up period.

Statistical Analyses

All analyses were performed with SPSS version 24 (SPSS Inc., Chicago, IL, USA). We compared demographic data using the Kruskal-Wallis test, or Chi-square test. The associations between BMI and progression to dementia over the follow-up period were estimated using Cox proportional hazard regression models and are shown as hazard ratios (HRs) with 95% confidence intervals (CIs). The multivariable models were as follows: First, we analyzed the associations without any adjustment. In Model 1, the independent effects of baseline BMI were evaluated after controlling for age, sex, and education. In Model 2, the CERAD-K total score, the presence of cognitive intervention, and the presence of each disease (hypertension, diabetes mellitus, hyperlipidemia, heart disease, or cerebrovascular disease) were added to Model 1. Finally, we divided the subjects into two groups by age (according to the median age), sex, the presence of cognitive intervention, and chronic diseases, separately. Statistical significance was defined as a *p*-value of 0.05. Values are presented as the mean ± standard deviation or frequency (percentage) as appropriate. Cumulative hazard curves according to BMI were derived from Model 2.

Ethics Statement

All participants voluntarily attended this study and gave written informed consent participate in the study. The Institutional Review Board of Catholic Medical Center approved this study protocol (KC17RESI0150).

RESULTS

Baseline Demographic Characteristics

The baseline demographic characteristics of the 388 MCI subjects according to BMI category are summarized in **Table 1**. At baseline, 24 subjects were underweight, 160 normal weight, 120 overweight, and 84 obese. The mean age was 74.5 years and women were predominant (66.2%). The mean follow-up duration from the diagnosis of MCI was 36.3 months. 152 subjects attended cognitive intervention programs.

Relationship Between BMI and the Progression to AD

Of the MCI subjects, 12 of 24 underweight subjects (54.2%), 40 of 160 normal weight subjects (25.0%), 17 of 120 overweight subjects (14.2%), and 9 of 84 obese subjects (10.7%) progressed to AD. Prior to adjustment for covariates, the results of the Cox proportional hazard model showed that the underweight group had a higher risk of progression to AD (hazard ratio [HR]: 2.09, 95% confidence interval [CI]: 1.11–3.92) relative to the normal weight group. Adjusting for all covariates (Model 2) accentuated the risk of progression to AD (HR: 2.38, 95% CI: 1.17–4.82) (**Table 2**, **Figure 1**).

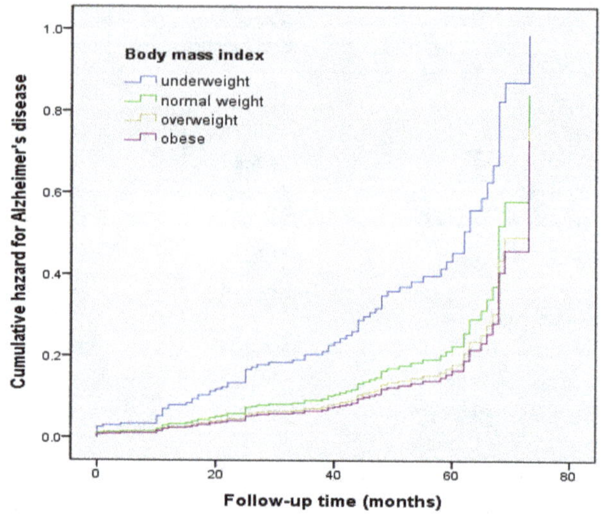

FIGURE 1 | Cumulative risk curves of the effects of baseline body mass index categories on progression to Alzheimer's disease. The figure was derived from model 2 (adjusted for age, sex, education, CERAD-K total score, cognitive intervention, hypertension, diabetes mellitus, hyperlipidemia, heart disease, and cerebrovascular disease).

Effects of Sex and Age on the Relationship Between BMI and Progression to AD

After stratifying by sex, underweight female had a higher risk of progression to AD (HR: 3.15, 95% CI: 1.40–7.10) than normal weight female in the fully adjusted model (Model 2). On the other hand, in male, there were no differences in the risk of progression to AD among the four BMI groups (**Table 3**).

Age was divided into two groups according to the median age. Stratification of the full model by age revealed that the four BMI groups had no differences in the risk of progression to AD in younger elderly group (age < 75), while the underweight group had a higher risk of progression to AD (HR: 3.52, 95% CI: 1.42–8.72) than the normal weight group in older elderly group (age ≥ 75) (**Table 4**).

Effects of Cognitive Intervention on the Relationship Between BMI and Progression to AD

Stratification of the full model by cognitive intervention revealed the negative effect of underweight to be limited to the non-intervention group (Model 2, **Table 5**). In the cognitive intervention group, the underweight group had no risk of progression to AD while the overweight group had a lower risk of progression to AD (HR: 0.37, 95% CI: 0.14–0.99) than the normal weight group. On the other hand, in group without cognitive intervention underweight group had a higher risk of progression to AD (HR: 3.06, 95% CI: 1.18–7.91) than the normal weight group.

Effects of Chronic Diseases on the Relationship Between BMI and Progression to AD

After stratifying by hypertension, underweight hypertensive group had a higher risk of progression to AD (HR: 4.71, 95% CI: 1.17–18.99) than normal weight hypertensive group in the fully adjusted model (Model 2). On the other hand, there were no differences in the risk of progression to AD among the four BMI groups in group without hypertension (**Table 6**).

After stratifying by DM, underweight non-diabetic group had a higher risk of progression to AD (HR: 2.35, 95% CI: 1.12–4.95) than normal weight non-diabetic group in the fully adjusted model (Model 2). On the other hand, there were no differences in the risk of progression to AD among the four BMI groups in group with DM. However, statistical power was very low because the sample size of underweight subjects with DM was too small ($N = 1$). Other chronic diseases such as hyperlipidemia, heart disease, and cerebrovascular disease did not affect the relationship between underweight and progression to AD in MCI subjects.

DISCUSSION

This is the first prospective clinical study to confirm the relationship between BMI and AD considering the heterogeneity of MCI subjects. Our major findings were as follows: First, underweight MCI subjects had a higher risk of progression to AD relative to the normal weight group. Second, the negative effects of underweight on progression to AD were even stronger in females, older elderly, the non-cognitive intervention group and the hypertensive group.

Our first finding that underweight MCI subjects had a higher risk of progression to AD is in line with previous findings [8, 9, 17]. There are various explanations about the relationship between underweight and AD. Aging itself is associated with weight loss; however, weight loss may be accelerated before diagnosis of AD [18]. In other words, weight loss may be either a potential cause of dementia or it may be an early manifestation of an underlying dementia. Lower BMI may reflect

TABLE 3 | Cox proportional hazard regression for risk of AD in MCI subjects according to baseline BMI stratified by sex (line No. 225).

	Unadjusted		**Model 1**		**Model 2**	
	Crude HR (95% CI)	***p*-value**	**Adjusted HR (95% CI)**	***p*-value**	**Adjusted HR (95% CI)**	***p*-value**
Males			$n = 129$			
BMI						
Underweight	1.01 (0.21–4.80)	0.992	0.91 (0.19–4.40)	0.906	0.52 (0.09–2.99)	0.465
Normal weight	Reference		Reference		Reference	
Overweight	0.77 (0.30–1.99)	0.585	0.75 (0.28–2.02)	0.573	0.60 (0.20–1.86)	0.379
Obese	0.75 (0.20–2.79)	0.665	0.92 (0.24–3.53)	0.899	1.20 (0.26–5.55)	0.818
Females			$n = 257$			
BMI						
Underweight	**2.58 (1.29–5.16)**	**0.008**	**2.57 (1.23–5.38)**	**0.012**	**3.15 (1.40–7.10)**	**0.006**
Normal weight	Reference		Reference		Reference	
Overweight	0.53 (0.25–1.11)	0.094	0.57 (0.27–1.21)	0.145	0.82 (0.37–1.84)	0.632
Obese	0.44 (0.18–1.07)	0.070	0.51 (0.21–1.24)	0.135	0.64 (0.25–1.63)	0.351

Model 1: Adjusted for age, sex, and education; Model 2: Adjusted for Model 1 plus CERAD-K total score, cognitive intervention, hypertension, diabetes mellitus, hyperlipidemia, heart disease, and cerebrovascular disease. AD, Alzheimer's disease; MCI, mild cognitive impairment; BMI, body mass index; HR, hazard ratio; CI, confidence interval. Statistically significant values are shown in bold.

TABLE 4 | Cox proportional hazard regression for risk of AD in MCI subjects according to baseline BMI stratified by age (<75, ≥75) (line No. 234).

	Unadjusted		**Model 1**		**Model 2**	
	Crude HR (95% CI)	***p*-value**	**Adjusted HR (95% CI)**	***p*-value**	**Adjusted HR (95% CI)**	***p*-value**
Age<75			$n = 198$			
BMI						
Underweight	**3.29 (1.04–10.45)**	**0.043**	2.90 (0.88–9.62)	0.082	0.81 (0.18–3.73)	0.788
Normal weight	Reference		Reference		Reference	
Overweight	0.55 (0.19–1.55)	0.256	0.58 (0.20–1.65)	0.309	0.47 (0.15–1.48)	0.197
Obese	0.63 (0.20–1.99)	0.429	0.69 (0.22–2.19)	0.530	0.48 (0.14–1.63)	0.238
Age≥75			$n = 183$			
BMI						
Underweight	1.63 (0.76–3.49)	0.212	1.77 (0.80–3.94)	0.160	**3.52 (1.42–8.72)**	**0.007**
Normal weight	Reference		Reference		Reference	
Overweight	0.70 (0.35–1.40)	0.315	0.79 (0.39–1.59)	0.505	1.17 (0.53–2.58)	0.693
Obese	0.54 (0.21–1.40)	0.204	0.54 (0.21–1.42)	0.214	0.93 (0.34–2.56)	0.893

Model 1: Adjusted for age, sex, education; Model 2: Adjusted for Model 1 plus CERAD-K total score, cognitive intervention, hypertension, diabetes mellitus, hyperlipidemia, heart disease, and cerebrovascular disease. AD, Alzheimer's disease; MCI, mild cognitive impairment; BMI, body mass index; HR, hazard ratio; CI, confidence interval. Statistically significant values are shown in bold.

a decrease in muscle mass or a decrease in fat. Some studies have shown that cognitive decline is associated with muscle loss [19, 20]. Poor nutritional status associated with reduced production of leptin, lack of vitamins, and essential fatty acids, can lead to oxidative damage to neuronal cells, and consequential acceleration of neurodegenerative processes [21]. Level of serum leptin, an adipocyte-derived peptide hormone have been lower in AD patients with BMI <20 compared to those with BMI >25 [22]. Another possible explanation is the degeneration of the mesial temporal cortex because limbic structures within the mesial temporal lobe are involved in appetite, feeding behaviors, memory, and emotional regulation all of which could potentially affected to body weight [23].

In our study, the association between underweight and progression to AD was restricted in females, and was not found in males. While these findings require further study and confirmation, one possible explanation for the observed gender difference may be hormonal factors. It is suggested that lower estrogen levels are potentially associated with AD in studies based on the association between estrogen replacement therapy in postmenopausal women [24, 25]. Because adipose tissue contributes to the production of estrogen, the circulating levels of estrogen are lower in women with less adipose tissue. Estrogens may affect cognition by binding to estrogen receptors that are located throughout the brain, especially in regions such as the hippocampus

TABLE 5 | Cox proportional hazard regression for risk of AD in MCI subjects according to baseline BMI stratified by cognitive intervention (line No. 251).

	Unadjusted		Model 1		Model 2	
	Crude HR (95% CI)	***p*-value**	**Adjusted HR (95% CI)**	***p*-value**	**Adjusted HR (95% CI)**	***p*-value**
Cognitive intervention-absent			*n* = 230			
BMI						
Underweight	**2.33 (1.07–5.09)**	**0.033**	**2.50 (1.09–5.69)**	**0.030**	**3.06 (1.18–7.91)**	**0.021**
Normal weight	Reference		Reference		Reference	
Overweight	0.89 (0.42–1.88)	0.7604	1.02 (0.47–2.18)	0.966	1.64 (0.71–3.78)	0.247
Obese	0.53 (0.20–1.39)	0.1946	0.62 (0.23–1.67)	0.347	0.87 (0.29–2.59)	0.803
Cognitive intervention-attended			*n* = 139			
BMI						
Underweight	1.91 (0.63–5.76)	0.250	1.74 (0.56–5.38)	0.338	3.59 (0.91–14.17)	0.068
Normal weight	Reference		Reference		Reference	
Overweight	**0.34 (0.14–0.82)**	**0.016**	**0.32 (0.13–0.80)**	**0.015**	**0.37 (0.14–0.99)**	**0.048**
Obese	0.47 (0.16–1.40)	0.172	0.50 (0.16–1.57)	0.237	0.51 (0.17–1.59)	0.249

Model 1: Adjusted for age, sex, and education; Model 2: Adjusted for Model 1 plus CERAD-K total score, cognitive intervention, hypertension, diabetes mellitus, hyperlipidemia, heart disease, and cerebrovascular disease. AD, Alzheimer's disease; MCI, mild cognitive impairment; BMI, body mass index; HR, hazard ratio; CI, confidence interval. Statistically significant values are shown in bold.

TABLE 6 | Cox proportional hazard regression for risk of AD in MCI subjects according to hypertension (line No. 265).

	Unadjusted		Model 1		Model 2	
	Crude HR (95% CI)	***p*-value**	**Adjusted HR (95% CI)**	***p*-value**	**Adjusted HR (95% CI)**	***p*-value**
Hypertension-no			*n* = 184			
BMI						
Underweight	1.90 (0.88–4.10)	0.105	1.78 (0.81–3.94)	0.154	1.94 (0.78–4.83)	0.153
Normal weight	Reference		Reference		Reference	
Overweight	0.54 (0.24–1.21)	0.133	0.53 (0.24–1.18)	0.119	0.41 (0.17–1.00)	0.050
Obese	0.25 (0.06–1.06)	0.060	0.27 (0.06–1.15)	0.077	0.25 (0.06–1.07)	0.062
Hypertension-yes			*n* = 197			
BMI						
Underweight	2.88 (0.90–9.21)	0.074	2.91 (0.80–10.60)	0.106	**4.71 (1.17–18.99)**	**0.030**
Normal weight	Reference		Reference		Reference	
Overweight	1.01 (0.41–2.47)	0.990	1.27 (0.51–3.15)	0.605	1.86 (0.68–5.04)	0.224
Obese	1.00 (0.39–2.57)	0.993	1.25 (0.47–3.29)	0.657	1.38 (0.49–3.85)	0.544

Model 1: Adjusted for age, sex, and education; Model 2: Adjusted for Model 1 plus CERAD-K total score, cognitive intervention, hypertension, diabetes mellitus, hyperlipidemia, heart disease, and cerebrovascular disease. AD, Alzheimer's disease; MCI, mild cognitive impairment; BMI, body mass index; HR, hazard ratio; CI, confidence interval. Statistically significant values are shown in bold.

and amygdala which are involved in learning and memory [26].

We also found that age affected the relationship between underweight and progression to AD in MCI subjects. In the older elderly group, underweight predicted higher progression to AD, but not in the younger elderly group. In previous studies, there was a difference in the effect of BMI on the onset of dementia according to age. Obesity in midlife is associated with incident AD [3, 5], whereas underweight in the elderly is associated with AD [6, 7]. This finding highlights the importance of stratifying subjects by age in studies of BMI and dementia and suggests that the older elderly should be considered a separate population from the larger majority of elderly younger than 75.

Our other finding was that the impact of BMI on the progression to AD was different according to the presence or absence of cognitive intervention. The effect of cognitive intervention may be explained by neuroplasticity. Neuroplasticity is defined as the brain's ability to adapt to changes in the environment through modification, reorganization, and creation of neural connections [27]. Many cognitive intervention programs attempt to enhance neuroplasticity of the brain. Therefore, cognitive intervention has a beneficial effect on cognitive decline in MCI subjects [28–30]. In the present study, cognitive intervention did not affect the progression of MCI to AD. However, we found that cognitive intervention affects the relationship between BMI and the progression to AD in MCI subjects. Underweight still increased the risk of progression to AD in the non-intervention group, while overweight had a protective effect on the progression to AD in the intervention group. It may be an inaccurate interpretation that cognitive intervention contributes to reducing the impact of underweight on the progression to AD, therefore further studies on the impact of cognitive intervention are needed.

Finally, we also found that the association between underweight and progression to AD was stronger in hypertensive group, and was not found in non-hypertensive group. In the study by Sakakura et al. leanness in hypertensive elderly patients was associated with poor cognitive function [31]. The mechanism of cognitive decline in lean hypertensive patients is not clear. However, it is well known that hypertension affects cognitive decline in elderly subjects [32, 33]. There are evidences that white matter medullary arterioles are vulnerable to hypertension, it can cause microvascular dysfunction and narrowing, which can lead to cerebral hypoperfusion [34, 35]. Recent study found that hypertension was associated with worse cognitive function and hippocampal hypometabolism in AD patients [36]. Because underweight and hypertension are risk factors for AD, MCI patients with underweight and hypertension may be highly likely to progress to AD.

This study has several limitations. First, we did not specify MCI diagnosis by amnestic MCI, non-amnestic MCI, single domain MCI, or multi-domain MCI. Second, amyloid imaging, CSF analysis, or pathological studies were not performed to determine on AD diagnosis. Third, the APOE genotype may modify the association between BMI and cognitive decline; however, we could not investigate this association because more than half of the participants did not undergo APOE genotyping. Fourth, this study only analyzed the presence or absence of cognitive intervention without taking the type of cognitive intervention and the duration of attendance into consideration. Fifth, we performed stratification analysis based on chronic diseases which may affect BMI, but we could not found the potential effects of chronic diseases such as DM on MCI and the progression to AD because of the small sample size. Furthermore, we did not investigate the treatment of chronic diseases. Sixth, Muscle loss is also known to be related to cognitive decline, but we could not consider sarcopenic obesity because we didn't investigate muscle mass. Finally, we did not measure longitudinal changes of BMI over time. Nonetheless, this study has several strengths. This study not only identified an effect of underweight on the progression to AD in MCI, but was also the first study to analyze the effects of sex, age, cognitive intervention, and chronic diseases on the relationship between BMI and progression to AD in MCI subjects. Other strength of this study is that the CERAD-K, which is a more accurate cognitive function assessment tool than the MMSE, was used to diagnose MCI and AD. Also, the CERAD-K total score and cognitive intervention attendance, which may affect progression to AD in MCI, were used covariates in this study, which was not done in previous studies. Furthermore, BMI is a biomarker that can be measured easily in clinical practice, so this outcome will be useful to clinicians.

In conclusion, although it is not known whether underweight is the cause of AD or preclinical symptom, these data indicate that low baseline BMI could be a useful marker for identifying individuals at increased risk for AD in MCI subjects. This result is stronger in females, older elderly, the non-cognitive intervention group, and the hypertensive group. Therefore, age and sex specific BMI control might be needed for delaying progression to AD in MCI subjects, and individuals who do not receive cognitive intervention or who have hypertension might need more BMI control.

AUTHOR CONTRIBUTIONS

CL planned the design and carried out the supervision of all parts of this study; SJ recruited participants, analyzed the data and drafted the manuscript; SY managed participants and collected the data; DK, CH, and HL collected the data and performed statistical analysis. All authors read and approved the final manuscript.

FUNDING

This research was supported by the Ministry of Trade, Industry and Energy (MOTIE, Korea) under Industrial Technology Innovation Program No. 10062378.

ACKNOWLEDGMENTS

We thank the members of Seocho Center for Dementia for collecting data.

REFERENCES

1. Mitchell AJ, Shiri-Feshki M. Rate of progression of mild cognitive impairment to dementia–meta-analysis of 41 robust inception cohort studies. *Acta Psychiatr Scand.* (2009) **119**:252–65. doi: 10.1111/j.1600-0447.2008.01326.x
2. Roberts R, Knopman DS. Classification and epidemiology of MCI. *Clin Geriatr Med.* (2013) **29**:753–72. doi: 10.1016/j.cger.2013.07.003
3. Whitmer RA, Gunderson EP, Barrett-Connor E, Quesenberry CP Jr, Yaffe K. Obesity in middle age and future risk of dementia: a 27 year longitudinal population based study. *BMJ* (2005) **330**:1360. doi: 10.1136/bmj.38446.466238.E0
4. Xu WL, Atti AR, Gatz M, Pedersen NL, Johansson B, Fratiglioni L. Midlife overweight and obesity increase late-life dementia risk: a population-based twin study. *Neurology* (2011) **76**:1568–74. doi: 10.1212/WNL.0b013e3182190d09
5. Fitzpatrick AL, Kuller LH, Lopez OL, Diehr P, O'Meara ES, Longstreth WT Jr, et al. Midlife and late-life obesity and the risk of dementia: cardiovascular health study. *Arch Neurol.* (2009) **66**:336–42. doi: 10.1001/archneurol.2008.582
6. Anstey KJ, Cherbuin N, Budge M, Young J. Body mass index in midlife and late-life as a risk factor for dementia: a meta-analysis of prospective studies. *Obes Rev.* (2011) **12**:e426–37. doi: 10.1111/j.1467-789X.2010.00825.x
7. Burns JM, Johnson DK, Watts A, Swerdlow RH, Brooks WM. Reduced lean mass in early Alzheimer disease and its association with brain atrophy. *Arch Neurol.* (2010) **67**:428–33. doi: 10.1001/archneurol.2010.38

8. Cova I, Clerici F, Maggiore L, Pomati S, Cucumo V, Ghiretti R, et al. Body mass index predicts progression of mild cognitive impairment to dementia. *Dement Geriatr Cogn Disord.* (2016) **41**:172–80. doi: 10.1159/000444216
9. Ye BS, Jang EY, Kim SY, Kim EJ, Park SA, Lee Y, et al. Unstable body mass index and progression to probable Alzheimer's disease dementia in patients with amnestic mild cognitive impairment. *J Alzheimers Dis.* (2015) **49**:483–91. doi: 10.3233/JAD-150556
10. Buschert V, Bokde AL, Hampel H. Cognitive intervention in Alzheimer disease. *Nat Rev Neurol.* (2010) **6**:508–17. doi: 10.1038/nrneurol.2010.113
11. Winblad B, Palmer K, Kivipelto M, Jelic V, Fratiglioni L, Wahlund LO, et al. Mild cognitive impairment–beyond controversies, towards a consensus: report of the International Working Group on Mild Cognitive Impairment. *J Intern Med.* (2004) **256**:240–6. doi: 10.1111/j.1365-2796.2004.01380.x
12. Lee JH, Lee KU, Lee DY, Kim KW, Jhoo JH, Kim JH, et al. Development of the Korean version of the consortium to establish a registry for Alzheimer's disease assessment packet (CERAD-K): clinical and neuropsychological assessment batteries. *J Gerontol B Psychol Sci Soc Sci.* (2002) **57**:P47–53. doi: 10.1093/geronb/57.1.P47
13. McKhann G, Drachman D, Folstein M, Katzman R, Price D, Stadlan EM. Clinical diagnosis of Alzheimer's disease: report of the NINCDS-ADRDA work group under the auspices of department of health and human services task force on Alzheimer's disease. *Neurology* (1984) **34**:939–44. doi: 10.1212/WNL.34.7.939
14. Thandassery RB, Appasani S, Yadav TD, Dutta U, Indrajit A, Singh K, et al. Implementation of the Asia-Pacific guidelines of obesity classification on the APACHE-O scoring system and its role in the prediction of outcomes of acute pancreatitis: a study from India. *Dig Dis Sci.* (2014) **59**:1316–21. doi: 10.1007/s10620-013-3000-7
15. Bhardwaj S, Misra A, Misra R, Goel K, Bhatt SP, Rastogi K, et al. High prevalence of abdominal, intra-abdominal and subcutaneous adiposity and clustering of risk factors among urban Asian Indians in North India. *PLoS ONE* (2011) **6**:e24362. doi: 10.1371/journal.pone.0024362
16. WHO Expert Consultation. Appropriate body-mass index for Asian populations and its implications for policy and intervention strategies. *Lancet* (2004) **363**:157–63. doi: 10.1016/S0140-6736(03)15268-3
17. Sobow T, Fendler W, Magierski R. Body mass index and mild cognitive impairment-to-dementia progression in 24 months: a prospective study. *Eur J Clin Nutr.* (2014) **68**:1216–9. doi: 10.1038/ejcn.2014.167
18. Johnson DK, Wilkins CH, Morris JC. Accelerated weight loss may precede diagnosis in Alzheimer disease. *Arch Neurol.* (2006) **63**:1312–7. doi: 10.1001/archneur.63.9.1312
19. Nourhashemi F, Andrieu S, Gillette-Guyonnet S, Reynish E, Albarede JL, Grandjean H, et al. Is there a relationship between fat-free soft tissue mass and low cognitive function? Results from a study of 7,105 women. *J Am Geriatr Soc.* (2002) **50**:1796–801. doi: 10.1046/j.1532-5415.2002.50507.x
20. Spauwen PJ, Murphy RA, Jonsson PV, Sigurdsson S, Garcia ME, Eiriksdottir G, et al. Associations of fat and muscle tissue with cognitive status in older adults: the AGES-Reykjavik Study. *Age Ageing* (2017) **46**:250–7. doi: 10.1093/ageing/afw219
21. Sergi G, De Rui M, Coin A, Inelmen EM, Manzato E. Weight loss and Alzheimer's disease: temporal and aetiologic connections. *Proc Nutr Soc.* (2013) **72**:160–5. doi: 10.1017/S0029665112002753
22. Power DA, Noel J, Collins R, O'Neill D. Circulating leptin levels and weight loss in Alzheimer's disease patients. *Dement Geriatr Cogn Disord.* (2001) **12**:167–70. doi: 10.1159/000051252
23. Grundman M, Corey-Bloom J, Jernigan T, Archibald S, Thal LJ. Low body weight in Alzheimer's disease is associated with mesial temporal cortex atrophy. *Neurology* (1996) **46**:1585–91. doi: 10.1212/WNL.46.6.1585
24. LeBlanc ES, Janowsky J, Chan BK, Nelson HD. Hormone replacement therapy and cognition: systematic review and meta-analysis. *JAMA* (2001) **285**:1489–99. doi: 10.1001/jama.285.11.1489
25. Waring SC, Rocca WA, Petersen RC, O'Brien PC, Tangalos EG, Kokmen E. Postmenopausal estrogen replacement therapy and risk of AD: a population-based study. *Neurology* (1999) **52**:965–70. doi: 10.1212/WNL.52.5.965
26. McEwen BS, Akama KT, Spencer-Segal JL, Milner TA, Waters EM. Estrogen effects on the brain: actions beyond the hypothalamus via novel mechanisms. *Behav Neurosci.* (2012) **126**:4–16. doi: 10.1037/a0026708
27. Kraft E. Cognitive function, physical activity, and aging: possible biological links and implications for multimodal interventions. *Neuropsychol Dev Cogn B Aging Neuropsychol Cogn.* (2012) **19**:248–63. doi: 10.1080/13825585.2011.645010
28. Belleville S. Cognitive training for persons with mild cognitive impairment. *Int Psychogeriatr.* (2008) **20**:57–66. doi: 10.1017/S104161020700631X
29. Kinsella GJ, Mullaly E, Rand E, Ong B, Burton C, Price S, et al. Early intervention for mild cognitive impairment: a randomised controlled trial. *J Neurol Neurosurg Psychiatry* (2009) **80**:730–6. doi: 10.1136/jnnp.2008.148346
30. Troyer AK, Murphy KJ, Anderson ND, Moscovitch M, Craik FI. Changing everyday memory behaviour in amnestic mild cognitive impairment: a randomised controlled trial. *Neuropsychol Rehabil.* (2008) **18**:65–88. doi: 10.1080/09602010701409684
31. Sakakura K, Hoshide S, Ishikawa J, Momomura S, Kawakami M, Shimada K, et al. Association of body mass index with cognitive function in elderly hypertensive Japanese. *Am J Hypertens* (2008) **21**:627–32. doi: 10.1038/ajh.2008.157
32. Kivipelto M, Helkala EL, Laakso MP, Hanninen T, Hallikainen M, Alhainen K, et al. Midlife vascular risk factors and Alzheimer's disease in later life: longitudinal, population based study. *BMJ* (2001) **322**:1447–51. doi: 10.1136/bmj.322.7300.1447
33. Peila R, White LR, Masaki K, Petrovitch H, Launer LJ. Reducing the risk of dementia: efficacy of long-term treatment of hypertension. *Stroke* (2006) **37**:1165–70. doi: 10.1161/01.STR.0000217653.01615.93
34. Hiroki M, Miyashita K, Oda M. Tortuosity of the white matter medullary arterioles is related to the severity of hypertension. *Cerebrovasc Dis.* (2002) **13**:242–50. doi: 10.1159/000057850
35. Faraco G, Iadecola C. Hypertension: a harbinger of stroke and dementia. *Hypertension* (2013) **62**:810–7. doi: 10.1161/HYPERTENSIONAHA.113.01063
36. Moonga I, Niccolini F, Wilson H, Pagano G, Politis M. Hypertension is associated with worse cognitive function and hippocampal hypometabolism in Alzheimer's disease. *Eur J Neurol.* (2017) **24**:1173–82. doi: 10.1111/ene.13374

16

Pathological Crying and Laughing in Motor Neuron Disease: Pathobiology, Screening, Intervention

*Eoin Finegan, Rangariroyashe H. Chipika, Stacey Li Hi Shing, Orla Hardiman and Peter Bede**

Computational Neuroimaging Group, Biomedical Sciences Institute, Trinity College Dublin, Dublin, Ireland

***Correspondence:**
Peter Bede
pbede@tcd.ie

Pathological crying and laughing (PCL) has significant quality-of-life implications in amyotrophic lateral sclerosis (ALS); it can provoke restrictive life-style modifications and lead to social isolation. Despite its high prevalence and quality of life implications, it remains surprisingly understudied. Divergent pathophysiological models have been proposed, centered on corticobulbar tract degeneration, prefrontal cortex pathology, sensory deafferentation, and impaired cerebellar gate-control mechanisms. Quantitative MRI techniques and symptom-specific clinical instruments offer unprecedented opportunities to elucidate the anatomical underpinnings of PCL pathogenesis. Emerging neuroimaging studies of ALS support the role of cortico–pontine–cerebellar network dysfunction in context-inappropriate emotional responses. The characterization of PCL-associated pathophysiological processes is indispensable for the development of effective pharmacological therapies.

Keywords: pathological crying and laughing, pseudobulbar affect, emotional lability, involuntary emotional expression disorder, motor neuron disease, amyotrophic lateral sclerosis, biomarkers, magnetic resonance imaging

INTRODUCTION

The terms “pathological crying and laughing,” “pseudobulbar affect,” “emotional lability,” and “involuntary emotional expression disorder” are often used interchangeably depending on geographical location and year of publication. Despite the differences in terminology, recurrent episodes of involuntary or exaggerated emotional expression, particularly in the form of crying and laughing, are common in several neurological conditions including, in order of prevalence: motor neuron disease (MND), traumatic brain injury (TBI), multiple sclerosis (MS), stroke, multiple system atrophy-cerebellar type (MSA-C), Alzheimer's disease (AD), and Parkinson's disease (PD) (1–6).

The disorder is particularly common in motor neuron diseases (MND): amyotrophic lateral sclerosis (ALS) and primary lateral sclerosis (PLS). Prevalence estimates vary, but between one quarter and one half of MND patients are thought to be affected (5, 7–11). While there is a paucity of studies comparing PCL prevalence across the spectrum of MND phenotypes, a recent study confirmed the relationship between clinical upper motor neuron dysfunction and PCL prevalence; PCL was most commonly identified in PLS and UMN-predominant patients (39%), followed by typical ALS (29%) and lower motor neuron (LMN) predominant groups (10%). Consistent with this pattern, there was a single case of PCL in a group of 12 patients with progressive muscular atrophy (PMA) (12). While the manifestations of the episodes may be congruent with the person's contemporary emotional state (10, 13, 14), the magnitude of emotional responses is disproportionate to the emotive stimulus and the social context. Such episodes may cause significant distress, embarrassment, and ultimately may lead to social withdrawal (15).

The primary objective of this review is to systematically appraise PCL-related studies in MND from a dual academic and clinical perspective. We outline established and emerging disease-models based on neuroimaging, neurosurgical and neurophysiological studies. The spectrum of clinical presentations, diagnostic challenges, functional impact, and treatment options are also discussed. We preferentially use the term "pathological crying and laughing" (PCL) in this review, in its broadest sense: encompassing the entire spectrum of presentations. Furthermore, while PCL in ALS is the primary focus of this review, we draw further information from PCL studies in other neurological conditions to discuss unifying, symptom-specific, pathophysiological concepts.

METHODS

A formal literature search was conducted using PubMed/Medline and Embase using the terms "pathological crying and laughing," "pseudobulbar affect," "emotional lability," involuntary emotional expression disorder" separately, and in combination with terms "amyotrophic lateral sclerosis," "motor neuron disease," "pseudobulbar palsy," "clinical trials," "treatment," and "pathology." Only articles in English, published between 1988 and October 2018 were included. A total of 220 articles met these criteria; these were systematically reviewed for information relating to diagnosis, disease-mechanisms, anatomical localization, and treatment options.

Historical Context and Terminology

The abundance of terms used to describe this syndrome epitomizes the tireless efforts to characterize the underpinnings of both physiological and pathological emotional expression. Charles Darwin observed in 1872 that "certain brain-diseases, as hemiplegia, brain-wasting, and senile decay, have a special tendency to induce weeping" (16). Oppenheim (17) used the term "pseudobulbar affect" (PBA), based on the important observation that the disorder commonly occurs in association with motor features of pseudobulbar palsy, a condition resulting from bilateral corticobulbar tract pathology. Although this association is still well-recognized (13, 18), the term PBA may be misleading; new evidence suggests that corticobulbar tract dysfunction alone is neither necessary, nor sufficient to cause PCL (19–23). "Emotional Lability" (EL) was described by Pierre-Marie as early as 1892, a term still commonly used in the literature (24). The term pathological crying and laughing (PCL) was used by Wilson in his influential essay of 1924, in which he introduced his unifying theory of the disorder (25). More recently, the term "involuntary emotional expression disorder" (IEED) has been proposed to encompass the wider range of emotional symptoms which may accompany the disorder (26).

Clinical Presentations, Diagnosis and Monitoring

A useful conceptualization of PCL is that symptoms may lie on a spectrum, (27) with infrequent, mood congruent but disproportionate episodes at one end, and frequent, mood incongruent episodes at the other. While there is considerable variability in episode type and character across patients, within individuals episodes tend to be consistent over time in terms of symptom type (i.e., uncontrolled laughing or crying), the context in which the episodes recur, the severity, duration, and the degree of voluntary control that the individual retains over the episodes (26, 28). The wide range of presentations coupled with the lack of unifying terminology, has hampered efforts to establish widely adopted diagnostic criteria. Several criteria have been proposed and later revised, reflecting evolving concepts of the PCL (29). *Poeck's* 1969 criteria (30), focus on episodes that are entirely situation inappropriate or unrelated to the patient's internal emotional state. Recent criteria are less restrictive, encompassing presentations across the entire spectrum (26, 27). Revised criteria proposed by Cummings et al. for "involuntary emotional expression disorder" (IEED) (26) are inclusive of episodes that are either disproportionate to the emotive stimulus or to the individual's internal emotional state. The episodes must represent a distinct change from the patient's emotional reactivity prior to the onset of a neurological disease. These criteria specifically require the exclusion of alternative causes for the symptoms; mood, facial tics, dystonia, or substance effects. More recently, Miller et al. proposed to include supportive features such as the presence of pseudobulbar signs and a proneness to anger (27). The latter reflects accruing observations from several studies (14, 23, 27, 31).

PCL needs to be carefully distinguished from mood disorders through careful clinical evaluation (1, 9, 32). A key difference is that crying in depression or excessive laughter in mania occur in the context of pervasive low or elevated mood, respectively (33). In the case of clinical depression, associated symptoms can also be identified such as anhedonia and insomnia (27, 34). Although some studies report an association between depression and PCL (12), more commonly, no significant association is found (8, 13, 35). The clinical distinction may be particularly challenging in cases where pathological crying co-exists with depressive symptoms (2, 36). Emerging evidence suggests that PCL may respond to selective serotonin reuptake

---

Abbreviations: AD, Alzheimer's disease; ALS, Amyotrophic lateral sclerosis; B.I.D., Bis in die/twice daily; CNS-LS, Center for Neurologic Study-lability scale; DxQ, Dextromethorphan-quinidine; EL, Emotional lability; ELQ, Emotional lability questionnaire; EMA, European Medicines Agency; FDA, US Food and Drug Administration; LMN, Lower motor neuron; MND, Motor neuron disease; MRI, Magnetic resonance imaging; MS, Multiple sclerosis; MSA-C, Multiple system atrophy-cerebellar type; NMDA, N-methyl-D-aspartate; PBA, Pseudobulbar affect; PC, Pathological crying; PCL, Pathological crying and laughing; PD, Parkinson's disease; PLACS, The pathological laughing and crying scale; PLS, Primary lateral sclerosis; PMA, Progressive muscular atrophy; SPECT, Single-photon emission computed tomography; SSRI, Selective serotonin re-uptake inhibitor; TBI, Traumatic brain injury; TCA, Tricyclic anti-depressant; UMN, Upper motor neuron.

inhibitors (SSRIs) within days, whereas depression typically only responds to pharmacological intervention after several weeks (37).

Similarly to the multitude of diagnostic criteria proposed for PCL, several screening and symptom severity scoring instruments have been developed. While not all of these have been extensively validated, these tools have been used in both academic research and clinical trials. The pathological laughing and crying scale (PLACS) was validated for use in stroke patients with "PBA" in 1993. The authors used it as an efficacy measure in a small placebo-controlled trial of nortriptyline; treatment was associated with symptom reduction (38). The Center for Neurologic Study-Lability Scale (CNS-LS) was introduced as a self-reported measure of "affective lability" in ALS (39). This short, self-administered questionnaire consists of 7 items; 4 relating to labile laughing and 3 relating to crying. The scale evaluates subjective burden of symptoms over the preceding week, in terms of episode burden and severity. While this scale relies on retrospective patient account, it has been shown to be an accurate indicator of episode frequency (40). The CNS-LS has been adopted as an efficacy measure in several recent clinical trials (41–44). Another assessment tool, the "emotional lability questionnaire" (ELQ) has also been validated in ALS. It extends the period over which symptoms are assessed from one up to four weeks prior to screening, which helps to capture patients who experience less frequent episodes (45, 46). In addition to PCL, it also includes a specific section on abnormal smiling. One of the strengths of the ELQ is that it includes the caregiver's perspective, which helps to identify lack of insight if significantly discordant scores are given by the patient and the carer. Interestingly, in ALS, there is significant agreement between patient and caregiver scores, indicating that patients are keenly aware of PCL symptoms (45). This concordance contrasts with behavioral deficits in ALS-FTD, where patient reports may differ substantially from caregivers reports (47).

Although screening instruments are valuable tools for identifying and monitoring PCL, they don't evaluate the impact of PCL on individual patients. There is evidence, that PCL impacts on the quality-of-life and social functioning of affected individuals (48) and may contribute to carer distress (49). There is a growing effort to understand the individualized experiences of patients with PCL (14, 35, 50, 51).

DISEASE MODELS

Traditional and Revised Hypotheses

The traditional PCL model, proposed by Wilson in 1924 has, until recently been the most widely accepted one (25). Under physiological circumstances, it contends, emotional expression is influenced by both voluntary motor and involuntary emotional centers. These pathways descend onto the medullary "facio-respiratory" centers, which mediate the facial movements and breathing patterns necessary to convey emotion. This model predicts that disruption of the descending voluntary inputs to the brainstem, such as may occur in pseudobulbar palsy, results in disinhibition of involuntary emotional influence on expression. In support of this model, Wilson cited cases of dissociated emotional and voluntary facial expression, such as the observation that some patients with pseudobulbar palsy are unable to make voluntary facial movements but can be observed to smile, laugh or cry in response to emotional stimuli. This phenomenon is usually termed "voluntary facial palsy" (52). The contrary, "mimic palsy" or "emotional facial palsy" is sometimes observed, in which a patient with entirely normal voluntary facial movements, exhibits a complete lack of movement on one side of the face when reacting to emotional stimuli (53).

Parvizi et al. highlighted several limitations of the traditional model (54). Patients with bilateral voluntary facial paralysis, as in Wilson's example do not seem to be excessively prone to PBA, as would be predicted by the "disinhibition" model. Furthermore, patients with severe PBA symptoms are usually able to voluntarily mimic laughing or crying, indicating that involuntary expression can occur alongside intact voluntary control.

The revised model of PCL draws on the increasing appreciation of the role of the cerebellum in cognitive processes (55, 56). This model suggests that the cerebellum plays a key role in gating and modulating emotional output in response to contextual cues from cortical and limbic areas (54). Modulation is believed to be mediated through cortico-ponto-cerebellar pathways. In normal motor control, the cerebellum is known to modulate motor output in response to multiple sensory inputs; disruption of these inputs produces motor modulation deficits, including dysmetria. The involuntary emotional expression resulting from disruption of cortico-ponto-cerebellar emotional circuits has, analogously been termed "affective dysmetria" (57).

Insights From Imaging and Neurophysiological Studies Across Neurological Diseases

Research over the past 30 years has led to a revision of the traditional model of PCL; studies have provided strong evidence to refute a simple causal relationship between PCL and corticobulbar tract dysfunction (58). Instead, a disruption within a widely dispersed network of emotional control appears to underlie the disorder. **Tables 1, 2** provide an overview of studies highlighting key anatomical regions implicated in the pathogenesis of PCL. An MRI-based lesion study in post-stroke pathological crying classified patients based on symptom severity (70). It found a positive pathoanatomical correlation between lesion size and location and pathological crying severity. Bilateral pontine infarcts were associated with greatest severity, while bilateral anterior hemispheric infarcts were associated with moderate PCL severity.

Among the likely neurotransmitters involved in the physiological expression of emotion, serotonin and glutamate have received particular attention (27, 71, 74). Evidence for dysfunction within these neurotransmitter pathways in PCL comes from the success of serotonergic (31, 38, 75), and anti-glutamatergic drugs (42) in PCL treatment. The selective serotonin re-uptake inhibitors (SSRIs) and tricyclic antidepressants (TCAs), are thought to work by increasing

TABLE 1 | Neuroanatomical regions implicated in PCL circuitry based on clinical observations.

References	Neurological condition	Terminology	*n*	Main study findings	Anatomical localization
CLINICAL CASES					
Parvizi et al. (3)	Cerebellar cyst	PC	1 PC+	Midline cerebellar cyst	Cerebellum (vermis)
Parvizi et al. (59)	MSA-C	PCL	PCL+: 1 PM and 9 clinical MSA-c	Pathological changes confined to cerebellum, basilar pons and olives	cerebellum and brainstem connections
Chattha et al. (60)	PD with STN-DBS	PBA	1 PBA+	Laughter with DBS stimulation of sub-thalamic nuclei	Basal ganglia: STN
Saini et al. (61)	CPM	PBA	1 PBA+	Basilar pons demyelination	CPC tracts: Pons
Martin et al. (62)	Anti-Yo cerebellar degeneration	PBA	1 PBA+	Breast cancer presenting as uncontrollable crying and motor cerebellar syndrome	Cerebellum
McCullagh et al. (20)	ALS	PCL	10 PCL + 8 PCL- 10 HC	Executive dysfunction in PCL+	Pre-motor frontal cortex
Palmieri et al. (45)	ALS	EL	29 EL+	Correlations: (1) bulbar disease and EL (2) bulbar disease and executive impairment. However, no correlation between PCL and cognitive changes	Extra-motor frontal lobe
Olney et al. (13)	ALS	PCL	21 PCL+, 14 PCL−	Laboratory study: PCL+ had impaired regulation of facial expression	Frontal cortex
Hübers et al. (63)	ALS	PCL	10 PCL+, 10 HC	PCL+ more susceptible to mood-incongruent stimuli than controls, PCL associated with emotional lability/suggestibility	Frontal cortex
NEUROSURGICAL CASES					
Krack et al. (64)	PD with STN-DBS	Mirthful laugh	2 PL+	Associated with DBS stimulation of bilateral STN in one patient and right STN in other	Basal ganglia: STN
Okun et al. (65)	PD post-thalamotomy	PBA	1 PBA+	Post-thalamotomy pathological laughing	Basal ganglia
Okun et al. (66)	PD with STN-DBS	PC	1 PC+	Pathological crying with DBS stimulation of left sub-thalamic nucleus	Basal ganglia: STN
Famularo et al. (67)	Cerebellar ependymoma	PL	1 PL+	PC as sole presenting feature of cerebellar vermis tumor abutting the floor of the fourth ventricle	Cerebellum (vermis)
Low et al. (68)	PD with STN-DBS	PC	1 PC+	Pathological crying with DBS stimulation in region of caudal internal capsule (without signs of PBP)	Internal capsule (caudal)
Wolf et al. (69)	PD with STN-DBS	PC	1 PC+	Pathological crying with DBS stimulation of sub-thalamic nuclei	Basal ganglia: STN

CPC, cortico-ponto-cerebellar pathways; CPM, Central Pontine Myelinolysis; Dx, Diagnosis; HC, Healthy control; MSA-C, Multiple system atrophy, cerebellar type; n, sample size; PBP,Pseudobulbar Palsy; PC, Pathological crying; PL, pathological laughing; PM, Post-mortem/Autopsy; SERT, Serotonin transporter; STN-DBS, Subthalamic nucleus, deep brain stimulation; UMN, Upper motor neuron; WM, White matter.

availability of serotonin at synapses in corticolimbic and cerebellar circuits (32).

A SPECT study found reduced brainstem serotonin receptor (SERT) densities in post-stroke PCL (71), providing further evidence of the role of serotonergic transmission in PCL. Serotonergic neurons from the raphe nuclei have widespread projections from the paramedian brainstem to cortical, subcortical, and cerebellar targets (76, 77). Also consistent with the serotonin hypothesis, lesions involving these nuclei and their projections are frequently associated with PCL (70). An MRI study of PBA in MS patients showed an association between symptoms and lesions in key regions: brainstem, bilateral inferior parietal, and medial frontal regions (23).

There is increasing recognition of the role of sensory deafferentation of the cerebellum in PCL (78). Evidence from neurophysiological studies in PCL suggests that the cerebellum may filter emotional output through a "gate-control" mechanism (79). At a cellular level, cerebellar Golgi cells may play a crucial role in gate-control. It has been demonstrated that Golgi cells, when activated from various peripheral inputs, show decreased firing rate, thereby reducing inhibition of granule cells (80). This finding, suggests, that rather than providing "gain-control," Golgi cells may act as a "context-specific gate" on transmission through the mossy fiber–granule cell pathway. A study of PCL in MSA-cerebellar type found a prevalence of 36% in this condition, in which clinically-significant cerebellar dysfunction is apparent (59).This prevalence estimate exceeds those of studies in idiopathic Parkinson's disease (5), suggesting that cerebellar pathology is linked to PCL in Parkinsonian disorders. Several neurological and neurosurgical case-reports have linked PCL to cerebellar pathology, especially in association with vermis pathology (3, 62, 67, 81). These studies support the cerebellar

TABLE 2 | Anatomical conclusions of neuroimaging studies in PCL.

References	Neurological condition	Terminology	*n*	Main study findings	Anatomical localization
Andersen et al. (70)	Stroke	PC	12 PC+	Isolated, bilateral pontine lesions in most severe cases; bilateral basal ganglia lesions in intermediate group; unilateral subcortical lesions in milder	Pons (raphe nuclei), Basal ganglia, Subcortical WM
Murai et al. (71)	Stroke	PC	6 PC+ 9 PC–	Reduced SERT binding ratios in midbrain/pons in PC	Brainstem (raphe nuclei)
Tateno et al. (72)	TBI	PCL	92 PCL+	PLC associated with traumatic frontal lobe lesions, particularly lateral left frontal lobe	Frontal lobes (esp. left lateral)
Ghaffar et al. (23)	MS	PBA	14 PBA+ 14 PBA–	Greater lesion volume in PBA subjects in brainstem; bilateral inferior parietal and medial inferior frontal; right medial superior frontal	Brainstem; Parietal lobes (bilateral inferior); frontal; basal ganglia
Floeter et al. (10)	ALS	PBA	22 PBA+ 25 PBA– 28 HC	PBA+ (vs. PBA-): reduced FA underlying left motor cortex, Increased MD underlying the frontotemporal cortex, the transverse pontine fibers, and MCP. IC pathology in both groups	widespread disruption of CPC tracts in PBA
Wang et al. (21)	Stroke	PCL	56 PCL+, 56 PCL–	PCL associated with pontine infarcts, particularly paramedian lesions	Pons
Christidi et al. (73)	ALS	PCL	28 PCL+ 28 PCL– 25 HC	PCL+ vs. PCL-: Reduced GM volume: left orbitofrontal cortex, frontal operculum, putamen; and bilateral frontal poles. WM pathology: decreased FA in left cingulum bundle, posterior corona radiata	Frontal cortex: left orbitofrontal; and operculum Cingulate WM

CPC, cortico-ponto-cerebellar pathways; CPM, Central Pontine Myelinolysis; Dx, Diagnosis; HC, Healthy control; MSA-C, Multiple system atrophy, cerebellar type; n, sample size; PBP, Pseudobulbar Palsy; PC, Pathological crying; PL, pathological laughing; PM, Post-mortem/Autopsy; SERT, Serotonin transporter; IC, Internal Capsule; STN-DBS, Subthalamic nucleus, deep brain stimulation; UMN, Upper motor neuron; WM, White matter.

gate-control theory of emotional expression, indicating that the disruption to cortico-ponto-cerebellar emotional circuitry may underlie this disorder.

Insights From PCL Studies in Motor Neuron Disease

Corticobulbar tract dysfunction in ALS has been linked to cognitive impairment, and in particular to executive dysfunction (82). A study of PCL in ALS found an association between PCL and poor performance in executive tasks, implicating pre-frontal cortical areas in the disorder (20). Other studies, in contrast have found no such associations (8, 45). Systematic studies of social cognition in patients with PCL are lacking. Despite the conflicting findings, evidence from imaging and neurophysiology studies support the involvement of frontal cortical dysfunction in PCL (73, 79).

Advanced neuroimaging techniques enable the characterization of symptom-specific structural (83, 84), and functional (85, 86) alterations, providing insights into disease mechanisms (87, 88). Given the high prevalence of PCL in MND, it provides unique opportunities to explore PCL-specific network alterations (58). Floeter et al. used MRI diffusion methods to explore the white matter signature of PCL in ALS and PLS (10). Both ALS and PLS patients exhibited considerable white matter pathology in the corticospinal tracts and the corpus callosum. PCL-associated white matter changes were identified in frontotemporal regions, transverse pontine fibers and the middle cerebellar peduncles. A recent multimodal MRI study by Christidi et al. used the CNS-LS to divide a large group of ALS patients into PCL-positive and PCL-negative groups (73). The PCL-positive group showed significant gray and white matter changes compared with the PCL-negative group. The gray matter assessment found reduced volume of left orbitofrontal cortex, operculum, putamen, and of bilateral frontal poles. White matter analyses revealed diffusion abnormalities in the left cingulum, the posterior corona radiata and in the left middle and bilateral inferior cerebellar peduncles. The finding of cerebellar involvement in PCL in ALS again implicates cerebellar dysfunction in the pathophysiology of PCL, across a range of neurological diseases. While it is challenging to detect cerebellar signs clinically in the presence of pyramidal and lower motor neuron degeneration in ALS, imaging studies suggest that cerebellar degeneration is an important feature of ALS pathology, which is likely to contribute to PCL (89–91).

THERAPEUTIC OPTIONS

Antidepressant Medication in the Management of PCL

Divergent pharmacological strategies have been explored in the management of PCL. SSRIs and TCAs are the most frequently used off-label medications (75). Surprisingly, we did not identify any placebo-controlled trial of any antidepressants for PCL in ALS. In the absence of robust clinical trial data in ALS, evidence from other neurological conditions, most-commonly stroke, is used to guide treatment. There have been positive results in small placebo-controlled trials of SSRIs including citalopram (92), fluoxetine, (31) sertraline (93) and of the TCA nortriptyline (38), in post-stroke PCL. Case-reports and uncontrolled trials reported symptom improvement with amitriptyline (94) and duloxetine (95) in ALS; memantine in AD (96); and mirtazapine in post-stoke PCL (97). A 2010 Cochrane review of treatments for "emotionalism" after stroke concluded that there is "suggestive but not definitive" evidence that antidepressants reduce frequency of symptoms, although it highlighted "several methodological deficiencies" in available studies (98).

Management of PCL in Motor Neuron Disease

In 2010, dextromethorphan/quinidine (Dx/Q) became the first FDA-approved treatment for PCL, following more than a decade of research into the potential benefits of the commonly-used anti-tussive for this indication (99). Dextromethorphan acts as a non-competitive glutamate antagonist on NMDA-receptors and as an agonist on sigma receptors (100). When administered alone, it is rapidly metabolized by first-pass metabolism through the cytochrome P450-2D6 system. The addition of the CYP-2D6 inhibitor, quinidine, dramatically increases the bioavailability of dextromethorphan (101). In 2004, a randomized, double-blinded study compared treatment with Dx/Q (30/30 mg twice daily) with dextromethorphan alone in ALS patients with PBA, defined by a CNS-LS score $\geq$13 (43). The combination not only reduced CNS-LS scores and episode frequency but also led to improvements in quality-of-life measures. Treatment-related side effects including nausea, dizziness, somnolence, and loose stools were relatively common however; about one quarter of patients withdrew from treatment, the majority within 1 week (102). A follow-up study in 2010 assessed whether a lower quinidine dose would reduce adverse effects relative to the earlier trial, while maintaining efficacy (42, 103) The study randomized ALS (n = 197) and MS (n = 129) patients with PBA to Dx/Q 30/10 mg BID, Dx/Q 20/10 mg BID or placebo BID. Both Dx/Q doses were found to reduce episode frequency, CNS-LS scores and to improve the likelihood of symptom remission compared to placebo. There was a lower discontinuation rate than in the earlier trial. It is interesting to note the considerable placebo response rate across efficacy endpoints in both trials. It must also be pointed-out that CYP450 2D6-poor metabolizers (104) were excluded from the efficacy and safety analyses raising questions about the requirement to screen for this phenotype prior to prescribing (105). Efficacy outcomes were also maintained in a 12-week open label extension study (106). A 52-week open-label study in 553 patients, including 199 patients with ALS, reported no serious drug-related adverse effects (75). However, clinicians must be cognizant of underlying cardiac conditions as quinidine can cause serious QT-interval prolongation (107).

Limitations of Currently Available Treatments

While the emergence of the first FDA-approved drug for PCL is an important advancement, the effective treatment of PCL remains challenging. Unfortunately, there have been no head-to-head trials of Dx/Q and any commonly used antidepressant. This knowledge-gap is particularly problematic given the current cost of Dx/Q, which may be prohibitive. Not only is the price of the approved combination product higher than alternative options, it is dramatically more expensive than the combined cost of its individual components (108). Finally, although Dx/Q was granted approval by the European Medicines Agency (EMA) in 2013, it was subsequently withdrawn by the manufacturer in 2016, on commercial grounds. (109, 110) A 2017 Cochrane review of "symptomatic treatments" in ALS highlighted emotional lability, as a symptom for which there is a "significant gap" in studies regarding the effectiveness of available treatments (111). There is a pressing and unmet need for robust clinical trials of antidepressants in the management of PCL. Finally, there is evidence that ALS patients and carers, lack awareness of the association between PCL and their underlying neurological condition (112), highlighting the importance of enquiring about PCL symptoms in patients with high-risk conditions, such as ALS.

CONCLUSIONS

Pathological crying and laughing is a shared symptom of many neurological conditions across infective, vascular, inflammatory, and neurodegenerative etiologies. Various terminologies have been used to encompass the heterogeneity of symptoms, which vary in severity, emotional congruity, frequency, and degree of control. After centuries of insightful observations, lesion studies and case reports, neuroimaging methods now provide long-awaited *in-vivo* insights into the specific pathophysiological mechanisms underlying the disorder. Patho-anatomical correlations indicate, that irrespective of the pathology (i.e., neurodegeneration, stroke, demyelination, TBI), the disorder occurs due to disruption in circuits involved in the initiation and modulation of emotional output. Key components of the network include sensori-motor cortical regions and their pontine and cerebellar connections. Further research is needed to elucidate the specific role of individual components within the network and their interactions. Effective symptomatic treatments are available; however, further studies are needed to establish individualized treatment strategies for patients experiencing impaired social or occupational functioning.

AUTHOR CONTRIBUTIONS

The manuscript was drafted by EF. RC, SLHS, OH and PB contributed to the conceptualization, editing, and revision of this paper.

ACKNOWLEDGMENTS

Peter Bede and the Computational Neuroimaging Group is supported by the Health Research Board (HRB-Ireland; HRB EIA-2017-019), the Andrew Lydon scholarship, the Irish Institute of Clinical Neuroscience IICN-Novartis Ireland Research Grant, the Iris O'Brien Foundation, and the Research Motor Neuron (RMN-Ireland) Foundation.

REFERENCES

1. Engelman W, Hammond FM, Malec JF. Diagnosing pseudobulbar affect in traumatic brain injury. *Neuropsychiatr Dis Treat.* (2014). 10:1903–10. doi: 10.2147/NDT.S63304
2. Patel N, Combs H, York M, Phan C, Jimenez-Shahed J. Pseudobulbar affect correlates with mood symptoms in parkinsonian disorders but not amyotrophic lateral sclerosis. *J Neuropsychiatry Clin Neurosci.* (2018). 30:214–9. doi: 10.1176/appi.neuropsych.17070131
3. Parvizi J, Schiffer R. Exaggerated crying and tremor with a cerebellar cyst. *J Neuropsychiatry Clin Neurosci.* (2007). 19:187–90. doi: 10.1176/jnp.2007.19.2.187
4. Vidovic V, Rovazdi MC, Kraml O, Kes VB. Pseudobulbar affect in multiple sclerosis patients. *Acta Clin Croat.* (2015). 54:159–63.
5. Brooks BR, Crumpacker D, Fellus J, Kantor D, Kaye RE. PRISM: a novel research tool to assess the prevalence of pseudobulbar affect symptoms across neurological conditions. *PLoS ONE.* (2013). 8:e72232. doi: 10.1371/journal.pone.0072232
6. Phuong L, Garg S, Duda JE, Stern MB, Weintraub D. Involuntary emotional expression disorder (IEED) in Parkinson's disease. *Parkinson Relat Disord.* (2009). 15:511–5. doi: 10.1016/j.parkreldis.2009.01.001
7. Work SS, Colamonico JA, Bradley WG, Kaye RE. Pseudobulbar affect: an under-recognized and under-treated neurological disorder. *Adv Ther.* (2011). 28:586–601. doi: 10.1007/s12325-011-0031-3
8. Lonergan K, Burke T, Pinto-Grau M, Vajda A, Heverin M, Dockree P, et al. Emotional lability in ALS: Delineating the relationship between lability, psychological status, cognition, and behavior. *Amyotr Later Scleros Frontotemp Degenerat.* (2016). 17:273. doi: 10.1080/21678421.2016.1232065/0016
9. Thakore NJ, Pioro EP. Laughter, crying and sadness in ALS. *J Neurol Neurosurg Psychiatry.* (2017). 88:825–31. doi: 10.1136/jnnp-2017-315622
10. Floeter MK, Katipally R, Kim MP, Schanz O, Stephen M, Danielian L, et al. Impaired corticopontocerebellar tracts underlie pseudobulbar affect in motor neuron disorders. *Neurology.* (2014). 83:620–7. doi: 10.1212/WNL.0000000000000693
11. Kuipers-Upmeijer J, De Jager AEJ, Hew JM, Snoek JW, Van Weerden TW. Primary lateral sclerosis: clinical, neurophysiological, and magnetic resonance findings. *J Neurol Neurosur.* (2001). 71:615–20. doi: 10.1136/jnnp.71.5.615
12. Thakore N, Pioro E. Prevalence, associations and course of depression in ALS: Observations from a large cohort. *Amyotrop Lateral Scleros Frontotemp Degenerat.* (2014) 15:55–6. doi: 10.3109/21678421.2014.960172/088
13. Olney NT, Goodkind MS, Lomen-Hoerth C, Whalen PK, Williamson CA, Holley DE, et al. Behaviour, physiology and experience of pathological laughing and crying in amyotrophic lateral sclerosis. *Brain.* (2011). 134:3455–66. doi: 10.1093/brain/awr297
14. Ahmed F, Murphy J, Lomen-Hoerth C. Utility of a new pseudobulbar questionnaire (PBAQ) for ALS. *Ann Neurol.* (2010). 68:S23–S4.
15. Wynn D, Kaye R, Hepner A. Impact of pseudobulbar affect on health and QoL. *Ann Neurol.* (2010). 68:S12.
16. Darwin C. *Chapter 6: Special Expressions of Man: Suffering and Weeping. The Expression of the Emotions in Man and Animals.* New York, NY: D. Appleton and Company (1872).
17. Oppenheim H. *Textbook of Nervous Diseases for Physicians and Students by Professor H. Oppenheim of Berlin: English trans-lation by Alexander Bruce.* London: T. N. Foulis Publisher (1911).
18. Tortelli R, Cortese R, Tursi M, D'Errico E, Muschitiello C, Capozzo R, et al. Frequency of pseudobulbar affect (PBA) in an incident ALS cohort: results from a population based registry. *Amyotrop Lateral Scler.* (2012). 13:128–9. doi: 10.3109/17482968.2012.721231/234
19. Ironside R. Disorders of laughter due to brain lesions1. *Brain.* (1956). 79:589–609. doi: 10.1093/brain/79.4.589
20. McCullagh S, Moore M, Gawel M, Feinstein A. Pathological laughing and crying in amyotrophic lateral sclerosis: an association with prefrontal cognitive dysfunction. *J Neurol Sci.* (1999). 169:43–8. doi: 10.1016/S0022-510X(99)00214-2
21. Wang G, Teng F, Chen Y, Liu Y, Li Y, Cai L, et al. Clinical features and related factors of poststroke pathological laughing and crying: a case-control study. *J Stroke Cerebrovasc Dis.* (2016). 25:556–64. doi: 10.1016/j.jstrokecerebrovasdis.2015.11.003
22. Asfora WT, DeSalles AA, Abe M, Kjellberg RN. Is the syndrome of pathological laughing and crying a manifestation of pseudobulbar palsy? *J Neurol Neurosurg Psychiatry.* (1989). 52:523–5. doi: 10.1136/jnnp.52.4.523
23. Ghaffar O, Chamelian L, Feinstein A. Neuroanatomy of pseudobulbar affect: a quantitative MRI study in multiple sclerosis. *J Neurol.* (2008). 255:406–12. doi: 10.1007/s00415-008-0685-1
24. Marie P. *Lec,ons Sur Les Maladies De La Moelle.* Paris: G Masson (1892).
25. Wilson SAK. Original papers. *Some Probl Neurol.* (1924). s1-4:299–333.
26. Cummings JL, Arciniegas DB, Brooks BR, Herndon RM, Lauterbach EC, Pioro EP, et al. Defining and diagnosing involuntary emotional expression disorder. *CNS Spectr.* (2006). 11:1–7. doi: 10.1017/S10928529000 26614
27. Miller A, Pratt H, Schiffer RB. Pseudobulbar affect: the spectrum of clinical presentations, etiologies and treatments. *Expert Rev Neurotherapeut.* (2011). 11:1077–88. doi: 10.1586/ern.11.68
28. Gallagher JP. Pathologic laughter and crying in ALS: A search for their origin. *Acta Neurol Scand.* (1989). 80:114–7. doi: 10.1111/j.1600-0404.1989.tb03851.x
29. Sauvé WM. Recognizing and treating pseudobulbar affect. *CNS Spectr.* (2016). 21:37–43. doi: 10.1017/S1092852916000791
30. Poeck K. Pathophysiology of emotional disorders associated with brain damage. In: Vinken P, Bruyn G, editors. *Handbook of Clinical Neurology.* Amsterdam (1969). p. 3–343.
31. Choi-Kwon S, Han SW, Kwon SU, Kang DW, Choi JM, Kim JS. Fluoxetine treatment in poststroke depression, emotional incontinence, and anger proneness: a double-blind, placebo-controlled study. *Stroke.* (2006). 37:156–61. doi: 10.1161/01.STR.0000190892.93663.e2
32. Ahmed A, Simmons Z. Pseudobulbar affect: prevalence and management. *Ther Clin Risk Manage.* (2013). 9:483–9. doi: 10.2147/TCRM.S53906
33. Arciniegas DB, Lauterbach EC, Anderson KE, Chow TW, Flashman LA, Hurley RA, et al. The differential diagnosis of pseudobulbar affect (PBA). Distinguishing PBA among disorders of mood and affect. Proceedings of a roundtable meeting. *CNS Spectr.* (2005). 10:1–14; quiz 5–6. doi: 10.1017/S1092852900026602
34. Lochead jD, Maguire GA, Nelson M. *Pseudobulbar Affect Versus Depression: Issues in Diagnosis and Treatment.* Psychiatric Times (2018) p. 35.
35. Adirim ZL, Caga J, Ramsey E, Zoing M, Mioshi E, Kiernan MC, et al. I can't help that i look sad: The experience of emotional lability in the ALS patient and caregiver. *Amyotrop Lateral Scleros Frontotemp Degenerat.* (2015). 16:34. doi: 10.3109/21678421.2015.1089039/0049
36. Calvert T, Knapp P, House A. Psychological associations with emotionalism after stroke. *J Neurol Neurosurg Psychiar.* (1998). 65:928–9. doi: 10.1136/jnnp.65.6.928
37. Iannaccone S, Ferini-Strambi L. Pharmacologic treatment of emotional lability. *Clin Neuropharmacol.* (1996). 19:532–5. doi: 10.1097/00002826-199619060-00008
38. Robinson RG, Parikh RM, Lipsey JR, Starkstein SE, Price TR. Pathological laughing and crying following stroke: validation of a measurement scale and a double-blind treatment study. *Am J Psychiatry.* (1993). 150:286–93. doi: 10.1176/ajp.150.2.286

39. Moore SR, Gresham LS, Bromberg MB, Kasarkis EJ, Smith RA. A self report measure of affective lability. *J Neurol Neurosurg Psychiatry.* (1997). 63:89–93. doi: 10.1136/jnnp.63.1.89
40. Smith RA, Berg JE, Pope LE, Thisted RA. Measuring pseudobulbar affect in ALS. *Amyotrop Lateral Scleros Other Motor Neuron Disord.* (2004). 5:99–102. doi: 10.1080/17434470410020058
41. Hammond FM, Alexander DN, Cutler AJ, D'Amico S, Doody RS, Sauve W, et al. PRISM II: an open-label study to assess effectiveness of dextromethorphan/quinidine for pseudobulbar affect in patients with dementia, stroke or traumatic brain injury. *BMC Neurol.* (2016). 16:89. doi: 10.1186/s12883-016-0609-0
42. Pioro EP, Brooks BR, Cummings J, Schiffer R, Thisted RA, Wynn D, et al. Dextromethorphan plus ultra low-dose quinidine reduces pseudobulbar affect. *Ann Neurol.* (2010). 68:693–702. doi: 10.1002/ana.22093
43. Brooks BR, Thisted RA, Appel SH, Bradley WG, Olney RK, Berg JE, et al. Treatment of pseudobulbar affect in ALS with dextromethorphan/quinidine: a randomized trial. *Neurology.* (2004). 63:1364–70. doi: 10.1212/01.WNL.0000142042.50528.2F
44. Panitch HS, Thisted RA, Smith RA, Wynn DR, Wymer JP, Achiron A, et al. Randomized, controlled trial of dextromethorphan/quinidine for pseudobulbar affect in multiple sclerosis. *Ann Neurol.* (2006). 59:780–7. doi: 10.1002/ana.20828
45. Palmieri A, Abrahams S, Soraru G, Mattiuzzi L, D'Ascenzo C, Pegoraro E, et al. Emotional lability in MND: relationship to cognition and psychopathology and impact on caregivers. *J Neurol Sci.* (2009). 278:16–20. doi: 10.1016/j.jns.2008.10.025
46. Newsom-Davis IC, Abrahams S, Goldstein LH, Leigh PN. The emotional lability questionnaire: a new measure of emotional lability in amyotrophic lateral sclerosis. *J Neurol Sci.* (1999). 169:22–5. doi: 10.1016/S0022-510X(99)00211-7
47. Woolley SC, Moore DH, Katz JS. Insight in ALS: Awareness of behavioral change in patients with and without FTD. *Amyotrop Lateral Scleros.* (2010). 11:52–6. doi: 10.3109/17482960903171110
48. Colamonico J, Formella A, Bradley W. Pseudobulbar affect: burden of illness in the USA. *Adv Ther.* (2012). 29:775–98. doi: 10.1007/s12325-012-0043-7
49. Goldstein LH, Atkins L, Landau S, Brown R, Leigh PN. Predictors of psychological distress in carers of people with amyotrophic lateral sclerosis: a longitudinal study. *Psychol Med.* (2006). 36:865–75. doi: 10.1017/S0033291706007124
50. Murphy J, Duong YN, Ahmed F, Lomen-Hoerth C. A new tool to measure pathological laughing and crying in ALS. *Amyotrop Lateral Scleros.* (2012). 13:165. doi: 10.3109/17482968.2012.721231/303
51. Young C, Aynsley G. ALS symptoms, disability and quality of life: literature review and model generation. *Amyotrop Lateral Scleros Frontotemp Degenerat.* (2014). 15:108–9. doi: 10.3109/21678421.2014.960178/097
52. Trepel M, Weller M, Dichgans J, Petersen D. Voluntary facial palsy with a pontine lesion. *J Neurol Neurosurg Psychiar.* (1996). 61:531–3. doi: 10.1136/jnnp.61.5.531
53. Hopf HC, Muller-Forell W, Hopf NJ. Localization of emotional and volitional facial paresis. *Neurology.* (1992). 42:1918–23. doi: 10.1212/WNL.42.10.1918
54. Parvizi J, Anderson SW, Martin CO, Damasio H, Damasio AR. Pathological laughter and crying: a link to the cerebellum. *Brain.* (2001). 124:1708–19. doi: 10.1093/brain/124.9.1708
55. Schmahmann JD, Sherman JC. The cerebellar cognitive affective syndrome. *Brain.* (1998). 121:561–79. doi: 10.1093/brain/121.4.561
56. Koziol LF, Budding D, Andreasen N, D'Arrigo S, Bulgheroni S, Imamizu H, et al. Consensus paper: the cerebellum's role in movement and cognition. *Cerebellum.* (2014). 13:151–77. doi: 10.1007/s12311-013-0511-x
57. Stoodley CJ, Schmahmann JD. Evidence for topographic organization in the cerebellum of motor control versus cognitive and affective processing. *Cortex.* (2010). 46:831–44. doi: 10.1016/j.cortex.2009.11.008
58. Bede P, Finegan E. Revisiting the pathoanatomy of pseudobulbar affect: mechanisms beyond corticobulbar dysfunction. *Amyotrop Lateral Scleros Frontotemp Degenerat.* (2018). 19:4–6. doi: 10.1080/21678421.2017.1392578
59. Parvizi J, Joseph J, Press DZ, Schmahmann JD. Pathological laughter and crying in patients with multiple system atrophy-cerebellar type. *Mov Disord.* (2007). 22:798–803. doi: 10.1002/mds.21348
60. Chattha PK, Greene PE, Ramdhani RA. Pseudobulbar laughter as a levodopa off phenomenon exacerbated by subthalamic deep brain stimulation. *J Clin Movement Disord.* (2015). 2:13. doi: 10.1186/s40734-015-0023-6
61. Saini M, Mamauag MJ, Singh R. Central pontine myelinolysis: a rare presentation secondary to hyperglycaemia. *Sing Med J.* (2015). 56:e71–3. doi: 10.11622/smedj.2015065
62. Martin AN, Dillon PM, Jones DE, Brenin DR, Lapides DA. Anti-Yo mediated paraneoplastic cerebellar degeneration associated with pseudobulbar affect in a patient with breast cancer. *Case Rep Oncol Med.* (2017). 2017:8120689. doi: 10.1155/2017/8120689
63. Hübers A, Kassubek J, Gron G, Gorges M, Aho-Oezhan H, Keller J, et al. Pathological laughing and crying in amyotrophic lateral sclerosis is related to frontal cortex function. *J Neurol.* (2016). 263:1788–95. doi: 10.1007/s00415-016-8201-5
64. Krack P, Kumar R, Ardouin C, Dowsey PL, McVicker JM, Benabid AL, et al. Mirthful laughter induced by subthalamic nucleus stimulation. *Movement Disord.* (2001). 16:867–75. doi: 10.1002/mds.1174
65. Okun MS, Heilman KM, Vitek JL. Treatment of pseudobulbar laughter after gamma knife thalamotomy. *Movement Disord.* (2002). 17:622–4. doi: 10.1002/mds.10174
66. Okun MS, Raju DV, Walter BL, Juncos JL, DeLong MR, Heilman K, et al. Pseudobulbar crying induced by stimulation in the region of the subthalamic nucleus. *J Neurol Neurosurg Psychiar.* (2004). 75:921–3. doi: 10.1136/jnnp.2003.016485
67. Famularo G, Corsi FM, Minisola G, De Simone C, Nicotra GC. Cerebellar tumour presenting with pathological laughter and gelastic syncope. *Eur J Neurol.* (2007). 14:940–3. doi: 10.1111/j.1468-1331.2007.01784.x
68. Low HL, Sayer FT, Honey CR. Pathological crying caused by high-frequency stimulation in the region of the caudal internal capsule. *Arch Neurol.* (2008). 65:264–6. doi: 10.1001/archneurol.2007.53
69. Wolf ME, Abdallat M, Blahak C, Krauss JK. Pathological crying induced by deep brain stimulation of the subthalamic nucleus in Parkinson's disease. *J Clin Neurosci.*(2017) 45:159–61. doi: 10.1016/j.jocn.2017.08.020
70. Andersen G, Ingeman-Nielsen M, Vestergaard K, Riis JO. Pathoanatomic correlation between poststroke pathological crying and damage to brain areas involved in serotonergic neurotransmission. *Stroke.* (1994). 25:1050–2. doi: 10.1161/01.STR.25.5.1050
71. Murai T, Barthel H, Berrouschot J, Sorger D, von Cramon DY, Muller U. Neuroimaging of serotonin transporters in post-stroke pathological crying. *Psychiatry Res.* (2003). 123:207–11. doi: 10.1016/S0925-4927(03)00065-9
72. Tateno A, Jorge RE, Robinson RG. Pathological Laughing and Crying Following Traumatic Brain Injury. *J Neuropsychiatry Clin Neurosci.* (2004). 16:426–34. doi: 10.1176/jnp.16.4.426
73. Christidi F, Karavasilis E, Ferentinos P, Xirou S, Velonakis G, Rentzos M, et al. Investigating the neuroanatomical substrate of pathological laughing and crying in amyotrophic lateral sclerosis with multimodal neuroimaging techniques. *Amyotrop Lateral Scleros Frontotemp Degenerat.* (2018). 19:12–20. doi: 10.1080/21678421.2017.1386689
74. Hornung JP. The human raphe nuclei and the serotonergic system. *J Chem Neuroanat.* (2003). 26:331–43. doi: 10.1016/j.jchemneu.2003.10.002
75. Formella A, Work S, Colamonico J, Kaye R. Use of antidepressants and atypical antipsychotics in patients with pseudobulbar affect. *J Manag Care Pharm.* (2011). 17:271.
76. Kerr CW, Bishop GA. Topographical organization in the origin of serotoninergic projections to different regions of the cat cerebellar cortex. *J Comparat Neurol.* (1991). 304:502–15. doi: 10.1002/cne.903040313
77. Bishop GA, Ho RH. The distribution and origin of serotonin immunoreactivity in the rat cerebellum. *Brain Res.* (1985). 331:195–207. doi: 10.1016/0006-8993(85)91545-8
78. Parvizi J, Coburn KL, Shillcutt SD, Coffey CE, Lauterbach EC, Mendez MF. Neuroanatomy of pathological laughing and crying: a report of the American Neuropsychiatric Association Committee on Research. *J Neuropsychiatry Clin Neurosci.* (2009). 21:75–87. doi: 10.1176/jnp.2009.21.1.75

79. Haiman G, Pratt H, Miller A. Brain responses to verbal stimuli among multiple sclerosis patients with pseudobulbar affect. *J Neurol Sci.* (2008). 271:137–47. doi: 10.1016/j.jns.2008.04.017
80. Holtzman T, Rajapaksa T, Mostofi A, Edgley SA. Different responses of rat cerebellar Purkinje cells and Golgi cells evoked by widespread convergent sensory inputs. *J Physiol.* (2006). 574:491–507. doi: 10.1113/jphysiol.2006.108282
81. Pollack IF, Polinko P, Albright AL, Towbin R, Fitz C. Mutism and pseudobulbar symptoms after resection of posterior fossa tumors in children. incidence and pathophysiology. *Neurosurgery.* (1995). 37:885–93. doi: 10.1227/00006123-199511000-00006
82. Abrahams S, Goldstein LH, Al-Chalabi A, Pickering A, Morris RG, Passingham RE, et al. Relation between cognitive dysfunction and pseudobulbar palsy in amyotrophic lateral sclerosis (1997). 62:464–72.
83. Bede P, Bokde A, Elamin M, Byrne S, McLaughlin RL, Jordan N, et al. Grey matter correlates of clinical variables in amyotrophic lateral sclerosis (ALS): a neuroimaging study of ALS motor phenotype heterogeneity and cortical focality. *J Neurol Neurosurg Psychiar.* (2013). 84:766–73. doi: 10.1136/jnnp-2012-302674
84. Bede P, Bokde AL, Byrne S, Elamin M, McLaughlin RL, Kenna K, et al. Multiparametric MRI study of ALS stratified for the C9orf72 genotype. *Neurology.* (2013). 81:361–9. doi: 10.1212/WNL.0b013e31829c5eee
85. Abrahams S, Goldstein LH, Simmons A, Brammer M, Williams SCR, Giampietro V, et al. Word retrieval in amyotrophic lateral sclerosis: a functional magnetic resonance imaging study. *Brain.* (2004). 127:1507–17. doi: 10.1093/Brain/Awh170.
86. Agosta F, Canu E, Valsasina P, Riva N, Prelle A, Comi G, et al. Divergent brain network connectivity in amyotrophic lateral sclerosis. *Neurobiol. Aging.* (2013). 34:419–27. doi: 10.1016/j.neurobiolaging.2012.04.015
87. Bede P, Hardiman O. Lessons of ALS imaging: pitfalls and future directions — a critical review. *NeuroImage.* (2014) 4:436–43. doi: 10.1016/j.nicl.2014.02.011
88. Bede P, Querin G, Pradat PF. The changing landscape of motor neuron disease imaging: the transition from descriptive studies to precision clinical tools. *Curr Opin Neurol.* (2018). 31:431–8. doi: 10.1097/WCO.0000000000000569
89. Bede P, Elamin M, Byrne S, McLaughlin RL, Kenna K, Vajda A, et al. Patterns of cerebral and cerebellar white matter degeneration in ALS. *J Neurol Neurosurg Psychiar.* (2015). 86:468–70. doi: 10.1136/jnnp-2014-308172
90. Prell T, Grosskreutz J. The involvement of the cerebellum in amyotrophic lateral sclerosis. *Amyotrop Lateral Scleros Frontotemp Degenerat.* (2013). 14:507–15. doi: 10.3109/21678421.2013.812661
91. Al-Sarraj S, King A, Troakes C, Smith B, Maekawa S, Bodi I, et al. p62 positive, TDP-43 negative, neuronal cytoplasmic and intranuclear inclusions in the cerebellum and hippocampus define the pathology of C9orf72-linked FTLD and MND/ALS. *Acta Neuropathol.* (2011). 122:691–702. doi: 10.1007/s00401-011-0911-2
92. Andersen G, Vestergaard K, Riis JO. Citalopram for post-stroke pathological crying. *Lancet.* (1993). 342:837–9. doi: 10.1016/0140-6736(93)92696-Q
93. Burns A, Russell E, Stratton-Powell H, Tyrell P, O'Neill P, Baldwin R. Sertraline in stroke-associated lability of mood. *Int J Geriatr Psychiatry.* (1999). 14:681–5.
94. Szczudlik A, Slowik A, Tomik B. [The effect of amitriptyline on the pathological crying and other pseudobulbar signs]. *Neurol Neurochirurg Polska.* (1995). 29:663–74.
95. Ferentinos P, Paparrigopoulos T, Rentzos M, Zouvelou V, Evdokimidis I. Duloxetine for pathological laughing and crying in amyotrophic lateral sclerosis. *Eur Neuropsychopharmacol.* (2009). 19:S409. doi: 10.1016/S0924-977X(09)70632-7
96. Prokšelj T, Jerin A, Kogoj A. Memantine may affect pseudobulbar affect in patients with Alzheimer's disease. *Acta Neuropsychiatr.* (2013). 25:361–6. doi: 10.1017/neu.2013.14
97. Kim SW, Shin IS, Kim JM, Lim SY, Yang SJ, Yoon JS. Mirtazapine treatment for pathological laughing and crying after stroke.*Clin Neuropharmacol.* (2005). 28:249–51. doi: 10.1097/01.wnf.0000185825.34819.ba
98. Hackett ML YM, Anderson CS, Horrocks JA, House A. Pharmaceutical interventions for emotionalism after stroke 2010. *Cochrane Database Syst Rev.* (2010) 17:CD003690. doi: 10.1002/14651858.CD003690.pub3
99. Smith RA. Dectromethorphan/quinidine: a novel dextromethorphan product for the treatment of emotional lability. *Expert Opin Pharmacother.* (2006). 7:2581–98. doi: 10.1517/14656566.7.18.2581
100. Rosen H. Dextromethorphan/quinidine sulfate for pseudobulbar affect. *Drugs Today.* (2008). 44:661–8. doi: 10.1358/dot.2008.44.9.1258664
101. Zhang Y, Britto MR, Valderhaug KL, Wedlund PJ, Smith RA. Dextromethorphan: enhancing its systemic availability by way of low-dose quinidine-mediated inhibition of cytochrome P4502D6. *Clin Pharmacol Ther.* (1992). 51:647–55. doi: 10.1038/clpt.1992.77
102. Smith RA, Brooks BR. Treatment of pseudobulbar affect in ALS. *Lancet Neurol.* (2005). 4:270. doi: 10.1016/S1474-4422(05)70058-2
103. Brooks B, Cummings J, Pioro E, Schiffer R, Wynn D, Hepner A. Pharmacokinetic/pharmacodynamic modeling of dextromethorphan/quinidine for a study in pseudobulbar affect. *Ann Neurol.* (2008). 64:S38–S. doi: 10.1002/ana.21502
104. Gaedigk A, Sangkuhl K, Whirl-Carrillo M, Klein T, Leeder JS. Prediction of CYP2D6 phenotype from genotype across world populations. *Genet Med.* (2016). 19:69. doi: 10.1038/gim.2016.80
105. Katz J. AVP-39: a successful randomized clinical trial on a supportive therapy for ALS. *Neurology.* (2004). 63:1345. doi: 10.1212/01.WNL.0000145385.55983.1E
106. Pioro E, Brooks B, Cummings J, Schiffer R, Wynn D, Hepner A, et al. Persistent efficacy of dextromethorphan (DM)/Quinidine (Q) for pseudobulbar affect (PBA): Results from a 12-Week, open-label extension (OLE) study. *Neurology.* (2010). 75:380. doi: 10.1212/WNL.0b013e3181e6e52d
107. Schoedel KA, Morrow SA, Sellers EM. Evaluating the safety and efficacy of dextromethorphan/quinidine in the treatment of pseudobulbar affect. *Neuropsychiatr Dis Treatment.* (2014). 10:1161–74. doi: 10.2147/NDT.S30713
108. Cruz MP. Nuedexta for the treatment of pseudobulbar affect: a condition of involuntary crying or laughing. *PT.* (2013). 38:325–8.
109. European Medicines Agency. *The Marketing Authorisation for Nuedexta has Been Withdrawn at the Request of the Marketing-Authorisation Holder 2016.* [30/10/2018]. Available online at: https://www.ema.europa.eu/en/medicines/human/EPAR/nuedexta#overview-section.
110. Motor Neurone Disease Association. *Neudexta; Withdrawal of Marketing Authorisation Mndassociation.org* Available online at: https://www.mndassociation.org/research/mnd-research-and-you/research-into-treatments/nuedexta/ (Accessed October 15, 2018).
111. Ng L KF, Young CA, Galea M. Symptomatic treatments for amyotrophic lateral sclerosis/motor neuron disease 2017. *Cochrane Database Syst Rev.* (2017) 1:CD011776. doi: 10.1002/14651858.CD011776.pub2
112. Wicks P, Frost J. ALS patients request more information about cognitive symptoms. *Eur J Neurol.* (2008). 15:497–500. doi: 10.1111/j.1468-1331.2008.02107.x

17

Lipid Biomarkers for Amyotrophic Lateral Sclerosis

Jose-Luis González De Aguilar [1,2*]

[1] *Université de Strasbourg, UMR_S1118, Strasbourg, France,*

[2] *INSERM, U1118, Mécanismes Centraux et Périphériques de la Neurodégénerescence, Strasbourg, France*

***Correspondence:**
Jose-Luis González De Aguilar
gonzalez@unistra.fr

Amyotrophic lateral sclerosis (ALS) is a fatal degenerative disease primarily characterized by the selective loss of upper and lower motor neurons. To date, there is still an unmet need for robust and practical biomarkers that could estimate the risk of the disease and its progression. Based on metabolic modifications observed at the level of the whole body, different classes of lipids have been proposed as potential biomarkers. This review summarizes investigations carried out over the last decade that focused on changes in three major lipid species, namely cholesterol, triglycerides and fatty acids. Despite some contradictory findings, it is becoming increasingly accepted that dyslipidemia, and related aberrant energy homeostasis, must be considered as essential components of the pathological process. Therefore, it is tempting to envisage dietary interventions as a means to counterbalance the metabolic disturbances and ameliorate the patient's quality of life.

Keywords: amyotrophic lateral sclerosis, biomarker, cholesterol, fatty acid, triglyceride

ALS AND THE NEED FOR BIOMARKERS

Amyotrophic lateral sclerosis (ALS) is a degenerative disease of upper and lower motor neurons mainly characterized by progressive muscle wasting, fasciculations, dysarthria, dysphagia, altered reflexes, and spasticity. It affects about 2 per 100,000 people per year, and usually appears at 40–70 years of age. A significant proportion of cases also presents cognitive or behavioral abnormalities typical of frontotemporal dementia (FTD). The etiology of ALS still remains elusive. About 90% of cases are considered as sporadic. The remaining 10% are inherited mostly in an autosomal dominant manner. Most familial cases can be explained by mutations in four major genes, including *C9ORF72*, *SOD1*, *FUS*, and *TARDBP*. Based on this genetic diversity, multiple pathogenic mechanisms have been implicated in triggering motor neuron degeneration, adding considerable complexity to the understanding of the disease (1).

From a clinical point of view, ALS is easily recognized in its full-blown presentation. However, the diagnostic process may be challenging at very early stages. The diagnosis is based on clinical examination, electrophysiological findings, medical history, and exclusion of confounding disorders. In practice, a correct diagnosis may take as long as 1 year (2). Moreover, disease progression is very heterogeneous. Death may occur between 1 and 5 years after diagnosis, but 20% of patients live longer than 5 years, and 10% survive for more than 10 years (3). Promising biomarkers of diagnosis and prognosis have been proposed based on advanced neurophysiological and neuroimaging techniques. However, many of these practices still lack validation and standardization between clinical centers, and they have been applied only to small cohorts of patients [(4–6), and references therein].

As far as molecular biomarkers are concerned, a great number of molecules have been isolated from patient material, including cerebrospinal fluid, blood and tissues, that recognized and/or monitored ALS with more or less accuracy [(7, 8), and references therein]. To date, changes in the amounts of neurofilament proteins found in cerebrospinal fluid and blood have been postulated as the most promising candidates [(9), and references therein]. However, these and other proposed molecular markers have not reached routine clinical application. Therefore, there is still an incontestable lack of robust and practical biomarkers that could facilitate an earlier diagnosis and improve the prognosis of ALS.

ALTERED ENERGY HOMEOSTASIS AND LIPID METABOLISM IN ALS

Amyotrophic lateral sclerosis was classically attributed to an intrinsic defect of upper and lower motor neurons. Now it is generally accepted that non-neuronal cells surrounding motor neurons, additional neuronal cell types, as well as other cells outside the nervous system participate actively in the pathological process [(10–12), and references therein]. In particular, compelling evidence has emerged over the last decade showing a characteristic imbalance between energy intake and consumption, which is associated with metabolic alterations at the level of the whole body of yet unexplained etiology [(13), and references therein]. Seminal studies revealed that many ALS patients show an increase in energy expenditure, or hypermetabolism, which could account, at least in part, for the decline of their nutritional status (14, 15). It was also recently reported that hypermetabolic patients have a worse prognosis than normometabolic ones (16), which could be related to a detrimental weight loss. In fact, patients that lost more than 5% of body mass at the time of diagnosis had an increased risk of death (17). In addition, a lower body mass index appeared to precede the symptomatic stage of the disease (18). Overall, these studies strongly support that the energy imbalance in ALS could contribute to the rapid deterioration of the patients.

The origin of the hypermetabolism in ALS is currently unknown, although recent studies have pointed to the altered function of hypothalamic neurons involved in the regulation of food intake and energy homeostasis (19, 20). From a therapeutic point of view, pioneering preclinical studies conducted on an ALS mouse model, which carries a mutation in the *Sod1* gene, provided part of the answer to this question. An increase in energy consumption occurs in these mice well-before the onset of the first motor symptoms. This is accompanied by a reduction of adiposity and lower levels of circulating leptin. Most importantly, these studies revealed that sustaining the hypermetabolic rate of ALS mice with a highly-energetic high-fat diet partially protected motor neurons and extended lifespan (21). Likewise, a higher premorbid intake of high-fat food was observed in ALS patients (18). Moreover, a moderate increase in fat mass over the course of the disease was associated with a decreased risk of death, and increasing circulating levels of leptin were positively associated with longer survival (17, 22). Although there is no conclusive evidence of a mechanistic link between the hypermetabolism present in ALS and altered levels of lipids, altogether, these studies suggest that the utilization of lipids as energy substrates could offer benefit, by counteracting an increased metabolic rate and compensating the associated weight loss. In this respect, several pilot studies reported positive effects of highly caloric fat supplements on ALS patients (23, 24). It was also shown that the administration of acetyl-L-carnitine, which supports the transport of fatty acids into mitochondria for being used as energy substrates, retarded the worsening of the patients (25). Recent research has made efforts to identify specific changes in lipid metabolism that could provide clues for future nutritional interventions, as well as serve as robust biomarkers for the disease. This review covers some of the most significant findings published during the last decade.

APOLIPOPROTEIN E AND THE RISK OF ALS

Apolipoprotein E (APOE) is a constituent of lipoprotein particles primarily involved in the transport of triglycerides and their clearance from the bloodstream. It is mainly synthesized in the liver but it is also produced by astrocytes in the brain, where APOE is the most important cholesterol carrier. The human *APOE* gene exists as three major alleles called ε2, ε3, and ε4. The identification of *APOE* ε4 as a risk factor for Alzheimer's disease represented a major breakthrough in the field [(26), and references therein]. On the contrary, most studies on ALS did not observe any association of *APOE* ε4 with an increased risk (27–30), excepted some recent findings (31). Additional reports showed complex interactions between particular *APOE* alleles and other genetic or physiopathological variables. Penco and collaborators identified a combination of seven genetic variants, inluding one affecting *APOE*, that distinguished between ALS patients and control subjects (32). It was also found that individuals who had suffered from head trauma in the adulthood were more prone to have ALS, and this association was stronger in the presence of *APOE* ε4 (33). In contrast, the frequency of *APOE* ε2, which is *a priori* neuroprotective, was higher in ALS patients that had practiced sport regularly (30). *APOE* ε2 also increased the risk of developing FTD in a cohort of patients with ALS (34). It must be noted, however, that the implication of *APOE* in the incidence of this form of dementia is rather controversial. The increase in the probability of having FTD was associated with *APOE* ε2 in some cases, and with *APOE* ε4 in other cases [(35), and references therein].

The influence of *APOE* on the course of ALS has also been contradictory. Initial reports revealed that *APOE* ε4 was associated with earlier age at onset but not with disease duration (27). However, follow-up studies failed to show any relationship between *APOE* ε4 and age at onset or rate of progression, although this allele was more frequent in men with bulbar-onset ALS (28). Parallel investigations did not find any association between the *APOE* genotype and age of onset, site of onset, rate of progression, cognitive impairment or survival (36). Overall, the implication of *APOE* in the incidence and progression of ALS is therefore not clearly established.

THE INTRIGUING CASE OF CHOLESTEROL

Cholesterol is an essential lipid molecule, which is transported through the bloodstream by several types of lipoprotein particles. In clinical practice, increased levels of total cholesterol or low-density lipoprotein cholesterol (LDL-c), in combination with decreased levels of high-density lipoprotein cholesterol (HDL-c), are indicative of a higher risk of atherosclerotic cardiovascular disease. In the case of ALS, hypercholesterolemia, as detected prior to the onset of motor symptoms, was initially associated with a lower risk (37). However, follow-up studies contradicted these findings. An increase in the premorbid intake of cholesterol was associated with a higher incidence of the disease, as shown after examination of dietary habits obtained from food frequency questionnaires (18). In addition, individuals with increased levels of LDL-c and a higher LDL-c/HDL-c ratio were more prone to develop ALS later (38). Finally, the analysis of GWAS databases revealed that particular alleles predisposing to elevated levels of LDL-c and total cholesterol appeared associated with an increased risk (39).

In many studies, the proportion of hypercholesterolemia individuals or the average contents of total cholesterol and LDL-c were shown to be higher in the ALS population and, in some cases, this increase was noticeable at the time of diagnosis (40–44). In agreement with these findings, a detailed analysis of circulating lipoprotein particles also showed increased levels of LDL-1, which is a LDL subfraction very enriched in cholesterol (44). Other reports, however, did not find clear-cut differences (45–48), or even revealed opposite results (49).

From a prognostic point of view, decreased levels of total cholesterol or LDL-c and a lower LDL-c/HDL-c ratio were associated with a severe respiratory impairment (42, 45). Contrasting with these findings, Delaye and collaborators did not observe any association between several cholesterol parameters and disease progression (44). Yet, most authors agree that hypercholesterolemia, present as elevated levels of total cholesterol and LDL-c or a higher LDL-c/HDL-c ratio, associates with longer survival. This association, however, did not reach significance after adjusting for potential confounding demographic and clinical factors (37, 40, 43, 49–51).

In addition to the biomarker potential of cholesterol *per se*, a few studies have focused on the implication of oxysterols, which are oxidized derivatives mainly involved in maintaining cholesterol homeostasis. Levels of several oxysterol metabolites, including 27-hydroxycholesterol, 24-hydroxycholesterol esters, and 3β,7α-dihydroxycholest-5-en-26-oic acid and other related compounds, were shown to be lower in ALS patients. These changes were detected in blood or cerebrospinal fluid, or both, and they were attributed to a deficit in the metabolism of excess cholesterol, which would result in subsequent toxicity in the brain (46, 52, 53). On the other hand, additional studies reported increased levels of 25-hydroxycholesterol in cerebrospinal fluid and serum of ALS patients. The accumulation of this toxic oxysterol derivative was associated, at least in serum, with a higher rate of disease progression (54).

THE ENERGIZING TRIGLYCERIDES IN ALS

Triglycerides are a primary source of energy for the body but, when accumulated in an excessive manner, they represent an important risk factor for cardiovascular disease. Triglyceride contents should be expected to change in ALS patients according to their characteristic high rate of energy expenditure. In this respect, the proportion of hypertriglyceridemia individuals was more important among ALS patients than in the normal population (55). Hypertriglyceridemia was also found in ALS women (42), and higher triglyceride levels were associated with a better functional status (48). Other reports, however, failed to reproduce these findings (40, 47, 48). Moreover, Blasco and collaborators identified a lipidomic signature in the cerebrospinal fluid of ALS patients, in which certain triglyceride species were found reduced at levels associated with a better prognosis (56). Finally, as in the case of cholesterol, hypertriglyceridemia was associated with longer survival, but this association appeared to have no effect after adjusting for confounding factors (47, 55).

THE ENTRANCE OF FATTY ACIDS ON STAGE

Fatty acids are lipid molecules key for sustaining the structural integrity of cell membranes, providing energy and serving in signaling pathways. They can be mainly transported through the bloodstream attached to a glycerol molecule (that is, in the form of triglycerides) or as non-esterified free fatty acids. The studies relating to the implication of fatty acids as biomarkers for ALS are scarce. Based on food frequency questionnaires, Fitzgerald and collaborators showed that a higher intake of ω3 polyunsaturated fatty acids, which are considered as neuroprotective factors, were associated with a reduced risk of ALS (57). Similar studies did not find the same association but rather reported a higher premorbid intake of *trans*- and saturated fatty acids associated with an increased risk (18). On average, the proportion of polyunsaturated fatty acids in the lipid fraction of clotted blood was decreased in ALS patients while that of monounsaturated fatty acids was concomitantly increased (58). Polyunsaturated fatty acids were also lower in the free fatty acid fraction of plasma (59). Finally, a higher palmitoleic/palmitic fatty acid ratio, indicative of increased adiposity, correlated with a better functional status, and was associated with longer survival (58).

CONCLUSION

Over the last decade, many lipid molecules have been proposed as promising biomarkers for ALS, but none of them has been translated into effective tools in clinical practice. There are several issues of concern that still need to be addressed. On the one hand, the etiology of ALS is multifactorial, and it is likely that the pathological process in subpopulations of patients, with different genetic and environmental backgrounds, is not the same. In the future, the use of cohorts of well-defined patients should improve statistical robustness. It would also be interesting to compare between patients with ALS and other patients suffering from mimic conditions. On the other hand, lipid changes at the level of the whole body can be affected by a myriad of factors, including genetic, nutritional, physical and pathological factors, which can introduce bias on the results. It is also noteworthy to mention that for those studies that used food frequency questionnaires to estimate food preferences and evaluate eating behavior, they depend, at least in part, on their interpretation probing the patient's perception of food intake, hence lacking sensitivity and objectiveness. Therefore, protocols and measurements need to be standardized between study centers.

Despite some conflicting findings, most studies presented in this review show important alterations of the circulating contents of cholesterol (and related lipoprotein particles), triglycerides and fatty acids, which occur prior to and over the course of ALS. These changes seem to reflect a metabolic environment, which would be appropriate to meet the high energy demands imposed by the increased metabolic rate present in the disease. The understanding of the mechanisms underlying this "low-grade dyslipidemia" is still insufficient but, from a clinical point of view, it leaves open the possibility for therapeutic nutritional intervention. In this respect, recent studies that analyzed the eating behavior of ALS patients revealed marked modifications in their food preferences. In particular, an increase in the intake of saturated fat and meat protein was associated with longer survival (60–62). Moreover, two clinical trials have been initiated, which aim at retarding disease progression by using high-caloric food supplements. The first trial (NCT02306590) is a randomized, parallel-group, double-blind study that compares between placebo and a treatment consisting of a high caloric fatty diet, which is equivalent to an additional intake of 45 g fat per day. The primary objective of this study is to evaluate the impact on survival. The second trial is a randomized, parallel-group, open label study that will determine the effects of a high-protein, high-energy supplement on the functional status of newly diagnosed ALS patients (NCT02152449). The results of these trials as well as the ongoing research on lipid biomarkers and on the understanding of their implication in ALS will certainly pave the way for developing new therapeutic tools.

AUTHOR CONTRIBUTIONS

The author confirms being the sole contributor of this work and has approved it for publication.

FUNDING

J-LG received funds from Association pour la Recherche sur la Sclérose Latérale Amyotrophique et autres Maladies du Motoneurone (ARSLA).

REFERENCES

1. van Es MA, Hardiman O, Chio A, Al-Chalabi A, Pasterkamp RJ, Veldink JH, et al. Amyotrophic lateral sclerosis. *Lancet.* (2017) 390:2084–98. doi: 10.1016/S0140-6736(17)31287-4
2. Cellura E, Spataro R, Taiello AC, La Bella V. Factors affecting the diagnostic delay in amyotrophic lateral sclerosis. *Clin Neurol Neurosurg.* (2012) 114:550–4. doi: 10.1016/j.clineuro.2011.11.026
3. Pupillo E, Messina P, Logroscino G, Beghi E, SLALOM Group. Long-term survival in amyotrophic lateral sclerosis: a population-based study. *Ann Neurol.* (2014) 75:287–97. doi: 10.1002/ana.24096
4. Vucic S, Ziemann U, Eisen A, Hallett M, Kiernan MC. Transcranial magnetic stimulation and amyotrophic lateral sclerosis: pathophysiological insights. *J Neurol Neurosurg Psychiatr.* (2013) 84:1161–70. doi: 10.1136/jnnp-2012-304019
5. Bede P, Hardiman O. Lessons of ALS imaging: pitfalls and future directions - a critical review. *Neuroimage Clin.* (2014) 4:436–43. doi: 10.1016/j.nicl.2014.02.011
6. Fatehi F, Grapperon AM, Fathi D, Delmont E, Attarian S. The utility of motor unit number index: a systematic review. *Neurophysiol Clin.* (2018) 48:251–9. doi: 10.1016/j.neucli.2018.09.001
7. Robelin L, Gonzalez De Aguilar JL. Blood biomarkers for amyotrophic lateral sclerosis: myth or reality? *Biomed Res Int.* (2014) 2014:525097. doi: 10.1155/2014/525097
8. Costa J, de Carvalho M. Emerging molecular biomarker targets for amyotrophic lateral sclerosis. *Clin Chim Acta.* (2016) 455:7–14. doi: 10.1016/j.cca.2016.01.011
9. Xu Z, Henderson RD, David M, McCombe PA. Neurofilaments as biomarkers for amyotrophic lateral sclerosis: a systematic review and meta-analysis. *PLoS ONE.* (2016) 11:e0164625. doi: 10.1371/journal.pone.0164625
10. Braak H, Brettschneider J, Ludolph AC, Lee VM, Trojanowski JQ, Del Tredici K. Amyotrophic lateral sclerosis - a model of corticofugal axonal spread. *Nat Rev Neurol.* (2013) 9:708–14. doi: 10.1038/nrneurol.2013.221
11. Lee J, Hyeon SJ, Im H, Ryu H, Kim Y, Ryu H. Astrocytes and microglia as non-cell autonomous players in the pathogenesis of ALS. *Exp Neurobiol.* (2016) 25:233–40. doi: 10.5607/en.2016.25.5.233
12. Loeffler JP, Picchiarelli G, Dupuis L, Gonzalez De Aguilar JL. The role of skeletal muscle in amyotrophic lateral sclerosis. *Brain Pathol.* (2016) 26:227–36. doi: 10.1111/bpa.12350
13. Dupuis L, Pradat PF, Ludolph AC, Loeffler JP. Energy metabolism in amyotrophic lateral sclerosis. *Lancet Neurol.* (2011) 10:75–82. doi: 10.1016/S1474-4422(10)70224-6
14. Desport JC, Preux PM, Magy L, Boirie Y, Vallat JM, Beaufrère B, et al. Factors correlated with hypermetabolism in patients with amyotrophic lateral sclerosis. *Am J Clin Nutr.* (2001) 74:328–34. doi: 10.1093/ajcn/74.3.328
15. Bouteloup C, Desport JC, Clavelou P, Guy N, Derumeaux-Burel H, Ferrier A, et al. Hypermetabolism in ALS patients: an early and persistent phenomenon. *J Neurol.* (2009) 256:1236–42. doi: 10.1007/s00415-009-5100-z
16. Jésus P, Fayemendy P, Nicol M, Lautrette G, Sourisseau H, Preux PM, et al. Hypermetabolism is a deleterious prognostic factor in patients with amyotrophic lateral sclerosis. *Eur J Neurol.* (2018) 25:97–104. doi: 10.1111/ene.13468
17. Marin B, Desport JC, Kajeu P, Jesus P, Nicolaud B, Nicol M, et al. Alteration of nutritional status at diagnosis is a prognostic factor for survival of amyotrophic lateral sclerosis patients. *J Neurol Neurosurg Psychiatr.* (2011) 82:628–34. doi: 10.1136/jnnp.2010.211474
18. Huisman MH, Seelen M, van Doormaal PT, de Jong SW, de Vries JH, van der Kooi AJ, et al. Effect of presymptomatic body mass index and consumption of fat and alcohol on amyotrophic lateral sclerosis. *JAMA Neurol.* (2015) 72:1155–62. doi: 10.1001/jamaneurol.2015.1584
19. Vercruysse P, Sinniger J, El Oussini H, Scekic-Zahirovic J, Dieterlé S, Dengler R, et al. Alterations in the hypothalamic melanocortin pathway in amyotrophic lateral sclerosis. *Brain.* (2016) 139:1106–22. doi: 10.1093/brain/aww004
20. Gorges M, Vercruysse P, Müller HP, Huppertz HJ, Rosenbohm A, Nagel G, et al. Hypothalamic atrophy is related to body mass index and age at

onset in amyotrophic lateral sclerosis. *J Neurol Neurosurg Psychiatr.* (2017) 88:1033–41. doi: 10.1136/jnnp-2017-315795

21. Dupuis L, Oudart H, René F, Gonzalez de Aguilar JL, Loeffler JP. Evidence for defective energy homeostasis in amyotrophic lateral sclerosis: benefit of a high-energy diet in a transgenic mouse model. *Proc Natl Acad Sci USA.* (2004) 101:11159–64. doi: 10.1073/pnas.0402026101
22. Nagel G, Peter RS, Rosenbohm A, Koenig W, Dupuis L, Rothenbacher D, et al. Adipokines, C-reactive protein and Amyotrophic Lateral Sclerosis - results from a population- based ALS registry in Germany. *Sci Rep.* (2017) 7:4374. doi: 10.1038/s41598-017-04706-5
23. Dorst J, Cypionka J, Ludolph AC. High-caloric food supplements in the treatment of amyotrophic lateral sclerosis: a prospective interventional study. *Amyotroph Lateral Scler Frontotemporal Degener.* (2013) 14:533–6. doi: 10.3109/21678421.2013.823999
24. Wills AM, Hubbard J, Macklin EA, Glass J, Tandan R, Simpson EP, et al. Hypercaloric enteral nutrition in patients with amyotrophic lateral sclerosis: a randomised, double-blind, placebo-controlled phase 2 trial. *Lancet.* (2014) 383:2065–72. doi: 10.1016/S0140-6736(14)60222-1
25. Beghi E, Pupillo E, Bonito V, Buzzi P, Caponnetto C, Chiò A, et al. Randomized double-blind placebo-controlled trial of acetyl-L-carnitine for ALS. *Amyotroph Lateral Scler Frontotemporal Degener.* (2013) 14:397–405. doi: 10.3109/21678421.2013.764568
26. Yu JT, Tan L, Hardy J. Apolipoprotein E in Alzheimer's disease: an update. *Annu Rev Neurosci.* (2014) 37:79–100. doi: 10.1146/annurev-neuro-071013-014300
27. Zetterberg H, Jacobsson J, Rosengren L, Blennow K, Andersen PM. Association of APOE with age at onset of sporadic amyotrophic lateral sclerosis. *J Neurol Sci.* (2008) 273:67–9. doi: 10.1016/j.jns.2008.06.025
28. Praline J, Blasco H, Vourc'h P, Garrigue MA, Gordon PH, Camu W, et al. APOE ε4 allele is associated with an increased risk of bulbar-onset amyotrophic lateral sclerosis in men. *Eur J Neurol.* (2011) 18:1046–52. doi: 10.1111/j.1468-1331.2010.03330.x
29. Govone F, Vacca A, Rubino E, Gai A, Boschi S, Gentile S, et al. Lack of association between APOE gene polymorphisms and amyotrophic lateral sclerosis: a comprehensive meta-analysis. *Amyotroph Lateral Scler Frontotemporal Degener.* (2014) 15:551–6. doi: 10.3109/21678421.2014.918149
30. Albani D, Pupillo E, Bianchi E, Chierchia A, Martines R, Forloni G, et al. The role of single-nucleotide variants of the energy metabolism-linked genes SIRT3, PPARGC1A and APOE in amyotrophic lateral sclerosis risk. *Genes Genet Syst.* (2016) 91:301–9. doi: 10.1266/ggs.16-00023
31. De Benedetti S, Gianazza E, Banfi C, Marocchi A, Lunetta C, Penco S, et al. Serum proteome in a sporadic amyotrophic lateral sclerosis geographical cluster. *Proteomics Clin Appl.* (2017) 11, 1–7 doi: 10.1002/prca.201700043
32. Penco S, Buscema M, Patrosso MC, Marocchi A, Grossi E. New application of intelligent agents in sporadic amyotrophic lateral sclerosis identifies unexpected specific genetic background. *BMC Bioinformatics.* (2008) 9:254. doi: 10.1186/1471-2105-9-254
33. Schmidt S, Kwee LC, Allen KD, Oddone EZ. Association of ALS with head injury, cigarette smoking and APOE genotypes. *J Neurol Sci.* (2010) 291:22–9. doi: 10.1016/j.jns.2010.01.011
34. Chiò A, Brunetti M, Barberis M, Iazzolino B, Montuschi A, Ilardi A, et al. The role of APOE in the occurrence of frontotemporal dementia in amyotrophic lateral sclerosis. *JAMA Neurol.* (2016) 73:425–30. doi: 10.1001/jamaneurol.2015.4773
35. Su WH, Shi ZH, Liu SL, Wang XD, Liu S, Ji Y. Updated meta-analysis of the role of APOE ε2/ε3/ε4 alleles in frontotemporal lobar degeneration. *Oncotarget.* (2017) 8:43721–32. doi: 10.18632/oncotarget.17341
36. Jawaid A, Poon M, Strutt AM, Rice LK, McDowell EJ, Salamone AR, et al. Does apolipoprotein E genotype modify the clinical expression of ALS? *Eur J Neurol.* (2011) 18:618–24. doi: 10.1111/j.1468-1331.2010.03225.x
37. Seelen M, van Doormaal PT, Visser AE, Huisman MH, Roozekrans MH, de Jong SW, et al. Prior medical conditions and the risk of amyotrophic lateral sclerosis. *J Neurol.* (2014) 261:1949–56. doi: 10.1007/s00415-014-7445-1
38. Mariosa D, Hammar N, Malmström H, Ingre C, Jungner I, Ye W, et al. Blood biomarkers of carbohydrate, lipid, and apolipoprotein metabolisms and risk of amyotrophic lateral sclerosis: a more than 20-year follow-up of the Swedish AMORIS cohort. *Ann Neurol.* (2017) 81:718–28. doi: 10.1002/ana.24936
39. Chen X, Yazdani S, Piehl F, Magnusson PKE, Fang F. Polygenic link between blood lipids and amyotrophic lateral sclerosis. *Neurobiol Aging.* (2018) 67:202.e1–202.e6. doi: 10.1016/j.neurobiolaging.2018.03.022
40. Dupuis L, Corcia P, Fergani A, Gonzalez De Aguilar JL, Bonnefont-Rousselot D, Bittar R, et al. Dyslipidemia is a protective factor in amyotrophic lateral sclerosis. *Neurology.* (2008) 70:1004–9. doi: 10.1212/01.wnl.0000285080.70324.27
41. Dedic SI, Stevic Z, Dedic V, Stojanovic VR, Milicev M, Lavrnic D. Is hyperlipidemia correlated with longer survival in patients with amyotrophic lateral sclerosis? *Neurol Res.* (2012) 34:576–80. doi: 10.1179/1743132812Y.0000000049
42. Ikeda K, Hirayama T, Takazawa T, Kawabe K, Iwasaki Y. Relationships between disease progression and serum levels of lipid, urate, creatinine and ferritin in Japanese patients with amyotrophic lateral sclerosis: a cross-sectional study. *Intern Med.* (2012) 51:1501–8. doi: 10.2169/internalmedicine.51.7465
43. Rafiq MK, Lee E, Bradburn M, McDermott CJ, Shaw PJ. Effect of lipid profile on prognosis in the patients with amyotrophic lateral sclerosis: Insights from the olesoxime clinical trial. *Amyotroph Lateral Scler Frontotemporal Degener.* (2015) 16:478–84. doi: 10.3109/21678421.2015.1062517
44. Delaye JB, Patin F, Piver E, Bruno C, Vasse M, Vourc'h P, et al. Low IDL-B and high LDL-1 subfraction levels in serum of ALS patients. *J Neurol Sci.* (2017) 380:124–7. doi: 10.1016/j.jns.2017.07.019
45. Chiò A, Calvo A, Ilardi A, Cavallo E, Moglia C, Mutani R, et al. Lower serum lipid levels are related to respiratory impairment in patients with ALS. *Neurology.* (2009) 73:1681–5. doi: 10.1212/WNL.0b013e3181c1df1e.
46. Wuolikainen A, Acimovic J, Lövgren-Sandblom A, Parini P, Andersen PM, Björkhem I. Cholesterol, oxysterol, triglyceride, and coenzyme Q homeostasis in ALS. Evidence against the hypothesis that elevated 27-hydroxycholesterol is a pathogenic factor. *PLoS ONE.* (2014) 9:e113619. doi: 10.1371/journal.pone.0113619
47. Huang R, Guo X, Chen X, Zheng Z, Wei Q, Cao B, et al. The serum lipid profiles of amyotrophic lateral sclerosis patients: a study from south-west China and a meta-analysis. *Amyotroph Lateral Scler Frontotemporal Degener.* (2015) 16:359–65. doi: 10.3109/21678421.2015.1047454
48. Barros ANAB, Dourado MET Jr, Pedrosa LFC, Leite-Lais L. Association of copper status with lipid profile and functional status in patients with amyotrophic lateral sclerosis. *J Nutr Metab.* (2018) 2018:5678698. doi: 10.1155/2018/5678698
49. Sutedja NA, van der Schouw YT, Fischer K, Sizoo EM, Huisman MH, Veldink JH, et al. Beneficial vascular risk profile is associated with amyotrophic lateral sclerosis. *J Neurol Neurosurg Psychiatr.* (2011) 82:638–42. doi: 10.1136/jnnp.2010.236752
50. Paganoni S, Deng J, Jaffa M, Cudkowicz ME, Wills AM. Body mass index, not dyslipidemia, is an independent predictor of survival in amyotrophic lateral sclerosis. *Muscle Nerve.* (2011) 44:20–4. doi: 10.1002/mus.22114
51. Blasco H, Patin F, Molinier S, Vourc'h P, Le Tilly O, Bakkouche S, et al. A decrease in blood cholesterol after gastrostomy could impact survival in ALS. *Eur J Clin Nutr.* (2017a) 71:1133–5. doi: 10.1038/ejcn.2017.54
52. Abdel-Khalik J, Yutuc E, Crick PJ, Gustafsson JÅ, Warner M, Roman G, et al. Defective cholesterol metabolism in amyotrophic lateral sclerosis. *J Lipid Res.* (2017) 58:267–78. doi: 10.1194/jlr.P071639
53. La Marca V, Maresca B, Spagnuolo MS, Cigliano L, Dal Piaz F, Di Iorio G, et al. Lecithin-cholesterol acyltransferase in brain: does oxidative stress influence the 24-hydroxycholesterol esterification? *Neurosci Res.* (2016) 105:19–27. doi: 10.1016/j.neures.2015.09.008
54. Kim SM, Noh MY, Kim H, Cheon SY, Lee KM, Lee J, et al. 25-Hydroxycholesterol is involved in the pathogenesis of amyotrophic lateral sclerosis. *Oncotarget.* (2017) 8:11855–67. doi: 10.18632/oncotarget.14416

55. Dorst J, Kuhnlein P, Hendrich C, Kassubek J, Sperfeld AD, Ludolph AC. Patients with elevated triglyceride and cholesterol serum levels have a prolonged survival in amyotrophic lateral sclerosis. *J Neurol.* (2011) 258:613–7. doi: 10.1007/s00415-010-5805-z

56. Blasco H, Veyrat-Durebex C, Bocca C, Patin F, Vourc'h P, Kouassi Nzoughet J, et al. Lipidomics reveals cerebrospinal-fluid signatures of ALS. *Sci Rep.* (2017b) 7:17652. doi: 10.1038/s41598-017-17389-9

57. Fitzgerald KC, O'Reilly ÉJ, Falcone GJ, McCullough ML, Park Y, Kolonel LN, et al. Dietary ω-3 polyunsaturated fatty acid intake and risk for amyotrophic lateral sclerosis. *JAMA Neurol.* (2014) 71:1102–10. doi: 10.1001/jamaneurol.2014.1214

58. Henriques A, Blasco H, Fleury MC, Corcia P, Echaniz-Laguna A, Robelin L, et al. Blood cell palmitoleate-palmitate ratio is an independent prognostic factor for amyotrophic lateral sclerosis. *PLoS ONE.* (2015) 10:e0131512. doi: 10.1371/journal.pone.0131512

59. Nagase M, Yamamoto Y, Miyazaki Y, Yoshino H. Increased oxidative stress in patients with amyotrophic lateral sclerosis and the effect of edaravone administration. *Redox Rep.* (2016) 21:104–12. doi: 10.1179/1351000215Y.0000000026

60. Ahmed RM, Caga J, Devenney E, Hsieh S, Bartley L, Highton-Williamson E, et al. Cognition and eating behavior in amyotrophic lateral sclerosis: effect on survival. *J Neurol.* (2016) 263:1593–603. doi: 10.1007/s00415-016-8168-2

61. Ahmed RM, Highton-Williamson E, Caga J, Thornton N, Ramsey E, Zoing M, et al. Lipid metabolism and survival across the frontotemporal dementia-amyotrophic lateral sclerosis spectrum: relationships to eating behavior and cognition. *J Alzheimers Dis.* (2018) 61:773–83. doi: 10.3233/JAD-170660

62. Kim B, Jin Y, Kim SH, Park Y. Association between macronutrient intake and amyotrophic lateral sclerosis prognosis. *Nutr Neurosci.* (2018) 1–8. doi: 10.1080/1028415X.2018.1466459

18

Biomarkers for Amyotrophic Lateral Sclerosis and Frontotemporal Dementia Associated with Hexanucleotide Expansion Mutations in *C9orf72*

Mary Kay Floeter[1*] *and Tania F. Gendron*[2]

[1] *National Institute of Neurological Disorders and Stroke, National Institutes of Health, Bethesda, MD, United States,*
[2] *Department of Neuroscience, Mayo Clinic, Jacksonville, FL, United States*

Correspondence:
Mary Kay Floeter
floeterm@ninds.nih.gov

Now that genetic testing can identify persons at risk for developing amyotrophic lateral sclerosis (ALS) many decades before symptoms begin, there is a critical need for biomarkers that signal the onset and progression of degeneration. The search for candidate disease biomarkers in patients with mutations in the gene *C9orf72* has included imaging, physiology, and biofluid measurements. In cross-sectional imaging studies, C9+ ALS patients display diffuse reductions of gray and white matter integrity compared to ALS patients without mutations. This structural imaging signature overlaps with frontotemporal dementia (FTD), reflecting the frequent co-occurrence of cognitive impairment, even frank FTD, in C9+ ALS patients. Changes in functional connectivity occur as critical components of the networks associated with cognition and behavior degenerate. In presymptomatic C9+carriers, subtle differences in volumes of subcortical structures and functional connectivity can be detected, often decades before the typical family age of symptom onset. Dipeptide repeat proteins produced by the repeat expansion mutation are also measurable in the cerebrospinal fluid (CSF) of presymptomatic gene carriers, possibly throughout their lives. In contrast, a rise in the level of neurofilament proteins in the CSF appears to presage the onset of degeneration in presymptomatic carriers in one longitudinal study. Cross-sectional studies indicate that neurofilament protein levels may provide prognostic information for survival in C9+ ALS patients. Longitudinal studies will be needed to validate the candidate biomarkers discussed here. Understanding how these candidate biomarkers change over time is critical if they are to be used in future therapeutic decisions.

Keywords: *C9orf72*, cortical thinning, diffusion tensor imaging, dipeptide repeat proteins, functional connectivity, motor neuron disease, neurofilament proteins, biomarker

INTRODUCTION

A repeat expansion mutation in the *C9orf72* gene is the most common cause of familial amyotrophic lateral sclerosis (ALS) in people of Northern European ancestry and accounts for 5-10% of sporadic ALS cases in Europe and the USA (1, 2). The *C9orf72* mutation (C9+) is also a common cause of familial frontotemporal dementia (FTD) (3). The clinical phenotype is often mixed, and many C9+ ALS patients have some degree of cognitive impairment, ranging from mild executive dysfunction to frank FTD (4). Because mutation carriers can be identified by genetic testing many decades before symptoms begin, there is considerable interest in biomarkers to identify when degeneration begins and to monitor disease progression. Currently, development of such biomarkers is at the early stage of identifying measures that differ in group comparisons. This review will discuss the current status of studies of non-invasive biomarkers such as imaging and physiology, and minimally invasive biomarkers derived from biofluids.

IMAGING STUDIES

There is particular interest in neuroimaging as a biomarker because it offers a way to visualize pathological changes in the brains of living patients. In autopsy studies, brains from C9+ patients exhibited the neuronal loss, gliosis, and TDP-43 inclusions characteristic of sporadic ALS and some FTD patients (5), as well as the nuclear RNA foci and cytoplasmic aggregates of dipeptide repeat (DPR) proteins specific to the *C9orf72* mutation (5, 6). The distribution of these pathologic findings differs between C9+ ALS and C9+ FTD patient brains (7, 8). The story emerging from neuroimaging studies is that the diversity of clinical phenotypes reflects the extent to which the most affected brain regions contribute to networks that underlie cognitive, behavioral, motor, and language function (9, 10).

Structural MRI—Gray Matter Atrophy

In structural MRI scans, C9+ ALS patients displayed extensive, relatively symmetric volume loss and cortical thinning compared to similarly aged healthy subjects (1, 11–14). Compared to C9– ALS patients (i.e., without the *C9orf72* mutation), C9+ ALS patients had greater atrophy of extra-motor cortical regions, particularly parieto-occipital cortical areas, including the cuneus and precuneus (11–13), and relatively less atrophy of the precentral motor cortex (13, 14). Correlations between volumetric changes and cognitive testing measures have led several investigators to conclude that the predominant gray matter imaging pattern in C9+ ALS patients is associated with cognitive changes (11–14). A similar pattern of diffuse, relatively symmetric cortical volume loss is found in C9+ FTD patients (15–19).

Several studies report more atrophy of subcortical structures in C9+ ALS than in C9– ALS patients. The topographic specificity of connections between these subcortical structures and specific cortical regions can lead to discrete functional deficits. Nearly all volumetric studies to date have reported thalamic atrophy in C9+ carriers. Thalamic atrophy has been reported in C9+ ALS patients (11–13), C9+ FTD patients (15, 16, 18–22), and presymptomatic C9+ carriers (23–26). Although C9+ ALS patients may have more thalamic atrophy compared to C9– ALS patients with a similar degree of cognitive impairment (11), the association between thalamic atrophy and cognitive impairment can be seen in FTD patients with other gene mutations (27) and C9– ALS patients with cognitive impairment (28). Because there is topographic specificity of corticothalamic circuits, degeneration of particular thalamic nuclei should produce different functional impairments. However, most MRI studies measured the hemi-thalamus in its entirety. Using a more refined segmentation scheme in a cohort of C9+ FTD patients, Lee and colleagues (20) found atrophy specifically in the medial pulvinar nucleus of the thalamus, a multisensory nucleus with connections to posterior parietal, prefrontal, and cingulate cortical areas (29). Schonecker and colleagues reported greater atrophy of motor sub-regions of the thalamus in symptomatic C9+ carriers (30).

Atrophy of other subcortical structures has also been reported. The cerebellum has been of particular interest because high levels of DPR proteins (8, 31, 32) and RNA foci were found in cerebellar Purkinje and granule cells in C9+ patients (33), and levels of cerebellar DPR proteins in C9+ ALS were correlated with cognitive impairment (31). While a pathological study reported no appreciable neuronal loss in the cerebellum (15), cerebellar atrophy has been reported in some, but not all, imaging studies. Detection differences largely reflect whether the whole cerebellum or focal cerebellar regions were measured. Changes in focal cerebellar regions, such as in lobule VIIa/crus I, were found in several studies of C9+ ALS and C9+ FTD patients (11, 17, 21, 27, 34). This region of the cerebellum has been mapped in functional MRI studies to cortical association networks, including the dorsolateral prefrontal cortex and parietal association areas that play a role in executive function (35). Volume loss has also been reported in various nuclei of the basal ganglia in C9+ ALS and C9+ FTD patients (20, 28, 36), a finding associated with cognitive and behavioral scores across the spectrum of ALS and FTD, and thought to result from disruption of corticostriatal circuits (37). Two studies also reported hippocampal atrophy in C9+ ALS (11, 38), a finding consistent with the occurrence of hippocampal sclerosis in some C9+ ALS-FTD brains (5) and memory deficits.

The diffuse nature of the brain atrophy, involving cortical and subcortical structures, has led to the suggestion that changes in ventricular volume be used to follow longitudinal disease progression in C9+ carriers (13, 17, 34) (**Figure 1**).

Pathological Correlates

The distribution of atrophy in structural MRI scans of C9+ ALS and FTD patients mirrors the distribution of neuronal loss and TDP-43 pathology in brains of C9+ ALS-FTD patients (5) and sporadic ALS and FTD patients (39). However, the relationship between these hallmarks of degeneration–neuronal loss, gliosis, and TDP-43 inclusions—and the RNA foci and DPR protein aggregates specific for the C9+ genotype is still evolving. Unlike TDP-43 pathology, which closely parallels neurodegeneration, the distribution of RNA foci (33) and DPR protein pathology do not (6–8, 33, 40, 41), although reports on the latter have been somewhat conflicting. A moderate association between the amount of poly(GA) dystrophic neurites and degeneration in the frontal cortex was observed (40), and inclusions of poly(GR), which is especially toxic in *in vitro* models (42), correlated with TDP-43 pathology and neurodegeneration in C9+ FTD-ALS brains (7, 41). Nevertheless, the presence of DPR protein aggregates and RNA foci did not lead to TDP-43 accumulation

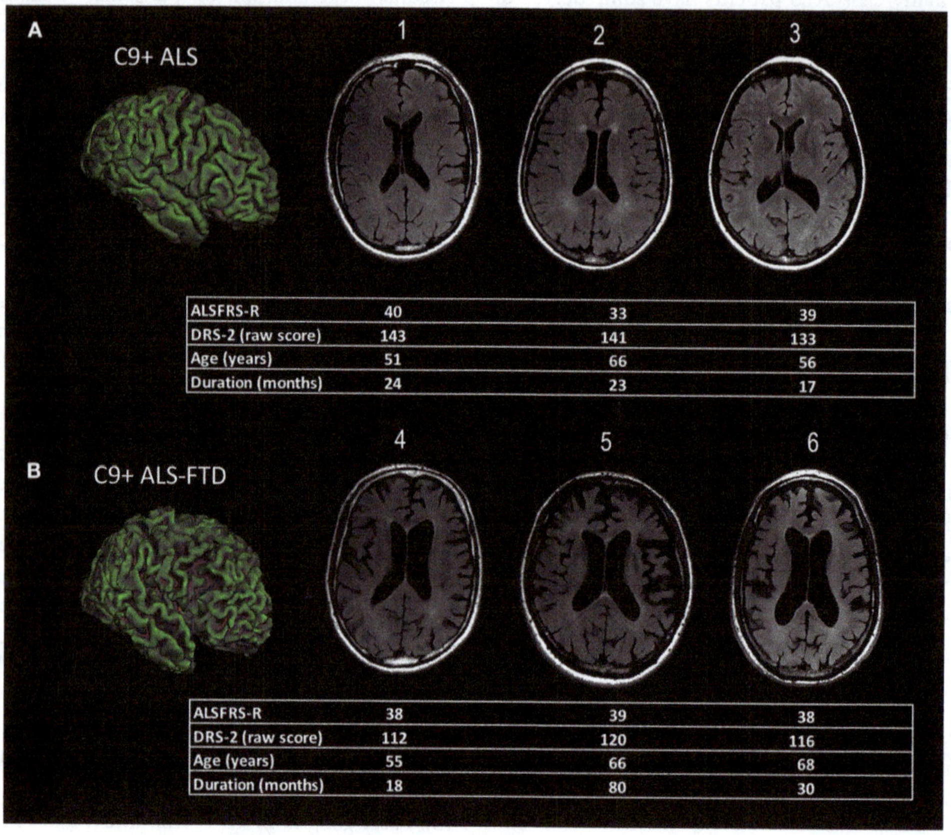

FIGURE 1 | Representative examples of diffuse cortical atrophy in MRI scans of ALS patients with *C9orf72* mutations. The demographic information and scores on motor and cognitive scales are listed below each patient's scan. **(A)** Compared to age-matched controls, mild ventricular enlargement was seen in C9+ patients 1, 2, and 3 who had ALS, but good cognitive function, as evidenced by their scores on the Mattis Dementia Rating Scale–2 (DRS-2). The surface rendering of one patient [left side of panel **(A)**] shows sulci in frontal lobe sulci are also mildly enlarged compared to the occipital lobe. **(B)** C9+ patients 4, 5, and 6 had ALS-FTD with a similar degree of motor dysfunction to those in panel **(A)**, as measured by their ALS functional rating scale revised (ALSFRS-R) scores, but marked cognitive impairment with low DRS-2 scores. There is marked enlargement of ventricles evident in axial slices, as well as enlargement of frontal and temporal sulci in the surface rendering at left of panel **(B)**.

in a neurologically healthy mosaic carrier (43), and DPR protein pathology with little, if any, TDP-43 pathology was observed in a c9FTD kindred with early intellectual disability (44) and three *C9orf72* mutation carriers who developed relatively rapid cognitive decline but died prematurely due to unrelated illness (45).

Diffusion Tensor Imaging of White Matter Tracts

In diffusion tensor imaging (DTI) studies, C9+ ALS patients showed more widespread loss of white matter integrity compared to healthy controls and C9− ALS patients, most commonly in the frontal white matter, as measured by decreased fractional anisotropy, increased radial diffusivity, or increased mean diffusivity (11, 12, 14, 38, 46). Several white matter tracts affected in C9+ ALS are not typically affected in cognitively intact C9− ALS patients, including the genu of the corpus callosum, anterior limbs of the internal capsule, thalamic radiations, and long association tracts such as the uncinate fasciculus, superior longitudinal fasciculus, and inferior longitudinal fasciculus (11, 12, 14, 38, 46). These frontal and association tracts were also affected in diffusion studies of C9+ FTD patients (17, 20, 36), and presymptomatic C9+ carriers in some studies (47). Motor tracts, including the corticospinal tract and motor segment of the corpus callosum, were affected in C9+ ALS patients compared to healthy controls (11, 46), but exhibited less disruption than in C9− ALS patients (14). In a group of C9+ carriers with a mixture of phenotypes, changes in diffusion indices of specific tracts correlated with clinical measures: frontal white matter correlated with lexical fluency and behavioral scores, and changes in motor tracts correlated with the ALS functional rating scale (46).

Unresolved Questions About Structural Imaging as a Biomarker

Several questions arise from the findings in structural MRI scans. First, does a genotype-specific C9+ MRI signature exist? To address this question, Westeneng and colleagues (38) identified a candidate "genotype-specific MRI signature" in a model comparing 92 volumetric and DTI variables in scans of 28 C9+ to 28 C9− ALS patients. Although 11 imaging variables identified a C9+ specific signature in the training dataset, nearly 20% of C9− ALS patients in a large validation dataset were classified as having the C9+ MRI signature. Misclassified patients scored more poorly on a measure of executive function, thus underscoring the close association between neuroanatomical atrophy patterns and clinical phenotypes. A second question is whether the volumetric differences in adult C9+ carriers arise during development or are a consequence of degeneration. This question was addressed in imaging studies comparing relatively young presymptomatic C9+ carriers (<age 40) to non-carriers from the same families. Although older presymptomatic C9+ carriers had clear evidence of atrophy compared to similarly-aged C9− family members, so did younger C9+ presymptomatic carriers when compared to C9− family members of the same age (24–26, 47, 48). Cortical and subcortical structures were smaller, particularly the thalamus, in younger C9+ carriers. The common genetic background of family members with and without the *C9orf72* mutation facilitated detection of small differences in these studies. Lee and colleagues found that smaller gray matter volumes occurred across a range of ages in presymptomatic C9+ carriers and had a similar age-related decline as in C9− controls, suggesting a developmental origin (47). Longitudinal studies in individual C9+ carriers before and after the onset of symptoms will be needed to truly determine whether congenitally small brain structures begin accelerated volume loss with the onset of degeneration in adulthood or whether the *C9orf72* mutation leads to slow, lifelong accumulation of subclinical pathology. Lastly, because the distribution of atrophy mirrors the distribution of TDP-43 in pathological studies (5), longitudinal structural imaging, in combination with clinical phenotyping, can be used to test hypotheses that TDP-43 pathology spreads through axonal connections. Pathological studies in sporadic ALS have led to the proposal that TDP-43 pathology spreads through corticofugal projections (49). In contrast, in behavioral-variant FTD, TDP-43 pathology has been proposed to spread from orbitofrontal cortex to posterior regions through axonal tracts (50).

Functional Connectivity

Changes in functional connectivity using task-based or resting state fMRI have been reported prior to development of clinical symptoms in patients with *GRN* or *MAPT* mutations at risk for FTD (51). Three studies examined changes in functional connectivity in resting state networks in C9+ carriers. One study in symptomatic carriers found that C9+ and C9− behavioral variant FTD patients had disruption of salience network connectivity that was associated with neuropsychiatric severity, as well as disruption of sensorimotor connectivity (20). The disruption of the salience network occurred with atrophy of different nodes within the salience network in individual patients (20). Disruption of the salience network and a network generated from a medial pulvinar nucleus seed was also observed in young presymptomatic C9+ carriers (47). Another study reported increased connectivity in the visual network of C9+ carriers with a mixture of motor and cognitive phenotypes compared to sporadic cases with similar phenotypes (11).

Proton Emission Tomography

Hypometabolism in the frontal lobes in FDG-PET studies is considered supportive of a clinical diagnosis of FTD (52). The few reports of PET imaging in C9+ carriers had slightly different findings. In one study, C9+ ALS patients had more widespread hypometabolism occurring in the cingulate, insula, caudate, and thalamus, with clusters of hypermetabolism in occipital, left precentral, left postcentral, and superior temporal cortex when compared to C9− ALS patients with or without FTD (53). In contrast, the other study reported that C9+ ALS and C9− ALS patients exhibited hypometabolism in peri-rolandic cortex; several prefrontal regions had hypometabolism in both groups, but C9+ ALS patients alone had focal hypometabolism in the thalamus and posterior cingulate cortex (54). One case study also reported frontal and temporal hypometabolism in a C9+ ALS patient who subsequently developed FTD (55). Another reported that amyloid imaging, but not FDG-PET, distinguished FTD from Alzheimer disease in a C9+ carrier (56).

PHYSIOLOGY

Physiological methods have been used to assess cortical function in C9+ carriers. Transcranial magnetic stimulation (TMS) is a non-invasive technique for assessing cortical excitability. Numerous TMS studies in sporadic ALS patients have provided evidence for hyperexcitability of the motor cortex early in disease (57), with loss of excitability at late stages (58). C9+ ALS patients were similarly found to have increased cortical excitability according to several different TMS indices, but presymptomatic C9+ carriers did not (59–61). Evoked potential measures have been used to explore particular cognitive functions in C9+ patients (62), but have not been routinely used to identify disease onset or severity. Electroimpedance myography (63) and Motor Unit Number Index (MUNIX) (64) are non-invasive methods that have been used to follow lower motor neuron dysfunction in ALS patients in clinical trials but, to date, have not been reported in C9+ ALS patients.

ENERGY METABOLISM

Patients with ALS develop defects in energy metabolism that include low body mass index (BMI), hypermetabolism, and hyperlipidemia (65, 66). While the contribution of dysregulated energy homeostasis to ALS pathogenesis remains to be resolved, such defects correlate with prognostic factors. For instance, weight loss and hypermetabolism are associated with faster disease progression and shorter survival in ALS (66–68). The cause of these metabolic changes is unknown, but may result from hypothalamic atrophy. Gorges et al. (69) have shown that the hypothalamus is atrophied in ALS patients and in presymptomatic ALS mutation carriers (the latter were comprised predominantly of C9+ individuals). Furthermore, they found a modest but significant correlation between hypothalamic volume and BMI, especially in patients with

TABLE 1 | Timeframes for detecting changes in selected candidate biomarkers in *C9orf72* carriers.

	Years prior to symptom onset	1 year prior to clinical symptoms	Early–mid stages of disease	Late stages of disease
CSF dipeptide repeat proteins	•	•	•	•
Functional connectivity salience network (fMRI)	•	•	•	•
Thalamic atrophy	•	•	•	•
CSF NfL		•	•	?
Cortical hyperexcitability (TMS)			•	?
Reduced integrity of frontal white matter and association tracts (DTI)		?	•	•
CSF pNfH		?	•	•
FDG-PET frontotemporal hypometabolism			•	•
Global loss of functional connectivity			•	•
Global volume loss–ventricular atrophy, subcortical atrophy			•	•
Diffuse cortical thinning			•	•
Diffuse loss of white matter integrity (DTI)			•	•

CSF, cerebrospinal fluid; DTI, diffusion tensor imaging; FDG-PET, fluoro-deoxyglucose proton emission tomography; fMRI, functional magnetic resonance imaging; pNfH, phosphorylated neurofilament heavy chain; NfL, Neurofilament light chain; TMS, transcranial magnetic stimulation. Question marks indicate measures needing further study.

familial ALS, and observed that anterior hypothalamic volumes correlate with age of disease onset (69). While these findings are not specific to C9+ carriers, they do suggest that hypothalamic atrophy, BMI, and disturbances in energy homeostasis could provide prognostic insight.

CSF AND BIOFLUID STUDIES

Fluid-based biomarker discovery efforts for ALS have most often been conducted using cerebrospinal fluid (CSF) due to its proximity to affected neuroanatomical regions. However, progress has been made using plasma and serum, and studies using urine and saliva are emerging (70). Among the more widely studied biomarker candidates are inflammatory mediators, metabolic markers and neurofilament proteins; the latter, however, have arguably garnered the most attention (70, 71). Neurofilament proteins, which include neurofilament heavy chain (NfH), neurofilament medium chain and neurofilament light chain (NfL), are abundantly and exclusively expressed in neurons where they form the neuronal cytoskeleton. Because neurofilament proteins are released from neurons upon axonal damage or degeneration, they are considered indicators of neuronal injury for various neurological disorders.

Neurofilament Proteins

In C9+ carriers, levels of CSF phosphorylated NfH (pNfH) were significantly higher in patients with ALS or FTD compared to asymptomatic individuals, and strongly associated with survival in patients with C9+ ALS (72). Notably, C9+ ALS patients had significantly higher pNFH levels than C9- ALS patients, which presumably reflected increased neurodegeneration, consistent with reports that patients with C9+ ALS develop greater brain atrophy, particularly in extra-motor regions, compared to C9- ALS patients (11–13). More diffuse degeneration may account for the shorter survival of C9+ ALS patients compared to C9- ALS patients (1, 72–75). Similar to pNfH, CSF NfL levels were elevated in symptomatic compared to presymptomatic C9+ carriers (76, 77), and higher NfL levels in symptomatic individuals correlated with greater disease severity and shorter survival (77). Furthermore, elevated CSF NfL in C9+ carriers was associated with lower gray matter volumes in the ventral and dorsomedial prefrontal cortex, ventral, and dorsal insula, anterior cingulate, caudate, medial thalamus, and other frontotemporoparietal regions (77).

These findings supporting CSF pNfH and NfL as prognostic markers for C9+ patients could significantly impact drug development. For instance, the heterogeneity of disease course in C9+ ALS could result in different proportions of fast and slow progressors in clinical treatment arms. Using pNfH and NfL levels as surrogates for progression rate could facilitate stratification of patients into balanced groups to reduce variability in treatment outcomes. Early evidence also suggests that NfL in CSF and serum can inform the potential phenoconversion of individuals from an asymptomatic to a symptomatic state (78). Through the study of individuals that carry a mutation in *C9orf72* or other ALS-associated genes, Benatar and colleagues found that NfL in asymptomatic mutation carriers was elevated above the range seen in healthy individuals as early as 12 months prior to the earliest clinical symptoms (78). Should these findings be validated in additional cohorts, NfL could provide insight on when neurodegeneration begins. This would facilitate the timely diagnosis of C9+ ALS, and increase the likelihood of enrolling patients in clinical trials at an early stage of disease when they are most likely to benefit from therapeutic intervention.

Dipeptide Repeat Proteins

In addition to prognostic biomarkers, markers of target engagement would improve the interpretation of clinical trials for C9+ ALS and FTD. As mentioned above, a characteristic neuropathological feature of C9+ ALS and FTD is the presence of neuronal inclusions formed of DPR proteins synthesized from expanded *C9orf72* repeats. One of these proteins, poly(GP), is abundantly expressed in the brain of C9+ carriers and is detected in CSF (72, 77, 79, 80). While several studies observed that CSF poly(GP) did not associate with age at disease onset, survival, or markers of neurodegeneration (e.g., CSF pNfH or NfL, or measures of brain atrophy) (72, 77, 79), poly(GP) shows promise as a pharmacodynamic biomarker (81).

Since RNA transcripts of expanded *C9orf72* repeats are believed to play a key role in C9+ ALS and FTD (82), therapeutic strategies that target *C9orf72* repeat RNA are being developed. Given that levels of poly(GP) correlated with levels of repeat-containing RNA in the cerebellum of C9+ carriers (31, 83), poly(GP) was investigated as a marker of target engagement for repeat RNA-based therapies. Antisense oligonucleotides (ASOs), small molecules and genetic modifiers that target *C9orf72* repeat RNA attenuated poly(GP) levels in various preclinical models including yeast, worms, mice, and C9+ ALS patient cell lines (81, 84, 85). For example, poly(GP) was detected in CSF of mice expressing an expanded *C9orf72* repeat in the brain, and CSF poly(GP) was decreased following treatment with a repeat RNA-targeting ASO. Of note, CSF poly(GP) levels correlated with DPR protein pathology, repeat RNA levels and RNA foci burden in the brains of mice (81). These data suggest that monitoring CSF poly(GP) before and during treatment of patients participating in clinical trials presents a feasible approach to gauge target engagement.

SUMMARY

The search for biomarkers of disease onset and progression in *C9orf72* repeat expansion carriers has yielded promising candidate biomarkers (**Table 1**). Clinically, cognitive, behavioral, and motor impairment occur on a continuum in patients with the *C9orf72* mutation. Non-invasive imaging studies in C9+ carriers have identified structural and functional changes in critical components of the networks associated with cognition and behavior. Early thalamic involvement has been detected in structural, functional, and metabolic imaging studies in C9+ carriers across different clinical phenotypes, in both prospective and retrospective studies. Diffusion changes in frontal white matter may also occur early in disease. These non-invasive imaging measures warrant further study in asymptomatic carriers as early markers of degeneration. Among the minimally invasive biomarker measures, CSF pNfH or NfL may allow identification of disease onset in asymptomatic carriers and forecast survival in symptomatic carriers (72, 77, 78). Now that *C9orf72* mutation carriers can be identified by genetic testing many decades before symptoms begin, and efforts to develop gene-directed therapy are underway, it is possible to imagine that biomarkers will play important roles in future therapeutic decisions. For example, in the future, persons known to carry the *C9orf72* mutation could undergo periodic screening with non-invasive tests such as MRI or physiology, followed by minimally invasive testing to measure CSF or blood biomarkers when findings suspicious for neurodegeneration arise.

AUTHOR CONTRIBUTIONS

MF and TG drafted sections of the manuscript and proofread the entire manuscript.

FUNDING

MF is supported by the intramural program of the National Institutes of Health, NINDS Z01 NS003146 for research on neurological disorders. This funding pays for the open access fee. TG's research is supported by the Muscular Dystrophy Association, the Target ALS Foundation, and the National Institutes of Health, NINDS P01 NS099114.

REFERENCES

1. Byrne S, Elamin M, Bede P, Shatunov A, Walsh C, Corr B, et al. Cognitive and clinical characteristics of patients with amyotrophic lateral sclerosis carrying a C9orf72 repeat expansion: a population-based cohort study. *Lancet Neurol.* (2012) 11:232–40. doi: 10.1016/S1474-4422(12)70014-5
2. Renton AE, Majounie E, Waite A, Simon-Sanchez J, Rollinson S, Gibbs JR, et al. A hexanucleotide repeat expansion in C9ORF72 is the cause of chromosome 9p21-linked ALS-FTD. *Neuron* (2011) 72:257–68. doi: 10.1016/j.neuron.2011.09.010
3. DeJesus-Hernandez M, Mackenzie IR, Boeve BF, Boxer AL, Baker M, Rutherford NJ, et al. Expanded GGGGCC hexanucleotide repeat in noncoding region of C9ORF72 causes chromosome 9p-linked FTD and ALS. *Neuron* (2011) 72:245–56. doi: 10.1016/j.neuron.2011.09.011
4. Rohrer JD, Isaacs AM, Mizielinska S, Mead S, Lashley T, Wray S, et al. C9orf72 expansions in frontotemporal dementia and amyotrophic lateral sclerosis. *Lancet Neurol.* (2015) 14:291–301. doi: 10.1016/S1474-4422(14)70233-9
5. Murray ME, DeJesus-Hernandez M, Rutherford NJ, Baker M, Duara R, Graff-Radford NR, et al. Clinical and neuropathologic heterogeneity of c9FTD/ALS associated with hexanucleotide repeat expansion in C9ORF72. *Acta Neuropathol.* (2011) 122:673–90. doi: 10.1007/s00401-011-0907-y
6. Mackenzie IR, Arzberger T, Kremmer E, Troost D, Lorenzl S, Mori K, et al. Dipeptide repeat protein pathology in C9ORF72 mutation cases: clinico-pathological correlations. *Acta Neuropathol.* (2013) 126:859–79. doi: 10.1007/s00401-013-1181-y
7. Sakae N, Bieniek KF, Zhang YJ, Ross K, Gendron TF, Murray ME, et al. Poly-GR dipeptide repeat polymers correlate with neurodegeneration and Clinicopathological subtypes in C9ORF72-related brain disease. *Acta Neuropathol Commun.* (2018) 6:63. doi: 10.1186/s40478-018-0564-7
8. Schludi MH, May S, Grasser FA, Rentzsch K, Kremmer E, Küpper C, et al. Distribution of dipeptide repeat proteins in cellular models and C9orf72 mutation cases suggests link to transcriptional silencing. *Acta Neuropathol.* (2015) 130:537–55. doi: 10.1007/s00401-015-1450-z
9. Bede P, Omer T, Finegan E, Chipika RH, Iyer PM, Doherty MA, et al. Connectivity-based characterisation of subcortical grey matter pathology in frontotemporal dementia and ALS: a multimodal neuroimaging study. *Brain Imaging Behav.* (in press). doi: 10.1007/s11682-018-9837-9
10. Sellami L, Bocchetta M, Masellis M, Cash DM, Dick KM, van Swieten J, et al. Distinct neuroanatomical correlates of neuropsychiatric symptoms in the three main forms of genetic frontotemporal dementia in the GENFI cohort. *J Alzheimers Dis.* (2018) 65:147–63. doi: 10.3233/JAD-180053

11. Agosta F, Ferraro PM, Riva N, Spinelli EG, Domi T, Carrera P, et al. Structural and functional brain signatures of C9orf72 in motor neuron disease. *Neurobiol Aging* (2017) 57:206–19. doi: 10.1016/j.neurobiolaging.2017.05.024
12. Bede P, Bokde AL, Byrne S, Elamin M, McLaughlin RL, Kenna K, et al. Multiparametric MRI study of ALS stratified for the C9orf72 genotype. *Neurology* (2013) 81:361–9. doi: 10.1212/WNL.0b013e31829c5eee
13. Floeter MK, Bageac D, Danielian LE, Braun LE, Traynor BJ, Kwan JY. Longitudinal imaging in C9orf72 mutation carriers: relationship to phenotype. *Neuroimage Clin.* (2016) 12:1035–43. doi: 10.1016/j.nicl.2016.10.014
14. Omer T, Finegan E, Hutchinson S, Doherty M, Vajda A, McLaughlin RL, et al. Neuroimaging patterns along the ALS-FTD spectrum: a multiparametric imaging study. *Amyotroph Lateral Scler Frontotemporal Degener.* (2017) 18:611–23. doi: 10.1080/21678421.2017.1332077
15. Irwin DJ, McMillan CT, Brettschneider J, Libon DJ, Powers J, Rascovsky K, et al. Cognitive decline and reduced survival in C9orf72 expansion frontotemporal degeneration and amyotrophic lateral sclerosis. *J Neurol Neurosurg Psychiatry* (2013) 84:163–9. doi: 10.1136/jnnp-2012-303507
16. Mahoney CJ, Beck J, Rohrer JD, Lashley T, Mok K, Shakespeare T, et al. Frontotemporal dementia with the C9ORF72 hexanucleotide repeat expansion: clinical, neuroanatomical and neuropathological features. *Brain* (2012) 135(Pt 3):736–50. doi: 10.1093/brain/awr361
17. Mahoney CJ, Downey LE, Ridgway GR, Beck J, Clegg S, Blair M, et al. Longitudinal neuroimaging and neuropsychological profiles of frontotemporal dementia with C9ORF72 expansions. *Alzheimers Res Ther.* (2012) 4:41. doi: 10.1186/alzrt144
18. McMillan CT, Russ J, Wood EM, Irwin DJ, Grossman M, McCluskey L, et al. C9orf72 promoter hypermethylation is neuroprotective: neuroimaging and neuropathologic evidence. *Neurology* (2015) 84:1622–30. doi: 10.1212/WNL.0000000000001495
19. Whitwell JL, Weigand SD, Boeve BF, Senjem ML, Gunter JL, DeJesus-Hernandez M, et al. Neuroimaging signatures of frontotemporal dementia genetics: C9ORF72, tau, progranulin and sporadics. *Brain* (2012) 135(Pt 3):794–806. doi: 10.1093/brain/aws001
20. Lee SE, Khazenzon AM, Trujillo AJ, Guo CC, Yokoyama JS, Sha SJ, et al. Altered network connectivity in frontotemporal dementia with C9orf72 hexanucleotide repeat expansion. *Brain* (2014) 137(Pt 11):3047–60. doi: 10.1093/brain/awu248
21. Cash DM, Bocchetta M, Thomas DL, Dick KM, van Swieten JC, Borroni B, et al. Patterns of gray matter atrophy in genetic frontotemporal dementia: results from the GENFI study. *Neurobiol Aging* (2018) 62:191–6. doi: 10.1016/j.neurobiolaging.2017.10.008
22. Sha SJ, Takada LT, Rankin KP, Yokoyama JS, Rutherford NJ, Fong JC, et al. Frontotemporal dementia due to C9ORF72 mutations: clinical and imaging features. *Neurology* (2012) 79:1002–11. doi: 10.1212/WNL.0b013e318268452e
23. Papma JM, Jiskoot LC, Panman JL, Dopper EG, den Heijer T, Donker Kaat L, et al. Cognition and gray and white matter characteristics of presymptomatic C9orf72 repeat expansion. *Neurology* (2017) 89:1256–64. doi: 10.1212/WNL.0000000000004393
24. Popuri K, Dowds E, Beg MF, Balachandar R, Bhalla M, Jacova C, et al. Gray matter changes in asymptomatic C9orf72 and GRN mutation carriers. *Neuroimage Clin.* (2018) 18:591–8. doi: 10.1016/j.nicl.2018.02.017
25. Rohrer JD, Nicholas JM, Cash DM, van Swieten J, Dopper E, Jiskoot L, et al. Presymptomatic cognitive and neuroanatomical changes in genetic frontotemporal dementia in the Genetic Frontotemporal dementia Initiative (GENFI) study: a cross-sectional analysis. *Lancet Neurol.* (2015) 14:253–62. doi: 10.1016/S1474-4422(14)70324-2
26. Walhout R, Schmidt R, Westeneng HJ, Verstraete E, Seelen M, van Rheenen W, et al. Brain morphologic changes in asymptomatic C9orf72 repeat expansion carriers. *Neurology* (2015) 85:1780–8. doi: 10.1212/WNL.0000000000002135
27. Bocchetta M, Gordon E, Cardoso MJ, Modat M, Ourselin S, Warren JD, et al. Thalamic atrophy in frontotemporal dementia - Not just a C9orf72 problem. *Neuroimage Clin.* (2018) 18:675–81. doi: 10.1016/j.nicl.2018.02.019
28. Bede P, Elamin M, Byrne S, McLaughlin RL, Kenna K, Vajda A, et al. Basal ganglia involvement in amyotrophic lateral sclerosis. *Neurology* (2013) 81:2107–15. doi: 10.1212/01.wnl.0000437313.80913.2c
29. Cappe C, Rouiller EM, Barone P. Multisensory anatomical pathways. *Hear Res.* (2009) 258:28–36. doi: 10.1016/j.heares.2009.04.017
30. Schonecker S, Neuhofer C, Otto M, Ludolph A, Kassubek J, Landwehrmeyer B, et al. Atrophy in the thalamus but not cerebellum is specific for C9orf72 FTD and ALS Patients - an atlas-based volumetric MRI study. *Front Aging Neurosci.* (2018) 10:45. doi: 10.3389/fnagi.2018.00045
31. Gendron TF, van Blitterswijk M, Bieniek KF, Daughrity LM, Jiang J, Rush BK, et al. Cerebellar c9RAN proteins associate with clinical and neuropathological characteristics of C9ORF72 repeat expansion carriers. *Acta Neuropathol.* (2015) 130:559–73. doi: 10.1007/s00401-015-1474-4
32. van Blitterswijk MM. DeJesus-Hernandez, Niemantsverdriet E, Murray ME, Heckman MG, Diehl NN, et al. Association between repeat sizes and clinical and pathological characteristics in carriers of C9ORF72 repeat expansions (Xpansize-72): a cross-sectional cohort study. *Lancet Neurol.* (2013) 12:978–88. doi: 10.1016/S1474-4422(13)70210-2
33. DeJesus-Hernandez M, Finch NA, Wang X, Gendron TF, Bieniek KF, Heckman MG, et al. In-depth clinico-pathological examination of RNA foci in a large cohort of C9ORF72 expansion carriers. *Acta Neuropathol.* (2017) 134:255–69. doi: 10.1007/s00401-017-1725-7
34. Whitwell JL, Boeve BF, Weigand SD, Senjem ML, Gunter JL, Baker MC, et al. Brain atrophy over time in genetic and sporadic frontotemporal dementia: a study of 198 serial magnetic resonance images. *Eur J Neurol.* (2015) 22:745–52. doi: 10.1111/ene.12675
35. Buckner RL, Krienen FM, Castellanos A, Diaz JC, and Yeo BT. The organization of the human cerebellum estimated by intrinsic functional connectivity. *J Neurophysiol.* (2011) 106:2322–45. doi: 10.1152/jn.00339.2011
36. Mahoney CJ, Simpson IJ, Nicholas JM, Fletcher PD, Downey LE, Golden HL, et al. Longitudinal diffusion tensor imaging in frontotemporal dementia. *Ann Neurol.* (2015) 77:33–46. doi: 10.1002/ana.24296
37. Machts J, Loewe K, Kaufmann J, Jakubiczka S, Abdulla S, Petri S, et al. Basal ganglia pathology in ALS is associated with neuropsychological deficits. *Neurology* (2015) 85:1301–9. doi: 10.1212/WNL.0000000000002017
38. Westeneng HJ, Walhout R, Straathof M, Schmidt R, Hendrikse J, Veldink JH, et al. Widespread structural brain involvement in ALS is not limited to the C9orf72 repeat expansion. *J Neurol Neurosurg Psychiatry* (2016) 87:1354–60. doi: 10.1136/jnnp-2016-313959
39. Geser F, Martinez-Lage M, Robinson J, Uryu K, Neumann M, Brandmeir NJ, et al. Clinical and pathological continuum of multisystem TDP-43 proteinopathies. *Arch Neurol.* (2009) 66:180–9. doi: 10.1001/archneurol.2008.558
40. Mackenzie IR, Frick P, Grässer FA, Gendron TF, Petrucelli L, Cashman NR, et al. Quantitative analysis and clinico-pathological correlations of different dipeptide repeat protein pathologies in C9ORF72 mutation carriers. *Acta Neuropathol.* (2015) 130:845–61. doi: 10.1007/s00401-015-1476-2
41. Saberi S, Stauffer JE, Jiang J, Garcia SD, Taylor AE, Schulte D, et al. Sense-encoded poly-GR dipeptide repeat proteins correlate to neurodegeneration and uniquely co-localize with TDP-43 in dendrites of repeat-expanded C9orf72 amyotrophic lateral sclerosis. *Acta Neuropathol.* (2018) 135:459–74. doi: 10.1007/s00401-017-1793-8
42. Flores BN, Dulchavsky ME, Krans A, Sawaya MR, Paulson HL, Todd PK, et al. Distinct C9orf72-associated dipeptide repeat structures correlate with neuronal toxicity. PLoS ONE (2016) 11:e0165084. doi: 10.1371/journal.pone.0165084
43. McGoldrick P, Zhang M, van Blitterswijk M, Sato C, Moreno D, Xiao S, et al. Unaffected mosaic C9orf72 case: RNA foci, dipeptide proteins, but upregulated C9orf72 expression. *Neurology* (2018) 90:e323–31. doi: 10.1212/WNL.0000000000004865
44. Proudfoot M, Gutowski NJ, Edbauer D, Hilton DA, Stephens M, Rankin J, et al. Early dipeptide repeat pathology in a frontotemporal dementia kindred with C9ORF72 mutation and intellectual disability. *Acta Neuropathol.* (2014) 127:451–8. doi: 10.1007/s00401-014-1245-7
45. Baborie A, Griffiths TD, Jaros E, Perry R, McKeith IG, Burn DJ, et al. Accumulation of dipeptide repeat proteins predates that of TDP-43 in frontotemporal lobar degeneration associated with hexanucleotide repeat expansions in C9ORF72 gene. *Neuropathol Appl Neurobiol.* (2015) 41:601–12. doi: 10.1111/nan.12178

46. Floeter MK, Danielian LE, Braun LE, Wu T. Longitudinal diffusion imaging across the C9orf72 clinical spectrum. *J Neurol Neurosurg Psychiatry* (2018) 89:53–60. doi: 10.1136/jnnp-2017-316799
47. Lee SE, Sias AC, Mandelli ML, Brown JA, Brown AB, Khazenzon AM, et al. Network degeneration and dysfunction in presymptomatic C9ORF72 expansion carriers. *Neuroimage Clin.* (2017) 14:286–97. doi: 10.1016/j.nicl.2016.12.006
48. Bertrand A, Wen J, Rinaldi D, Houot M, Sayah S, Camuzat A, et al. Early cognitive, structural, and microstructural changes in presymptomatic C9orf72 carriers younger than 40 years. *JAMA Neurol.* (2018) 75:236–45. doi: 10.1001/jamaneurol.2017.4266
49. Braak H, Brettschneider J, Ludolph AC, Lee VM, Trojanowski JQ, Del Tredici K. Amyotrophic lateral sclerosis-a model of corticofugal axonal spread. *Nat Rev Neurol.* (2013) 9:708–14. doi: 10.1038/nrneurol.2013.221
50. Brettschneider J, Del Tredici K, Irwin DJ, Grossman M, Robinson JL, Toledo JB, et al. Sequential distribution of pTDP-43 pathology in behavioral variant frontotemporal dementia (bvFTD). *Acta Neuropathol.* (2014) 127:423–39. doi: 10.1007/s00401-013-1238-y
51. Dopper EG, Rombouts SA, Jiskoot LC, den Heijer T, de Graaf JR, de Koning I, et al. Structural and functional brain connectivity in presymptomatic familial frontotemporal dementia. *Neurology* (2014) 83:e19–26. doi: 10.1212/WNL.0000000000000583
52. Shivamurthy VK, Tahari AK, Marcus C, Subramaniam RM. Brain FDG PET and the diagnosis of dementia. AJR *Am J Roentgenol.* (2015) 204:W76–85. doi: 10.2214/AJR.13.12363
53. Cistaro A, Pagani M, Montuschi A, Calvo A, Moglia C, Canosa A, et al. The metabolic signature of C9ORF72-related ALS: FDG PET comparison with nonmutated patients. *Eur J Nucl Med Mol Imaging* (2014) 41:844–52. doi: 10.1007/s00259-013-2667-5
54. Van Laere K, Vanhee A, Verschueren J, De Coster L, Driesen A, Dupont P, et al. Value of 18fluorodeoxyglucose-positron-emission tomography in amyotrophic lateral sclerosis: a prospective study. *JAMA Neurol.* (2014) 71:553–61. doi: 10.1001/jamaneurol.2014.62
55. Adeli A, Savica R, Lowe VJ, Vemuri P, Knopman DS, Dejesus-Hernandez M, et al. The GGGGCC repeat expansion in C9ORF72 in a case with discordant clinical and FDG-PET findings: PET trumps syndrome. *Neurocase* (2014) 20:110–20. doi: 10.1080/13554794.2012.732090
56. Martikainen MH, Gardberg M, Jansson L, Röyttä M, Rinne JO, Kaasinen V. Brain F-FDG and C-PiB PET findings in two siblings with FTD/ALS associated with the C9ORF72 repeat expansion. *Neurocase* (2014) 20:150–7. doi: 10.1080/13554794.2012.741252
57. Vucic S, Kiernan MC. Transcranial magnetic stimulation for the assessment of neurodegenerative disease. *Neurotherapeutics* (2017) 14:91–106. doi: 10.1007/s13311-016-0487-6
58. Triggs WJ, Menkes D, Onorato J, Yan RS, Young MS, Newell K, et al. Transcranial magnetic stimulation identifies upper motor neuron involvement in motor neuron disease. *Neurology* (1999) 53:605–11. doi: 10.1212/WNL.53.3.605
59. Geevasinga N, Menon P, Nicholson GA, Ng K, Howells J, Kril JJ, et al. Cortical function in asymptomatic carriers and patients with C9orf72 amyotrophic lateral sclerosis. *JAMA Neurol.* (2015) 72:1268–74. doi: 10.1001/jamaneurol.2015.1872
60. Schanz O, Bageac D, Braun L, Traynor BJ, Lehky TJ, Floeter MK. Cortical hyperexcitability in patients with C9ORF72 mutations: relationship to phenotype. *Muscle Nerve* (2016) 54:264–9. doi: 10.1002/mus.25047
61. Williams KL, Fifita JA, Vucic S, Durnall JC, Kiernan MC, Blair IP, et al. Pathophysiological insights into ALS with C9ORF72 expansions. *J Neurol Neurosurg Psychiatry* (2013) 84:931–5. doi: 10.1136/jnnp-2012-304529
62. Iyer PM, Mohr K, Broderick M, Gavin B, Burke T, Bede P, et al. Mismatch negativity as an indicator of cognitive sub-domain dysfunction in amyotrophic lateral sclerosis. *Front Neurol.* (2017) 8:395. doi: 10.3389/fneur.2017.00395
63. Rutkove SB, Caress JB, Cartwright MS, Burns TM, Warder J, David WS, et al. Electrical impedance myography correlates with standard measures of ALS severity. *Muscle Nerve* (2014) 49:441–3. doi: 10.1002/mus.24128
64. Neuwirth C, Barkhaus PE, Burkhardt C, Castro J, Czell D, de Carvalho M, et al. Tracking motor neuron loss in a set of six muscles in amyotrophic lateral sclerosis using the Motor Unit Number Index (MUNIX): a 15-month longitudinal multicentre trial. *J Neurol Neurosurg Psychiatry* (2015) 86:1172–9. doi: 10.1136/jnnp-2015-310509
65. Dupuis L, Pradat PF, Ludolph AC, Loeffler JP. Energy metabolism in amyotrophic lateral sclerosis. *Lancet Neurol.* (2011) 10:75–82. doi: 10.1016/S1474-4422(10)70224-6
66. Steyn FJ, Ioannides ZA, van Eijk RPA, Heggie S, Thorpe KA, Ceslis A, et al. Hypermetabolism in ALS is associated with greater functional decline and shorter survival. *J Neurol Neurosurg Psychiatry* (2018) 89:1016–23. doi: 10.1136/jnnp-2017-317887
67. Jawaid A, Murthy SB, Wilson AM, Qureshi SU, Amro MJ, Wheaton M, et al. A decrease in body mass index is associated with faster progression of motor symptoms and shorter survival in ALS. *Amyotroph Lateral Scler.* (2010) 11:542–8. doi: 10.3109/17482968.2010.482592
68. Peter RS, Rosenbohm A, Dupuis L, Brehme T, Kassubek J, Rothenbacher D, et al. Life course body mass index and risk and prognosis of amyotrophic lateral sclerosis: results from the ALS registry Swabia. *Eur J Epidemiol.* (2017) 32:901–8. doi: 10.1007/s10654-017-0318-z
69. Gorges M,Vercruysse, Muller HP, Huppertz HJ, Rosenbohm A, Nager G, et al. Hypothalamic atrophy is related to body mass index and age at onset in amyotrophic lateral sclerosis. *J Neurol Neurosurg Psychiatry* (2017) 88:1033–41. doi: 10.1136/jnnp-2017-315795
70. Vu LT, Bowser R. Fluid-based biomarkers for amyotrophic lateral sclerosis. *Neurotherapeutics* (2017) 14:119–134. doi: 10.1007/s13311-016-0503-x
71. Khalil M, Teunissen CE, Otto M, Piehl F, Sormani MP, Gattringer T, et al. Neurofilaments as biomarkers in neurological disorders. *Nat Rev Neurol.* (2018) 14:577–89. doi: 10.1038/s41582-018-0058-z
72. Gendron TF, Daughrity LM, Heckman MG, Diehl NN, Wuu J, et al. Phosphorylated neurofilament heavy chain: a biomarker of survival for C9ORF72-associated amyotrophic lateral sclerosis. *Ann Neurol.* (2017) 82:139–46. doi: 10.1002/ana.24980
73. Floeter MK, Traynor BJ, Farren J, Braun LE, Tierney M, Wiggs EA, et al. Disease progression in C9orf72 mutation carriers. *Neurology* (2017) 89:234–41. doi: 10.1212/WNL.0000000000004115
74. García-Redondo A, Dols-Icardo O, Rojas-García R, Esteban-Pérez J, Cordero-Vázquez P, Muñoz-Blanco JL, et al. Analysis of the C9orf72 gene in patients with amyotrophic lateral sclerosis in Spain and different populations worldwide. *Hum Mutat.* (2013) 34:79–82. doi: 10.1002/humu.22211
75. Umoh ME, Fournier C, Li Y, Polak M, Shaw L, Landers JE, et al. Comparative analysis of C9orf72 and sporadic disease in an ALS clinic population. *Neurology* (2016) 87:1024–30. doi: 10.1212/WNL.0000000000003067
76. Meeter LH, Dopper EG, Jiskoot LC, Sanchez-Valle R, Graff C, Benussi L, et al. Neurofilament light chain: a biomarker for genetic frontotemporal dementia. *Ann Clin Transl Neurol.* (2016) 3:623–36. doi: 10.1002/acn3.325
77. Meeter LHH, Gendron TF, Sias AC, Jiskoot LC, Russo SP, Donker Kaat L, et al. Poly(GP), neurofilament and grey matter deficits in C9orf72 expansion carriers. *Ann Clin Transl Neurol.* (2018) 5:583–97. doi: 10.1002/acn3.559
78. Benatar M, Wuu J, Andersen PM, Lombardi V, Malaspina A. Neurofilament light: a candidate biomarker of presymptomatic amyotrophic lateral sclerosis and phenoconversion. *Ann Neurol.* (2018) 84:130–9. doi: 10.1002/ana.25276
79. Lehmer C, Oeckl P, Weishaupt JH, Volk AE, Diehl-Schmid J, Schroeter ML, et al. Poly-GP in cerebrospinal fluid links C9orf72-associated dipeptide repeat expression to the asymptomatic phase of ALS/FTD. *EMBO Mol Med.* (2017) 9:859–68. doi: 10.15252/emmm.201607486
80. Su Z, Zhang Y, Gendron TF, Bauer PO, Chew J, Yang WY, et al. Discovery of a biomarker and lead small molecules to target r(GGGGCC)-associated defects in c9FTD/ALS. *Neuron* (2014) 83:1043–50. doi: 10.1016/j.neuron.2014.07.041
81. Gendron TF, Chew J, Stankowski JN, Hayes LR, Zhang YJ, Prudencio M, et al. Poly(GP) proteins are a useful pharmacodynamic marker for C9ORF72-associated amyotrophic lateral sclerosis. *Sci Transl Med.* (2017) 9:eaai7866. doi: 10.1126/scitranslmed.aai7866
82. Gendron TF, Petrucelli L. Disease mechanisms of C9ORF72 repeat expansions. *Cold Spring Harb Perspect Med.* (2018) 8:a024224. doi: 10.1101/cshperspect.a024224

83. van Blitterswijk M, Gendron TF, Baker MC, M. DeJesus-Hernandez, Finch NA, Brown PH, et al. Novel clinical associations with specific C9ORF72 transcripts in patients with repeat expansions in C9ORF72. *Acta Neuropathol.* (2015) 130:863–76. doi: 10.1007/s00401-015-1480-6
84. Jiang J, Zhu Q, Gendron TF, Saberi S, McAlonis-Downes M, Seelman A, et al. Gain of toxicity from ALS/FTD-linked repeat expansions in C9ORF72 is alleviated by antisense oligonucleotides targeting GGGGCC-containing RNAs. *Neuron* (2016) 90:535–50. doi: 10.1016/j.neuron.2016.04.006
85. Kramer NJ, Carlomagno Y, Zhang YJ, Almeida S, Cook CN, Gendron TF, et al. Spt4 selectively regulates the expression of C9orf72 sense and antisense mutant transcripts. *Science* (2016) 353:708–12. doi: 10.1126/science.aaf7791

19

Predictive Factors for Early Initiation of Artificial Feeding in Patients with Sporadic Creutzfeldt-Jakob Disease

*Pei-Chen Hsieh, Han-Tao Li, Chun-Wei Chang, Yih-Ru Wu and Hung-Chou Kuo**

Department of Neurology, Linkou Chang Gung Memorial Hospital, College of Medicine, Chang Gung University, Taipei, Taiwan

Correspondence:
Hung-Chou Kuo
kuo0426@adm.cgmh.org.tw

Background: Akinetic mutism has often been used as the predictor of sporadic Creutzfeldt-Jacob disease (sCJD) endpoints, but it may be difficult for general physcians to assess. Nasogastric (NG) tube insertion is indicated for many neurodegenerative diseases with a clinical course of swallowing failure, and can be more easily identified than akinetic mutism by general physicians. Therefore, the aim of this study was to identify whether there are predictive factors for early initiation of artificial feeding in patients with sCJD who require enteral nutrition due to swallowing failure.

Methods: We retrospectively reviewed the medical records of all patients diagnosed with probable sCJD who were admitted to the neurology ward at a medical center in Taiwan from January 2002 to July 2017. We used Pearson's chi-squared test to detect the correlation of initial symptoms, neurological signs, brain magnetic resonance imaging (MRI), electroencephalography (EEG), and increased levels of 14-3-3 protein in cerebrospinal fluid (CSF) analysis. The Cox proportional hazards model was used to detect prognostic factors for early initiation of NG tube insertion in sCJD patients.

Results: The onset age ranged from 51 to 83 years, and mostly ranged from 60 to 79 years. Akinetic mutism was correlated with pyramidal tract signs, myoclonus, and extrapyramidal signs. Furthermore, myoclonus was revealed to be associated with pyramidal tract signs. Multivariate Cox regression analysis showed that myoclonus and elevated CSF levels of 14-3-3 protein are predictive of early NG insertion.

Conclusions: Increased levels of 14-3-3 protein in CSF and the presence of myoclonus at diagnosis are predictive of early swallowing difficulty and indicate rapid deterioration in probable sCJD. In addition to akinetic mutism, early initiation of artificial feeding can be used to predict early deterioration in sCJD.

Keywords: creutzfeldt-jakob disease, artificial feeding, pognosis, myoclonus, akinetic mutism

INTRODUCTION

The annual global incidence rate of sporadic Creutzfeldt-Jakob disease (sCJD) is approximately 1–1.5 cases per million people (1). In Taiwan, the incidence rate is 0.55 cases per million people per year. The pathogenesis of sCJD remains unclear. There are variable clinical symptoms and signs in sCJD. The median survival duration for patients with sCJD is 4–6 months (2, 3), but Asian populations may have longer survival (4, 5). Longer survival has been associated with younger age, female gender, absence of CSF 14-3-3 protein and type 2a prion protein, sharp-wave complexes on EEG, and MV form in codon 129 PRNP human gene (6, 7). Survival has been found to be prolonged in patients who received tube feeding after they reached the state of akinetic mutism (8).

Our patients were genotyped at codon 129 of the PRNP gene and all were methionine homozygotes (MM) from 1998 to 2007, and the type was referred to as myoclonic type of sCJD (5, 9). sCJD is a rapidly progressive dementia that leads to decreased level of consciousness and cortical impairment which causes unsafe swallowing. The use of a nasogastric (NG) tube is a risk factor for mortality in advanced dementia (10–12). The initiation of artificial feeding indicates that patients have lost the ability to perform activities of daily living (ADL) and the disease has progressed to the final stage (13, 14). Although other studies have used akinetic mutism as the predictor for sCJD endpoints, it is difficult for general physicians to assess in patients whose consciousness level is impaired (4, 15, 16). Dysphagia is used for prognosis in spinal and bulbar muscular atrophy but there is a lack of reliable clinical markers for dysphagia assessment (17–19). The requirement for initiation of feeding tube insertion is easier to identify than detection of swallowing failure by a general physician or even a caregiver.

Although tube feeding may prolong survival in sCJD, the initiation time of artificial feeding may be a more suitable endpoint than akinetic mutism. Therefore, the goal of this study was to determine if there are predictive factors for early NG tube feeding.

METHODS

We retrospectively reviewed the medical charts of all patients diagnosed with probable sCJD and admitted to the neurology ward from January 2002 to July 2017 at Chang Gung Memorial Hospital. All of the cases were submitted by physicians who diagnose sCJD and were reviewed by the neurology, neuroradiology, and neuropathology experts of the CJD Surveillance Unit (CJDSU) at the Taiwan Neurological Society. We had a total of 35 probable sCJD patients. We included patients whose initial symptoms occurred within 2 months of admission and who could have a neurological examination with a Glasgow coma scale (GCS) score of 15 out of 15. We excluded a patient who had a history of progressive supranuclear palsy that made it difficult to identify initial neurological symptoms. Data were collected at baseline included gender, age, time of admission, cerebrospinal fluid (CSF) with 14-3-3 proteins, presence of high signal on diffusion-weighted images of magnetic resonance imaging (MRI), periodic sharp wave complex (PSWC) in electroencephalography (EEG) findings, NG tube insertion time, initial presentation, and abnormal neurological examination at admission. Results of CSF 14-3-3 protein assay data were obtained through collaboration with the Taiwan Prion Disease Pathology Surveillance Center. Clinical signs and symptoms that were assessed by neurologists included cognitive impairment (memory impairment, visual spatial dysfunction, apraxia, aphasia, and akinetic mutism), visual disturbance (visual field defect, visual hallucination, complex visual disturbance), cerebellar disturbance (ataxic gait, limbs dysmetria), pyramidal dysfunction (hemiparesis, spasticity, hyperreflexia, positive Babinski sign), extrapyramidal dysfunction (rigidity, bradykinesia, dystonia, dyskinesia), myoclonus, and seizure. NG tube insertion was performed when a patient was assessed by a clinical physician as having decreased level of consciousness or severe cognitive impairment that caused poor intake. The date of NG insertion was recorded according to medical record. The protocol was approved by the institutional review board of Chang Gung Memorial Hospital (IRB No.: 201701320B0).

Statistical Analysis

The time from admission to NG insertion of all patients were compared with age, sex, neurological signs, the elevation of CSF 14-3-3 protein, and brain MRI findings. Four patients did not have the records of NG insertion times because of loss to follow-up. We used Pearson's test was used to estimate the correlation of initial symptoms, clinical neurological signs, MRI image findings, and 14-3-3 proteins in CSF. For the cumulative incidence of NG tube insertion, the Kaplan–Meier method was used for overall analysis and each of the above features was stratified. The Cox proportional hazards model was used to identify the prognostic factors for the duration from onset to

TABLE 1 | Baseline demographic and clinical characteristics of sCJD patients.

Patients with sCJD	***n* = 30**	**(%)**
SEX		
Female	12	43
Male	18	57
Age of Onset ± SD (year)	67.7 ± 9.3	
Median (year)	68.5	
Range (year)	51-83	
AGE AT DIAGNOSIS (YEAR)		
40–49	0	
50–59	6	20
60–69	12	40
70–79	9	28
80–89	3	10
Initial symptom to admission ± SD (day)	27.5 ± 12	
CLINICAL MANIFESTATIONS AT DISEASE ONSET (%)		
Cognitive impairment	10	33
Visual disturbance	11	37
Gait disturbance	11	37
Speech disturbance	8	27
Increased 14-3-3 protein in CSF (%)	22/30	73
PSWC in Initial EEG (%)	10/30	33
BRAIN MRI FINDINGS		
Cortical involvement	14/30	47
Cortical and basal ganglia involvement	16/30	53

CSF, Cerebrospinal fluid; EEG, electroencephalography; MRI, magnetic resonance imaging; PSWC, periodic sharp wave complex; sCJD, sporadic Creutzfeldt-Jakob disease.

NG tube dependence, and the backward selection method in multivariate analysis was used to assess the independent effects of the investigated factors. Statistical significance was selected using the selection method at $P < 0.05$ in univariate regression analyses. We used the Wald test to estimate hazard ratios (HRs) and 95% confidence intervals (CIs), and we used Pearson's chi-squared test to detect the correlation of neurological signs at admission, imaging findings, 14-3-3 proteins in CSF, and initial PSWC on EEG. Statistical analyses were performed using SPSS version 22.

RESULTS

Thirty patients with probable sCJD admitted from January 2002 to July 2017 were included in the study. Basic characteristics are summarized in **Table 1**. The onset age ranged from 51 to 83 years, and mostly ranged from 60 to 79 years. The median age at diagnosis was 68.5 years. Female patients accounted for 43% of the patients in this study. Increased levels of CSF 14-3-3 protein were found in 22 of 30 patients. The PSWC of initial EEG was 33%. Among all patients, 47% had the characteristic brain MRI findings indicating cortical ribbon signs and 53% had the MRI findings indicating both cortical and basal ganglia involvement (**Table 1**). The initial symptoms of cognitive impairment, visual disturbance, unsteadiness, and speech disturbance were present in 43, 37, 37, and 27% of the patients, respectively. The most common neurological sign during admission was visual spatial dysfunction, which was followed by myoclonus and cerebellar and extrapyramidal dysfunction (**Figure 1**).

Correlations Among Variables at Diagnosis

The Pearson's x^2 test was used to assess correlation between neurological signs and variables, and the variables included basal ganglia and cortical involvement on brain MRI, PSWC on initial EEG, increased 14-3-3 protein in CSF, sex, and age. In addition, the neurological signs were also compared with each other. Both basal ganglia and cortical involvement on brain MRI were significantly correlated with akinetic mutism ($P < 0.01$). Akinetic mutism was correlated with abnormal pyramidal and extrapyramidal signs and myoclonus. Furthermore, myoclonus was associated with pyramidal tract signs. **Figure 2** shows correlations between investigative tests and neurological signs and between variables at diagnosis. An

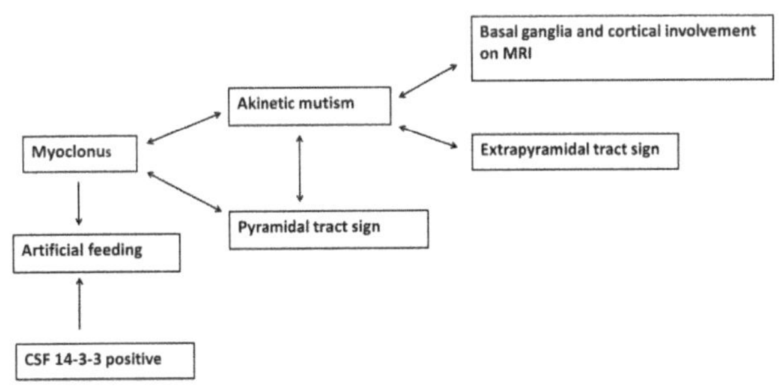

FIGURE 2 | The association between neurological signs and brain MRI findings as well as myoclonus and detectable 14-3-3 protein in CSF leading to early artificial feeding in sporadic Creutzfeldt-Jakob disease.

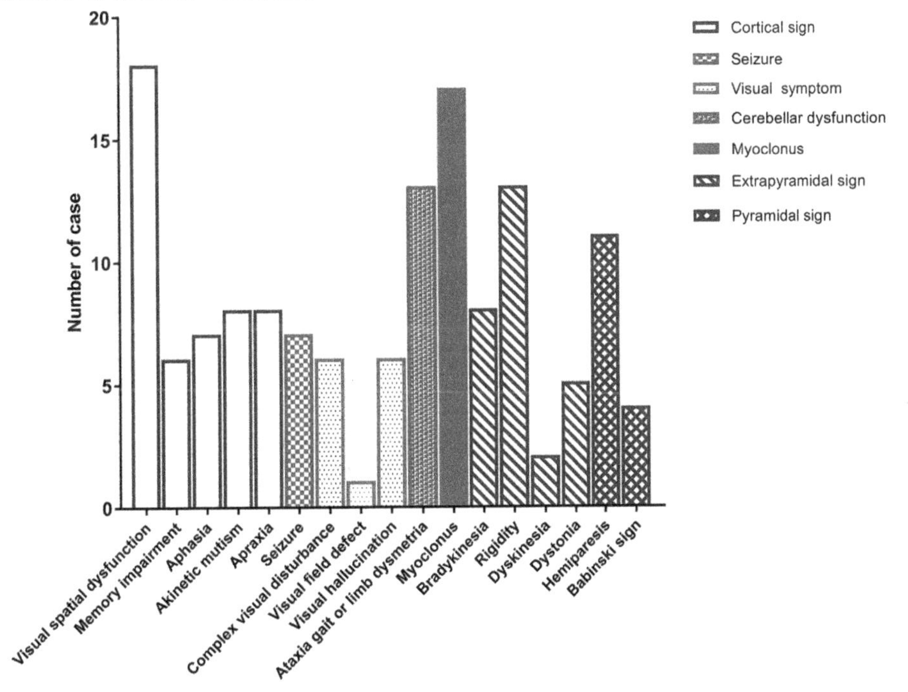

FIGURE 1 | The initial neurological signs of patients with sporadic Creutzfeldt-Jakob disease at first hospitalization.

association was revealed between myoclonus, akinetic mutism, and pyramidal tract dysfunction. Furthermore, myoclonus and detectable CSF 14-3-3 protein might lead to early use of artificial feeding.

Relationships Between Clinical Signs and Symptoms and NG Tube Insertion Time

The median time of NG tube insertion was 46.4 days after the onset of the initial symptom. **Table 2** shows a univariate Cox regression analysis of gender, age, PSWC in EEG, MRI with both basal ganglia and cortical involvement, elevation of CSF 14-3-3 protein, and neurological signs during initial hospitalization. The result demonstrated significant differences in the CSF 14-3-3 protein, myoclonus, pyramidal dysfunction, extrapyramidal dysfunction, and akinetic mutism. These were attributed to NG tube insertion. Patients with increased 14-3-3 protein in CSF were found to have 6.5 times higher risk of early NG tube insertion. No significant differences were found in the characteristic findings of sCJD on EEG and brain MRI with both cortex and basal ganglia involvement. The median periods from first hospitalization to NG tube insertion in myoclonus and CSF analysis were 10 and 19 days, respectively. **Figure 3** shows the cumulative incidences of artificial feeding in sCJD patients with (3A) myoclonus and (3B) 14-3-3 protein in CSF.

DISCUSSION

Swallowing requires coordination of multiple bulbar muscles and relatively clear consciousness (14). NG tube insertion is globally used for many neurological patients who suffer from swallowing failure and poor nutrition, and swallowing failure indicates that the patient's condition has reached the end of life in many neurodegenerative diseases (13). Therefore, NG tube feeding is a predictive factor of mortality in advanced dementia (12). On the other hand, feeding tube insertion increases the survival of CJD patients due to better supportive care (8).

Creutzfeldt-Jacob disease is a prion disease that can present as irreversible rapidly progressive dementia, accompanied by myoclonus, pyramidal tract, extrapyramidal tract, or cerebellar involvement (20). Most of the patients with decreased level of consciousness or severe cognitive dysfunction need NG tube feeding for nutrition support during disease progression. In Chinese culture and Taiwan's health insurance system, the majority of patients receive intensive life-sustaining treatment, and some even continue the treatment until there is irreversible advanced neurological disorder. Unlike akinetic mutism, NG tube insertion makes it easier for clinical physicians to detect patients with severe neurodegenerative disease. Furthermore, the time until death of patients with NG tube feeding can be influenced by underlying comorbidities such as aspiration pneumonia or other infectious diseases. NG tube insertion caused by swallowing failure is an early sign of poor outcome in patients with dementia syndromes. Increased 14-3-3 protein in CSF has been considered as an indicator of rapid neuronal damage (7). Our study found that the presence of myoclonus and elevated levels of CSF 14-3-3 protein led to a rapid deterioration of the patient's condition and the consequent need for enteral nutrition. According to Nakatani et al. akinetic mutism is the neurological symptom of sCJD endpoint. Cerebellar disturbance and psychiatric symptoms increase the risk of akinetic mutism. Myoclonus is a potential contributing factor of akinetic mutism and exercise-induced seizures, and myoclonus and myoclonic seizures are associated with pyramidal dysfunction (16). In our study, akinetic mutism was associated

TABLE 2 | Univariate and multivariate regression analyses of the day of nasogastric tube insertion.

Variables	HR	Univariate *P*-value	95% CI		HR	Multivariate *P*-value	95% CI	
			Lower	Upper			Lower	Upper
Gender: male	1.29	0.539	0.574	2.887				
Age at diagnosis > 65 (years)	1.40	0.426	0.613	3.180				
PWSC in EEG	1.76	0.203	0.738	4.181				
Cortical and basal ganglia involvement	1.77	0.188	0.767	4.117				
Increase in CSF 14-3-3 protein	2.85	0.039**	1.056	7.669	6.529	0.003**	1.928	22.109
CLINICAL SIGNS								
Myoclonus	5.61	0.001**	2.027	15.511	18.51	< 0.001**	4.875	70.279
Cognitive dysfunction	0.55	0.430	0.126	2.417				
Pyramidal dysfunction	4.08	0.007**	1.466	11.356				
Extrapyramidal dysfunction	2.72	0.029*	1.109	6.658				
Cerebellar sign	1.07	0.868	0.474	2.419				
Cortical visual dysfunction	0.98	0.953	0.423	2.249				
Akinetic mutism	4.19	0.009**	1.438	12.215				
Seizure	1.73	0.287	0.632	4.706				

*EEG, electroencephalography; MRI, magnetic resonance imaging; PSWC, periodic sharp wave complex; *$p < 0.05$, **$p < 0.01$.*

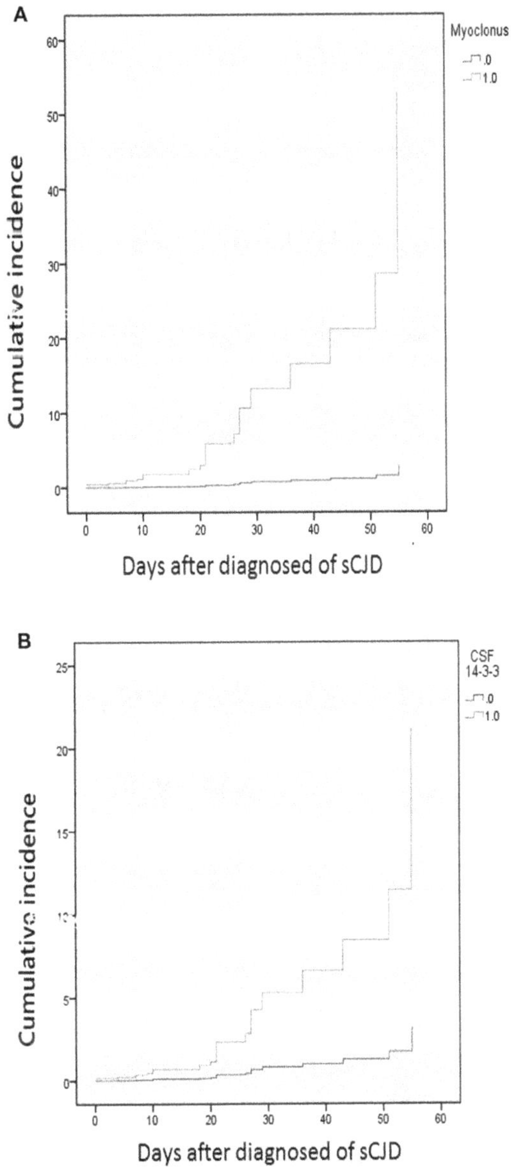

FIGURE 3 | Stratified cumulative incidence of artificial feeding in **(A)** myoclonus and **(B)** 14-3-3 protein in CSF at diagnosis of sporadic Creutzfeldt-Jakob disease.

with both cortical and basal ganglia involvement on brain MRI, pyramidal dysfunction, myoclonus, and extrapyramidal signs, indicating that neocortex and subcortical structures may be severely involved when akinetic mutism occurs. Therefore, since myoclonus, akinetic mutism, and pyramidal tract dysfunction are closely related, we may predict that the risk of swallowing failure increases when a patient presents with myoclonus.

Myoclonus in sCJD can present as irregular or rhythmic positive and negative jerky movements (21–23). It occurs in 82–100% of CJD patients and can be a focal or generalized pattern during the disease course, especially in the majority of advanced forms of all genotypes (24, 25). The presence of myoclonus has been considered to originate in the brainstem or thalamus area (15). Periodic rhythmic synchronized myoclonus has been suspected due to a hyperexcitable cortico-subcortical loop (26, 27). Furthermore, myoclonus occurred more frequently and earlier in MM type at codon 129 of the prion protein gene compared to other codon 129 polymorphism (9, 28). This genotype was considered to have the shortest survival compared to MV and VV forms of the human PRNP gene (7, 9). According to Iwasaki et al. CJD patients who have early onset of myoclonus, rapid disease progression to the akinetic mutism state, and PSWC on EEG were associated with relatively poor prognosis (8).

In conclusion, the dependence on artificial feeding could be a time point to predict the prognosis for CJD patients. The presence of myoclonus in CJD patients increases the risk of the need for artificial feeding and indicates an early irreversible dependence in daily activities.

AUTHOR CONTRIBUTIONS

P-CH wrote the initial manuscript and statistical analysis. H-TL collected data of all of the sCJD patients. P-CH, C-WC, Y-RW, and H-CK involve in conception and design and analysis and interpretation of data. H-CK also gave revision of manuscript for important intellectual content.

ACKNOWLEDGMENTS

This study was partially supported by a grant from Chang Gung Memorial Hospital, Taipei, Taiwan (CMRPG3G0431).

REFERENCES

1. World Health Organization. *WHO Manual for Surveillance of Human Transmissible Spongiform Encephalopathies Including Variant Creutzfeldt-Jakob Disease* (2003). Geneva: World Health Organization.
2. Parchi P, Giese A, Capellari S, Brown P, Schulz-Schaeffer W, Windl O, et al. Classification of sporadic Creutzfeldt-Jakob disease based on molecular and phenotypic analysis of 300 subjects. *Ann Neurol.* (1999) 46:224–33.
3. Ladogana A, Puopolo M, Croes EA, Budka H, Jarius C, Collins S, et al. Mortality from Creutzfeldt-Jakob disease and related disorders in Europe, Australia, and Canada. *Neurology* (2005) 64:1586–91. doi: 10.1212/01.WNL.0000160117.56690.B2
4. Nagoshi K, Sadakane A, Nakamura Y, Yamada M, Mizusawa H. Duration of prion disease is longer in Japan than in other countries. *J Epidemiol.* (2011) 21:255–62. doi: 10.2188/jea.JE20100085
5. Lu CJ, Sun Y, Chen SS. Incidence of Creutzfeldt-Jakob disease in Taiwan: a prospective 10-year surveillance. *Eur J Epidemiol.* (2010) 25:341–7. doi: 10.1007/s10654-010-9446-4
6. Puopolo M, Ladogana A, Almonti S, Daude N, Bevivino S, Petraroli R, et al. Mortality trend from sporadic Creutzfeldt-Jakob disease (CJD) in Italy, 1993-2000. *J Clin Epidemiol.* (2003) 56:494–9. doi: 10.1016/S0895-4356(02)00606-6
7. Pocchiari M, Puopolo M, Croes EA, Budka H, Gelpi E, Collins S, et al. Predictors of survival in sporadic Creutzfeldt-Jakob disease and other

human transmissible spongiform encephalopathies. *Brain* (2004) 127:2348–59. doi: 10.1093/brain/awh249

8. Iwasaki Y, Akagi A, Mimuro M, Kitamoto T, Yoshida M. Factors influencing the survival period in Japanese patients with sporadic Creutzfeldt-Jakob disease. *J Neurol Sci.* (2015) 357:63–8. doi: 10.1016/j.jns.2015.06.065
9. Iwasaki Y. Creutzfeldt-Jakob disease. *Neuropathology* (2017) 37:174–88. doi: 10.1111/neup.12355
10. Sarkar P, Cole A, Scolding NJ, Rice CM. Percutaneous endoscopic gastrostomy tube insertion in neurodegenerative disease: a retrospective study and literature review. *Clin Endosc.* (2017) 50:270–8. doi: 10.5946/ce.2016.106
11. Mitchell SL, Kiely DK, Lipsitz LA. The risk factors and impact on survival of feeding tube placement in nursing home residents with severe cognitive impairment. *Arch Intern Med.* (1997) 157:327–32.
12. Alvarez-Fernandez B, García-Ordoñez MA, Martínez-Manzanares C, Gómez-Huelgas R. Survival of a cohort of elderly patients with advanced dementia: nasogastric tube feeding as a risk factor for mortality. *Int J Geriatr Psychiatry* (2005) 20:363–70. doi: 10.1002/gps.1299
13. Mitchell SL, Teno JM, Kiely DK, Shaffer ML, Jones RN, Prigerson HG, et al. The clinical course of advanced dementia. *N Engl J Med.* (2009) 361:1529–38. doi: 10.1056/NEJMoa0902234
14. Harwood RH. Feeding decisions in advanced dementia. *J R Coll Physicians Edinb.* (2014) 44:232–7. doi: 10.4997/JRCPE.2014.310
15. Iwasaki Y, Mimuro M, Yoshida M, Kitamoto T, Hashizume Y. Survival to akinetic mutism state in Japanese cases of MM1-type sporadic Creutzfeldt-Jakob disease is similar to Caucasians. *Eur J Neurol.* (2011) 18:999–1002. doi: 10.1111/j.1468-1331.2010.03185.x
16. Nakatani E, Kanatani Y, Kaneda H, Nagai Y, Teramukai S, Nishimura T, et al. Specific clinical signs and symptoms are predictive of clinical course in sporadic Creutzfeldt-Jakob disease. *Eur J Neurol.* (2016) 23:1455–62. doi: 10.1111/ene.13057
17. Banno H, Katsuno M, Suzuki K, Tanaka S, Suga N, Hashizume A, et al. Swallowing markers in spinal and bulbar muscular atrophy. *Ann Clin Transl Neurol.* (2017) 4:534–43. doi: 10.1002/acn3.425
18. Kertscher B, Speyer R, Palmier M, Plant C. Bedside screening to detect oropharyngeal dysphagia in patients with neurological disorders: a systematic review. *Dysphagia* (2014) 29:204–12. doi: 10.1007/s00455-013-9490-9
19. Walshe M. Oropharyngeal dysphagia in neurodegenerative disease. *J Gastroenterol Hepatol Res.* (2014) 3:1265–71. doi: 10.6051/j.issn.2224-3992.2014.03.408-2
20. Ironside JW, Ritchie DL, Head MW. Prion diseases. *Handb Clin Neurol.* (2017) 145:393–403. doi: 10.1002/9780470015902.a0000426
21. Panzica F, Canafoglia L, Franceschetti S, Binelli S, Ciano C, Visani E, et al. Movement-activated myoclonus in genetically defined progressive myoclonic epilepsies: EEG-EMG relationship estimated using autoregressive models. *Clin Neurophysiol.* (2003) 114:1041–52. doi: 10.1016/S1388-2457(03)00066-X
22. Shibasaki H, Motomura S, Yamashita Y, Shii H, Kuroiwa Y. Periodic synchronous discharge and myoclonus in Creutzfeldt-Jakob disease: diagnostic application of jerk-locked averaging method. *Ann Neurol.* (1981) 9:150–6. doi: 10.1002/ana.410090208
23. Shibasaki, H. Neurophysiological classification of myoclonus. *Neurophysiol Clin.* (2006) 36:267–9. doi: 10.1016/j.neucli.2006.11.004
24. Brown P, Cathala F, Castaigne P, Gajdusek C. Creutzfeldt-Jakob disease: clinical analysis of a consecutive series of 230 neuropathologically verified cases. *Ann Neurol.* (1986) 20:597–602. doi: 10.1002/ana.410200507
25. Burger LJ, Rowan AJ, Goldensohn ES. Creutzfeldt-Jakob disease. An electroencephalographic study. *Arch Neurol.* (1972) 26:428–33.
26. Binelli S, Agazzi P, Canafoglia L, Scaioli V, Panzica F, Visani E, et al. Myoclonus in Creutzfeldt-Jakob disease: polygraphic and video-electroencephalography assessment of 109 patients. *Mov Disord.* (2010) 25:2818–27. doi: 10.1002/mds.23397
27. Shibasaki H, Neshige R, Hashiba Y. Cortical excitability after myoclonus: jerk-locked somatosensory evoked potentials. *Neurology* (1985) 35:36–41.
28. Hashimoto T, Iwahashi T, Ishii W, Yamamoto K, Ikeda S. EEG-EMG polygraphic study of dystonia and myoclonus in a case of Creutzfeldt-Jakob disease. *Epilepsy Behav Case Rep.* (2015) 4:30–2. doi: 10.1016/j.ebcr.2015.05.002

20

Split-Hand Syndrome in Amyotrophic Lateral Sclerosis: Differences in Dysfunction of the FDI and ADM Spinal Motoneurons

Zhi-Li Wang[1], Liying Cui[1,2], Mingsheng Liu[1], Kang Zhang[1], Shuangwu Liu[1] and Qingyun Ding[1]*

[1] *Department of Neurology, Peking Union Medical College Hospital, Chinese Academy of Medical Sciences, Beijing, China,*
[2] *Neurosciences Center, Chinese Academy of Medical Sciences, Beijing, China*

***Correspondence:**
Liying Cui
pumchcuily@sina.com

The F-wave test allows for the non-invasive assessment of spinal motoneuron excitability. We investigated the difference in spinal motoneuron dysfunction between the first dorsal interosseous (FDI) and abductor digit minimi (ADM) muscles by investigating F-waves and to assess the contribution of spinal mechanisms to split-hand syndrome in patients with amyotrophic lateral sclerosis (ALS). Sixty-five consecutive ALS patients and twenty age- and gender-matched healthy controls (HCs) were enrolled. Motor nerve conduction studies and F-waves were performed bilaterally on median and ulnar nerves in all subjects. HCs revealed prominently longer F-wave latencies, lower chronodispersion, mean F-wave amplitude, and mean and maximal F/M amplitude ratio ($P < 0.001$) in the FDI compared to the ADM. However, no significant differences in almost all F-wave parameters between the FDI and ADM were observed in ALS patients with affected hands except the minimal and mean F-wave latency. These data suggest that excitability is greatly changed in the spinal motoneurons innervating the FDI. Furthermore, the mean F-wave amplitude ($r = 0.454$, $P = 0.002$) of the FDI was significantly correlated with the FDI/ADM CMAP amplitude ratio in ALS patients with affected hands but not of the ADM. Our findings suggested that the dysfunction of spinal motoneurons between the FDI and ADM was different in ALS, and spinal motoneuron dysfunction was associated with development of the split-hand phenomenon.

Keywords: amyotrophic lateral sclerosis, F-wave, motor neuron, split-hand, first dorsal interosseous muscle, motor neuron disease

INTRODUCTION

Amyotrophic lateral sclerosis (ALS) is a rapidly progressive neurodegenerative disorder involving both upper and lower motor neurons (LMNs) and is often characterized by muscle weakness and atrophy, especially the small hand muscles. Dissociated atrophy of intrinsic hand muscles as an early and specific clinical feature of ALS, termed the split-hand sign, refers to preferential weakness and wasting of the abductor pollicis brevis (APB) and first dorsal interosseous (FDI) muscles with relative sparing of the abductor digit minimi (ADM) (Kuwabara et al., 1999, 2008; Wilbourn, 2000; Eisen and Kuwabara, 2012; Eisen et al., 2017). Menon et al. (2014b) reported that the split-hand sign was often evident in 62% of patients at the time of visiting and in 95% at follow-up.

Although the thenar complex muscles (APB/FDI) and hypothenar muscles (ADM) constituting the split-hand are innervated through the same spinal segments (C8 and T1), the FDI and ADM, which are differentially affected, share ulnar innervation (Weber et al., 2000; Kuwabara et al., 2008; Eisen and Kuwabara, 2012). Corticomotoneuronal input and spinal/peripheral mechanisms have been suggested to be involved (Weber et al., 2000; Bae et al., 2009; Eisen and Kuwabara, 2012; Shibuya et al., 2013; Menon et al., 2014b; Eisen et al., 2017), and cortical dysfunction is considered as the likely pathophysiological mechanism underlying the split-hand phenomenon, while axonal dysfunction may appear as a downstream process (Menon et al., 2014a,b). The spinal mechanisms underlying the development of split-hand in ALS remain controversial. For example, Cengiz et al. (2018) reported no significant difference in cutaneous silent period measurements between the ADM and FDI, suggesting no role of spinal cord excitability changes in split-hand syndrome. However, Wilbourn (2000) reported the finding of split-hand in ALS in 1992, as well as in other diseases with only LMN dysfunction, and suggested that the lesion responsible for the ALS split-hand was at the level of the cervical anterior horn cell (Schelhaas et al., 2003). Further, Fang et al. (2016) found differences between the dysfunction of spinal motoneurons innervating the APB and the ADM in ALS. Thus, in the present study, we examined the hypothesis that spinal mechanisms contribute to split-hand in ALS.

The F-wave is a late response that reflects antidromic activation of motoneurons. Previous studies have shown that F-waves were not only used to assess changes in the excitability of spinal motoneurons (Espiritu et al., 2003; Lin and Floeter, 2004; Argyriou et al., 2006) but also as a probe to determine the activity of the motor cortex (Mercuri et al., 1996; Rivner, 2008). A direct comparison of the F-wave variables of the FDI and ADM innervated by the same nerve and the same spinal segments may provide more valuable information on the excitability changes of the spinal motoneuron pool and shed light on the complex mechanisms of split-hands. To date, the characteristics of multiple F-wave variables in the FDI have not been assessed in healthy subjects and ALS in previous studies. Therefore, the aims of this study were to (1) identify the characteristics of F-waves of the FDI, and (2) to ascertain the difference in spinal motoneuron dysfunction between the FDI and ADM in patients with ALS and HCs and to clarify the spinal pathophysiology of split-hand.

MATERIALS AND METHODS

Subjects

Sixty-five consecutive patients diagnosed as having definite, probable and laboratory-supported probable sporadic ALS according to the revised El Escorial criteria were included in this study. All patients were recruited at the department of neurology in Peking Union Medical College Hospital between December 2017 and November 2018. Patients with ALS complicated by diabetic neuropathy, alcohol abuse, carpal tunnel syndrome, cervical myelopathy, and other neurological disorders were excluded. Control data were obtained from 20 age- and gender-matched healthy volunteers, whose nerve condition studies were normal. In each patient the muscle strength was assessed using the Medical Research Council (MRC) score, and a total MRC score was calculated for the following muscle groups assessed bilaterally: shoulder abduction, elbow flexion, elbow extension, wrist dorsiflexion, finger abduction, thumb abduction, hip flexion, knee extension, and ankle dorsiflexion (Menon et al., 2014b). The maximum possible total MRC score was 90. The clinical status of each patient was evaluated with the ALS Functional Rating Scale-Revised (ALSFRS-R) and upper motor neuron (UMN) score, as previous studies described (Cedarbaum et al., 1999; Grapperon et al., 2014). Two groups were established from the ALS patients, an affected hand group with wasting and weakness in the intrinsic hand muscles, where the data from the more affected hands were analyzed (45 patients), and an unaffected hand group, where the data for bilateral hands were analyzed in this group (20 patients). The hand was considered to be unaffected if the intrinsic hand muscles contained APB, FDI and ADM of normal strength; no wasting or weakness; and the nerve conduction studies (NCSs) were within normal limits. The hands of the healthy controls (HCs) were analyzed bilaterally. To estimate the influence of UMN involvement in the split-hand phenomenon, two subgroups were formed from ALS patients in the affected hand group, designated as the P group (pyramidal signs) and the NP group (no pyramidal signs). A more conservative but robust criterion for UMN lesion was used in the present study, requiring both increased tendon reflexes and positive Hoffman's sign in defining the presence of pyramidal lesion in the arm (de Carvalho et al., 2002). The study was approved by the Peking Union Medical College Hospital Clinical Research Ethics Committee (Beijing, China), and all participants provided signed informed consent.

Nerve Conduction Studies

All patients underwent routine NCSs and electromyography (EMG) using an EMG machine (Medtronic-Dantec Electronics, Skovlunde, Denmark). A peak-to-peak amplitude of maximal compound muscle action potential (CMAP) was elicited by using supramaximal (120%) surface stimulation of the median and ulnar nerves at the wrist and recorded from the APB, FDI and ADM muscles according to previously described standard methods (Stimulus duration: 0.1 ms; Filter setting: 20 Hz–10 kHz Gain: 200 μV/division; Sweep speed: 5 ms/division). Specifically, for FDI recording, the active electrode (G1) was placed on its belly and the reference electrode (G2) at the medial aspect of the proximal interphalangeal joint of the index finger (Kuwabara et al., 2008). The distance between the cathode and active (G1) recording electrodes for ADM muscles was 6.5 cm, while the distance between the cathode and active (G1) electrode for the FDI muscle was 8–10 cm. There was no evidence of conduction block or M response temporal dispersion in ALS patients. The skin temperature was maintained above 32°C. The following parameters were obtained: distal motor latency (DML), motor conduction velocity (MCV), CMAP amplitude (peak-to-peak), and the FDI/ADM CMAP amplitude ratio.

F-Wave Studies

The F-waves of ulnar nerves were recorded with surface electrodes attached to the skin over the FDI and ADM muscles, the same position as in motor nerve conduction studies (de Carvalho et al., 2002; Kim, 2011). One hundred consecutive supramaximal (120%) percutaneous stimuli were delivered to the ulnar nerve at the wrist at a frequency of 1 Hz with the cathode proximal to the anode (Filters setting: 20 Hz–3 kHz; amplifier gain: 200 μV/division). A peak-to-peak deflection from baseline of at least 40 μV was accepted as an F-wave (Peioglou-Harmoussi et al., 1985). The following F-wave variables were measured in the FDI and ADM: the minimum, mean and maximum latency corrected according to the subject's height (FLmin/H, FLmax/H, FLmean/H) (ms/m); chronodispersion; persistence; mean and maximum F-wave amplitude (peak-to-peak); mean and maximum F/M amplitude ratio (average or maximum peak-to-peak amplitude of F-waves expressed as a percentage of maximum distal CMAP amplitude); and the number of repeater F-waves. The repeater F-waves were identified as having the same shape, latency, and amplitude, and were calculated by the following indices as described by Chroni et al. (Chroni et al., 2012): index repeating neuron (index RN) (number of repeating neuron/ number of traces with different F-wave shapes in a series of 100 stimuli × 100), and index repeater F-waves (index Freps) (total number of F-wave repeaters/total number of traces with F-waves in the same nerve × 100). Due to the nature of the applied F-wave technique, which requires recording of a significant number of F-waves, we only examined the FDI and ADM muscles with strength of MRC of 2 or higher. And nerves without F-waves or the CAMP amplitude ≤ 2.0 mV were excluded from our analysis.

Statistical Analysis

All analyses were performed using SPSS for windows version 24.0 (SPSS, IBM, Chicago, IL, United States). Normality was checked by the Shapiro–Wilk test. Normally distributed data are expressed as the mean ± SD and were compared using one-way ANOVA and the Student-Newman-Keuls (SNK) test. Mean values of measured variables between the FDI and ADM within the same group were compared using Student's *t*-test. Non-normally distributed data are expressed as the medians (IQR) and were compared using the Kruskal–Wallis *H*-test. Once the null hypothesis was rejected, pairwise comparisons of the groups were tested using the Mann–Whitney *U*-test and Bonferroni correction with a significance level of $P < 0.017$. The relationship between the F-wave parameters and FDI/ADM CAMP amplitude ratio was assessed using Pearson's correlation and Spearman's rank correlation test. For comparison of the frequency distribution of categorical variables (gender and disease onset), the χ^2 test was used. The level of statistical significance was established at $P < 0.05$.

RESULTS

The clinical profiles of the ALS patients and HCs are presented in **Table 1**. Among the ALS groups, all patients studied herein had a clinically predominant LMN syndrome and none had a pure UMN syndrome. The total MRC scores were higher in the unaffected hand group than the affected hand group. Disease duration, UMN score and ALSFRS-R were not significantly different between the affected hand and unaffected hand groups. The age at examination, gender ratio, and height were comparable between patients and controls.

Table 2 summarizes the overall comparisons between motor conduction values obtained from the ulnar nerves (FDI and ADM) of both patients with ALS and HCs. In HCs, the mean CMAP amplitude in FDI was greater than that in ADM, and the mean FDI/ADM CMAP amplitude ratio was calculated as 1.38. A significant reduction of FDI/ADM CMAP amplitude ratio (0.9 ± 0.3) was observed in the affected hand group compared with HCs, confirming that the split-hand phenomenon was evident in the present ALS patients (Kuwabara et al., 2008).

The results of F-wave variables are displayed in **Table 3**. When the FDI and ADM were compared in HCs, the FDI showed

TABLE 1 | Clinical profile of participants.

Parameters	Affected hand (A, *n* = 45)	Unaffected hand (B, *n* = 20)	HCs (C, *n* = 20)	*P*-value		
				A vs. C	B vs. C	A vs. B
Age (year)	53.42 ± 8.82 (34–66)	51.20 ± 9.71 (35–69)	52.4 ± 9.13 (39–73)	>0.05	>0.05	> 0.05
Gender (male:female)	25:20	7:13	11:9	>0.05	>0.05	> 0.05
Height (cm)	165.84 ± 8.57	163.85 ± 7.56	166.3 ± 8.18	>0.05	>0.05	> 0.05
Disease duration (months)	14.73 ± 8.89 (3–45)	11.70 ± 6.97 (4–27)	NA	NA	NA	0.158
Disease onset (bulbar: upper limbs: lower limbs)	9:28:8	9:3:8	NA	NA	NA	0.002
Total MRC scores	73.44 ± 10.27 (43–88)	83.35 ± 6.78 (67–90)	NA	NA	NA	< 0.001
UMN scores	39.24 ± 14.03 (4–64)	32.10 ± 12.87 (5–54)	NA	NA	NA	0.057
ALSFRS-R	40.44 ± 4.18 (28–47)	42.30 ± 2.76 (36–46)	NA	NA	NA	0.099

HCs, healthy controls; MRC, Medical Research Council; UMN, upper motor neuron; ALSFRS-R, amyotrophic lateral sclerosis functional rating scale-revised; NA, not applicable.

TABLE 2 | Results of nerve conduction studies and split-hand.

Parameters	Affected hand (A, *n* = 45)	Unaffected hand (B, *n* = 40)	HCs (C, *n* = 40)	*P*-value		
				A vs. C	B vs. C	A vs. B
DML (ms)						
FDI	3.60 ± 0.40	3.45 ± 0.38	3.42 ± 0.32	**0.005**	0.519	0.089
ADM	2.47 ± 0.45	2.20 ± 0.26	2.19 ± 0.25	**0.001**	0.784	**0.002**
CMAP amplitude (mV)						
FDI	7.05 ± 4.31	17.91 ± 4.73	17.78 ± 3.77	**< 0.001**	0.825	**< 0.001**
ADM	7.49 ± 3.41	13.31 ± 2.80	14.62 ± 2.85	**< 0.001**	0.027	**< 0.001**
FDI/ADM CMAP amplitude ratio	0.90 ± 0.30	1.42 ± 0.28	1.38 ± 0.21	**< 0.001**	0.593	**< 0.001**
MCV (m/s)						
FDI	56.99 ± 4.53	60.11 ± 1.94	60.18 ± 1.45	**< 0.001**	0.159	**< 0.001**
ADM	55.89 ± 3.66	60.12 ± 1.22	60.20 ± 1.46	**< 0.001**	0.102	**< 0.001**

DML, distal motor latency; FDI, first dorsal interosseous; ADM, abductor digit minimi; CMAP, compound muscle action potential; MCV, motor conduction velocity; HCs, healthy controls. All data are expressed as the mean ± SD. Values with significant differences printed in bold characters.

TABLE 3 | Results of F-wave variables in the ALS patients and the healthy controls.

Parameters	Affected hand (A, *n* = 45)	Unaffected hand (B, *n* = 40)	HCs (C, *n* = 40)	*P*-value		
				A vs. C	B vs. C	A vs. B
Minimal F latency (ms/m)						
FDI	16.37 ± 0.95**	15.84 ± 0.71**	15.13 ± 0.46**	**< 0.001**	**< 0.001**	0.022
ADM	15.62 ± 0.92**	14.93 ± 0.79**	14.50 ± 0.47**	**< 0.001**	**0.016**	**< 0.001**
Maximal F latency (ms/m)						
FDI	18.93 ± 1.78	17.70 ± 0.92*	16.74 ± 0.57**	**< 0.001**	**< 0.001**	**< 0.001**
ADM	18.59 ± 1.70	16.99 ± 0.89*	15.13 ± 0.46**	**< 0.001**	**< 0.001**	**< 0.001**
Mean F latency (ms/m)						
FDI	17.41 ± 1.15*	16.53 ± 0.72**	15.82 ± 0.54**	**< 0.001**	**< 0.001**	**< 0.001**
ADM	16.80 ± 1.03*	15.81 ± 0.84**	15.17 ± 0.52**	**< 0.001**	**< 0.001**	**< 0.001**
F-wave chronodispersion (ms)						
FDI	4.22 ± 2.27	3.04 ± 0.95*	2.49 ± 0.55*	**< 0.001**	**0.001**	**0.004**
ADM	4.91 ± 2.31	3.34 ± 0.70*	2.88 ± 0.66*	**< 0.001**	**0.003**	**< 0.001**
F-wave persistence (%)						
FDI	62 (41)	96.5 (9.25)*	100 (0.75)	**< 0.001**	**< 0.001**	**< 0.001**
ADM	71 (54.5)	99 (1)*	100 (0)	**< 0.001**	**0.002**	**< 0.001**
Mean F-wave amplitude (μV)						
FDI	269 (216.5)	178.5 (127.25)*	174.5 (90.75)**	**0.002**	0.648	**0.015**
ADM	266 (199.5)	257.5 (124)*	264.5 (126.5)**	> 0.05	> 0.05	> 0.05
Mean F/M amplitude ratio (%)						
FDI	3.99 (5.96)	1.04 (0.6)**	1.03 (0.57)**	**< 0.001**	0.950	**< 0.001**
ADM	3.76 (3.47)	2.13 (1.23)**	1.85 (0.80)**	**< 0.001**	0.258	**< 0.001**
Maximal F/M amplitude ratio (%)						
FDI	11.97 (9.72)	3.37 (3.28)*	2.80 (1.82)**	**< 0.001**	0.020	**< 0.001**
ADM	10.01 (11.51)	5.86 (4.09)*	4.33 (2.52)**	**< 0.001**	0.017	**< 0.001**
Index RN (%)						
FDI	16.67 (23.07)	1.62 (3.23)**	0 (0)	**< 0.001**	**< 0.001**	**< 0.001**
ADM	18.18 (29.81)	0 (1.79)**	0 (0)	**< 0.001**	0.017	**< 0.001**
Index Freps (%)						
FDI	55.81 (51.57)	4.12 (13.33)**	0 (0)	**< 0.001**	**< 0.001**	**< 0.001**
ADM	50 (59.12)	0 (3.77)**	0 (0)	**< 0.001**	0.017	**< 0.001**

*HCs, healthy controls; FDI, first dorsal interosseous; ADM, abductor digit minimi. Normally distributed data are expressed as the mean ± SD, and non-normally distributed data are expressed as the medians (IQR). Values with significant differences printed in bold characters. **P <0.001, *P <0.05, between the FDI and the ADM in each group. For comparisons of F-wave variables among affected hand group, unaffected hand and healthy control group, Bonferroni correction with a significance level of P < 0.017.*

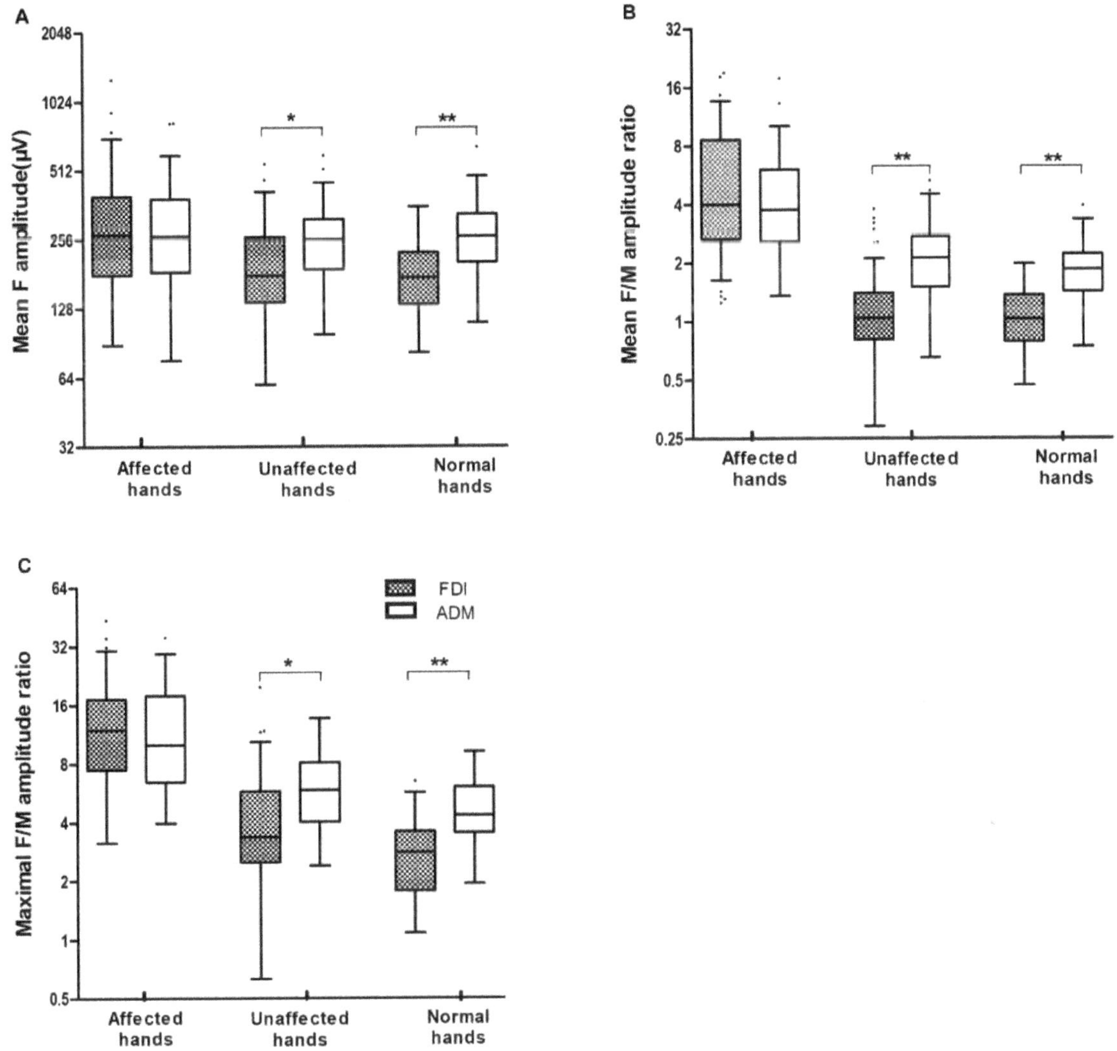

FIGURE 1 | The mean F-wave amplitude **(A)**, and the mean and maximal F/M amplitude ratios **(B,C)**, recorded over the FDI and ADM muscles were significantly increased in ALS patients with affected hands compared with those with unaffected hands. When the FDI and ADM were compared in HCs and the unaffected hand group, the FDI showed a noticeably lower mean F-wave amplitude, and a lower mean and maximal F/M amplitude ratios, than for the ADM. By contrast, there were no differences in F-wave measurements between the FDI and ADM in the affected hand group. $^{**}P < 0.001$; $^{*}P < 0.05$. The numerical data on the Y-axis were logarithmically transformed (Log2).

noticeably longer F-wave latencies and lower chronodispersion, mean F-wave amplitude, and mean and maximal F/M amplitude ratios than the ADM. This trend was similar in the unaffected hand group (**Figures 1A–C**). In contrast, no differences between the FDI and ADM for F-wave measurements were observed in the affected hand group except the FLmin/H and FLmean/H. Concerning the F-wave variables in the unaffected hand group, the F-wave latencies, persistence, chronodispersion of the FDI and ADM and index RN, and index Freps of the FDI were significantly changed compared to controls, along with the relative normal mean F-wave amplitude, mean and maximal F/M amplitude ratios of the FDI and ADM and index RN and index Freps of the FDI (column B vs. C). **Table 4** shows the comparison of F-wave parameters in ALS patients with pronounced split-hands between subgroups of those with (P) and without (NP) pyramidal signs. No difference was observed between the P and NP groups. Additionally, the difference between the FDI and ADM was not significant in both groups.

The results of the correlation analysis conducted between the F-wave parameters and FDI/ADM CMAP amplitude ratio displayed in **Supplementary Table S1**. Combining these parameters, it was evident that the F-wave amplitude ($r = 0.454$, $P = 0.002$) of the FDI was significantly correlated with the FDI/ADM CMAP amplitude ratio in the affected hand group, but not with the ADM. There was no significant correlation between other F-wave variables in both the ADM and FDI and the FDI/ADM CMAP amplitude ratio in the affected hand group of ALS patients. No significant relation was observed between the F-wave variables and FDI/ADM CMAP amplitude ratios in the unaffected hand group and HCs.

TABLE 4 | Comparison of F-wave parameters in ALS patients with split-hands between subgroups of those with (P) and without (NP) pyramidal signs.

Parameters	P group (*n* = 21)	NP group (*n* = 24)	*P*-value
F-wave persistence (%)			
FDI	62 (40)	59 (42.75)	0.637
ADM	84 (50)	52.5 (60)	0.255
Mean F-wave amplitude (μV)			
FDI	219 (180)	310.5 (286)	0.481
ADM	209 (162)	326.5 (181.25)	0.062
Mean F/M amplitude ratio (%)			
FDI	3.47 (3.01)	5.03 (7.39)	0.387
ADM	2.89 (1.74)	4.26 (3.41)	0.055
Maximal F/M amplitude ratio (%)			
FDI	11 (8.97)	15.2 (18.11)	0.106
ADM	9.09 (7.65)	13.47 (12.10)	0.116

FDI, first dorsal interosseous; ADM, abductor digit minimi; P, with pyramidal signs; NP, without pyramidal signs; Non-normally distributed data are expressed as the medians (IQR).

DISCUSSION

Results Related to the Changes in ALS

Our NCSs variables of the FDI and ADM and F-wave values of the ADM in HCs and patients with ALS showed a close resemblance to the previous findings (Peioglou-Harmoussi et al., 1985; Kuwabara et al., 2008; Buschbacher et al., 2015; Fang et al., 2016). In the present study, ALS patients with an unaffected hand did not show significant changes in DML, CMAP amplitude, or MCV recorded over the FDI and ADM in contrast with HCs. While a significantly decreased CMAP amplitude was associated with increased DML and slowed MCV in both the FDI and ADM were observed in our patients with affected hands. These findings are compatible with the chronic denervation/reinnervation process, and are associated with the pathophysiological changes in ALS (de Carvalho et al., 2002; Argyriou et al., 2006).

We used F-waves as an indicator of dysfunction of spinal motoneurons. The F-wave amplitudes are related to the excitability of spinal motoneurons and axonal compensatory reinnervation (Argyriou et al., 2006; Hachisuka et al., 2015). Specifically, the F/M amplitude ratio was used as a quantified index of the proportion of the motoneuron pool, as this measure is minimally influenced by muscle wasting (Argyriou et al., 2006). In ALS patients, the mean F-wave amplitude, and mean and maximal F/M amplitude ratios, were increased in the FDI and ADM. Similar findings were reported and inferred that both anterior horn cell hyperexcitability (Argyriou et al., 2006) and the formation of large post-reinnervation motor units due to LMN dysfunction (Drory et al., 2001) are important factors. In the present study, ALS patients also showed reduced F-wave persistence and increased repeater F-waves. Similar changes were reported in post-polio syndrome (PPS) (Hachisuka et al., 2015). Both F-wave persistence and repeater-F waves are influenced by the number of functional LMNs and motoneuron excitability. A low F-wave persistence indicates loss of function of LMNs and decreased excitability of the motoneuron pool (de Carvalho et al., 2002; Argyriou et al., 2006; Rivner, 2008). With respect to the mechanism of production of repeater F-waves in PPS, it was proposed that loss of motoneurons or decreased excitability of some anterior horn cells caused the remaining anterior horn cells with increased excitability to produce more frequent repeated backfiring (Hachisuka et al., 2015). This underlying pathophysiology in PPS may also explain the increased repeater F-waves in ALS (Chroni et al., 2012; Hachisuka et al., 2015). In addition, the F-wave latencies and chronodispersion were markedly prolonged in our ALS group. However, the F-wave latencies commonly thought to be influenced by height and preferential loss of fast-conduction neurons and the chronodispersion represent the conduction velocity of the motor neurons recruited, which are valuable markers of the conduction properties of motor axons (Fisher, 1998; Espiritu et al., 2003; Rivner, 2008). Their prolongation may be related to axonal degeneration, demyelination secondary to proximal axonal swellings or loss of fast conducting fibers (Argyriou et al., 2006; Hachisuka et al., 2015). As such, analyzing F-waves, especially the amplitude, mean and maximal F/M amplitude ratios, persistence, and the repeater F-waves, may provide an indicator of changes in spinal motoneuron pool excitability (Espiritu et al., 2003; Lin and Floeter, 2004). Intriguingly, we note that F-wave latencies and chronodispersion prolongation, persistence decline and repeater F-waves increase progressively early in patients with unaffected hands, suggesting early dysfunction of motor axons and LMNs in ALS and that subtle subclinical alterations may be reliably assessed by F-wave test.

Results Related to Split-Hand Syndrome

Our study shows a significantly decreased FDI/ADM CMAP amplitude ratio (<0.9) in ALS patients, and this finding reflects the split-hand phenomenon in ALS (Kuwabara et al., 2008; Menon et al., 2013) and presents evidence of LMN involvement. Further, there was a higher CMAP amplitude of the FDI and a lower amplitude of F-waves compared with the ADM in HCs, which has not been previously reported. The reduction in F-wave amplitude is often caused by damage to the LMNs and decreased motor neuron excitability (Taniguchi et al., 2008). The lower amplitude of F-waves, and the lower mean and maximal F/M amplitude ratios in the FDI compared with the ADM of HCs, is likely caused by physiological differences in the excitability of their motoneuron pools, and may relate to central impulses in favor of inhibition in the FDI (Menon et al., 2014c). Similar physiological differences, including lower mean F-wave amplitude, and lower mean and maximal F/M amplitude ratios, in the FDI, compared with the ADM, were also observed in ALS patients with unaffected hands. In addition, compared with the ADM, lower F-wave persistence and increased repeater F-waves were observed in the FDI in the unaffected hands group. These findings suggest a greater degree of spinal motoneuron hypoexcitability and loss of function of LMNs in the FDI. However, patterns of F-wave measurements changes in this study, especially those parameters detecting excitability of the spinal motoneuron pool (F-wave persistence, amplitudes, mean and maximal F/M amplitude ratio and repeater F-waves), were similar in FDI and ADM in ALS patients with affected hands. The absence of differences in F-wave variables between the FDI and ADM in ALS may imply a significantly enhanced excitability of spinal motoneurons innervating the FDI. We also found a significant correlation between F-wave amplitude in the FDI with the FDI/ADM CMAP amplitude ratio, but not with the ADM, suggesting that the different changes in spinal motoneuron excitability between the FDI and ADM were associated with development of the split-hand phenomenon in ALS.

At the segment spinal motoneuron level, the excitability of the motoneuron pool may be affected by the excitatory and inhibitory central nervous system (Mastaglia and Carroll, 1985; de Carvalho et al., 2002). To further clarify the impact of UMN activity drive on the excitability of the anterior horn cells in ALS patients with split-hand, we examined the F-wave parameters in our subgroup, including persistence, amplitude, and the F/M amplitude ratio, which presumptively are influenced by the corticospinal tract and cortical activity (Lin and Floeter, 2004; Rivner, 2008; Hara et al., 2010). However, we found no differences in F-waves between the P and the NP subgroups or between the FDI and ADM subgroups. The differences in segmental motoneuron excitability were not closely correlated to UMN involvement in our study. Thus, we suspect that the pathophysiology of the split-hand may also have spinal mechanisms.

Our study has some limitations. This was exploratory research with a small sample size. Thus, more patients and follow-up studies are required to confirm our findings on spinal motoneuron excitability associated with split-hand syndrome in ALS. Because of the stimulation of the ulnar at the wrist, the distance from the stimulus site to the target muscle is considerably longer for the FDI than for the ADM. The comparison of F-wave latencies in the FDI and ADM may be of less value. Owing to the predominant involvement of LMN in ALS, signs of pyramidal lesions may be difficult to detect. Moreover, we defined pyramidal lesions in the upper limbs requiring both increased tendon reflexes in the arm and Hoffman's sign, which may lack sensitivity. So, subclinical or possible involvement of UMN cannot be excluded in the NP group, and because of the relative small sample size, the results of F-wave parameters between the P and NP subgroup need to be verified in a larger population of ALS patients. Moreover, F-waves do not allow for accurate measurement of changes in UMN excitability influenced on spinal motoneurons, and a reliable method is needed for further studies. Combining transcranial magnetic stimulation (TMS) with the F-wave test investigates the UMN involvement and spinal motoneuron excitability at the same time and on the same patient groups could elucidate the pathophysiological basis of the split-hand in ALS.

In summary, the present study draws attention to a particular pattern of F-wave abnormalities in the FDI and ADM. Spinal motoneurons innervating the FDI have physiologically greater inhibitory modulation than the ADM, and in ALS, the enhanced excitability is more prominent in spinal motoneurons innervating the FDI that is consistent with the split-hand sign. Although cortical mechanisms could also be involved, we propose that spinal motoneurons dysfunction is associated with the development of the split-hand syndrome.

AUTHOR CONTRIBUTIONS

Z-LW, ML, and LC designed the experiments and/or interpreted the data. Z-LW and QD performed the experiments and analyzed the data. ML, SL, and KZ contributed to reagents, materials, and analysis tools. Z-LW and LC drafted the manuscript.

FUNDING

This study was funded by the National Key Research and Development Program of China (Grant Nos. 2016YFC0905100 and 2016YFC0905103) and the Chinese Academy of Medical Sciences (CAMS) Innovation Fund for Medical Sciences (CIFMS) (Grant Nos. 2016-I2M-1-002 and 2016-I2M-1-004).

REFERENCES

1. Argyriou, A. A., Polychronopoulos, P., Talelli, P., and Chroni, E. (2006). F wave study in amyotrophic lateral sclerosis: assessment of balance between upper and lower motor neuron involvement. *Clin. Neurophysiol.* 117, 1260–1265. doi: 10.1016/j.clinph.2006.03.002
2. Bae, J. S., Sawai, S., Misawa, S., Kanai, K., Isose, S., and Kuwabara, S. (2009). Differences in excitability properties of FDI and ADM motor axons. *Muscle Nerve* 39, 350–354. doi: 10.1002/mus.21107
3. Buschbacher, R. M., Bayindir, O., Malec, J., and Akyuz, G. (2015). Ulnar motor study to first dorsal interosseous: best reference electrode position and normative data. *Muscle Nerve* 52, 231–233. doi: 10.1002/mus.24524
4. Cedarbaum, J. M., Stambler, N., Malta, E., Fuller, C., Hilt, D., Thurmond, B., et al. (1999). The ALSFRS-R: a revised ALS functional rating scale that incorporates assessments of respiratory function. BDNF ALS Study Group (Phase III). *J. Neurol. Sci.* 169, 13–21. doi: 10.1016/S0022-510X(99) 00210-5
5. Cengiz, B., Mercan, M., and Kuruoglu, R. (2018). Spinal excitability changes do not influence the mechanisms of split-hand syndrome in amyotrophic lateral sclerosis. *Muscle Nerve* 58, 503–508. doi: 10.1002/mus. 26123
6. Chroni, E., Tendero, I. S., Punga, A. R., and Stalberg, E. (2012). Usefulness of assessing repeater F-waves in routine studies. *Muscle Nerve* 45, 477–485. doi: 10.1002/mus.22333
7. de Carvalho, M., Scotto, M., Lopes, A., and Swash, M. (2002). F-Waves and the corticospinal lesion in amyotrophic lateral sclerosis. *Amyotroph. Lateral Scler. Other Motor Neuron Disord.* 3, 131–136. doi: 10.1080/146608202760834139
8. Drory, V. E., Kovach, I., and Groozman, G. B. (2001). Electrophysiologic evaluation of upper motor neuron involvement in amyotrophic lateral sclerosis. *Amyotroph. Lateral Scler. Other Motor Neuron Disord.* 2, 147–152.
9. Eisen, A., Braak, H., Del Tredici, K., Lemon, R., Ludolph, A. C., and Kiernan, M. C. (2017). Cortical influences drive amyotrophic lateral sclerosis. *J. Neurol. Neurosurg. Psychiatry* 88, 917–924. doi: 10.1136/jnnp-2017-315573
10. Eisen, A., and Kuwabara, S. (2012). The split hand syndrome in amyotrophic lateral sclerosis. *J. Neurol. Neurosurg. Psychiatry* 83, 399–403. doi: 10.1136/jnnp-2011- 301456
11. Espiritu, M. G., Lin, C. S., and Burke, D. (2003). Motoneuron excitability and the F wave. *Muscle Nerve* 27, 720–727. doi: 10.1002/mus.10388
12. Fang, J., Cui, L., Liu, M., Guan, Y., Li, X., Li, D., et al. (2016). Differences in dysfunction of thenar and hypothenar motoneurons in amyotrophic

lateral sclerosis. *Front. Hum. Neurosci.* 10:99. doi: 10.3389/fnhum.2016.00099

13. Fisher, M. A. (1998). The contemporary role of F-wave studies. F-wave studies: clinical utility. *Muscle Nerve* 21, 1098–1101. doi: 10.1002/(SICI)1097-4598(199808)21:83.3.CO;2-F
14. Grapperon, A. M., Verschueren, A., Duclos, Y., Confort-Gouny, S., Soulier, E., Loundou, A. D., et al. (2014). Association between structural and functional corticospinal involvement in amyotrophic lateral sclerosis assessed by diffusion tensor MRI and triple stimulation technique. *Muscle Nerve* 49, 551–557. doi: 10.1002/mus.23957
15. Hachisuka, A., Komori, T., Abe, T., and Hachisuka, K. (2015). Repeater F-waves are signs of motor unit pathology in polio survivors. *Muscle Nerve* 51, 680–685. doi: 10.1002/mus.24428
16. Hara, M., Kimura, J., Walker, D. D., Taniguchi, S., Ichikawa, H., Fujisawa, R., et al. (2010). Effect of motor imagery and voluntary muscle contraction on the F wave. *Muscle Nerve* 42, 208–212. doi: 10.1002/mus.21667
17. Kim, D. H. (2011). Ulnar nerve conduction study of the first dorsal interosseous muscle in korean subjects. *Ann. Rehabil. Med.* 35, 658–663. doi: 10.5535/arm. 2011.35.5.658
18. Kuwabara, S., Mizobuchi, K., Ogawara, K., and Hattori, T. (1999). Dissociated small hand muscle involvement in amyotrophic lateral sclerosis detected by motor unit number estimates. *Muscle Nerve* 22, 870–873. doi: 10.1002/(SICI)1097- 4598(199907)22:7<870::AID-MUS9>3.0.CO;2-O
19. Kuwabara, S., Sonoo, M., Komori, T., Shimizu, T., Hirashima, F., Inaba, A., et al. (2008). Dissociated small hand muscle atrophy in amyotrophic lateral sclerosis: frequency, extent, and specificity. *Muscle Nerve* 37, 426–430. doi: 10.1002/mus. 20949
20. Lin, J. Z., and Floeter, M. K. (2004). Do F-wave measurements detect changes in motor neuron excitability? *Muscle Nerve* 30, 289–294. doi: 10.1002/mus.20110 Mastaglia, F. L., and Carroll, W. M. (1985). The effects of conditioning stimuli on the F-response. *J. Neurol. Neurosurg. Psychiatry* 48, 182–184. doi: 10.1136/jnnp. 48.2.182
21. Menon, P., Kiernan, M. C., and Vucic, S. (2014a). ALS pathophysiology: insights from the split-hand phenomenon. *Clin. Neurophysiol.* 125, 186–193. doi: 10. 1016/j.clinph.2013.07.022
22. Menon, P., Kiernan, M. C., and Vucic, S. (2014b). Cortical dysfunction underlies the development of the split-hand in amyotrophic lateral sclerosis. *PLoS One* 9:e87124. doi: 10.1371/journal.pone.0087124
23. Menon, P., Kiernan, M. C., and Vucic, S. (2014c). Cortical excitability differences in hand muscles follow a split-hand pattern in healthy controls. *Muscle Nerve* 49, 836–844. doi: 10.1002/mus.24072
24. Menon, P., Kiernan, M. C., Yiannikas, C., Stroud, J., and Vucic, S. (2013). Split-hand index for the diagnosis of amyotrophic lateral sclerosis. *Clin. Neurophysiol.* 124, 410–416. doi: 10.1016/j.clinph.2012.07.025
25. Mercuri, B., Wassermann, E. M., Manganotti, P., Ikoma, K., Samii, A., and Hallett, M. (1996). Cortical modulation of spinal excitability: an F-wave study. *Electroencephalogr. Clin. Neurophysiol.* 101, 16–24. doi: 10.1016/0013-4694(95)00164-6
26. Peioglou-Harmoussi, S., Fawcett, P. R., Howel, D., and Barwick, D. D. (1985). F-responses: a study of frequency, shape and amplitude characteristics in healthy control subjects. *J. Neurol. Neurosurg. Psychiatry* 48, 1159–1164. doi: 10.1136/jnnp.48.11.1159
27. Rivner, M. H. (2008). The use of F-waves as a probe for motor cortex excitability. *Clin. Neurophysiol.* 119, 1215–1216. doi: 10.1016/j.clinph.2008.01.103
28. Schelhaas, H. J., van de Warrenburg, B. P., Kremer, H. P., and Zwarts, M. J. (2003). The "split hand" phenomenon: evidence of a spinal origin. *Neurology* 61, 1619–1620. doi: 10.1212/01.WNL.0000096009.50213.6C
29. Shibuya, K., Misawa, S., Nasu, S., Sekiguchi, Y., Mitsuma, S., Beppu, M., et al. (2013). Split hand syndrome in amyotrophic lateral sclerosis: different excitability changes in the thenar and hypothenar motor axons. *J. Neurol. Neurosurg. Psychiatry* 84, 969–972. doi: 10.1136/jnnp-2012- 304109
30. Taniguchi, S., Kimura, J., Yanagisawa, T., Okada, F., Yamada, T., Taniguchi, S., et al. (2008). Rest-induced suppression of anterior horn cell excitability as measured by F waves: comparison between volitionally inactivated and control muscles. *Muscle Nerve* 37, 343–349. doi: 10.1002/mus.20936
31. Weber, M., Eisen, A., Stewart, H., and Hirota, N. (2000). The split hand in ALS has a cortical basis. *J. Neurol. Sci.* 180, 66–70. doi: 10.1016/S0022-510X(00)00430-5 Wilbourn, A. J. (2000). The "split hand syndrome". *Muscle Nerve* 23:138. doi:10.1002/(SICI)1097-4598(200001)23:1<138::AID-MUS22>3.0.CO;2-7

21

Clinical Measures of Bulbar Dysfunction in ALS

Yana Yunusova[1,2,3]*, *Emily K. Plowman*[4], *Jordan R. Green*[5,6], *Carolina Barnett*[7,8] *and Peter Bede*[9]

[1] Department of Speech Language Pathology, University of Toronto, Toronto, ON, Canada, [2] Hurvitz Brain Sciences Research Program, Sunnybrook Research Institute, Toronto, ON, Canada, [3] Volcal Tract Visualization Lab, Toronto Rehabilitation Institute, University Health Network, Toronto, ON, Canada, [4] Swallowing Systems Core, Department of Speech, Language, and Hearing Sciences, University of Florida, Gainesville, FL, United States, [5] Department of Communication Sciences and Disorders, MGH Institute of Health Professions, Boston, MA, United States, [6] Speech and Hearing Biosciences and Technology Program, Harvard University, Cambridge, MA, United States, [7] Division of Neurology, Department of Medicine, University of Toronto and University Health Network, Toronto, ON, Canada, [8] Institute of Health Policy, Management and Evaluation, Dalla Lana School of Public Health, University of Toronto, Toronto, ON, Canada, [9] Computational Neuroimaging Group, Academic Unit of Neurology, Trinity College Dublin, Dublin, Ireland

***Correspondence:**
Yana Yunusova
yana.yunusova@utoronto.ca

Bulbar impairment represents a hallmark feature of Amyotrophic Lateral Sclerosis (ALS) that significantly impacts survival and quality of life. Speech and swallowing dysfunction are key contributors to the clinical heterogeneity of ALS and require well-timed and carefully coordinated interventions. The accurate clinical, radiological and electrophysiological assessment of bulbar dysfunction in ALS is one of the most multidisciplinary aspects of ALS care, requiring expert input from speech-language pathologists (SLPs), neurologists, otolaryngologists, augmentative alternative communication (AAC) specialists, dieticians, and electrophysiologists—each with their own evaluation strategies and assessment tools. The need to systematically evaluate the comparative advantages and drawbacks of various bulbar assessment instruments and to develop integrated assessment protocols is increasingly recognized. In this review, we provide a comprehensive appraisal of the most commonly utilized clinical tools for assessing and monitoring bulbar dysfunction in ALS based on the COnsensus-based Standards for the selection of health Measurement INstruments (COSMIN) evaluation framework. Despite a plethora of assessment tools, considerable geographical differences exist in bulbar assessment practices and individual instruments exhibit considerable limitations. The gaps identified in the literature offer unique opportunities for the optimization of existing and development of new tools both for clinical and research applications. The multicenter validation and standardization of these instruments will be essential for guideline development and best practice recommendations.

Keywords: amyotrophic lateral sclerosis, Bulbar ALS, outcome assessment (Health Care), dysphagia, dysarthria, COSMIN

INTRODUCTION

ALS is a relentlessly progressive neurodegenerative disease with considerable clinical heterogeneity compared to other neurodegenerative conditions. Bulbar impairment (oro-motor, dysarthria and dysphagia) is a hallmark feature of the disease and has been associated with the condition since its earliest descriptions (1). While only approximately 30% of patients exhibit bulbar symptoms at onset, the majority of patients develop speech and swallowing difficulties with disease progression.

Bulbar signs and symptoms play an important role in the diagnosis of ALS and pose unique management challenges. Bulbar presentation has been associated with shorter survival (2, 3), faster functional decline (4), reduced quality of life (5–7) and increased multidisciplinary support needs (8, 9). Dysarthria has been consistently associated with low mood, withdrawal from activities and social isolation (10, 11). Dysphagia in ALS may lead to weight loss, malnutrition, dehydration, aspiration pneumonia, hospitalization and reduced quality of life (12, 13). Despite these important sequelae, bulbar impairment in ALS is relatively understudied, and the research literature is sparse (14). Proxies of bulbar impairment are underrepresented among outcome measures in clinical trials (15). Validated diagnostic, monitoring and prognostic markers of bulbar dysfunction are lacking and clinical assessment practices vary considerably across various centers (16).

Assessment measures are broadly classified as "diagnostic" when their primary purpose is to confirm the diagnosis, exclude mimics, or classify individual patient according to disease-onset. Some measures have been optimized to characterize symptom severity, while other indices are primarily used to monitor longitudinal change. Depending on the primary purpose of a measure, it is subject to a specific set of requirements defined by the COnsensus-based Standards for the selection of health Measurement INstruments (COSMIN) guidelines (17). These require that, in order to reliably integrate assessment tools into clinical practice, their measurement properties need to be firmly established relative to their primary purpose. All tests need to be assessed for validity and reliability (reproducibility). Diagnostic and screening tests should also be evaluated for their detection abilities (i.e., sensitivity/specificity). Discriminative measures need to be able to detect group differences and measures proposed to track longitudinal change need to be assessed for their ability to capture progressive changes.

The objective of this paper is to provide a review of established bulbar measures in ALS from a diagnostic, screening and disease monitoring perspective. This work is not intended as an exhaustive review of all available measures of bulbar impairment in ALS but as a summary of the current state of the field and its most pressing needs.

Abbreviations: AAC, augmentative alternative communication; ALS, Amyotrophic Lateral Sclerosis; ALSFRS-R, Amyotrophic Lateral Sclerosis—Functional Rating Scale—Revised; ALSSS, ALS Severity Scale; CNS-BFS, Center for Neurologic Study-Bulbar Function Scale; COSMIN, COnsensus-based Standards for the selection of health Measurement Instruments; CNE, Cranial nerve exam; DDK, dysdiadochokinesis; EAT-10, Eating Assessment Tool-10; EIM, electrical impedance myography; EMG, electromyography; FLAIR, Fluid-attenuated inversion recovery; FDA, Frenchay Dysarthria Assessment; FEES, fiberoptic evaluation of swallowing; FSE, Videofluoroscopic swallowing evaluation; FT9, Fine'til 9; GRE/SWI, gradient recalled echo/susceptibility weighted imaging; IOPI, Iowa Oral Performance Instrument; KPa, kilopascal; LMN, lower motor neuron; MAIP, maximum anterior isometric pressure; MiToS, Milano-Torino staging; MR, magnetic resonance; MRI, magnetic resonance imaging; MUNE, Motor Unit Number Estimation; MTP, maximum tongue pressure; MUNIX, Motor unit number index; MUPs, motor unit potentials; NdSSS, Neuromuscular Disease Clinical Status Scale; OSS, Oral Secretion Scale; SCM, sternocleidomastoid; SLPs, speech-language pathologists; SSS, Sialorrhea Scoring Scale; SIT, Sentence Intelligibility Test; syl/sec, syllables per second; T1 W, T1 weighted; UMN, upper motor neuron; WPM, words-per-minute.

TOOLS FOR DIAGNOSING AND SCREENING FOR BULBAR ALS

Table 1 provides a summary of tools primarily used for the diagnosis of bulbar dysfunction in ALS highlighting their main advantages and limitations.

Cranial Nerve Exam (CNE)

Clinical evidence of upper motor neuron (UMN) and lower motor neuron (LMN) degeneration is required for the diagnosis of ALS. With regards to bulbar impairment, clinical UMN signs include pathological reflexes (e.g., brisk jaw jerk, gag, and other facial reflexes) (18) and LMN signs encompass muscle weakness, atrophy and fasciculations in the jaw, face, tongue and palate (33). Although the clinical neurological examination remains "the best way to localize neurodegeneration *in vivo* and to follow the process in real time," (34) and the reliability of CNE has been evaluated in various neurologic populations (21, 35), the quantitative psychometric profile of CNE i.e., inter and intra-later reliability, sensitivity, specificity, and responsiveness, have not been systematically evaluated in ALS to date. This represents a research priority for the standardization of assessments.

Needle EMG

The role of electromyography (EMG) in ALS is the confirmation of acute and chronic denervation. The former may be evidenced by fibrillations, positive sharp waves and fasciculation potentials, which in the tongue are not readily detectable since complete relaxation is difficult to achieve (22). Polyphasic motor unit potentials (MUPs) with prolonged duration, increased amplitude and decreased recruitment are suggestive of chronic denervation. Quantitative motor unit action potential analysis in subclinical bulbar involvement is thought to be superior to peak ratio interference pattern analysis (36). Depending on local protocols, the genioglossus is the most commonly assessed muscle (37), but the evaluation of the sternocleidomastoid (38), masseter, temporalis, frontalis (39), mentalis (40), and trapezius (22) muscles have also been proposed to resolve diagnostic uncertainty. While Motor Unit Number Estimation (MUNE) techniques (41, 42), such as MUNIX (43) have been extensively utilized to quantify motor neuron loss in the limbs, they have only been relatively recently adopted to assess the denervation of the tongue (44) and further development is required for their acceptance to clinical practice.

Clinical Neuroimaging

While brain imaging is not required to establish the diagnosis of ALS, MRI is commonly used as part of the diagnostic work-up to rule out alternative neurological conditions which may mimic ALS (45, 46). In bulbar onset patients the careful evaluation of the brain stem for structural, neoplastic, vascular, inflammatory and infiltrative processes is particularly important. Pathological processes superior to the brainstem; demyelination, neurovascular syndromes, neurosarcoidosis, leukodystrophies, malignancies, and neurodegenerative conditions may also manifest in bulbar symptoms if involving the corticobulbar tracts or the bulbar segments of the motor cortex. A number

TABLE 1 | Tools for diagnosis of bulbar signs or ALS.

Tool	Description	Advantages	Limitations	Recommendations
1. Cranial Nerve Examination	Bulbar motor UMN and LMN signs: weakness, fasciculations, atrophy, tone, reflexes	Well established; (18) easy to perform; reliability of items established in stroke, (19) structural disorders (20) and mixed neurological populations; (21) validated with respect to detection of dysphagia with VFSE	Not sufficiently standardized, subjective; measurement properties have not been evaluated in ALS	Individual items and the test as a whole require further standardization and better testing of measurement properties
2. Needle EMG, Genioglossus, Sternocleidomastoid (SCM), Trapezius	Indicates acute and chronic denervation in selected muscles, LMN changes	Well established, helpful in the exclusion of mimics able to detect subclinical involvement; can be quantitative	Invasive, not well standardized across clinics, requires substantial training, low sensitivity due to difficulty with relaxation (tongue<SCM<trapezius); (22) commonly qualitative	Requires further standardization and establishment of quantitative measures
3. Clinical MRI of bulbar regions (e.g., brainstem, bulbar region of the PMC)	The clinical role of MRI is to rule out neurological mimics, tongue and pharyngeal pathology	Widely available, noninvasive, potentially sensitive to prodromal stages of bulbar disease	Qualitative, not formally assessed with respect to clinical utility in the diagnosis of early stages of bulbar disease	Requires further research effort in establishing clinical utility
4. Auditory perceptual assessment of dysarthria types	Detection of UMN vs. LMN signs in speech/ voice tasks; rating specified dimensions of voice/ speech quality on a Likert scale	Well-established method in dysarthria assessment in SLP	Specific set of ALS-relevant items is not established; (23, 24) may not be equally sensitive to all dysarthria severities; requires specialized training; not well utilized in neurology; lengthy; low reliability for some items (25)	Items require further identification and standardization in ALS as well as better testing of measurement properties
5. Frenchay Dysarthria Assessment	Comprehensive assessment of bulbar structure and function (goals and item overlap with #1 and #4)	Well-established method in dysarthria assessment in SLP; reliability is established (26)	Relatively lengthy; not specific to ALS; validation is limited	Items require further identification and standardization as well as better testing of measurement properties
6. Videofluoroscopic Swallowing Exam (VFSE)	"Gold standard" dysphagia assessment to directly visualize swallow safety and efficiency	Well established in ALS; showed sensitivity to prodromal stage of dysphagia and sensitivity to change (27–29)	Requires expensive instrumentation and highly trained personnel; involves radiation exposure (minimal); need for a separate and additional test	Recommended clinically in patients demonstrated high risk of dysphagia to diagnose and test impact of strategies for treatment planning
7. EAT-10	Screening tool for dysphagia; 10 items; self-administered, symptom-based	Validated and reliability assessed in a large non-ALS cohort; differentiated safe vs. unsafe swallowers in ALS; cut-off of 8 or higher indicates high likelihood of dysphagia (3.1 times); sensitivity 86%, specificity 76%; (30) quick and easy, low administrative burden for scoring	Subjective; may not be sensitive to early disease stages	Recommended for use in clinic as a screener for the presence of dysphagia in ALS.
8. 3oz Swallow Test	Screening tool for dysphagia; 3oz of water given to patient in a cup; Pass / Fail; fail includes inability to drink without stopping, cough or throat clear, "wet" voice	Validated in general patient populations with very high sensitivity but poor specificity; quick and easy to use	Not validated in ALS; may miss patients with sensory deficits (silent aspirators) and early signs of dysphagia, (31) could also overestimate dysphagia risk due to "maximum performance" nature of test	Requires further standardization as well as better testing of measurement properties
9. Voluntary Cough	Screening tool for airway defense physiologic capacity using airflow spirometry or peak cough flow meter	Objective, instrumental; validity, reliability, sensitivity (up to 90%) and specificity (up to 82%), depending on the measure, relative to VFS, have been established in ALS (32)	Requires instrumentation and a trained examiner; voluntary cough is mediated differently neurologically to a reflexive cough; effort dependent	Recommended for use in clinic as a screener to index airway defense capacity to expel tracheal aspirate or secretions in ALS

of extrapyramidal and cerebellar conditions may also present with localization-specific (ataxic, hypokinetic, hyperkinetic) dysarthria and imaging has a role to rule out gross striatal, nigral and cerebellar pathologies. The incidental identification of tongue tumors on MRI in patients with suspected ALS has also been reported (47). A number of radiological cues have been associated with ALS, such as high signal along the pyramidal tracts on T2 weighted or FLAIR imaging, low signal in the precentral gyrus on GRE/SWI, isolated motor cortex atrophy on T1W, but these qualitative visual cues are not specific to ALS and are not sensitive for diagnostic or monitoring purposes (48). Quantitative imaging studies of ALS on the other hand have successfully captured the cortical (UMN) components of bulbar dysfunction in a somatotopic distribution (49, 50) and characterized the pathological substrate of pseudobulbar affect (51, 52). With relentless methodological (53) and conceptual advances in neuroimaging (54), the establishment of multicenter data repositories (55) and the increasing availability of 7 Tesla systems (56), the anatomical underpinnings of bulbar dysfunction are likely to be characterized in further detail.

Auditory-Perceptual Dysarthria Evaluation and Frenchay Dysarthria Assessment

"The Mayo Clinic" method of dysarthria categorization involves auditory-perceptual evaluation of specific voice and speech features during a passage reading, phonation of /a/, and oral dysdiadochokinesis (DDK) with /pa, /ta/, /ka/, and /pataka/ (57–59). The identification of "harsh," "strained," or "strangled" voice quality, slow speaking rate and "excess and equal" stress pattern during passage reading and DDK are typically linked to UMN dysfunction and "spastic dysarthria." "Breathy" or weak voice, hypernasality, nasal emissions, and articulatory imprecision without changes in speaking rate are classically associated with LMN dysfunction and "flaccid dysarthria." ALS is typically characterized by mixed spastic-flaccid dysarthria presenting with articulatory imprecision, hypernasality, harshness, slow rate and prosodic abnormalities. Although the reliability of observational assessments have been repeatedly questioned (10), protocol standardization, assessor training, and reference samples are thought to improve assessment reliability (60). Despite these efforts, auditory-perceptual assessment remains surprisingly underutilized, requiring standardization of practices, psychometric evaluation and multi-center validation in ALS.

Tools like the Frenchay Dysarthria Assessment (FDA) (26) are particularly well-suited for diagnostic purposes as they can comprehensively assess both structure and function of the bulbar musculature through a combination of CNE items and the auditory-perceptual dysarthria assessment. However, FDA was not specifically developed for ALS, and the evaluation of its measurement properties in ALS is lacking. DDK, which is included in CNE, FDA and perceptual dysarthria assessments, is commonly used to track disease progression, and has shown high sensitivity but low specificity for detecting bulbar signs in the prodromal phase of bulbar ALS (61, 62). With further optimization, DDK may have a diagnostic potential, particularly if certain performance constrains are imposed or its complexity is increased (63, 64).

Dysphagia Diagnosis and Screening

Videofluoroscopic swallowing evaluation (VFSE) remains the gold standard of dysphagia assessment in most neurological conditions allowing the direct visualization of swallowing safety and efficiency i.e., aspiration and the presence of residue, respectively. In ALS however, VFSE is underutilized (16) due to a number of factors such as the presumed lack of therapeutic relevance, lack of access to equipment or perceived patient burden etc. A number of screening tools have been recently evaluated for the early identification of those at risk for dysphagia in ALS. Currently, the Eating Assessment Tool-10 (EAT-10) demonstrated good sensitivity and adequate specificity for detecting aspiration in ALS (30), while instrumental measures of airflow during voluntary cough showed excellent sensitivity and specificity to detect aspiration (32). The bedside 3oz water swallow test is also extensively utilized, but its measurement properties in ALS are still unknown. There is a general consensus among SLPs that patients who fail dysphagia screening should be further evaluated by instrumental techniques to directly visualize the swallowing process using VFSE or fiberoptic evaluation of swallowing (FEES) techniques (65). This is an important consideration given the high incidence of "silent" aspiration in this patient population. Instrumental assessments, not only confirm the diagnosis of dysphagia, but inform on swallowing safety, help to identify the specific etiology of dysphagia, and guide therapeutic strategies that can be tested during the instrumental exam by directly visualizing their impact.

TOOLS FOR DISEASE MONITORING—STAGING AND LONGITUDINAL TRACKING

Certain bulbar measures have been optimized to track the decline of bulbar function in individual patients and entire cohorts. **Table 2** summarizes proposed bulbar monitoring tools in ALS.

Bulbar Monitoring (Overall)

A recent clinical practice survey of ALS care in the United States revealed that the Revised ALS—Functional Rating Scale (ALSFRS-R) bulbar sub-score, clinician or patient administered, represented the only measure routinely used to evaluate bulbar dysfunction in the clinical setting (16). It contains only 3 questions to address changes in speech, swallowing and salivation that are each merely rated on a four-point ordinal scale. While the total ALSFRS-R score is thought to have excellent reliability, the measurement properties of the individual sub-scores (e.g., bulbar) have not been specifically evaluated to date (66, 67, 91, 92). The Center for Neurologic Study-Bulbar Function Scale (CNS-BFS) is a 15-item questionnaire of bulbar involvement which has recently been validated against the ALSFRS-R and "timed" speech and swallowing tasks, and has already been successfully utilized in a clinical trial (71, 72). However, the CNS-BFS still needs to be validated against VFSE.

The Appel scale is one of the best characterized tools to track ALS-associated impairment and functional decline (73). Other clinician-administered instruments include the Norris (74), Tuffs (93), and Charing Cross (94) scales, but their original

TABLE 2 | Tools to measure bulbar dysfunction severity and disease progression.

Tool	Description	Advantages	Limitations	Recommendations
1. ALSFRS-R, bulbar sub-score	Tracks bulbar disease progression; 3 "bulbar" questions; 0 (no function)–4 (normal function)	Quick and easy to perform; patient and caregiver versions available; well validated as a total score; (66) recent studies suggest using "domain-specific" subscores instead of a total score; (67, 68) declines linearly; an accepted end point in clinical trials	Limited assessment of bulbar dysfunction; symptom report; may underestimate sisease severity; (69) changes relatively late in the disease; skewed to detection of the LMN impairment (70)	Recommended for use in clinic and clinical trials but caution due to limited nature of bulbar assessment
2. Center for Neurologic Study-Bulbar Function Scale (CNS-BFS)	Reports solely on bulbar symptoms, 21 questions regarding speech, swallowing and salivation	Validated-high criterion and construct validity, (71) good reliability, responsive to change over time and improved in a clinical trial (72)	Symptom report; potentially not sensitive to early phases of the disease; need further validation against VFSE	Recommended for bulbar evaluation in clinic and clinical trials
3. Appel scale	Includes 5-point ratings of functional status of speech and swallowing (scores 6–30) and bulbar disease progression	Reliable; responsive to disease progression (linear decline); the composite score distinguishes slow from fast progressors, predicts survival, provides bases for clinical classification with management recommendations depending on severity (73)	Validation is limited to date; includes only 2 questions related to bulbar function—1 speech and 1 swallowing	Requires further evaluation of measurement properties; limited for the assessment of bulbar dysfunction
4. Norris scale	34-item ranking system; (74) 6 items in the "bulbar" category (i.e., chew, swallow, speak, jaw jerk, atrophy face/ tongue, lability) on a 3-point scale for each item	Quick and easy to administer; includes a range of bulbar items; has been used in clinical trials (75)	All items (functional and non-functional) rated equally; 3-point scale might be too coarse to detect change; limited information on the development and validation of the tool; responsiveness not established	Requires further evaluation of measurement properties; limited for the assessment of bulbar dysfunction
5. ALS Severity Scale (ALSSS)	10-point staging scale; was designed to supports management/rehabilitation practices in ALS; includes 1 speech and 1 swallowing item (0 to 10)	Easy to perform; clear description of each stage; adequate reliability; sig correlations with timed tests and speech intelligibility; responsive to change over time (76)	Ordinal scale; includes only 1 speech and 1 swallowing item	Requires further evaluation of measurement properties
6. Neuromuscular Disease Clinical Status Scale (NdSSS)	8-stage dysphagia severity scale to track the development of symptoms of dysphagia over time	Quick and easy to administer by a trained clinician; reliability, concurrent validity relative to other scales and responsiveness reported (77) and adequate	Focused predominantly on description of intake/ diet; not validated against VFSE	Although promising, requires further evaluation of measurement properties in other cultures
7. Oral Secretion Scale (OSS)	5-point scale to evaluate the severity of sialorrhea in ALS	Quick and easy to administer; validated against ALSFRS-R bulbar subscore and SSS; adequate reliability; can be used by different professions (78)	Floor effect in the more severely involved individuals; responsiveness not assessed; not linked to dysphagia outcomes	Recommended for evaluation of severity of sialorrhea in clinic and in clinical trials
8. Sialorrhea Scoring Scale (SSS)	9-point scale to evaluate the severity of sialorrhea	Quick and easy to administer; validated against ALSFRS-R bulbar subscore and OSS; adequate reliability; can be used by different professions; better spread of scores across the severity range compared to OSS (78)	Responsiveness not assessed; reliability was somewhat lower than for OSS; not linked to dysphagia outcomes	Recommended for evaluation of severity of sialorrhea in clinic and in clinical trials

(Continued)

TABLE 2 | Continued

Tool	Description	Advantages	Limitations	Recommendations
9. Sentence Intelligibility Test—Speech Intelligibility and Speaking rate	% of words understood by a listener during a sentence transcription task, and number of words produced per minute (WPM)	Easy to perform; supported by software; validated in multiple studies with respect to ALSSS (79) and ALSFRS-R; decline in rate to 125 WPM predicts intelligibility drop and is used to time AAC interventions; WPM changes linearly with disease progression (80, 81)	Requires a trained SLP; requires a trained transcriber; low sensitivity to early bulbar disease; (61) declines over 12% in sentence intelligibility and 37 WPM are outside of measurement error (82)	Speaking rate is recommended to be tracked during clinic in order to plan AAC interventions for those at risk for loss of speech intelligibility
10. Timed tests: Speech and pause durations in a passage*	A passage reading task (e.g., Bamboo) (83) allows a separation between speaking and pause events; gives a detailed picture of the components of speaking rate	Easy to perform; allows practice to minimize reading errors; distinguished patients with ALS with bulbar and respiratory signs; (84) showed sensitivity to change in a drug trial (85)	Currently requires time consuming, by-hand measurements; requires training; measurement properties (e.g., responsiveness, measurement error) are not well established; bulbar effects need further differentiation from respiratory and cognitive effects	Requires further standardization as well as better testing of measurement properties; subsequently would benefit from automation
11. Times tests: DDK*	A syllable repetition task (pa; ta; ka; pa-ta-ka) in syllables per second (syl/sec) that is used to detect slowing of the oral movements	Easy to perform; clinicians are familiar with the task; easily measured instrumentally; free of cognitive-linguistic effects; distinguishes slow from fast progressors; (86) cut off 4.6 syl/s 91% sensitivity and 54% specificity in detecting bulbar signs in pre-symptomatic patients (61)	Requires training/ modeling and maximum effort from patients; measurement properties are not fully established (e.g., responsiveness; error of measurement)	Requires further standardization as well as better testing of measurement properties; subsequently would benefit from automation
12. Maximum Tongue Pressure (MTP)*	A measure of tongue strength using a commercially available devices	Affordable easy to use clinical tool; validated against ALSFRS-R bulbar subscore and VFSE; cut off <21 KPa has sensitivity 80% and specificity 100% for detecting bulbar dysfunction on ALSFRS-R (87) and oral dysphagia; adequate reliability; independent prognostic factor of survival (88)	Requires training of the clinician and patient prior to measurement—results are placement dependent; (89) requires max effort; insufficient data on responsiveness; (90) not associated with dysarthria and speech intelligibility loss	Requires further standardization as well as testing of measurement properties

**May be used for diagnostic purposes.*

development, optimization and validation studies can be difficult to acquire and subsequently, their performance is relatively difficult to judge. The ability of these instruments to represent specific stages and their potential to track progressive bulbar impairment is largely unknown. A number of global ALS staging systems have been developed recently, such as the King's clinical staging system, the Milano-Torino (MiToS) functional staging, the Fine'til 9 (FT9) framework (95, 96), but bulbar impairment is just a small component of these instruments. Among the staging tools, the ALS Severity Scale (ALSSS) is particularly noteworthy, as it uses a 10-point scale for two bulbar functions, speech and swallowing. It was designed to guide rehabilitation efforts in ALS and, and pending formal psychometric evaluation, it may prove to be particularly useful (97).

Functional Monitoring of Dysphagia and Oral Secretion Scales

The Neuromuscular Disease Clinical Status Scale (NdSSS), which focuses solely on dysphagia, underwent one of the most rigorous psychometric evaluations to date. This tool exhibited excellent inter- and intra- rater reliability and correlated well with the functional oral intake scale (77). It has not been validated against VFSE yet, and given the potential for considerable geographical differences in oral intake, it is unclear how this tool may be validated around the world. While there are several tools to assess sialorrhea in ALS, such as the Oral Secretion Scale (OSS) and Sialorrhea Scoring Scale (SSS) available (78), these also need comprehensive psychometric evaluation and validation.

Functional Monitoring of Dysarthria

"Speech intelligibility" refers to the degree to which a speaker is understood by a listener, and "speaking rate" refers to speaking speed. Although both of these measures can be assessed on a 5 or 7-point Likert scale (49), the Sentence Intelligibility Test (SIT) is often preferred by SLPs, as it provides a more fine-grained estimate of speech intelligibility (i.e., percent of words transcribed correctly) and speaking rate (i.e., number of words produced per minute) (98). Speech intelligibility is considered abnormal when it falls below 97%, and speaking rate is considered abnormal below 160 words-per-minute (WPM) (99, 100). Speech intelligibility is a general indicator of the severity of dysarthria and it declines relatively late in the course of the disease (101). Speaking rate typically declines prior to significant changes in speech intelligibility, and it changes more linearly with symptom duration than speech intelligibility. Therefore, speaking rate is particularly useful in monitoring bulbar impairment longitudinally (102, 103). A speaking rate of 125 WPM or less is the recommended cut off for to trigger referral to the augmentative and alternative communication services (99).

Digital speech recordings and automated analyses can provide new opportunities for in-depth, observer-independent evaluations, especially during a passage reading and syllable repetition (DDK) tasks. In passage reading tasks, such as the Bamboo Passage, which has been specifically developed to support automatic analyses, certain phrases are semi-automatically identified, and speech duration and pause intervals can be accurately quantified (83). The measures derived from this analysis e.g., percentage pause time, mean phrase duration etc. have been identified to be sensitive to the prodromal stages of bulbar dysfunction (61) and also showed to detect response to pharmaceutical interventions such as dextromethorphan/quinidine (Nuedexta) therapy (85). A recent longitudinal study suggested that the main advantage of the DDK tasks may be in their ability to reliably distinguish slow- and fast-progressors (86).

Physiological Monitoring

Muscle strength testing in ALS has been initially performed using force transducers (strain gauges) (104, 105) and later with pressure bulbs via the Iowa Oral Performance Instrument (IOPI) (IOPI Medical LLC) or TPM-01 (JMS, Hiroshima). Lingual pressure testing using the IOPI revealed adequate reliability of a maximum tongue pressure estimate (MTP, or maximum anterior isometric pressure, MAIP) but not for the measure of endurance (89). Only one study assessed longitudinal changes in MTP in ALS to date (90) and reported its decline in patients with bulbar onset within 3 months and for those with spinal onset within 6 months. Tongue strength has also been shown to be an independent predictor of survival (88); however, formal psychometric evaluation is awaited to determine the MTP's utility to measure progressive changes over time.

DISCUSSION

In order to firmly establish the clinical utility of specific bulbar instruments and their potential as outcome measures in clinical trials, their measurement properties need to be comprehensively characterized. Among the diagnostic dysphagia instruments, screening tools, such as EAT-10 and voluntary cough (30, 32) have been well evaluated. Among speech measures, only DDK rate came close to demonstrating diagnostic utility (61). The remaining tools require extensive evaluation with regards to their diagnostic accuracy. While a large number of novel assessment tools have been proposed to track the progression of bulbar impairment, only the ALSFRS-R, the CNS-BFS and some bulbar staging systems (e.g., NdSSS, OSS, SSS) meet at least basic measurement requirements. Most existing disease monitoring tools lack the ability to capture subtle progressive changes, which is indispensable for disease tracking tools. Robust systematic psychometric evaluation is needed to improve the currently available clinical, academic and pharmacological-trial assessment tools.

Despite the gaps in the current literature and the limitations of current clinical trial designs, we are likely to witness considerable advances in standardized bulbar assessments and the emergence of purpose-designed, disease-specific, well-validated bulbar assessment tools. Emerging technologies such as quantitative neuroimaging, muscle ultrasound, electrical impedance myography (EIM), high-resolution manometry, videomanofluoroscopy, and speech acoustic monitoring are likely to soon complement our armamentarium of clinical tools. A number of promising imaging techniques have already been utilized to characterize the pathological substrate of bulbar impairment in ALS including diffusion tensor imaging (106, 107), cortical thickness measurements (50, 108, 109), morphometry-type analyses (49, 110), magnetization transfer ratio imaging (106), MR spectroscopy (111), MRI intensitometry (112), and task-based functional MRI (113, 114). Despite these advances, MRI-derived metrics remain underutilized in the clinical setting and as outcome measures in pharmacological trials. This is in sharp contrast with clinical trials in Multiple Sclerosis, where MRI plays an established role as a key outcome measure in phase III clinical trials (115). Muscle ultrasound may capture tongue fasciculations in the absence of fasciculation potentials on EMG and the combination of ultrasound and EMG may help the detection of early denervation (116). Likewise, EIM shows promise in detecting changes in the structural composition of the tongue in ALS and may evolve into an important tool to detect early bulbar involvement (117, 118). High-resolution manometry and videomanofluoroscopy may provide unique insights into the dynamics of bolus movement and swallowing pressures enabling early detection of bulbar dysfunction and thus, timely interventions (119, 120). Acoustic analysis of speech has been proposed as a means for the objective assessment of bulbar impairment for over two decades, but until recently extracting these measure has been extremely time consuming. Recent developments in automatic audio and video analysis methods and smart phone technologies make speech analysis technologically feasible, enabling observer-independent multiparametric analyses (121–123). These emerging methodologies will need careful development, optimization and evaluation according to established methodological guidelines (e.g., COSMIN framework).

CONCLUSIONS

Recent advances in neuroimaging, development of staging systems, patient-reported outcome measures and the emergence of novel instrumental speech and swallowing assessment techniques promise novel insights into bulbar dysfunction in ALS. However, in order for these methods to be integrated into routine clinical practice and pharmacological trials, they have to be rigorously evaluated with respect to their measurement properties, diagnostic performance and longitudinal tracking abilities. The establishment of large international collaborations and relentless biomarker research efforts give cause for optimism for the development of validated bulbar assessments, which in turn will contribute to best practice recommendations, enable well-timed clinical interventions and facilitate accurate patient stratification in clinical trials.

AUTHOR CONTRIBUTIONS

YY and PB reviewed references, drafted the manuscript, and generated the tables. EP provided expert opinion on dysphagia assessments and edited the drafts of the manuscript. JG provided expert opinion on dysarthria assessments and edited the drafts of the manuscript. CB provided expert opinion on measurement development and edited the drafts of the manuscript.

FUNDING

This work was supported by NIH R01DC01729 grant. Peter Bede is supported by the Health Research Board (HRB–Ireland; HRB EIA-2017-019), the Irish Institute of Clinical Neuroscience IICN–Novartis Ireland Research Grant, the Iris O'Brien Foundation, and the Research Motor Neuron (RMN-Ireland) Foundation.

ACKNOWLEDGMENTS

We wish to thank Nicholas Wasylyk for his help with literature search and data extraction.

REFERENCES

1. Clarke JL, Jackson JH. On a case of muscular atrophy, with disease of the spinal cord and medulla oblongata. *Med Chirurg Transac.* (1867) 50:489–98.1. doi: 10.1177/095952876705000122
2. Chio A, Logroscino G, Hardiman O, Swingler R, Mitchell D, Beghi E, et al. Prognostic factors in ALS: a critical review. *Amyotroph Lateral Scler.* (2009) 10:310–23. doi: 10.3109/17482960802566824
3. Elamin M, Bede P, Montuschi A, Pender N, Chio A, Hardiman O. Predicting prognosis in amyotrophic lateral sclerosis: a simple algorithm. *J Neurol.* (2015) 262:1447–54. doi: 10.1007/s00415-015-7731-6
4. Daghlas I, Lever TE, Leary E. A retrospective investigation of the relationship between baseline covariates and rate of ALSFRS-R decline in ALS clinical trials. *Amyotroph Lateral Scler Frontotemporal Degener.* (2018) 19:206–11. doi: 10.1080/21678421.2017.1418001
5. Hecht M, Hillemacher T, Grasel E, Tigges S, Winterholler M, Heuss D, et al. Subjective experience and coping in ALS. *Amyotroph Lateral Scler Other Motor Neuron Disord.* (2002) 3:225–31. doi: 10.1080/146608202760839009
6. Mitsumoto H, Del Bene M. Improving the quality of life for people with ALS: the challenge ahead. *Amyotroph Lateral Scler Other Motor Neuron Disord.* (2000) 1:329–36. doi: 10.1080/146608200300079464
7. Bach JR. Amyotrophic lateral sclerosis. Communication status and survival with ventilatory support. *Am J Phys Med Rehabil.* (1993) 72:343–9. doi: 10.1097/00002060-199312000-00002
8. Rooney J, Byrne S, Heverin M, Tobin K, Dick A, Donaghy C, et al. A multidisciplinary clinic approach improves survival in ALS: a comparative study of ALS in Ireland and Northern Ireland. *J Neurol Neurosurg Psychiatry* (2014) 86:496–501. doi: 10.1136/jnnp-2014-309601
9. Van den Berg JP, Kalmijn S, Lindeman E, Veldink JH, de Visser M, Van der Graaff MM, et al. Multidisciplinary ALS care improves quality of life in patients with ALS. *Neurology* (2005) 65:1264–7. doi: 10.1212/01.wnl.0000180717.29273.12
10. Tomik B, Guiloff RJ. Dysarthria in amyotrophic lateral sclerosis: a review. *Amyotroph Lateral Scler.* (2010) 11:4–15. doi: 10.3109/17482960802379004
11. Watts CR, Vanryckeghem M. Laryngeal dysfunction in Amyotrophic Lateral Sclerosis: a review and case report. *BMC Ear Nose Throat Disord.* (2001) 1:1. doi: 10.1186/1472-6815-1-1
12. Hardiman O, Al-Chalabi A, Chio A, Corr EM, Logroscino G, Robberecht W, et al. Amyotrophic lateral sclerosis. *Nat Rev Dis Primers* (2017) 3:17071. doi: 10.1038/nrdp.2017.72
13. Tabor L, Gaziano J, Watts S, Robison R, Plowman EK. Defining swallowing-related quality of life profiles in individuals with amyotrophic lateral sclerosis. *Dysphagia* (2016) 31:376–82. doi: 10.1007/s00455-015-9686-2
14. Waito AA, Valenzano TJ, Peladeau-Pigeon M, Steele CM. Trends in research literature describing dysphagia in motor neuron diseases (MND): a scoping review. *Dysphagia* (2017) 32:734–47. doi: 10.1007/s00455-017-9819-x
15. Miller RG, Munsat TL, Swash M, Brooks BR. Consensus guidelines for the design and implementation of clinical trials in ALS. World Federation

of Neurology committee on Research. *J Neurol Sci.* (1999) 169:2–12. doi: 10.1016/S0022-510X(99)00209-9
16. Plowman EK, Tabor LC, Wymer J, Pattee G. The evaluation of bulbar dysfunction in amyotrophic lateral sclerosis: survey of clinical practice patterns in the United States. *Amyotroph Lateral Scler Frontotemporal Degener.* (2017) 18:351–7. doi: 10.1080/21678421.2017.1313868
17. Mokkink LB, Terwee CB, Patrick DL, Alonso J, Stratford PW, Knol DL, et al. The COSMIN checklist for assessing the methodological quality of studies on measurement properties of health status measurement instruments: an international Delphi study. *Q Life Res.* (2010) 19:539–49. doi: 10.1007/s11136-010-9606-8
18. Tremolizzo L, Susani E, Lunetta C, Corbo M, Ferrarese C, Appollonio I. Primitive reflexes in amyotrophic lateral sclerosis: prevalence and correlates. *J Neurol.* (2014) 261:1196–202. doi: 10.1007/s00415-014-7342-7
19. McCullough GH, Wertz RT, Rosenbek JC, Mills RH, Ross KB, Ashford JR. Inter- and intrajudge reliability of a clinical examination of swallowing in adults. *Dysphagia* (2000) 15:58–67. doi: 10.1007/s004550010002
20. Chow W, Brandt M, Dworschak-Stokan A, Doyle P, Matic D, Husein M. Validation of the mirror-fogging test as a screening tool for velopharyngeal insufficiency. *Open Otorhinolaryngol J.* (2015) 8:15–21. doi: 10.2174/1874428101508010015
21. Koch I, Ferrazzi A, Busatto C, Ventura L, Palmer K. Cranial nerve examination for neurogenic dysphagia patients. *Otolaryngology* (2017) 7:4. doi: 10.4172/2161-119X.1000319
22. Sonoo M, Kuwabara S, Shimizu T, Komori T, Hirashima F, Inaba A, et al. Utility of trapezius EMG for diagnosis of amyotrophic lateral sclerosis. *Muscle Nerve* (2009) 39:63–70. doi: 10.1002/mus.21196
23. Van der Graaff M, Kuiper T, Zwinderman A, Van de Warrenburg B, Poels P, Offeringa A, et al. Clinical identification of dysarthria types among neurologists, residents in neurology and speech therapists. *Eur Neurol.* (2009) 61:295–300. doi: 10.1159/000206855
24. Kearns KP, Simmons NN. Interobserver reliability and perceptual ratings: More than meets the ear. *J Speech Lang Hear Res.* (1988) 31:131–6. doi: 10.1044/jshr.3101.131
25. Bunton K, Kent RD, Duffy JR, Rosenbek JC, Kent JF. Listener agreement for auditory-perceptual ratings of dysarthria. *J Speech Lang Hear Res.* (2007) 50:1481–95. doi: 10.1044/1092-4388(2007/102)
26. Enderby P. Frenchay dysarthria assessment. *Br J Disord Commun.* (1980) 15:165–73. doi: 10.3109/13682828009112541
27. Briani C, Marcon M, Ermani M, Costantini M, Bottin R, Iurilli V, et al. Radiological evidence of subclinical dysphagia in motor neuron disease. *J Neurol.* (1998) 245:211–6. doi: 10.1007/s004150050207
28. Wright R, Jordan C. Videofluoroscopic evaluation of dysphagia in motor neurone disease with modified barium swallow. *Palliat Med.* (1997) 11:44–8. doi: 10.1177/026921639701100105
29. Higo R, Tayama N, Nito T. Longitudinal analysis of progression of dysphagia in amyotrophic lateral sclerosis. *Auris Nasus Larynx* (2004) 31:247–54. doi: 10.1016/j.anl.2004.05.009
30. Plowman EK, Tabor LC, Robison R, Gaziano J, Dion C, Watts SA, et al. Discriminant ability of the Eating Assessment Tool-10 to detect aspiration in individuals with amyotrophic lateral sclerosis. *Neurogastroenterol Motility* (2016) 28:85–90. doi: 10.1111/nmo.12700
31. Mari F, Matei M, Ceravolo MG, Pisani A, Montesi A, Provinciali L. Predictive value of clinical indices in detecting aspiration in patients with neurological disorders. *J Neurol Neurosurg Psychiatry* (1997) 63:456–60. doi: 10.1136/jnnp.63.4.456
32. Plowman EK, Watts SA, Robison R, Tabor L, Dion C, Gaziano J, et al. Voluntary cough airflow differentiates safe versus unsafe swallowing in amyotrophic lateral sclerosis. *Dysphagia* (2016) 31:383–90. doi: 10.1007/s00455-015-9687-1
33. Brooks BR, Miller RG, Swash M, Munsat TL. El escorial revisited: revised criteria for the diagnosis of amyotrophic lateral sclerosis. *Amyotroph Lateral Scler Other Motor Neuron Disord.* (2000) 1:293–9. doi: 10.1080/146608200300079536
34. Ravits JM, La Spada AR. ALS motor phenotype heterogeneity, focality, and spread: deconstructing motor neuron degeneration. *Neurology* (2009) 73:805–11. doi: 10.1212/WNL.0b013e3181b6bbbd
35. McCullough GH, Rosenbek JC, Wertz RT, McCoy S, Mann G, McCullough K. Utility of clinical swallowing examination measures for detecting aspiration post-stroke. *J Speech Lang Hear Res.* (2005) 48:1280–93. doi: 10.1044/1092-4388(2005/089)
36. Finsterer J, Erdorf M, Mamoli B, Fuglsang-Frederiksen A. Needle electromyography of bulbar muscles in patients with amyotrophic lateral sclerosis: evidence of subclinical involvement. *Neurology* (1998) 51:1417–22. doi: 10.1212/WNL.51.5.1417
37. Tankisi H, Otto M, Pugdahl K, Fuglsang-Frederiksen A. Spontaneous electromyographic activity of the tongue in amyotrophic lateral sclerosis. *Muscle Nerve* (2013) 48:296–8. doi: 10.1002/mus.23781
38. Li J, Petajan J, Smith G, Bromberg M. Electromyography of sternocleidomastoid muscle in ALS: a prospective study. *Muscle Nerve* (2002) 25:725–8. doi: 10.1002/mus.10115
39. Pan H, Jian F, Lin J, Chen N, Zhang Z, Wang Y, et al. Needle electromyography of the frontalis muscle in patients with amyotrophic lateral sclerosis. *Muscle Nerve* (2016) 54:1093–6. doi: 10.1002/mus.25236
40. Preston DC, Shapiro BE, Raynor EM, Kothari MJ. The relative value of facial, glossal, and masticatory muscles in the electrodiagnosis of amyotrophic lateral sclerosis. *Muscle Nerve* (1997) 20:370–2. doi: 10.1002/(SICI)1097-4598(199703)20:3<370::AID-MUS18>3.0.CO;2-4
41. Gooch CL, Pullman SL, Shungu DC, Ulug AM, Chane S, Gordon PH, et al. Motor unit number estimation (MUNE) in diseases of the motor neuron: utility and comparative analysis in a multimodal biomarker study. *Suppl Clin Neurophysiol.* (2009) 60:153–62. doi: 10.1016/S1567-424X(08)00015-9
42. de Carvalho M, Barkhaus PE, Nandedkar SD, Swash M. Motor unit number estimation (MUNE): where are we now? *Clin Neurophysiol.* (2018) 129:1507–16. doi: 10.1016/j.clinph.2018.04.748
43. Neuwirth C, Barkhaus PE, Burkhardt C, Castro J, Czell D, de Carvalho M, et al. Tracking motor neuron loss in a set of six muscles in amyotrophic lateral sclerosis using the Motor Unit Number Index (MUNIX): a 15-month longitudinal multicentre trial. *J Neurol Neurosurg Psychiatry* (2015) 86:1172–9. doi: 10.1136/jnnp-2015-310509
44. McIlduff C, Boegle A, Qi K, Rutkove S. Motor unit number estimation recording from the tongue: a pilot study. *Neurology* (2017) 88(Suppl. 16):P4.113.
45. Traynor BJ, Codd MB, Corr B, Forde C, Frost E, Hardiman O. Amyotrophic lateral sclerosis mimic syndromes: a population-based study. *Arch Neurol.* (2000) 57:109–13. doi: 10.1001/archneur.57.1.109
46. Turner MR, Talbot K. Mimics and chameleons in motor neurone disease. *Pract Neurol.* (2013) 13:153–64. doi: 10.1136/practneurol-2013-000557
47. Volanti P, Mannino M, Piccoli T, La Bella V. Carcinoma of the tongue and bulbar-onset amyotrophic lateral sclerosis: unusual differential diagnosis. *Neurol Sci.* (2007) 28:151–3. doi: 10.1007/s10072-007-0809-x
48. Bede P, Hardiman O. Lessons of ALS imaging: Pitfalls and future directions—a critical review. *NeuroImage Clin.* (2014) 4:436–43. doi: 10.1016/j.nicl.2014.02.011
49. Bede P, Bokde A, Elamin M, Byrne S, McLaughlin RL, Jordan N, et al. Grey matter correlates of clinical variables in amyotrophic lateral sclerosis (ALS): a neuroimaging study of ALS motor phenotype heterogeneity and cortical focality. *J Neurol Neurosurg Psychiatry.* (2013) 84:766–73. doi: 10.1136/jnnp-2012-302674
50. Schuster C, Kasper E, Machts J, Bittner D, Kaufmann J, Benecke R, et al. Focal thinning of the motor cortex mirrors clinical features of amyotrophic lateral sclerosis and their phenotypes: a neuroimaging study. *J Neurol.* (2013) 260:2856–64. doi: 10.1007/s00415-013-7083-z
51. Christidi F, Karavasilis E, Ferentinos P, Xirou S, Velonakis G, Rentzos M, et al. Investigating the neuroanatomical substrate of pathological laughing and crying in amyotrophic lateral sclerosis with multimodal neuroimaging techniques. *Amyotroph Lateral Scler Frontotemporal Degener.* (2018) 19:12–20. doi: 10.1080/21678421.2017.1386689
52. Bede P, Finegan E. Revisiting the pathoanatomy of pseudobulbar affect: mechanisms beyond corticobulbar dysfunction. *Amyotroph Lateral Scler Frontotemporal Degener.* (2018) 19:4–6. doi: 10.1080/21678421.2017.1392578
53. Querin G, El Mendili MM, Bede P, Delphine S, Lenglet T, Marchand-Pauvert V, et al. Multimodal spinal cord MRI offers accurate

diagnostic classification in ALS. *J Neurol Neurosurg Psychiatry* (2018) 89:1220–1. doi: 10.1136/jnnp-2017-317214

54. Bede P, Querin G, Pradat PF. The changing landscape of motor neuron disease imaging: the transition from descriptive studies to precision clinical tools. *Curr Opin Neurol.* (2018) 31:431–8. doi: 10.1097/WCO.0000000000000569
55. Muller HP, Turner MR, Grosskreutz J, Abrahams S, Bede P, Govind V, et al. A large-scale multicentre cerebral diffusion tensor imaging study in amyotrophic lateral sclerosis. *J Neurol Neurosurg Psychiatry.* (2016) 87:570–9. doi: 10.1136/jnnp-2015-311952
56. Atassi N, Xu M, Triantafyllou C, Keil B, Lawson R, Cernasov P, et al. Ultra high-field (7tesla) magnetic resonance spectroscopy in Amyotrophic Lateral Sclerosis. *PLoS ONE* (2017) 12:e0177680. doi: 10.1371/journal.pone.0177680
57. Darley FL, Aronson AE, Brown JR. Clusters of deviant speech dimensions in the dysarthrias. *J Speech Lang Hear Res.* (1969) 12:462–96. doi: 10.1044/jshr.1203.462
58. Darley FL, Aronson AE, Brown JR. Differential diagnostic patterns of dysarthria. *J Speech Lang Hear Res.* (1969) 12:246–69. doi: 10.1044/jshr.1202.246
59. Duffy J. *Motor Speech Disorders: Substrates, Differential Diagnosis, and Management.* St. Louis, MO: Elsevier (2013).
60. Kent RD. Hearing and believing: some limits to the auditory-perceptual assessment of speech and voice disorders. *Am J Speech Lang Pathol.* (1996) 5:7–23. doi: 10.1044/1058-0360.0503.07
61. Allison KM, Yunusova Y, Campbell TF, Wang J, Berry JD, Green JR. The diagnostic utility of patient-report and speech-language pathologists' ratings for detecting the early onset of bulbar symptoms due to ALS. *Amyotroph Lateral Scler Frontotemporal Degener.* (2017) 18:358–66. doi: 10.1080/21678421.2017.1303515
62. Rong P, Yunusova Y, Richburg B, Green JR. Automatic extraction of abnormal lip movement features from the alternating motion rate task in amyotrophic lateral sclerosis. *Int J Speech Lang Pathol.* (2018). doi: 10.1080/17549507.2018.1485739. [Epub ahead of print].
63. Mefferd AS, Green JR, Pattee G. A novel fixed-target task to determine articulatory speed constraints in persons with amyotrophic lateral sclerosis. *J Commun Disord.* (2012) 45:35–45. doi: 10.1016/j.jcomdis.2011.09.002
64. Goonetilleke A, Guiloff RJ. Accuracy, reproducibility and variability of quantitative assessments of bulbar and respiratory function in motor neurone disease. *J Neurol Sci.* (1994) 124(Suppl.):64–6. doi: 10.1016/0022-510X(94)90181-3
65. Onesti E, Schettino I, Gori MC, Frasca V, Ceccanti M, Cambieri C, et al. Dysphagia in amyotrophic lateral sclerosis: impact on patient behavior, diet adaptation, and riluzole management. *Front Neurol.* (2017) 8:94. doi: 10.3389/fneur.2017.00094
66. Cedarbaum JM, Stambler N, Malta E, Fuller C, Hilt D, Thurmond B, et al. The ALSFRS-R: a revised ALS functional rating scale that incorporates assessments of respiratory function. *J Neurol Sci.* (1999) 169:13–21. doi: 10.1016/S0022-510X(99)00210-5
67. Franchignoni F, Mora G, Giordano A, Volanti P, Chio A. Evidence of multidimensionality in the ALSFRS-R Scale: a critical appraisal on its measurement properties using Rasch analysis. *J Neurol Neurosurg Psychiatry* (2013) 84:1340–5. doi: 10.1136/jnnp-2012-304701
68. Rooney J, Burke T, Vajda A, Heverin M, Hardiman O. What does the ALSFRS-R really measure? A longitudinal and survival analysis of functional dimension subscores in amyotrophic lateral sclerosis. *J Neurol Neurosurg Psychiatry* (2017) 88:381–5. doi: 10.1136/jnnp-2016-314661
69. Voustianiouk A, Seidel G, Panchal J, Sivak M, Czaplinski A, Yen A, et al. ALSFRS and appel ALS scores: discordance with disease progression. *Muscle Nerve* (2008) 37:668–72. doi: 10.1002/mus.20977
70. Gordon PH, Cheng B, Katz IB, Mitsumoto H, Rowland LP. Clinical features that distinguish PLS, upper motor neuron–dominant ALS, and typical ALS. *Neurology* (2009) 72:1948–52. doi: 10.1212/WNL.0b013e3181a8269b
71. Smith RA, Macklin EA, Myers KJ, Pattee GL, Goslin KL, Meekins GD, et al. Assessment of bulbar function in amyotrophic lateral sclerosis: Validation of a self-report scale (Center for Neurologic Study Bulbar Function Scale). *Eur J Neurol.* (2018) 25:907–e66. doi: 10.1111/ene.13638
72. Smith R, Pioro E, Myers K, Sirdofsky M, Goslin K, Meekins G, et al. Enhanced bulbar function in amyotrophic lateral sclerosis: the Nuedexta treatment trial. *Neurotherapeutics* (2017) 14:762–72. doi: 10.1007/s13311-016-0508-5
73. Appel V, Stewart S, Smith G, Appel SH. A rating scale for amyotrophic lateral sclerosis: description and preliminary experience. *Ann Neurol.* (1987) 22:328–33. doi: 10.1002/ana.410220308
74. Norris FH, Calanchini PR, Fallat RJ, Panchari S, Jewett B. The administration of guanidine in amyotrophic lateral sclerosis. *Neurology* (1974) 24:721–8. doi: 10.1212/WNL.24.8.721
75. Lacomblez L, Bouche P, Bensimon G, Meininger V. A double-blind, placebo-controlled trial of high doses of gangliosides in amyotrophic lateral sclerosis. *Neurology* (1989) 39:1635–7. doi: 10.1212/WNL.39.12.1635
76. Haverkamp LJ, Appel V, Appel SH. Natural history of amyotrophic lateral sclerosis in a database population. Validation of a scoring system and a model for survival prediction. *Brain* (1995) 118:707–19. doi: 10.1093/brain/118.3.707
77. Wada A, Kawakami M, Liu M, Otaka E, Nishimura A, Liu F, et al. Development of a new scale for dysphagia in patients with progressive neuromuscular diseases: the Neuromuscular Disease Swallowing Status Scale (NdSSS). *J Neurol.* (2015) 262:2225–31. doi: 10.1007/s00415-015-7836-y
78. Abdelnour-Mallet M, Tezenas Du Montcel S, Cazzolli PA, Assouline A, Pointon C, Leveque N, et al. Validation of robust tools to measure sialorrhea in amyotrophic lateral sclerosis: a study in a large French cohort. *Amyotroph Lateral Scler Frontotemporal Degener.* (2013) 14:302–7. doi: 10.3109/21678421.2012.735238
79. Ball LJ, Willis A, Beukelman DR, Pattee GL. A protocol for identification of early bulbar signs in amyotrophic lateral sclerosis. *J Neurol Sci.* (2001) 191:43–53. doi: 10.1016/S0022-510X(01)00623-2
80. Makkonen T, Ruottinen H, Puhto R, Helminen M, Palmio J. Speech deterioration in amyotrophic lateral sclerosis (ALS) after manifestation of bulbar symptoms. *Int J Lang Commun Disord.* (2018) 53:385–92. doi: 10.1111/1460-6984.12357
81. Nishio M, Niimi S. Changes over time in dysarthric patients with amyotrophic lateral sclerosis (ALS): A study of changes in speaking rate and maximum repetition rate (MRR). *Clin Linguist Phonet.* (2009) 14:485–97. doi: 10.1080/026992000750020323
82. Stipancic KL, Yunusova Y, Berry JD, Green JR. Minimally detectable change and minimal clinically important difference of a decline in sentence intelligibility and speaking rate for individuals with amyotrophic lateral sclerosis. *J Speech Lang Hear Res.* (2018) 61:2757–71. doi: 10.1044/2018_JSLHR-S-17-0366
83. Green JR, Beukelman DR, Ball LJ. Algorithmic estimation of pauses in extended speech samples of dysarthric and typical speech. *J Med Speech Lang Pathol.* (2004) 12:149–54.
84. Yunusova Y, Graham NL, Shellikeri S, Phuong K, Kulkarni M, Rochon E, et al. Profiling speech and pausing in amyotrophic lateral sclerosis (als) and frontotemporal dementia (ftd). *PLoS ONE* (2016) 11:e0147573. doi: 10.1371/journal.pone.0147573
85. Green JR, Allison KM, Cordella C, Richburg BD, Pattee GL, Berry JD, et al. Additional evidence for a therapeutic effect of dextromethorphan/quinidine on bulbar motor function in patients with amyotrophic lateral sclerosis: a quantitative speech analysis. *Br J Clin Pharmacol.* (2018) 84:2849–56. doi: 10.1111/bcp.13745
86. Rong P, Yunusova Y, Green JR (eds). Speech intelligibility decline in individuals with fast and slow rates of ALS progression. In: *INTERSPEECH.* Dresden (2015).
87. Hiraoka A, Yoshikawa M, Nakamori M, Hosomi N, Nagasaki T, Mori T, et al. Maximum tongue pressure is associated with swallowing dysfunction in ALS patients. *Dysphagia* (2017) 32:542–7. doi: 10.1007/s00455-017-9797-z
88. Weikamp JG, Schelhaas HJ, Hendriks JC, de Swart BJ, Geurts AC. Prognostic value of decreased tongue strength on survival time in patients with amyotrophic lateral sclerosis. *J Neurol.* (2012) 259:2360–5. doi: 10.1007/s00415-012-6503-9
89. Adams V, Mathisen B, Baines S, Lazarus C, Callister R. Reliability of measurements of tongue and hand strength and endurance using the Iowa

Oral Performance Instrument with elderly adults. *Disabil Rehabil.* (2015) 37:389–95. doi: 10.3109/09638288.2014.921245
90. Easterling C, Antinoja J, Cashin S, Barkhaus PE. Changes in tongue pressure, pulmonary function, and salivary flow in patients with amyotrophic lateral sclerosis. *Dysphagia* (2013) 28:217–25. doi: 10.1007/s00455-012-9436-7
91. Kaufmann P, Levy G, Montes J, Buchsbaum R, Barsdorf AI, Battista V, et al. Excellent inter-rater, intra-rater, and telephone-administered reliability of the ALSFRS-R in a multicenter clinical trial. *Amyotroph Lateral Scler.* (2007) 8:42–6. doi: 10.1080/17482960600888156
92. Gordon PH, Miller RG, Moore DH. ALSFRS-R. *Amyotroph Lateral Scler Other Motor Neuron Disord.* (2004) 5(Suppl 1):90–3. doi: 10.1080/17434470410019906
93. Smith RA, Melmed S, Sherman B, Frane J, Munsat TL, Festoff BW. Recombinant growth hormone treatment of amyotrophic lateral sclerosis. *Muscle Nerve* (1993) 16:624–33. doi: 10.1002/mus.880160608
94. Guiloff RJ, Goonetilleke A. Natural history of amyotrophic lateral sclerosis. Observations with the charing cross amyotrophic lateral sclerosis rating scales. *Adv Neurol.* (1995) 68:185–98.
95. Fang T, Al Khleifat A, Stahl DR, Lazo La Torre C, Murphy C, Young C, et al. Comparison of the King's and MiToS staging systems for ALS. *Amyotroph Lateral Scler Frontotemporal Degener.* (2017) 18:227–32. doi: 10.1080/21678421.2016.1265565
96. Thakore NJ, Lapin BR, Kinzy TG, Pioro EP. Deconstructing progression of amyotrophic lateral sclerosis in stages: a Markov modeling approach. *Amyotroph Lateral Scler Frontotemporal Degener.* (2018) 19:483–94. doi: 10.1080/21678421.2018.1484925
97. Hillel AD, Miller RM, Yorkston K, McDonald E, Norris FH, Konikow N. Amyotrophic lateral sclerosis severity scale. *Neuroepidemiology* (1989) 8:142–50. doi: 10.1159/000110176
98. Beukelman D, Yorkston K, Hakel M, Dorsey M. *Speech Intelligibility Test.* Lincoln, NE: Madonna Rehabilitation Hospital (2007).
99. Beukelman D, Fager S, Nordness A. Communication support for people with ALS. *Neurol Res Int.* (2011) 2011:714693. doi: 10.1155/2011/714693
100. Yorkston KM, Hammen VL, Beukelman DR, Traynor CD. The effect of rate control on the intelligibility and naturalness of dysarthric speech. *J Speech Hear Disord.* (1990) 55:550–60. doi: 10.1044/jshd.5503.550
101. Yorkston K, Strande E, Miller R, Hillel A, Smith K. Speech deterioration in amyotrophic lateral sclerosis: Implications for the timing of intervention. *J Med Speech Lang Pathol.* (1993) 1:35–46.
102. Ball LJ, Beukelman DR, Pattee GL. Timing of speech deterioration in people with amyotrophic lateral sclerosis. *J Med Speech Lang Pathol.* (2002) 10:231–5.
103. Rong P, Yunusova Y, Wang J, Green JR. Predicting early bulbar decline in amyotrophic lateral sclerosis: a speech subsystem approach. *Behav Neurol.* (2015) 2015:183027. doi: 10.1155/2015/183027
104. Langmore SE, Lehman ME. Physiologic deficits in the orofacial system underlying dysarthria in amyotrophic lateral sclerosis. *J Speech Lang Hear Res.* (1994) 37:28–37. doi: 10.1044/jshr.3701.28
105. DePaul R, Brooks BR. Multiple orofacial indices in amyotrophic lateral sclerosis. *J Speech Lang Hear Res.* (1993) 36:1158–67. doi: 10.1044/jshr.3606.1158
106. Borsodi F, Culea V, Langkammer C, Khalil M, Pirpamer L, Quasthoff S, et al. Multimodal assessment of white matter tracts in amyotrophic lateral sclerosis. *PLoS ONE* (2017) 12:e0178371. doi: 10.1371/journal.pone.0178371
107. Schuster C, Elamin M, Hardiman O, Bede P. The segmental diffusivity profile of amyotrophic lateral sclerosis associated white matter degeneration. *Eur J Neurol.* (2016) 23:1361–71. doi: 10.1111/ene.13038
108. Chen ZY, Liu MQ, Ma L. Cortical thinning pattern of bulbar- and spinal-onset amyotrophic lateral sclerosis: a surface-based morphometry study. *Chin Med Sci J.* (2018) 33:100–6. doi: 10.24920/11812
109. Walhout R, Westeneng HJ, Verstraete E, Hendrikse J, Veldink JH, van den Heuvel MP, et al. Cortical thickness in ALS: towards a marker for upper motor neuron involvement. *J Neurol Neurosurg Psychiatry* (2014) 86:288–94. doi: 10.1136/jnnp-2013-306839
110. Chen ZY, Liu MQ, Ma L. Gray matter volume changes over the whole brain in the bulbar- and spinal-onset amyotrophic lateral sclerosis: a voxel-based morphometry study. *Chin Med Sci J.* (2018) 33:20–8. doi: 10.24920/11804
111. Vora M, Kumar S, Sharma S, Sharma S, Makhaik S, Sood RG. Advanced magnetic resonance neuroimaging in bulbar and limb onset early amyotrophic lateral sclerosis. *J Neurosci Rural Pract.* (2016) 7:102–8. doi: 10.4103/0976-3147.165423
112. Hartung V, Prell T, Gaser C, Turner MR, Tietz F, Ilse B, et al. Voxel-based MRI intensitometry reveals extent of cerebral white matter pathology in amyotrophic lateral sclerosis. *PLoS ONE* (2014) 9:e104894. doi: 10.1371/journal.pone.0104894
113. Kollewe K, Munte TF, Samii A, Dengler R, Petri S, Mohammadi B. Patterns of cortical activity differ in ALS patients with limb and/or bulbar involvement depending on motor tasks. *J Neurol.* (2011) 258:804–10. doi: 10.1007/s00415-010-5842-7
114. Mohammadi B, Kollewe K, Samii A, Krampfl K, Dengler R, Munte TF. Decreased brain activation to tongue movements in amyotrophic lateral sclerosis with bulbar involvement but not Kennedy syndrome. *J Neurol.* (2009) 256:1263–9. doi: 10.1007/s00415-009-5112-8
115. Filippi M, Horsfield MA, Ader HJ, Barkhof F, Bruzzi P, Evans A, et al. Guidelines for using quantitative measures of brain magnetic resonance imaging abnormalities in monitoring the treatment of multiple sclerosis. *Ann Neurol.* (1998) 43:499–506. doi: 10.1002/ana.410430414
116. Misawa S, Noto Y, Shibuya K, Isose S, Sekiguchi Y, Nasu S, et al. Ultrasonographic detection of fasciculations markedly increases diagnostic sensitivity of ALS. *Neurology* (2011) 77:1532–7. doi: 10.1212/WNL.0b013e318233b36a
117. Shellikeri S, Yunusova Y, Green JR, Pattee GL, Berry JD, Rutkove SB, et al. Electrical impedance myography in the evaluation of the tongue musculature in amyotrophic lateral sclerosis. *Muscle Nerve* (2016) 52:584–91. doi: 10.1002/mus.24565
118. McIlduff CE, Yim SJ, Pacheck AK, Rutkove SB. Optimizing electrical impedance myography of the tongue in amyotrophic lateral sclerosis. *Muscle Nerve* (2017) 55:539–43. doi: 10.1002/mus.25375
119. Noh EJ, Park MI, Park SJ, Moon W, Jung HJ. A case of amyotrophic lateral sclerosis presented as oropharyngeal dysphagia. *J Neurogastroenterol Motility* (2010) 16:319–22. doi: 10.5056/jnm.2010.16.3.319
120. Takasaki K, Umeki H, Enatsu K, Kumagami H, Takahashi H. Evaluation of swallowing pressure in a patient with amyotrophic lateral sclerosis before and after cricopharyngeal myotomy using high-resolution manometry system. *Auris Nasus Larynx* (2010) 37:644–7. doi: 10.1016/j.anl.2010.02.003
121. Norel R, Pietrowicz M, Agurto C, Rishoni S, Cecchi G. Detection of amyotrophic lateral sclerosis (ALS) via acoustic analysis. *bioRxiv [preprint]* (2018). doi: 10.21437/Interspeech.2018-2389
122. Wang J, Kothalkar PV, Cao B, Heitzman D. (eds). Towards automatic detection of amyotrophic lateral sclerosis from speech acoustic and articulatory samples. In: *INTERSPEECH.* San Francisco, CA (2016). doi: 10.21437/Interspeech.2016-1542
123. Bandini A, Green JR, Taati B, Orlandi S, Zinman L, Yunusova Y. Automatic detection of amyotrophic lateral sclerosis (ALS) from video-based analysis of facial movements: speech and non-speech tasks. In: *13th IEEE International Conference on Automatic Face & Gesture Recognition (FG 2018).* X'ian (2018). doi: 10.1109/FG.2018.00031

22

Magnetic Resonance Spectroscopy in ALS

*Sanjay Kalra**

Division of Neurology, Department of Medicine, Neuroscience and Mental Health Institute, University of Alberta, Edmonton, AB, Canada

Correspondence:
Sanjay Kalra
sanjay.kalra@ualberta.ca

Proton magnetic resonance spectroscopy (MRS) provides a means of measuring cerebral metabolites relevant to neurodegeneration *in vivo*. In amyotrophic lateral sclerosis (ALS), neurochemical changes reflecting neuronal loss or dysfunction (decreased N-actylaspartate [NAA]) is most significant in the motor cortex and corticospinal tracts. Other neurochemical changes observed include increased myo-inositol (mIns), a putative marker of gliosis. MRS confirmation of involvement of non-motor regions such as the frontal lobes, thalamus, basal ganglia, and cingulum are consistent with the multi-system facet of motor neuron disease with ALS being part of a MND-FTD spectrum. MRS-derived markers exhibit an encouraging discriminatory ability to identify patients from healthy controls, however more data is needed to determine its ability to assist with the diagnosis in early stages when upper motor neuron signs are limited, and in distinguishing from disease mimics. Longitudinal change of NAA and mIns do not appear to be reliable in monitoring disease progression. Technological advances in hardware and high field scanning are increasing the number of accessible metabolites available for interrogation.

Keywords: biomarker, magnetic resonance spectroscopy, neuroimaging, amyotrophic lateral sclerosis, neurodegeneration

BACKGROUND AND TECHNICAL CONSIDERATIONS

Magnetic resonance imaging has emerged as a promising tool to provide a biomarker in neurological and psychiatric disorders. Routine structural MRI is not helpful in this regard in ALS as signal intensity and gross volume changes in T1 and T2 weighted images is not apparent in the vast majority of cases (1). Advanced imaging and post-processing methods are necessary to reveal pathology that is not evident to the naked eye. Numerous studies have demonstrated the potential of MRS in research and clinical care in brain disorders, including ALS. Results have been consistent amongst investigators using different methods to quantify key metabolites such as NAA, and renewed interest along with advancing technology are leading to studies probing previously inaccessible chemicals such as Gama-aminobutyric acid (GABA).

With routine structural MRI, the abundance and microenvironment of protons is quantified resulting in essentially images of the distribution of water since it is the most abundant proton-rich molecule. The most basic MRS experiment quantifies instead protons in molecules other than water. The experiment is usually a measurement from a defined volume (rather than the whole brain), and produces a spectrum rather than an image. Different peaks in the spectrum arise from different protons and their microenvironment. The positioning along the x-axis of peaks is dependent on the spin frequency of the protons contributing to the peak, with the area under the peak dependent on the number of protons. Small shifts in frequency can occur due to magnetic field perturbations arising from nearby molecules, leading to a change the shape of a peak (singlets, doublets, triplets, etc.). The frequency of a peak and its splitting structure are key elements used in the identification of the metabolite from where the peak arises.

Images can be produced from metabolites such as NAA, however these are of much lower resolution than structural MRI (which is essentially MRS of water) because of the very low concentrations of such molecules. The lower concentration of the target metabolites also means that MRS scans are comparatively longer than routine structural imaging. Rather than a structural evaluation, MRS is a means of quantifying neurochemistry in the brain of low abundance metabolites. MR spectra can be obtained using other nuclei, including phosphorus, fluorine, carbon, and sodium. These typically require alternate hardware (e.g., specific RF coils) to that typically available with clinical and clinical research systems used for proton MRS.

Metabolites

The metabolites that are visible and quantifiable is dependent on a number of factors, and requires a sufficient concentration typically in the range of micromoles/gm. Spectral resolution and SNR must be sufficient to accurately identify and quantify individual peaks, and this is determined by many factors including B0 field strength and homogeneity, acquisition sequence (PRESS, STEAM, MEGA-PRESS, etc.), and TE, amongst others. Higher field strengths and lower TE in general give access to more metabolites.

There are a number of metabolites detectable using contemporary methods that have relevance in neurological disease (**Figure 1**). N-acetylaspartate (NAA), along with a small contribution from N-acetylaspartylglutamate, is localized only in neurons and their processes, and thus NAA serves as a marker of neuronal integrity. The total creatine peak arises from metabolites (creatine plus phosphocreatine) involved in energy metabolism. Total choline (choline, phosphorylcholine, glycerophosphorylcholine) is a marker of membrane turnover. Increased levels are reported with cell proliferation, both neuronal and glial.

Beyond NAA, there are a number of metabolites that can be measured which are of particular relevance to neurodegeneration in ALS. Myo-inositol (mIns) has a preferential distribution in glial cells, and is as such a putative glial marker. Glutamate is the primary CNS excitatory neurotransmitter. It is difficult to separate using routine MRS techniques from glutamine, and is thus may be expressed as "Glx." GABA is the primary inhibitory neurotransmitter in the brain. Glutathione functions as an antioxidant. Glutamate, GABA, and glutathione can be measured at ultrahigh field (7 T), or high field (3 T) using advanced spectral editing methods.

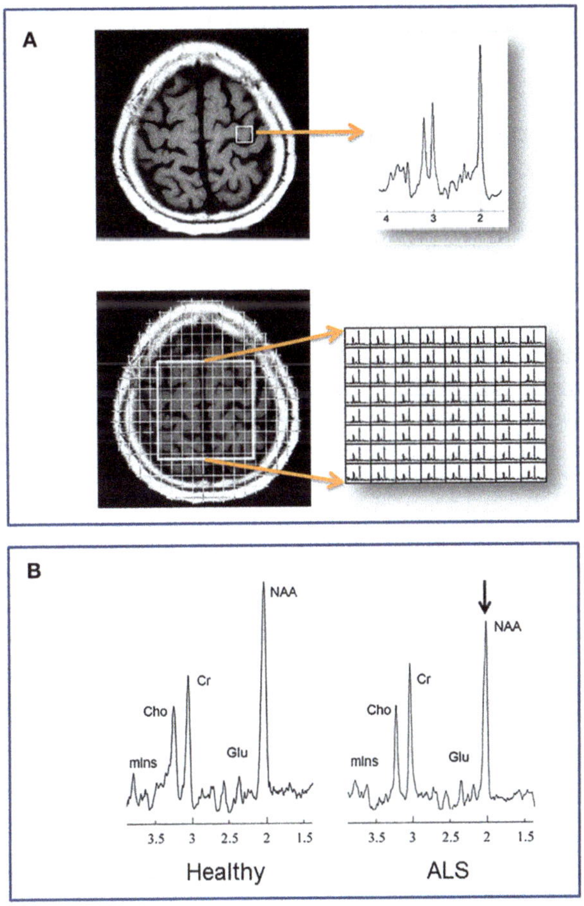

FIGURE 1 | (A) Localization methods. Neurochemical data are acquired from specified volumes during a single MRS scan. A single spectrum is recorded in single voxel spectroscopy (SVS), such as from the left precentral gyrus in the example at top. With magnetic resonance spectroscopic imaging (MRSI) multiple spectra are acquired, such as from a 2 dimensional plane centered over the central sulcus in the example at bottom. **(B)** A representative spectrum from the motor cortex of a healthy individual compared to one from a patient with ALS. N-acetylaspartate is reduced in ALS, reflecting reduced neuronal integrity. Cho, choline; Cr, creatine; Glu, glutamate; mIns, myo-inositol; NAA, N-acetylaspartate.

Acquisition

MRS can be performed using the same hardware systems as for structural imaging. The lowest field strength advised, and indeed what many papers to date report experiments from, are studies at 1.5 T. The benefits of high field imaging include access to more metabolites, shorter acquisition times, and higher spatial resolution. The former comes from increased SNR and increased chemical shift dispersion. The benefit is particularly relevant to detecting metabolites that have very low concentration or a complex resonance peak structure such as glutamate and GABA.

Unlike whole-brain structural imaging the location from where a spectrum is acquired usually must be pre-defined. Traditional localization schemes to define where spectra are acquired, include single voxel spectroscopy (SVS) and multivoxel spectroscopic imaging (MRSI) (**Figure 1**). In the former, a single spectrum is acquired from a discrete volume of interest (VOI), such as the motor cortex, internal capsule, etc. With MRSI, individual spectra are acquired from multiple regions within a 2-dimensional slab or a 3-dimensional volume. These volumes are positioned at the time of scanning, and the acquired spectra within the volume are selected after processing. Critical steps during data acquisition, but beyond the scope of this review, are water and lipid suppression, and shimming to minimize local field inhomogeneity.

Data Post-processing and Quantification

Post-processing of data includes a number of steps (e.g., residual water suppression, Fourier transformation, phase correction), with ultimately the production of spectral peaks. These are baseline corrected and fitted. The area under a fitted peak correlates with the number of protons contributing to the signal and thus metabolite density. Processing and quantification is available on MRI consoles, or with stand-alone software such as LCModel (2).

It is paramount to be aware that a metabolite resonance reflects its contributing protons throughout the voxel being sampled, including all cell and tissue types (neurons, glia, gray matter, white matter) and compartments (intracellular, extracellular). The derivation of absolute concentrations (i.e., mmol/L) requires additional MR experiments and processes to correct, for example, partial volume effects, coil loading, field inhomogeneity, and relaxation effects with a potential concern to data reliability. Resonance signals are thus often reported as a ratio to a reference metabolite, such as Cr or Cho (NAA/Cr); this inherently performs the aforementioned correction, however it requires the assumption that the reference metabolite is stable in the disease under question. Normalization with a water signal is used by some as an alternative and obviates the issue of whether Cr or Cho are unchanged, though comes with its own issues.

Recent Advances

High and Ultrahigh Field Imaging, and "New Metabolites"

Within the last decade, research and clinical MR systems have transitioned from a low field of 1.5 T to a high field of 3 T. Studies at the latter are becoming common place, with studies at the ultrahigh field of 7 T emerging.

The benefits of high field imaging include access to more metabolites, shorter acquisition times, and higher spatial resolution. The former comes from increased SNR and increased chemical shift dispersion; this is particularly relevant to metabolites that have very low concentration or complex resonance peak structure such as glutamate, GABA, and mIns. Higher field systems are accompanied by a number of challenges that require attention for successful spectroscopy experiments: greater main (B0) and applied RF (B1) field inhomogeneity and chemical shift mis-registration, altered T1 and T2 relaxation times, greater safety concerns, and higher purchase and operating costs (3).

3D MRSI and Automated Quantification

Single voxel spectroscopy and MRSI constrain the acquisition of data from small and discrete regions (volume of interest). These spatial restrictions are necessary, in part, for optimization of field homogeneity. Thus, MRS scans demand an additional level of knowledge, expertise, and experience from the MR technologist required for accurate positioning of the VOI. Larger sampling of the brain can be done with multislice MRSI (4–6), or 3D MRSI (7), however these further increase acquisition times. Echo-planar spectroscopic imaging (EPSI) has been an exciting development as it permits high resolution volumetric (whole brain) spectroscopic imaging in a single acquisition within a clinically acceptable timeframe (8). It has been applied in ALS to study the neurochemistry of the CST in its 3-dimensional extent (9, 10), and of multiple spatially discrete areas (11, 12).

RESULTS

At the time of writing, a general survey reveals there have been just over 60 papers published describing human proton MRS experiments in ALS, with inclusion of ~1,400 patients with ALS or related motor neuron disease (primary lateral sclerosis, progressive muscular atrophy). The majority of papers have interrogated neurochemistry of the motor system, namely the primary motor cortex and corticospinal tract. Published works also report findings in "extra-motor" regions including the prefrontal cortex, subcortical gray, brainstem, and spinal cord. Longitudinal MRS studies are few, as they are with other imaging modalities. With few exceptions, studies published since 2011 have been done at high field (3 T) or ultrahigh field (7 T).

Participants in studies have consisted of patients meeting El Escorial Criteria for ALS with combined upper and lower motor neuron signs. The number of MND participants in each study range from 7 to 169, with many studies having 10–30. Some have included subjects with no UMN signs (PMA) (6, 11, 13–16) generally showing the expected correlation of more normal NAA in such subjects. All studies have been conducted at a single center, except for a prospective multicenter study conducted at 4 sites in the Canadian ALS Neuroimaging Consortium [ClinicalTrials.gov # NCT02405182 and in press (Neurology: Clinical Practice)].

Cross-Sectional

Motor Cortex

The regional focus of most studies has been on the motor cortex or CST. NAA ratios to Cr, Cho, or Cr+Cho are reduced in the precentral gyrus (4–6, 12, 13, 15, 17–39). A decline in absolute quantities of NAA (14, 16, 21, 22, 31, 40–43) corroborate these observations of reduced ratios of NAA. A gradient effect can be observed when spectra are acquired from the motor cortex and regions immediately surrounding it, such that less prominent reductions are present in the postcentral gyrus and premotor areas compared to the precentral gyrus (13, 25).

Corticospinal Tract

The corticospinal tract has been interrogated using various methods. One group found reduced NAA/Cr+Cho) in the centrum semioval (CSO) and internal capsule combined, but not individually in these two regions (4). In part contrary to this, a study using a coronal MRSI method in the plane of the CST found reduced NAA/Cr in the precentral gyrus and corona radiata, but normal levels in the internal capsule and cerebral peduncle (44). Another found reduced NAA/Cr in both the motor cortex and

IC (32). NAA of the entire CST was found to be reduced using a whole-brain 3D spectroscopic acquisition protocol (9, 10).

Extra-Motor Regions

The presence of frontotemporal lobar degeneration (FTLD) is supported by reduced NAA indices in various frontal regions including the dorsolateral (11, 23) and mesial prefrontal (19, 45) cortices. Mesial prefrontal cortex neurochemistry is abnormal in patients who for the most part are not cognitively impaired, suggesting MRS may be more sensitive to detecting FTLD than clinical measures (45). "Extra-motor" degeneration was similarly demonstrated in the mid-cingulate gyrus (34), thalamus (34, 46), and basal ganglia (46). As expected, NAA is normal in the parietal and occipital lobes (5, 11, 23, 25, 26, 33, 40) and cerebellum (14).

Brainstem

Reductions in NAA indices are described by most (21, 43, 47, 48) but not all studies (33) that have examined the brainstem.

Spinal Cord

MRS of the upper cervical spinal cord revealed substantially reduced NAA ratios 25–40% in patients with ALS (49, 50). Notably, a single voxel was used enclosing the breadth of the cord. Thus, the spectrum included contributions from both white matter tracts and the anterior horn and other cells in the gray matter. One group extended their methods to investigate neurochemical changes in asymptomatic SOD1+ individuals (51). They found comparably reduced NAA/Cr and NAA/mIns in asymptomatic (39.7% and 18.0%) and patients with ALS (41.2% and 24.0%) compared to healthy controls, inferring the presence of neurochemical changes early in the disease and even before symptoms or signs are present.

Other Metabolites

Reflective of astrogliosis, mIns is increased in the motor cortex (29, 40, 43, 48, 52, 53). The NAA/mIns ratio may be a more robust marker of degeneration as it reflects the combined pathology of decreased neuronal integrity and gliosis with the individual metabolite levels becoming abnormal in opposite directions in the motor cortex (16, 29, 48) and mesial prefrontal cortex (45).

Given one of the putative pathophysiological mechanisms is excitotoxicity, one may have expected Glu to be increased. However, results have been conflicting for the motor cortex where it (or Glx) were normal (16, 21, 43, 52), increased (32), or decreased (40). Studies at 7 T where its quantification may be more precise were conflicting with levels in the motor cortex normal (48) or increased (53). Glx was increased in the medulla (54) along with a negative correlation with the ALSFRS bulbar subscore. Later studies of the pons revealed normal pontine Glu or Glx (43, 48). MRS measurements of the inhibitory neurotransmitter GABA in the motor cortex have been reported to be reduced using the MEGA-PRESS technique at 3T (43, 55), but normal using a STEAM sequence at 7T (53). As discussed above MRS measurements will largely reflect the intracellular metabolic rather than synaptic neurotransmitter pool; as such, reductions may simply be the result of neuronal loss.

Initial findings of decreased glutathione in the primary motor cortex (35) which would have been supportive of a role for oxidative stress in the pathogenesis of ALS were not replicated by subsequent studies at 3 T or 7 T (48, 53).

Diagnostic Accuracy

A number of studies have assessed the discriminatory power of NAA and its ratios in the motor cortex to separate ALS patients from healthy controls. Sensitivity ranges from 53 to 100%, specificity ranges from 37 to 100%, with the average amongst the studies ~80% for both. MRS improves the accuracy when combined DTI assessment of the corticospinal tract (56, 57) or of signal change on structural imaging (36, 56).

Longitudinal

A number of studies suggest a decline in NAA indices over varying intervals; interpretation of these reports is difficult due to small numbers of patients (5, 19, 22, 52, 58, 59).

In a more rigorous design, longitudinal change in absolute NAA and its ratio to Cr and Cho were measured every 3 months out to 1 year. Changes were seen in the motor cortex and outside the motor cortex over 3 and 9 months, respectively depending on the El Escorial designation, but overall did not follow a consistent pattern (27). In a treatment trial of growth hormone, the placebo arm of 20 patients did not have any change in motor cortex NAA/(Cho+Cr) at 0, 6, or 12 months (60).

In a larger study of 43 patients, 30 had at least one follow up scan on a 3 month interval, demonstrating a non-significant ($p = 0.06$) decline in motor cortex NAA/Cr (6).

Recently, longitudinal neurochemical observations were made at 7 T at 6 and 12 months. Motor cortex NAA/mIns declined and pontine Glx increased. In a sub group analysis, this pattern of neurochemical change was not present in those whose upper limb and bulbar function did not deteriorate over time (61).

Correlations

The presence of correlations with an imaging finding provides a degree of biological validity to the imaging metric. Not surprisingly, NAA indices are more reduced in patients with a greater severity of UMN findings on neurological examination (13–15, 20, 28, 31, 40, 52), however this is not always the case (48). As a measure of UMN function, finger tapping has the advantage of being objective and providing a continuous measure. Correlations with tapping have been reported in a number (4, 6, 16, 18, 39), but not all, (44) studies. A few studies have also noted a correlation with the El Escorial criteria (15, 27, 48). Reports are conflicting with respect to associations with disease duration, progression rate, or disability as quantified by ALSFRS-R. With respect to the latter this is not surprising given that disability is largely driven by muscular weakness which in turn is dependent considerably on LMN status.

The evaluation of neurochemical associations with cognitive or behavioral impairment is limited in ALS. As would be expected dorsolateral prefrontal cortex NAA/Cr correlates with cognitive measures of executive function, including verbal fluency (11) and the Wisconsin Card Sorting Test (23). However, mesial prefrontal cortex NAA/mIns did not correlate with the Addenbrook Cognitive Examination or verbal fluency (45); this may have been due to the localization of the voxel (mesial rather than dorsolateral) or that the ACE may not be an optimal cognitive screening measure in ALS (62).

The marked clinical heterogeneity of patients with ALS makes prognostication a difficult task, yet this would be extremely helpful in clinic for counseling patients and to assist as an enrichment strategy in clinical trials. MRS was the first neuroimaging modality to reveal an association of cerebral degeneration with survival. Reduced motor cortex NAA/Cho was the strongest predictor of shorter survival, followed by older age and shorter symptom duration (30).

MONITORING TREATMENT

There have been several studies evaluating treatment effects using MRS. The commencement of riluzole, an antiglutamatergic agent, is accompanied by an increase in NAA/Cr in the motor cortex observed at 1 day (63) and 3 weeks (58) after its initiation. Increases in NAA/Cr suggest the existence of a population of metabolically dysfunctional neurons amenable to treatment. This supposition is supported by the observation of maintained NAA/Cr levels in ALS patients in contrast to a decline in NAA/Cr in healthy controls who received creatine supplementation (24). Changes in NAA/Cr were not observed with gabapentin (25), intrathecal BDNF (26), or minocycline (64). Preliminary observations have also been made on the Glx signal with creatine supplementation (24, 65). In contrast to the studies discussed thus far, there have been reports from studies that have performed sub-analyses on patients comparing those who are taking riluzole to those who are riluzole-naïve (43, 48); these have had varying results.

CONCLUSIONS AND FUTURE DIRECTIONS

What has MRS delivered in the field of ALS thus far, and what is needed?

Cross sectional changes reflecting cerebral neuronal impairment (abnormal NAA indices) are consistently present, and with reasonable accuracy in discriminating patients from controls in group analysis. However, with regards to diagnostic utility, a biomarker of cerebral degeneration will be most helpful in the clinic for patients presenting with LMN signs but insufficient UMN signs; MRS data (as for much of the neuroimaging field) is lacking for such patients. In the more immediate future, MRS should be able to play a part in addressing phenotypic heterogeneity, as associations have been demonstrated with various behavioral measures. Future studies addressing diagnostic potential and heterogeneity would benefit from larger sample sizes, deep phenotyping, inclusion of disease mimics, incorporation of other imaging modalities (e.g., DTI), and incorporation of biofluids for correlative and validation analyses. Of note, there is very little known of the association of cerebral neurochemicals with cognitive impairment in ALS.

There is sensitivity to measuring longitudinal change in metabolites that appears best observed with time intervals of at least 3 months. However, there is considerable variability, which currently prohibits its use as a biomarker of disease progression. The experience of MRS to date of assessing response to therapy has been largely proof of principle. Progress in this area has been hampered in part by the lack of robust disease modifying therapies upon which to frame spectroscopy experiments. Inclusion of MRS in phase II clinical trials may provide opportunities validating metabolites as measures of disease progression, target engagement, or therapeutic response.

The feasibility for MRS to be applied for clinical and routinely for research applications, especially for multicenter efforts and to allow inter-study comparison of results, will require refinement, optimization, and standardization of acquisition and processing protocols, in parallel with greater user expertise. Reference to general (66) and ALS-specific guidelines (67) are starting points for such an endeavor. The advent of whole brain MRSI combined with automated quantification is a significant advancement that could facilitate the modality's uptake to more research labs and eventually clinics.

Advances in technology (higher fields, new sequences) are already permitting the quantification of previously undetectable disease-relevant metabolites and of anatomical regions previously inaccessible (spinal cord). This will continue to provide opportunities for exploring biological insights *in vivo* and for evaluating novel disease markers that may meet the desperate need of a biomarker in ALS.

AUTHOR CONTRIBUTIONS

The author confirms being the sole contributor of this work and has approved it for publication.

REFERENCES

1. Filippi M, Agosta F, Abrahams S, Fazekas F, Grosskreutz J, Kalra S, et al. EFNS guidelines on the use of neuroimaging in the management of motor neuron diseases. *Eur J Neurol.* (2010) 17:526–e20. doi: 10.1111/j.1468-1331.2010.02951.x
2. Provencher SW. Estimation of metabolite concentrations from localized *in vivo* proton NMR spectra. *Magn ResonMed.* (1993) 30:672–9. doi: 10.1002/mrm.1910300604
3. Vargas MI, Martelli P, Xin L, Ipek O, Grouiller F, Pittau F, et al. Clinical neuroimaging using 7 T MRI: challenges and prospects. *J Neuroimaging.* (2018) 28:5–13. doi: 10.1111/jon.12481
4. Rooney WD, Miller RG, Gelinas D, Schuff N, Maudsley AA, Weiner MW. Decreased N-acetylaspartate in motor cortex and corticospinal tract in ALS. *Neurology.* (1998) 50:1800–5. doi: 10.1212/WNL.50.6.1800
5. Suhy J, Miller RG, Rule R, Schuff N, Licht J, Dronsky V, et al. Early detection and longitudinal changes in amyotrophic lateral sclerosis by (1)H MRSI. *Neurology.* (2002) 58:773–9. doi: 10.1212/WNL.58.5.773
6. Mitsumoto H, Ulug AM, Pullman SL, Gooch CL, Chan S, Tang MX, et al. Quantitative objective markers for upper and lower motor neuron dysfunction in ALS. *Neurology.* (2007) 68:1402–10. doi: 10.1212/01.wnl.0000260065.57832.87
7. Yin H, Lim CC, Ma L, Gao Y, Cai Y, Li D, et al. Combined MR spectroscopic imaging and diffusion tensor MRI visualizes corticospinal

tract degeneration in amyotrophic lateral sclerosis. J *Neurol.* (2004) 251:1249–54. doi: 10.1007/s00415-004-0526-9
8. Ebel A, Soher BJ, Maudsley AA. Assessment of 3D proton MR echo-planar spectroscopic imaging using automated spectral analysis. *Magn Reson Med.* (2001) 46:1072–8. doi: 10.1002/mrm.1301
9. Govind V, Sharma KR, Maudsley AA, Arheart KL, Saigal G, Sheriff S. Comprehensive evaluation of corticospinal tract metabolites in amyotrophic lateral sclerosis using whole-brain 1H MR spectroscopy. *PLoS ONE.* (2012) 7:e35607. doi: 10.1371/journal.pone.0035607
10. Stagg CJ, Knight S, Talbot K, Jenkinson M, Maudsley AA, Turner MR. Whole-brain magnetic resonance spectroscopic imaging measures are related to disability in ALS. *Neurology.* (2013) 80:610–5. doi: 10.1212/WNL.0b013e318281ccec
11. Quinn C, Elman L, McCluskey L, Hoskins K, Karam C, Woo JH, et al. Frontal lobe abnormalities on MRS correlate with poor letter fluency in ALS. *Neurology.* (2012) 79:583–8. doi: 10.1212/WNL.0b013e3182635720
12. Verma G, Woo JH, Chawla S, Wang S, Sheriff S, Elman LB, et al. Whole-brain analysis of amyotrophic lateral sclerosis by using echo-planar spectroscopic imaging. *Radiology.* (2013) 267:851–7. doi: 10.1148/radiol.13121148
13. Pioro EP, Antel JP, Cashman NR, Arnold DL. Detection of cortical neuron loss in motor neuron disease by proton magnetic resonance spectroscopic imaging *in vivo*. *Neurology.* (1994) 44:1933–8. doi: 10.1212/WNL.44.10.1933
14. Gredal O, Rosenbaum S, Topp S, Karlsborg M, Strange P, Werdelin L. Quantification of brain metabolites in amyotrophic lateral sclerosis by localized proton magnetic resonance spectroscopy. *Neurology.* (1997) 48:878–81. doi: 10.1212/WNL.48.4.878
15. Kaufmann P, Pullman SL, Shungu DC, Chan S, Hays AP, Del Bene ML, et al. Objective tests for upper motor neuron involvement in amyotrophic lateral sclerosis (ALS). *Neurology.* (2004) 62:1753–7. doi: 10.1212/01.WNL.0000125182.17874.59
16. van der Graaff MM, Lavini C, Akkerman EM, Majoie C, Nederveen AJ, Zwinderman AH, et al. MR spectroscopy findings in early stages of motor neuron disease. *AJNR AmJNeuroradiol.* (2010) 31:1799–806. doi: 10.3174/ajnr.A2217
17. Jones AP, Gunawardena WJ, Coutinho CM, Gatt JA, Shaw IC, Mitchell JD. Preliminary results of proton magnetic resonance spectroscopy in motor neurone disease (amytrophic lateral sclerosis). *J Neurol Sci.* (1995) 129 (Suppl):85–9. doi: 10.1016/0022-510X(95)00072-A
18. Giroud M, Walker P, Bernard D, Lemesle M, Martin D, Baudouin N, et al. Reduced brain N-acetyl-aspartate in frontal lobes suggests neuronal loss in patients with amyotrophic lateral sclerosis. *Neurol Res.* (1996) 18:241–3. doi: 10.1080/01616412.1996.11740412
19. Strong MJ, Grace GM, Orange JB, Leeper HA, Menon RS, Aere C. A prospective study of cognitive impairment in ALS. *Neurology.* (1999) 53:1665–70. doi: 10.1212/WNL.53.8.1665
20. Chan S, Shungu DC, Douglas-Akinwande A, Lange DJ, Rowland LP. Motor neuron diseases: comparison of single-voxel proton MR spectroscopy of the motor cortex with MR imaging of the brain. *Radiology.* (1999) 212:763–9. doi: 10.1148/radiology.212.3.r99au35763
21. Bradley WG, Bowen BC, Pattany PM, Rotta F. 1H-magnetic resonance spectroscopy in amyotrophic lateral sclerosis. *J Neurol Sci.* (1999) 169:84–6. doi: 10.1016/S0022-510X(99)00221-X
22. Pohl C, Block W, Karitzky J, Traber F, Schmidt S, Grothe C, et al. Proton magnetic resonance spectroscopy of the motor cortex in 70 patients with amyotrophic lateral sclerosis. *Arch Neurol.* (2001) 58:729–35. doi: 10.1001/archneur.58.5.729
23. Abe K, Takanashi M, Watanabe Y, Tanaka H, Fujita N, Hirabuki N, et al. Decrease in N-acetylaspartate/creatine ratio in the motor area and the frontal lobe in amyotrophic lateral sclerosis. *Neuroradiology.* (2001) 43:537–41. doi: 10.1007/s002340000521
24. Vielhaber S, Kaufmann J, Kanowski M, Sailer M, Feistner H, Tempelmann C, et al. Effect of creatine supplementation on metabolite levels in ALS motor cortices. *Exp Neurol.* (2001) 172:377–82. doi: 10.1006/exnr.2001.7797
25. Kalra S, Cashman NR, Caramanos Z, Genge A, Arnold DL. Gabapentin therapy for amyotrophic lateral sclerosis: lack of improvement in neuronal integrity shown by MR spectroscopy. *AJNR Am J Neuroradiol.* (2003) 24:476–80.
26. Kalra S, Genge A, Arnold D. A prospective, randomized, placebo-controlled evaluation of corticoneuronal response to intrathecal BDNF therapy in ALS using magnetic resonance spectroscopy: feasibility and results. *Amyotroph Lateral Scler Other Motor Neuron Disord.* (2003) 4:22–6. doi: 10.1080/14660820301179
27. Rule RR, Suhy J, Schuff N, Gelinas DF, Miller RG, Weiner MW. Reduced NAA in motor and non-motor brain regions in amyotrophic lateral sclerosis: a cross-sectional and longitudinal study. *Amyotroph Lateral Scler Other Motor Neuron Disord.* (2004) 5:141–9. doi: 10.1080/14660820410017109
28. Wang S, Poptani H, Woo JH, Desiderio LM, Elman LB, McCluskey LF, et al. Amyotrophic lateral sclerosis: diffusion-tensor and chemical shift MR imaging at 3.0 T. *Radiology.* (2006) 239:831–8. doi: 10.1148/radiol.2393050573
29. Kalra S, Hanstock CC, Martin WR, Allen PS, Johnston WS. Detection of cerebral degeneration in amyotrophic lateral sclerosis using high-field magnetic resonance spectroscopy. *Arch Neurol.* (2006) 63:1144–8. doi: 10.1001/archneur.63.8.1144
30. Kalra S, Vitale A, Cashman NR, Genge A, Arnold DL. Cerebral degeneration predicts survival in amyotrophic lateral sclerosis. *J Neurol Neurosurg Psychiatry.* (2006) 77:1253–5. doi: 10.1136/jnnp.2006.090696
31. Nelles M, Block W, Traber F, Wullner U, Schild HH, Urbach H. Combined 3T diffusion tensor tractography and 1H-MR spectroscopy in motor neuron disease. *AJNR Am J Neuroradiol.* (2008) 29:1708–14. doi: 10.3174/ajnr.A1201
32. Han J, Ma L. Study of the features of proton MR spectroscopy ((1)H-MRS) on amyotrophic lateral sclerosis. *J Magn Reson Imaging.* (2010) 31:305–8. doi: 10.1002/jmri.22053
33. Sivak S, Bittsansky M, Kurca E, Turcanova-Koprusakova M, Grofik M, Nosal V, et al. Proton magnetic resonance spectroscopy in patients with early stages of amyotrophic lateral sclerosis. *Neuroradiology.* (2010) 52:1079–85. doi: 10.1007/s00234-010-0685-6
34. Sudharshan N, Hanstock C, Hui B, Pyra T, Johnston W, Kalra S. Degeneration of the mid-cingulate cortex in amyotrophic lateral sclerosis detected *in vivo* with MR spectroscopy. *AJNR Am J Neuroradiol.* (2011) 32:403–7. doi: 10.3174/ajnr.A2289
35. Weiduschat N, Mao X, Hupf J, Armstrong N, Kang G, Lange DJ, et al. Motor cortex glutathione deficit in ALS measured *in vivo* with the J-editing technique. *Neurosci Lett.* (2014) 570:102–7. doi: 10.1016/j.neulet.2014.04.020
36. Cervo A, Cocozza S, Sacca F, Giorgio SM, Morra VB, Tedeschi E, et al. The combined use of conventional MRI and MR spectroscopic imaging increases the diagnostic accuracy in amyotrophic lateral sclerosis. *Eur J Radiol.* (2015) 84:151–7. doi: 10.1016/j.ejrad.2014.10.019
37. Liu C, Jiang R, Yi X, Zhu W, Bu B. Role of diffusion tensor imaging or magnetic resonance spectroscopy in the diagnosis and disability assessment of amyotrophic lateral sclerosis. *J Neurol Sci.* (2015) 348:206–10. doi: 10.1016/j.jns.2014.12.004
38. Vora M, Kumar S, Sharma S, Sharma S, Makhaik S, Sood RG. Advanced magnetic resonance neuroimaging in bulbar and limb onset early amyotrophic lateral sclerosis. *J Neurosci Rural Pract.* (2016) 7:102–8. doi: 10.4103/0976-3147.165423
39. Wang Y, Li X, Chen W, Wang Z, Xu Y, Luo J, et al. Detecting neuronal dysfunction of hand motor cortex in ALS: a MRSI study. *Somatosens Mot Res.* (2017) 34:15–20. doi: 10.1080/08990220.2016.1275544
40. Bowen BC, Pattany PM, Bradley WG, Murdoch JB, Rotta F, Younis AA, et al. MR imaging and localized proton spectroscopy of the precentral gyrus in amyotrophic lateral sclerosis. *AJNR Am J Neuroradiol.* (2000) 21:647–58.
41. Sarchielli P, Pelliccioli GP, Tarducci R, Chiarini P, Presciutti O, Gobbi G, et al. Magnetic resonance imaging and 1H-magnetic resonance spectroscopy in amyotrophic lateral sclerosis. *Neuroradiology.* (2001) 43:189–97. doi: 10.1007/s002340000472
42. Schuff N, Rooney WD, Miller R, Gelinas DF, Amend DL, Maudsley AA, et al. Reanalysis of multislice (1)H MRSI in amyotrophic lateral sclerosis. *Magn Reson Med.* (2001) 45:513–6. doi: 10.1002/1522-2594(200103)45:3<513::AID-MRM1067>3.0.CO;2-D
43. Foerster BR, Pomper MG, Callaghan BC, Petrou M, Edden RA, Mohamed MA, et al. An imbalance between excitatory and inhibitory neurotransmitters in amyotrophic lateral sclerosis revealed by use of

3-T proton magnetic resonance spectroscopy. *JAMA Neurol.* (2013) 70:1009–16. doi: 10.1001/jamaneurol.2013.234

44. Pyra T, Hui B, Hanstock C, Concha L, Wong JC, Beaulieu C, et al. Combined structural and neurochemical evaluation of the corticospinal tract in amyotrophic lateral sclerosis. *Amyotroph Lateral Scler.* (2010) 11:157–65. doi: 10.3109/17482960902756473
45. Usman U, Choi C, Camicioli R, Seres P, Lynch M, Sekhon R, et al. Mesial prefrontal cortex degeneration in amyotrophic lateral sclerosis: a high-field proton MR spectroscopy study. *AJNR Am J Neuroradiol.* (2011). doi: 10.3174/ajnr.A2590
46. Sharma KR, Saigal G, Maudsley AA, Govind V. 1H MRS of basal ganglia and thalamus in amyotrophic lateral sclerosis. NMR Biomed. (2011) 24:1270–6. doi: 10.1002/nbm.1687
47. Cwik VA, Hanstock CC, Allen PS, Martin WR. Estimation of brainstem neuronal loss in amyotrophic lateral sclerosis with *in vivo* proton magnetic resonance spectroscopy. *Neurology.* (1998) 50:72–7. doi: 10.1212/WNL.50.1.72
48. Cheong I, Marjanska M, Deelchand DK, Eberly LE, Walk D, Oz G. Ultra-high field proton MR spectroscopy in early-stage amyotrophic lateral sclerosis. *Neurochem Res.* (2017) 42:1833–44. doi: 10.1007/s11064-017-2248-2
49. Carew JD, Nair G, Pineda-Alonso N, Usher S, Hu X, Benatar M. Magnetic resonance spectroscopy of the cervical cord in amyotrophic lateral sclerosis. *Amyotroph Lateral Scler.* (2011) 12:185–91. doi: 10.3109/17482968.2010.515223
50. Ikeda K, Murata K, Kawase Y, Kawabe K, Kano O, Yoshii Y, et al. Relationship between cervical cord 1H-magnetic resonance spectroscopy and clinoco-electromyographic profile in amyotrophic lateral sclerosis. *Muscle Nerve.* (2013) 47:61–7. doi: 10.1002/mus.23467
51. Carew JD, Nair G, Andersen PM, Wuu J, Gronka S, Hu X, et al. Presymptomatic spinal cord neurometabolic findings in SOD1-positive people at risk for familial ALS. *Neurology.* (2011) 77:1370–5. doi: 10.1212/WNL.0b013e318231526a
52. Block W, Karitzky J, Traber F, Pohl C, Keller E, Mundegar RR, et al. Proton magnetic resonance spectroscopy of the primary motor cortex in patients with motor neuron disease: subgroup analysis and follow-up measurements. *Arch Neurol.* (1998) 55:931–6. doi: 10.1001/archneur.55.7.931
53. Atassi N, Xu M, Triantafyllou C, Keil B, Lawson R, Cernasov P, et al. Ultra high-field (7tesla) magnetic resonance spectroscopy in Amyotrophic Lateral Sclerosis. *PLoS ONE.* (2017) 12:e0177680. doi: 10.1371/journal.pone.0177680
54. Pioro EP, Majors AW, Mitsumoto H, Nelson DR, Ng TC. 1H-MRS evidence of neurodegeneration and excess glutamate + glutamine in ALS medulla. *Neurology.* (1999) 53:71–9. doi: 10.1212/WNL.53.1.71
55. Foerster BR, Callaghan BC, Petrou M, Edden RA, Chenevert TL, Feldman EL. Decreased motor cortex gamma-aminobutyric acid in amyotrophic lateral sclerosis. *Neurology.* (2012) 78:1596–600. doi: 10.1212/WNL.0b013e3182563b57
56. Charil A, Corbo M, Filippi M, Kesavadas C, Agosta F, Munerati E, et al. Structural and metabolic changes in the brain of patients with upper motor neuron disorders: a multiparametric MRI study. *Amyotroph Lateral Scler.* (2009) 10:269–79. doi: 10.3109/17482960902777339
57. Foerster BR, Carlos RC, Dwamena BA, Callaghan BC, Petrou M, Edden RA, et al. Multimodal MRI as a diagnostic biomarker for amyotrophic lateral sclerosis. *Ann Clin Transl Neurol.* (2014) 1:107–14. doi: 10.1002/acn3.30
58. Kalra S, Cashman NR, Genge A, Arnold DL. Recovery of N-acetylaspartate in corticomotor neurons of patients with ALS after riluzole therapy. *Neuroreport.* (1998) 9:1757–61. doi: 10.1097/00001756-199806010-00016
59. Unrath A, Ludolph AC, Kassubek J. Brain metabolites in definite amyotrophic lateral sclerosis: a longitudinal proton magnetic resonance spectroscopy study. *J Neurol.* (2007) 254:1099–106. doi: 10.1007/s00415-006-0495-2
60. Sacca F, Quarantelli M, Rinaldi C, Tucci T, Piro R, Perrotta G, et al. A randomized controlled clinical trial of growth hormone in amyotrophic lateral sclerosis: clinical, neuroimaging, and hormonal results. *J Neurol.* (2012) 259:132–8. doi: 10.1007/s00415-011-6146-2
61. Cheong I, Deelchand DK, Eberly LE, Marjanska M, Manousakis G, Guliani G, et al. Neurochemical correlates of functional decline in amyotrophic lateral sclerosis. *J Neurol Neurosurg Psychiatry.* (2018) 90:294–301. doi: 10.1136/jnnp-2018-318795
62. Chenji S, Mah D, Johnston W, Camicioli R, Fisher N, Kalra S. Utility of the addenbrooke's cognitive examination in amyotrophic lateral sclerosis. *Can J Neurol Sci.* (2018) 45:527–32. doi: 10.1017/cjn.2018.68
63. Kalra S, Tai P, Genge A, Arnold DL. Rapid improvement in cortical neuronal integrity in amyotrophic lateral sclerosis detected by proton magnetic resonance spectroscopic imaging. *J Neurol.* (2006) 253:1060–3. doi: 10.1007/s00415-006-0162-7
64. Khiat A, D'Amour M, Souchon F, Boulanger Y. MRS study of the effects of minocycline on markers of neuronal and microglial integrity in ALS. *Magn Reson Imaging.* (2010) 28:1456–60. doi: 10.1016/j.mri.2010.06.032
65. Atassi N, Ratai EM, Greenblatt DJ, Pulley D, Zhao Y, Bombardier J, et al. A phase I, pharmacokinetic, dosage escalation study of creatine monohydrate in subjects with amyotrophic lateral sclerosis. *Amyotroph Lateral Scler.* (2010) 11:508–13. doi: 10.3109/17482961003797130
66. Oz G, Alger JR, Barker PB, Bartha R, Bizzi A, Boesch C, et al. Clinical proton MR spectroscopy in central nervous system disorders. *Radiology.* (2014) 270:658–79. doi: 10.1148/radiol.13130531
67. Turner MR, Grosskreutz J, Kassubek J, Abrahams S, Agosta F, Benatar M, et al. Towards a neuroimaging biomarker for amyotrophic lateral sclerosis. *Lancet Neurol.* (2011) 10:400–3. doi: 10.1016/S1474-4422(11)70049-7

23

Longitudinal Alterations of Alpha-Synuclein, Amyloid Beta, Total and Phosphorylated Tau in Cerebrospinal Fluid and Correlations between their Changes in Parkinson's Disease

*Mahsa Dolatshahi[1], Shayan Pourmirbabaei[1], Aida Kamalian[1], Amir Ashraf-Ganjouei[1], Mehdi Yaseri[2] and Mohammad H. Aarabi[1]**

[1] *Faculty of Medicine, Tehran University of Medical Sciences, Tehran, Iran,*

[2] *Department of Epidemiology and Biostatistics, School of Public Health, Tehran University of Medical Sciences, Tehran, Iran*

***Correspondence:**
Mohammad Aarabi
mohammadhadiarabi@gmail.com

Background: Parkinson's disease (PD) is characterized by proteinopathies and these proteinopathies seem to interact synergistically and lead to protein aggregations and changes in protein cerebrospinal fluid (CSF) levels. In this study, we aimed to explore the longitudinal changes of CSF a lpha-synuclein (α-syn), total tau (t-tau), phosphorylated tau (p-tau), and beta-amyloid ($A\beta_{1-42}$) and their relationships with each other and with baseline clinical entities like REM sleep behavior disorder (RBD), cognitive impairment, motor symptoms, and olfaction dysfunction.

Method: One hundred and twelve non-demented PD patients and 110 controls were recruited from Parkinson's Progression Markers Initiative (PPMI).We used a linear mixed model within groups to assess longitudinal protein changes over 6 and 12 months and a random regression coefficient within the linear mixed model to investigate the correlation between proteins and their baseline clinical characteristics.

Results: P-tau was lower in PDs only at baseline, but during a year, p-tau increased more rapidly in PDs than controls. $A\beta_{1-42}$ was not significantly different between groups at any separate timepoint; however, when assessed longitudinally, $A\beta_{1-42}$ showed significant changes in both groups. Conversely, t-tau and α-syn differed significantly between groups, but their longitudinal changes were not significant in either of the groups. Moreover, all proteins' baseline levels, except p-tau, could determine estimated longitudinal tau changes. Baseline RBDSQ scores but not UPDRS III, MoCA, or UPSIT scores were predictive of longitudinal increase in α-syn levels.

Conclusion: Longitudinal changes in levels of CSF proteins are related to each other and could help researchers further understand PD pathology. In addition, RBD seems to be a potential prognostic factor for PD progression. However, in order to reach a consensus, longer follow-up times are required.

Keywords: Parkinson's disease, Cerebrospinal fluid (CSF), Longitudinal, alpha-synuclein, tau, beta-amyloid

INTRODUCTION

As the life expectancy of population increases, neurodegenerative diseases like Parkinson's disease (PD) become the spotlight in medicine (1). PD is characterized by several pathological mechanisms like lysosomal damage, oxidative stress, and most importantly protein aggregation. The main form of proteinopathy in PD has long been considered to be synucleinopathy, i.e., intraneuronal inclusions of alpha-synuclein in the form of Lewy bodies and Lewy neurites. However, recent research has indicated the accompanying role of other AD-associated proteinopathies like tauopathy and beta-amyloidopathy (2).

Moreover, it is known that PD symptoms progress heterogeneously (3) which can be mainly attributed to the variations in the predominant pathological mechanisms (4, 5). These variations can make a great difference in manifestations of PD symptoms such as cognitive dysfunction and contribute to disease heterogeneity. For example, concomitant AD-pathology (tau and beta-amyloid aggragations) is a more common observation in PD dementia (PDD) (6, 7). On the other hand, recently it has been revealed that the predominant clinical manifestations which patients are presented with at baseline might be a predictor for progression of disease, both from a pathophysiological and clinical point of view. More importantly, these differences in the type and severity of underlying proteinopathies determine the most effective therapeutic procedure for each person, which is the cornerstone of personalized medicine. Thus, clinicians would benefit from a method to detect the main pathological pathways leading to dopaminergic neuron loss and PD symptoms in each individual, in association with their different clinical entities, for both diagnostic and curative purposes (8, 9).

On the other hand, many studies have reached the notion that mutual interactions between different proteins promote the aggregation of these proteins *in vivo* and accelerate cognitive dysfunction (10). Most notably, alpha-synuclein induces polymerization, and aggregation of tau and thereby promotes the formation of intracellular amyloid–tau inclusions (11, 12). It also engages in cross-seeding with tau proteins so they tend to co-exist in intracellular inclusions (13).

Importantly, these proteinopathies are mirrored in changes of CSF protein concentrations, which can be easily measured in clinic. Unfortunately, despite the large number of studies, the diagnostic utility of CSF biomarkers has been unsatisfactory (14).

Numerous studies have assessed the concentration of CSF biomarkers in PD. However, most of these studies were cross-sectional and just a few studies assessed longitudinal changes of CSF markers and lead to inconsistant results. These cross-sectional studies have mostly shown decreased CSF levels of alpha-synuclein (α-syn) in PD and other synucleinopathies compared to healthy controls (15–20). In addition, the levels of Alzheimer's disease (AD) biomarkers such as total tau (t-tau), phosphorylated tau (p-tau), and beta-amyloid 1-42 ($A\beta_{1-42}$) have been previously shown to be decreased or normal in PD patients (17–21). Apart from the mentioned findings, there has been some different observations. For example, in the study conducted by Montine et al., one third of non-demented PD patients and half of PDD patients showed higher CSF tau levels compared to healthy controls (17). Moreover, the study of Parkinson Progression Markers Initiative (PPMI) (200 healthy controls and 400 PDs) showed non-significantly changed levels of $A\beta_{1-42}$ compared to controls at baseline (20). Specific patterns of changes in levels of these proteins in different groups of PD patients with various PD symptoms have been observed, which are reviewed elsewhere (22, 23).

Longitudinal studies that evaluated longitudinal changes of CSF proteins (α-syn, t-tau, p-tau, and $A\beta_{1-42}$) levels in PD patients have reached heterogeneous results e.g., the study conducted by Hall et al. has shown significantly increasing levels of all proteins except $A\beta_{1-42}$ during a two-year follow-up, in which increase of p-tau was associated with motor symptoms aggravation and cognitive decline (21). Another study done by Majbour et al. revealed no significant change in levels of t-tau, p-tau, $A\beta_{40}$, and $A\beta_{42}$ but an increase in total and oligomeric α-syn levels and a decrease in serine129 phosphorylated α-syn during a two-year follow-up (24). The study conducted by Stewart et al. has shown a decline in alpha-synuclein over a 2-year follow-up in patients of DATATOP cohort who received medication, which was associated with an improvement in cognitive abilities but was not correlated with motor symptoms (25). On the other hand, a recent study by Forland et al. showed nonsignificant changes of CSF alpha-synuclein in a 4-year follow-up (26). Another study done by Boungiorno et al. has shown a longitudinal decline in CSF Aβ but an increase in t-tau levels during 18 months, which were not significantly associated with cognitive decline (27). On the whole, these studies have shown quite inconsistent results regarding longitudinal changes of CSF proteins.

Thus, it seems that conducting studies with a large sample size in ongoing cohorts with drug-naïve cases like PPMI can be helpful in interpretation of these heterogeneous results and complementing our knowledge about this cohort. Furthermore, investigating the correlations between baseline levels of proteins and their changes in association with clinical manifestations facilitates estimation of patients' prognoses and can lead to a better understanding of PD pathogenesis.

In this study, we used a relatively large sample size in recent-onset, drug-naive, non-demented patients recruited from PPMI cohort to investigate the longitudinal changes in CSF protein levels and also their association with each other, with baseline levels of each protein, and also the clinical entities. These longitudinal assessments might elucidate the interaction between pathological mechanisms during disease progression and whether they have any associations with heterogeneous clinical manifestations.

METHODS

Participants

The participants of this study were recruited from the Parkinson Progression Markers Initiative (PPMI) database freely available at http://www.ppmi-info.org/. PPMI cohort comprises 400 recently

Abbreviations: CSF, cerebrospinal fluid; PD, Parkinson's disease; HC, healthy controls; α-syn, alpha-synuclein; Aβ, beta-amyloid; t-tau, total tau; p-tau, phosphorylated tau.

diagnosed PD and 200 healthy subjects followed longitudinally for biomarker assessment at 21 clinical sites using standard data acquisition protocols (28). The PPMI study was approved by the Institutional Review Board of all participating sites and all participants were given written informed consent before inclusion in the study. PD subjects of PPMI study were recruited at disease threshold, meaning that they had been diagnosed within 2 years while they were drug-naïve at baseline. The clinical criteria for PD diagnosis included asymmetric resting tremor and/or asymmetric bradykinesia. In addition, all subjects underwent dopamine transporter (DAT) imaging and DAT deficit was considered necessary for PD diagnosis. The subjects were assessed for motor symptoms using Unified Parkinson's Disease Rating Scale part III (UPDRS III), cognitive impairment using Montreal Cognitive Assessment (MoCA). REM sleep Behavior Disorder (RBD) and olfaction dysfunction were assessed using REM Sleep Behavior Disorder Screening Questionnaire (RBDSQ) and University of Pennsylvania Smell Identification Test (UPSIT), respectively. Healthy subjects were required to have no significant neurologic dysfunction, no first-degree family member with PD and MoCA >26 (2011). In PPMI cohort longitudinal data for CSF samples were available only for a portion of the patients. Thus, we selected the subjects for which longitudinal CSF data were available at baseline (BL), the second visit (V02) i.e., 6 months after recruitment, and the fourth visit (V04) i.e., one year after recruitment. We excluded the patients who met the criteria for PD dementia (PDD) at baseline and those who had recently received medications to have a clinically homogenous sample. In the end, 112 PD patients and 110 matched healthy subjects with the above-mentioned properties were included in the study. Complementary data on disease duration, age, gender, and UPDRS III score at different time points is provided in Supplementary Tables 1–4.

CSF Samples Collection and Analysis

CSF was collected by using standardized lumbar puncture procedures. CSF was collected into siliconized polypropylene tubes and the first 1–2 mL of CSF of sent to the site's local laboratory for routine testing for cell count, total protein level, and glucose level. An additional 15–20 mL of CSF was transferred into 15-mL conical propylene tubes at room temperature, mixed gently, centrifuged at 2,000 g for 10 min at room temperature, and transferred into 1.5-mL pre-cooled siliconized polypropylene aliquot tubes followed by immediate freezing on dry ice. The frozen aliquots of CSF were shipped overnight to the PPMI Biorepository Core Laboratories on dry ice and then thawed, aliquoted into 0.5-mL siliconized polypropylene tubes, refrozen once, and stored at −80°C. The coded frozen aliquots of CSF were transferred from the PPMI Biorepository Core laboratories to the University of Pennsylvania and to Covance for analyses. CSF Aβ1-42, t-tau and p-tau were measured using the xMAP-Luminex platform with INNOBIA AlzBio3 immunoassay kit-based reagents (Fujirebio-Innogenetics, Ghent, Belgium). CSF α-syn and CSF hemoglobin levels were analyzed using appropriate commercially available sandwich type ELISA kits (Covance, Dedham, MA) [2011; (19, 20)].

Statistical Analysis

We used Kolmogorov-Smirnov test as well as a Q-Q plot to check for the normal distribution of data. To present data, we used mean, standard deviation, median, and range. To find the difference between the two groups during the study period, we used the Mann-Whitney test. To assess the changes within each group (PD, controls) considering the correlation of measurements (CSF protein concentrations, age, disease duration), we used a linear mixed model within each group. In this analysis, multiple comparison corrections were performed by Bonferroni method. Other linear mixed models with the interaction of time and groups were used to test the difference of trends in parameters during the study course between the two groups. Correlation of different parameters and their changes during the study course was assessed with Pearson correlation. To adjust for the probable confounding effect of age, sex, and disease duration (in PD group) we used partial correlation coefficient. Finally, to evaluate the effect of baseline values of biomarkers on their own changes and the changes of other biomarkers, we used a two-step procedure: in the first step, we obtained the estimated mean change of each parameter on each subject with the use of random regression coefficients of a linear mixed model. In the next step, we used correlation coefficient to evaluate the relation of these estimations with baseline values of all parameters. Also, the correlation of different biomarkers' estimated changes was calculated. All statistical analyses were performed by R (R Foundation for Statistical Computing, Vienna, Austria), http://www.R-project.org/. A p-value of < 0.05 was considered statistically significant.

RESULTS

Demographics

Demographics and clinical scores of study participants and their comparison are given in **Table 1**. UPDRS III, MoCA, and UPSIT scores were significantly lower in PD compared to controls at baseline and after a year (for MoCA and UPDRS III). MoCA and UPDRS III scores were significantly lower at V04 compared to baseline in PD patients. However, in controls, only MoCA scores were lower at V04 compared to baseline. RBDSQ scores, however, not only showed no difference between PD and control groups, but also they were not different at baseline compared to V04.

On the whole, age and disease duration were correlated with levels of some CSF biomarkers at different time points in PD and controls.

Values of $A\beta_{1-42}$ were correlated with age in the control group and levels of t-tau showed correlation with age in PD group at all time points. Percentage of changes in levels of t-tau and $A\beta_{1-42}$ were correlated with age in both groups.

Baseline values of p-tau and t-tau in PD groups were correlated with disease duration. Also, percentage of changes of p-tau and $A\beta_{1-42}$ during 6 months was correlated with disease duration. Percentage of changes during one year, only for t-tau and $A\beta_{1-42}$, was correlated with disease duration.

TABLE 1 | Demographics and clinical tests including Unified Parkinson's Disease Rating Scale part III (UPDRS III), Montreal Cognitive Assessment (MoCA), REM sleep Behavior Disorder Questionnaire (RBDSQ), and University of Pennsylvania Smell Identification Test (UPSIT) scores at Baseline (BL) and after a year, visit 04 (V04) in Parkinson's disease (PD) and control subjects.

	PD (n = 112)	Control (n = 110)	P-value (PD, control) [two-sample t-test]	P-value (BL, V04) [paired sample t-test]
Age (years) (mean ± SD)	60.89 ± 10.46	61.54 ± 10.03	0.6381[a]	–
Gender (Male Number/ %)	80M/71.42%	69M/62.72%	0.2465[b]	–
Disease duration (months) (mean ± SD)	14.23 ± 14.08	–	–	–
UPDRS III (BL) (mean ± SD)	19.15 ± 8.16	2.41 ± 1.39	0.0000[a]	0.0027[c](*PD*)
UPDRS III (V04) (mean ± SD)	22.98 ± 10.52	3.12 ± 1.92	0.0000[a]	0.1555[c](*control*)
MoCA (BL) (mean ± SD)	27.03 ± 2.10	28.22 ± 1.06	0.0000[a]	0.0031[c](*PD*)
MoCA (V04) (mean ± SD)	26.34 ± 2.42	27.29 ± 2.10	0.0023[a]	0.0000[c](*control*)
RBDSQ (BL) (mean ± SD)	4.17 ± 2.89	3.95 ± 2.89	0.5358[a]	0.3394[c](*PD*)
RBDSQ (V04) (mean ± SD)	3.99 ± 2.82	3.60 ± 2.99	0.6371[a]	0.5694[c](*control*)
UPSIT baseline (mean ± SD)	20.77 ± 8.03	33.99 ± 4.69	0.0000[a]	–

n, number; SD, standard deviation.
[a]p-values obtained by independent samples t-test.
[b]p-values obtained by chi-square independence test.
[c]p-values obtained by paired samples t-test (difference between clinical scores at baseline and after 1-year follow-up).

Difference Between PD and Control in Biomarker Levels at Different Time Points

The levels of α-syn and t-tau were significantly lower in PD group than controls at baseline, after six months, and after one year. P-tau level was significantly lower in PD group at baseline, but not after 6 months and one year. Levels of $A\beta_{1-42}$ showed no significant difference between the two groups at any time point. (**Table 2**).

Longitudinal Changes Over 6 Months and One Year in CSF Biomarker Levels in PD and Control Groups

The levels of α-syn showed no significant change after 6 months and one year in neither of the groups. P-tau level had not significantly changed after 6 months in either group; however, its level had significantly risen after one year in PD group but not in controls. T-tau showed no significant change after 6 months and one year in control. T-tau levels had decreased significantly after 6 months in PD group, but no significant change was observed from baseline to visit 4 (after one year). $A\beta_{1-42}$ had not significantly changed after 6 months, but it had significantly increased after one year in both control and PD groups.

On the whole, the pattern of changes (increase or decrease) of biomarkers was not different between controls and PD group, except for total tau for which there was a different pattern of change between the two groups. Also, the trend of changes based on interaction analysis of time and group, within the linear mixed model, was not significantly different between the two groups. (**Table 2**, **Figure 1**).

Correlation Between Levels of Different CSF Biomarkers at Different Time Points

None of the CSF biomarkers showed any significant correlation with each other in control group when adjusted for age and sex although several significant correlations were observed in control group when not adjusted. Correlations between levels of the same biomarker at different time points were significant in the PD group whether adjustment for age, gender, and disease duration was done or not. However, there were some exceptions for t-tau.

Correlation of Baseline Values of Each Biomarker With Estimated Changes of Different Biomarkers During Study Period

Baseline values of all biomarkers were correlated with their own estimated changes, except for p-tau. Additionally, baseline values of all biomarkers were correlated with estimated changes of t-tau and baseline values of α-syn correlated to estimated changes of $A\beta_{1-42}$ (P = 0.002). (**Table 3**, **Figure 2**).

Correlation of Estimated Changes of Different Biomarkers During Study Period With Each Other

Estimated changes of p-tau and t-tau were positively correlated to each other ($P = 0.002$). Moreover, estimated changes of p-tau and $A\beta_{1-42}$ were correlated positively ($P < 0.001$). (**Table 3**, **Figure 3**).

Correlation of Baseline Values of MoCA, RBDSQ, UPSIT, and UPDRS III Scores With Estimated Changes of Different Biomarkers During Study

Using linear mixed models for changes of p-tau, t-tau, α-syn, and Aβ CSF levels, with interaction of baseline UPDRS III, RBDSQ, UPSIT, and MoCA scores, no significant association between these clinical scores with estimated

TABLE 2 | Biomarker changes in PD and control group within a linear mixed model.

Parameter	**Control**		**PD**		**Group difference**	**P of trend with interaction of time and group**
	Mean ± SD	**Median (range)**	**Mean ± SD**	**Median (range)**	$P^{\dagger}$	**diff**$^{\$}$
α-synuclein						0.950
Value at baseline	2,163 ± 976	1,950 (593 to 5,238)	1,783 ± 700	1,704 (333 to 5,174)	0.007	
Value at 6 months	2,196 ± 924	2,070 (659 to 5,209)	1,822 ± 700	1,770 (680 to 4,659)	0.001	
Crude change till 6 months	33 ± 623	7 (-1,913 to 2,258)	40 ± 317	34 (−674 to 837)	0.948	
Change% till 6 months	8 ± 37	0 (−61 to 257)	6 ± 27	2 (−40 to 192)	0.943	
P§-within linear mixed model till 6 months	1.000		0.774			
Value at 1 year	2,166 ± 964	2,037 (729 to 5,295)	1,812 ± 712	1,700 (782 to 4,633)	0.004	
Crude change till 1 year	3 ± 589	−5 (−2,292 to 1,748)	30 ± 406	11 (−1,612 to 1,284)	0.872	
Change% till 1 year	5 ± 34	0 (−55 to 161)	6 ± 31	1 (−46 to 202)	0.737	
P§-within linear mixed model till 1 year	1.000		1.000			
P-tau						0.654
Value at baseline	17 ± 9	14 (6 to 59)	15 ± 8	12 (6 to 40)	0.032	
Value at 6 months	16 ± 8	13 (6 to 53)	15 ± 9	11 (5 to 56)	0.221	
Crude change till 6 months	−1 ± 9	0 (−24 to 39)	0 ± 10	0 (−22 to 40)	0.421	
Change% till 6 months	0 ± 0	0 (−2 to 1)	0 ± 1	0 (−2 to 2)	0.433	
P§-within linear mixed model till 6 months	0.983		1.000			
Value at 1 year	20 ± 13	16 (6 to 90)	19 ± 11	15 (5 to 58)	0.622	
Crude change till 1 year	3 ± 15	1 (−30 to 75)	4 ± 13	3 (−27 to 47)	0.365	
Change% till 1 year	0 ± 1	0 (−2 to 4)	0 ± 1	0 (−2 to 3)	0.256	
P§-within linear mixed model till 1 year	0.094		0.003			
T-tau						0.240
Value at baseline	52 ± 26	45 (18 to 188)	45 ± 18	39 (22 to 121)	0.047	
Value at 6 months	51 ± 24	45 (17 to 181)	43 ± 18	37 (16 to 135)	0.002	
Crude change till 6 months	−1 ± 9	0 (−27 to 35)	−2 ± 6	−2 (−15 to 22)	0.037	
Change% till 6 months	0 ± 0	0 (−1 to 2)	0 ± 0	0 (−2 to 2)	0.006	
P§-within linear mixed model till 6 months	1.000		0.007			
Value at 1 year	53 ± 27	45 (19 to 216)	44 ± 18	39 (19 to 129)	0.002	
Crude change till 1 year	1 ± 10	1 (−28 to 40)	−1 ± 6	−1 (−28 to 15)	0.047	
Change% till 1 year	0 ± 0	0 (−1 to 3)	0 ± 0	0 (−1 to 2)	0.025	
P§-within linear mixed model till 1 year	0.893		0.459			
$A\beta_{1-42}$						0.785
Value at baseline	368 ± 103	379 (89 to 680)	362 ± 84	368 (140 to 627)	0.561	
Value at 6 months	374 ± 100	374 (98 to 610)	364 ± 95	374 (129 to 687)	0.245	
Crude change till 6 months	6 ± 54	5 (−230 to 152)	2 ± 52	4 (−122 to 205)	0.404	
Change% till 6 months	0 ± 3	0 (−18 to 8)	0 ± 4	0 (−28 to 19)	0.484	
P§-within linear mixed model till 6 months	0.835		1.000			
Value at 1 year	388 ± 106	392 (95 to 691)	382 ± 105	379 (144 to 733)	0.376	
Crude change till 1 year	20 ± 64	20 (−265 to 190)	20 ± 71	6 (−161 to 317)	0.370	
Change% till 1 year	1 ± 4	1 (−12 to 16)	1 ± 4	0 (−8 to 14)	0.428	
P§-within linear mixed model till 1 year	0.022		0.043			

† *P-value of comparing the groups at each timepoint based on Mann-Whitney test; however, the 95% Confidence Intervals are based on t-statistics.*
§ *Longitudinal changes within the liner mixed model in each group, multiple comparison correction performed by Bonferroni method.*
$ *Comparison between the trend of changes in groups based on interaction analysis of time and group, within a linear mixed model.*

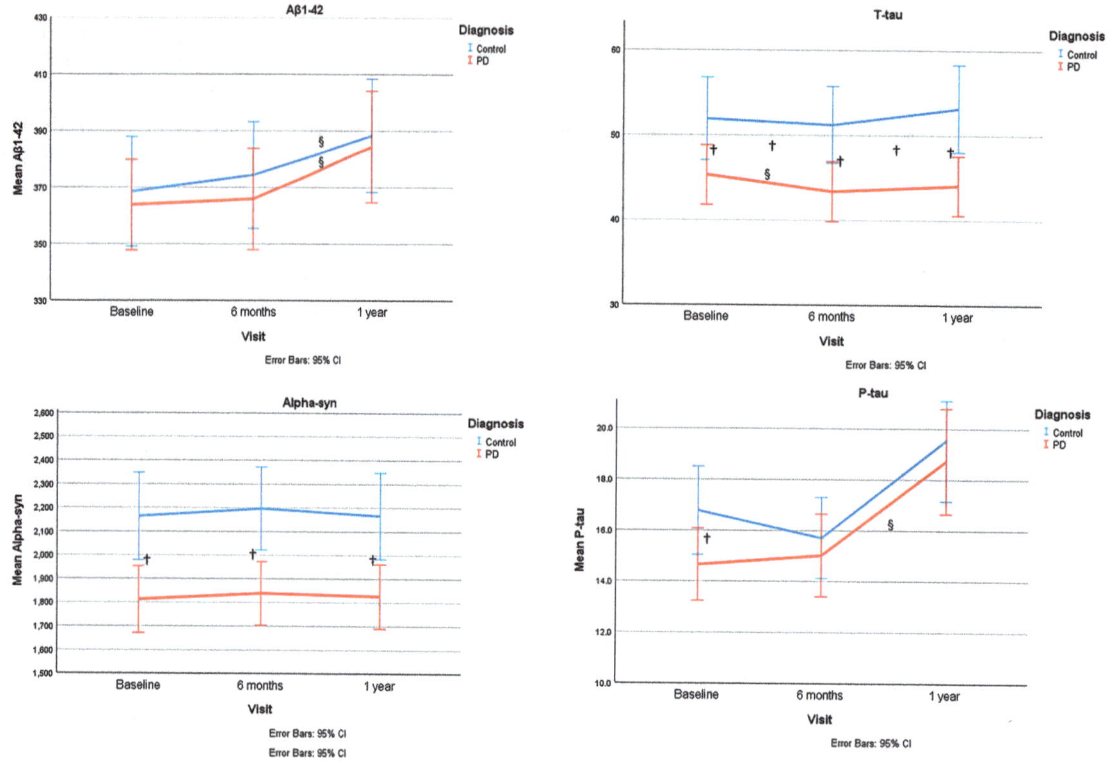

FIGURE 1 | Representation of α-syn, P-tau, T-tau, and Aβ 1-42 levels at different time points and the trend of changes during study period. [§]shows significant changes during time within each group within a linear mixed model. [†]shows the significant group differences for CSF levels of markers at each time point or their changes (from baseline to 6 months or from baseline to 1 year).

changes of each CSF marker was observed except for the significant correlation between estimated changes in alpha-synuclein level and RBDSQ scores ($p = 0.0013$) (data not shown).

DISCUSSION

In this study, we explored baseline levels and longitudinal changes of CSF markers and evaluated their association with each other in drug-naïve, non-demented PD patients of PPMI cohort who were at the early stage of their disease. In addition, we evaluated the power of baseline clinical scores (UPDRS III, MoCA, UPSIT, RBDSQ) in prediction of longitudinal changes of CSF markers in PD patients. In brief, all CSF markers were lower in PDs compared to controls except $A\beta_{1-42}$ at baseline, which was similar to the results of the previously mentioned cross-sectional study in PPMI cohort. In longitudinal assessment, $A\beta_{1-42}$ and p-tau concentrations showed an increase in PD patients with the former also increasing in control subjects. Correlations between baseline concentrations of each of the CSF markers with their own estimated changes were significant except for p-tau. Furthermore, longitudinal changes of p-tau levels were positively correlated to t-tau and $A\beta_{1-42}$ longitudinal changes.

Difference Between PD and Control in Biomarker Levels at Different Time Points and Their Changes During Time

This study has shown a reduced level of α-syn and t-tau at all time-points and p-tau only at baseline in patients' CSF compared to healthy controls'. This observation is in line with the most recent studies (16, 20, 21); however, some studies observed higher or unchanged CSF t-tau or p-tau levels in PD patients (17, 29–31).

P-tau levels were significantly lower in the PD group compared to controls and rose significantly during the 1-year follow-up time, only in the PD group. Therefore, the p-tau level differences between PD and control groups vanished at the 6-month and one-year time points. On the other hand, t-tau levels were different between the two groups at all time points despite their non-significant longitudinal changes. In the study by Boungiorno et al., t-tau but not p-tau longitudinal increase was significant. Hall et al., however, found an increase in both. Thus, due to the high rate of p-tau changes during the disease course, at least in some time points, there would be an overlap with p-tau levels in controls, which challanges its diagnostic value. Thus, we hypothesize that CSF t-tau is a better candidate as a diagnostic tool than p-tau, which needs to be further investigated.

Our study does not provide the means to discover the underlying mechanism of these protein level differences;

TABLE 3 | The correlation and regression coefficient of estimated changes and baseline values with estimated change of different factors during study periods, obtained within linear mixed model.

Estimated		**Estimated changes per year***				**Baseline values**			
Change per year*		**α-synuclein**	**P-tau**	**T-tau**	**Aβ42**	**α-synuclein**	**P-tau**	**T-tau**	**Aβ42**
α-synuclein	r		0.015	0.092	0.096	−0.310	−0.036	−0.125	0.042
	B		0.309	27.400	0.429	−0.020	−0.211	−0.306	0.022
	P		0.871	0.335	0.314	0.001	0.708	0.190	0.663
P-tau	r	0.015		−0.220	0.387	0.129	0.030	0.228	−0.068
	B	0.001		−3.286	0.087	0.000	0.009	0.028	−0.002
	P	0.871		0.020	0.000	0.175	0.750	0.016	0.476
T-tau	r	0.092	−0.220		−0.159	−0.762	−0.399	−0.983	−0.193
	B	0.000	−0.015		−0.002	0.000	−0.008	−0.008	0.000
	P	0.335	0.020		0.094	0.000	0.000	0.000	0.041
Aβ1-42	r	0.096	0.387	−0.159		0.297	−0.052	0.127	0.635
	B	0.021	1.731	−10.599		0.004	−0.068	0.070	0.075
	P	0.314	0.000	0.094		0.002	0.587	0.182	0.000

r, Correlation coefficient.
B, Linear regression coefficient.
**Estimated changes were calculated for each subject based on the regression coefficient of each subject within a linear mixed model.*
The correlations were assessed between different biomarkers in the study. One single biomarker could not have a correlationship with itself and they were marked black.

however, we speculate that at the very early stages of PD, i.e., at our baseline, there is an accumulation of toxic p-tau in form of neurofibrillary tangles (NFTs) in neurons, which causes absorption of more functional tau molecules from extracellular space as a compensatory mechanism in order to reverse back the function of neuronal trafficking. The similar mechanisms are the case for α-syn. In contrast, it has been shown that due to the altered processing of α-syn and occasionally increased transcription of SNCA gene, neurons secrete exosomal α-syn and propagate PD pathology (32, 33). Maybe, the observed changes of α-syn in different studies vary based on the weight of such mechanisms. This phenomenon causes a decrease in t-tau, p-tau, and α-syn levels in CSF. In later phases of the disease, due to axonal damage, p-tau and α-syn molecules accumulated in form of NFTs and Lewy bodies are released into CSF and the levels of p-tau and α-syn will increase. However, α-syn longitudinal changes are not significant in the time points we have studied, which is in line with some of the previous studies (26). One theory is that in PD the accelerated injury to neuronal plasma membrane which causes an increase in CSF α-syn, is contradicted by the more α-syn intracellular accumulation (34). Thus, variability in rates of axonal degeneration is one of the important factors in this regard and probably α-syn change is not an appropriate diagnostic tool for PD (35). We reckon that levels of t-tau and α-syn might have already fallen in earlier stages (because of absorption of these molecules into neurons as a compensation) and in the follow-up time due to the floor effect, no longitudinal decrease could be observed, although heterogeneity in disease duration makes such assumptions non-applicable. Maybe, longer follow-up times could allow significant longitudinal changes.

It is worthy of note that in AD, CSF tau levels are elevated from the earliest phases of the disease (36, 37) except for the subgroups of patients with the concomitant alpha-synucleinopathy, i.e., Dementia with Lewy Bodies (DLB) (37). This common observation in synucleinopathies might refer to the colocalization of tau molecules with α-syn, which contributes to their reduction in CSF.

On the other hand, $A\beta_{1-42}$ levels were not significantly different between the two groups at any time point although significant longitudinal increase of $A\beta_{1-42}$ was observed in both groups. However, the study done by Buongiorno et al. has shown the opposite, i.e., a decrease in Aβ levels during 18 months, which was associated with cognitive decline in non-demented PD patients (27). In addition, in the study done by Hall et al. the changes in Aβ levels in PD patients with long disease durations were non-significant during 2 years. Herein, we checked for levels of whole CSF Aβ ($A\beta_{1-42}$) in contrast to the mentioned study, which evaluated the level of $A\beta_{42}$, and this might explain the discrepancies in results. The progressive reduction of $A\beta_{1-42}$ levels in other studies (both in AD and PD) can be mainly attributed to its extracellular accumulation but we can not justify the observed increase in $A\beta_{1-42}$ in our study.

On the whole, it seems that the difference in clinical and pathophysiological characteristics contributes to variability in disease progression and different results of such studies.

Variables which affect the results of these studies include the rate of axonal damage, clinical endophenotypes, the stage of the disease, and whether compensatory mechanisms are working properly. For instance, it is shown that significantly increased levels of CSF α-syn and t-tau is a common phenomenon in the ones who develop PD dementia (PDD) (16). This is similar to the observation of increased α-syn and t-tau in AD patients compared to healthy controls (36–38). Herein, we excluded the patients fulfilling the criteria for PDD at baseline, and this might explain the reason why t-tau and α-syn did not increase during

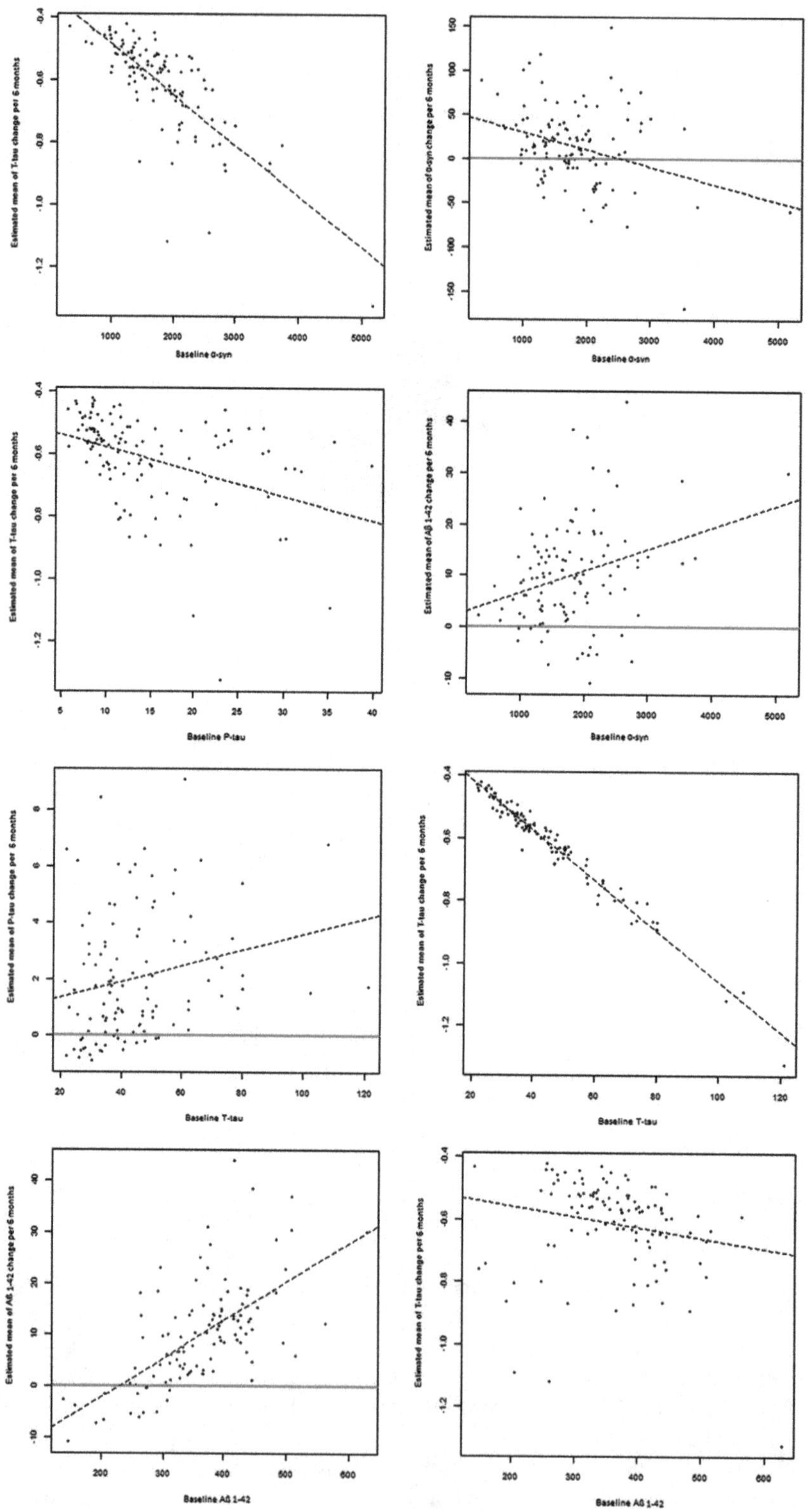

FIGURE 2 | Significant correlations between baseline CSF levels of α-syn, P-tau, T-tau, and $A\beta_{1-42}$ with estimated changes of α-syn, P-tau, T-tau, and $A\beta_{1-42}$.

the course of the disease in our sample. Moreover, it seems that as the disease duration increases, higher levels of α-syn in patients compared to HC is encountered in CSF samples as opposed to the lower levels of this protein in early-stage PD cases such as ours. This is in line with the previous longitudinal assessment done by Hall et al. in which despite significant increases in all

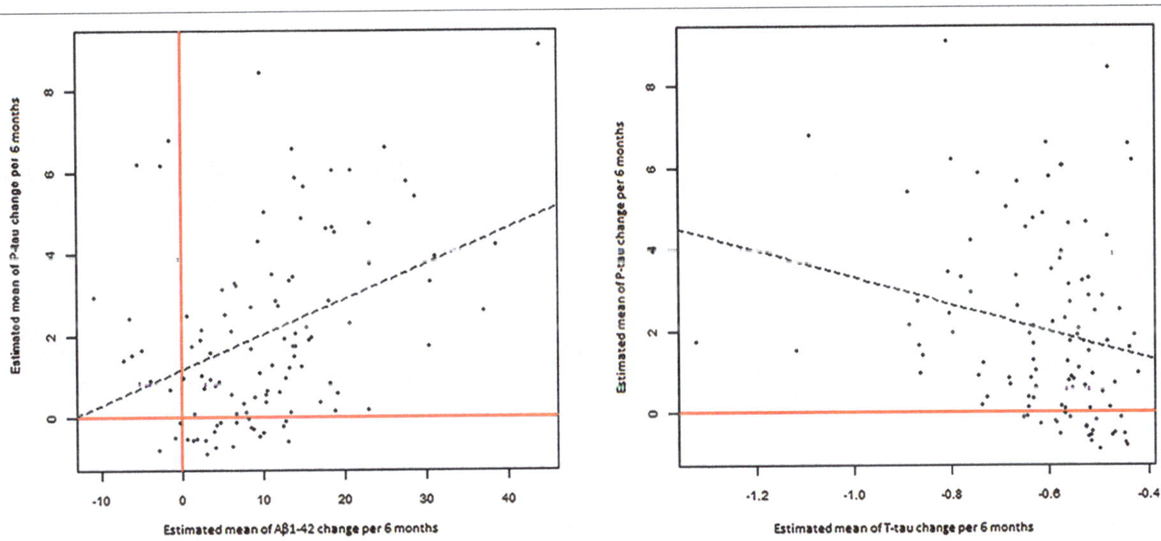

FIGURE 3 | Significant correlations between estimated changes in CSF levels of α-syn, P-tau, T-tau, and Aβ 1- 42.

CSF markers except $A\beta_{42}$, non-significantly changed level of CSF proteins in patients with short disease duration (<5 years from diagnosis) and controls were observed (21). Similarly, all patients in our study had short disease duration (<2 years) and also due to shorter follow-up time in our study, the time required for significant changes in some of the biomarkers was not provided.

Correlation Between Levels of Different CSF Biomarkers at Different Time Points and Between Their Estimated Changes

This study showed the correlation between different CSF markers adjusted for age and gender at different time points in PD patients. No significant correlation found in control group when adjusted for age and gender. In addition, lower baseline levels of p-tau, t-tau, and α-syn were correlated with lower rate of estimated decrease of t-tau within a linear mixed model.

The disappearance of any association between CSF biomarkers in controls after adjusting for age and gender made us infer that any observed correlation between protein concentrations in healthy people was confounded by age and gender. However, in PD group correlations remained significant after this adjustment; meaning that there must be a pathological and disease-specific link between these proteinopathies. Therefore, we suspect that any correlation observed between levels of different biomarkers in control cases of previous PPMI studies was the result of not adjusting them for age and gender (20).

Probably the most distinctive part of this study was the assessment of correlation between "estimated" changes of biomarkers within a linear mixed model and baseline values of different biomarkers. Lower p-tau, t-tau, and α-syn levels at baseline were predictive of the higher rate of t-tau level decrease in the next year. The power of lower α-syn levels at baseline for estimation of lower rate of *t*-tau decrease might be due to lower baseline α-syn CSF levels being associated with more toxic α-syn accumulation in Lewy bodies. Actually, accumulation of α-syn in Lewy body has a seeding effect on tau oligomerization and accumulation (11–13). In addition, accumulation of tau itself propagates its accumulation in neurofibrillary tangles. These protein accumulations (α-syn and tau) inhibit release of tau into CSF (39). Although, these phenomena necessitate more tau absorption into neurons as a compensatory mechanism, in later stages such mechanisms do not seem to function and there is lower rate of decrease in tau levels (making these changes were not significant in a one-year follow-up due to the floor effect or short follow-up time).

On the other hand, lower levels of $A\beta_{1-42}$ were predictive of the lower rate of tau decrease in CSF. We suppose that lower level of CSF $A\beta_{1-42}$ means more accumulation of Aβ in extracellular amyloid plaques and lead to lower free (intracellular) Aβ level, which is necessary for tau phosphorylation and accumulation (40).

On the whole, these results show that changes of t-tau CSF levels may be the convergence point of PD pathology. However, because amyloidopathy and synucleinopathy have opposing effects on the rate of CSF tau level changes, assessing CSF t-tau levels can not reflect the severity of underlying proteinopathies and thus, the rate of t-tau CSF level changes may be quite small and need a long time to change. Therefore, in short follow-up times, like in our study, its changes would not be significant.

Another finding was that lower CSF α-syn levels at baseline were predictive of slower $A\beta_{1-42}$ increase after one year. One explanation is that α-syn accumulation propagates Aβ accumulations and its lower CSF concentrations. For instance, a recent study has shown that non-amyloid beta component of human alpha-synuclein oligomers induces the formation of new Aβ oligomers (41).

Correlation Between Baseline Clinical Entities of PD Patients and Longitudinal Changes of CSF Markers

It has been suggested that Rapid Eye Movement (REM) sleep Behavior Disorder (RBD) can be a clue to early diagnosis of neurodegenerative diseases (42), specifically it can help with early detection of PD (19, 43, 44). Affliction of brainstem structures which control REM sleep with alpha-synuclein protein inclusions in early phases of PD seems to be the underlying mechanism responsible for RBD (45).

In this study, we detected significant increase in CSF levels of alpha-synuclein in PD-RBD patients. Although a previous cross-sectional study in PD patients have revealed no association between CSF alpha-synuclein levels and RBD (46), prior investigations have revealed that CSF Prion Proteins (PrPs) are significantly elevated in PD patients with RBD compared to PD patients without sleep disorders (47), which might be suggestive of accelerated neuronal degeneration in PD-RBD patients and thus, introduce RBD as potentially the most appropriate clinical predictive marker of neuronal degeneration and disease progression in PD, as shown previously (48).

Importantly, changes in other CSF protein levels were not associated with UPDRS III, MoCA, and UPSIT scores. This might refer to the fact that motor symptoms, cognitive impairment, and olfaction dysfunction are not appropriate predictors of progression of neuronal degeneration in PD patients. In this study we have not assessed progression of different PD symptoms in association with the baseline clinical scores and it is worthy of note that although these CSF biomarkers pattern of changes in patients with various clinical entities at baseline might elucidate the speed of neurodegeneration to some extent, it does not necessarily mean that clinical manifestations progress is in line with CSF marker changes. However, it might help identify the speed of neurodegeneration at a molecular level and design more targeted therapies.

CONCLUSION

Although there are some positive points to this study like recruitment of drug-naïve patients, it suffers from some limitations like short follow-up time. To reach a more comprehensive conclusion, further longitudinal assessments regarding the predictive role of CSF proteins and their different species in patients at different stages of the disease and with longer follow-ups are suggested.

In addition, the patients in this study were quite heterogeneous in terms of disease duration which renders this study to some limitations; for instance, the patterns of CSF protein changes of different subgroups at different disease stages may be different.

In addition, in the manuscript we have assumed that lower CSF concentration of proteins is due to their accumulation in extracellular and intracellular spaces. This assumption might not be the case and several undiscovered mechanisms may play a role in determining the CSF concentrations of these proteins. There are some other limitations such as various degrees of CSF concentrations due to altered states of hydration and the position of proteins in a caudo-rostral column from the lumbar region to the cerebral origin. Moreover, clinical application of the difficult and invasive procedure of lumbar puncture to determine CSF markers as a way to follow-up the patients suffering from neurodegenerative diseases seems unlikely and such studies may just help enlighten the pathological mechanisms of proteinopathies.

In sum, it seems that α-syn, t-tau, p-tau, and Aβ play a role in PD pathology and have bidirectional interactions with each other, which mostly converge on tau pathology and lead to changes of CSF tau levels. Most noticeably, colocalization of α-syn and t-tau molecules in intracellular inclusions cause a reduction in CSF α-syn and t-tau levels, in contrast to AD without synucleinopathies which is associated with higher levels of CSF tau.

Importantly, among the clinical measures we applied, only RBD was predictive of α-syn increase during time. This might refer to the fact that evaluating patients for RBD at baseline is far more important than motor, olfaction, or cognitive assessment for prognostic purposes.

We suggest that different subtypes of PD patients progress heterogeneously. Thus, conducting similar studies in patient subtypes with various clinical symptoms and genetic, epigenetic, and environmental predispositions may be helpful.

In addition, most of the studies have shown the role of lower Aβ levels at baseline in predicting cognitive decline in the future (49). However, recently, predictive roles for tau levels in cognitive decline have been shown in other neurodegenerative diseases like Alzheimer's disease (50) and Huntington's disease (51). This observation in AD has been attributed to the later position of tau in the preclinical phase of the disease. To the best of our knowledge, there has been no evidence about the temporality of changes in tau and Aβ pathology in PD, i.e., whether CSF tau levels start to rise (or maybe fall) in later stages of the disease compared to Aβ or not. Thus, it seems that conducting longitudinal studies are necessary to discover whether changes in Aβ or tau is a more appropriate predictor of cognitive decline in the future.

INFORMED CONSENT

Informed consent was obtained from all individual participants included in the study.

AUTHOR CONTRIBUTIONS

MD, MA, AA-G, SP, AK contributed to the conception and design of the study; MY, AA-G, MD, SP contributed to data collection and analysis; and MD, SP, AK, AA-G contributed to writing the manuscript.

ACKNOWLEDGMENTS

This work was funded by grants from the Michael J Fox Foundation for Parkinson's Research, the W Garfield Weston Foundation, and the Alzheimer's Association, the Canadian Institutes for Health Research, and the Natural Sciences and Engineering Research Council of Canada. We thank Christian Beckmann and Simon Eickhoff for their advice on data analysis. Data used in this article were obtained from the Parkinsons Progression Markers Initiative (PPMI) database (www.ppmi-info.org/data). For up-to-date information on the study, visit www.ppmi-info.org. PPMI is sponsored and partially funded by the Michael J Fox Foundation for Parkinsons Research and funding partners, including AbbVie, Avid Radiopharmaceuticals, Biogen, Bristol-Myers Squibb, Covance, GE Healthcare, Genentech, GlaxoSmithKline (GSK), Eli Lilly and Company, Lundbeck, Merck, Meso Scale Discovery (MSD), Pfizer, Piramal Imaging, Roche, Servier, and UCB (http://www.ppmi-info.org/about-ppmi/who-we-are/study-sponsors/).

REFERENCES

1. Rodriguez M, Rodriguez-Sabate C, Morales I, Sanchez A, Sabate M. Parkinson's disease as a result of aging. *Aging Cell* (2015) 14:293–308. doi: 10.1111/acel.12312
2. Bourdenx M, Koulakiotis NS, Sanoudou D, Bezard E, Dehay B, Tsarbopoulos A. Protein aggregation and neurodegeneration in prototypical neurodegenerative diseases: Examples of amyloidopathies, tauopathies and synucleinopathies. *Prog Neurobiol.* (2015) 155:171–93. doi: 10.1016/j.pneurobio.2015.07.003.
3. Thenganatt MA, Jankovic J. Parkinson disease subtypes. *JAMA Neurol.* (2014) 71:499–504. doi: 10.1001/jamaneurol.2013.6233
4. Halliday GM, Holton JL, Revesz T, Dickson DW. Neuropathology underlying clinical variability in patients with synucleinopathies. *Acta Neuropathol.* (2011) 122:187–204. doi: 10.1007/s00401-011-0852-9
5. Petrou M, Dwamena BA, Foerster BR, MacEachern MP, Bohnen NI, Muller ML, et al. Amyloid deposition in Parkinson's disease and cognitive impairment: a systematic review. *Mov Disord.* (2015) 30:928–35. doi: 10.1002/mds.26191
6. Sabbagh MN, Adler CH, Lahti TJ, Connor DJ, Vedders L, Peterson LK, et al. Parkinson disease with dementia: comparing patients with and without Alzheimer pathology. *Alzheimer Dis Assoc Disord.* (2009) 23:295–7. doi: 10.1097/WAD.0b013e31819c5ef4
7. Irwin DJ, White MT, Toledo JB, Xie SX, Robinson JL, Van Deerlin V, et al. Neuropathologic substrates of Parkinson disease dementia. *Ann Neurol.* (2012) 72:587–98. doi: 10.1002/ana.23659
8. Smirnova L, Harris G, Delp J, Valadares M, Pamies D, Hogberg HT, et al. A LUHMES 3D dopaminergic neuronal model for neurotoxicity testing allowing long-term exposure and cellular resilience analysis. *Arch Toxicol.* (2015) 90:2725–43. doi: 10.1007/s00204-015-1637-z
9. Bellou V, Belbasis L, Tzoulaki I, Evangelou E, Ioannidis JP. Environmental risk factors and Parkinson's disease: an umbrella review of meta-analyses. *Parkinsonism Relat Disord.* (2016) 23:1–9. doi: 10.1016/j.parkreldis.2015.12.008
10. Clinton LK, Blurton-Jones M, Myczek K, Trojanowski JQ, LaFerla FM. Synergistic Interactions between Abeta, tau, and alpha-synuclein: acceleration of neuropathology and cognitive decline. *J Neurosci.* (2010) 30:7281–9. doi: 10.1523/JNEUROSCI.0490-10.2010
11. Waxman EA, Giasson BI. Induction of intracellular tau aggregation is promoted by alpha-synuclein seeds and provides novel insights into the hyperphosphorylation of tau. *J Neurosci.* (2011) 31:7604–18. doi: 10.1523/JNEUROSCI.0297-11.2011
12. Oikawa T, Nonaka T, Terada M, Tamaoka A, Hisanaga S, Hasegawa M. Alpha-synuclein fibrils exhibit gain of toxic function, promoting tau aggregation and inhibiting microtubule assembly. *J Biol Chem.* (2016) 291:15046–56. doi: 10.1074/jbc.M116.736355
13. Sengupta U, Guerrero-Munoz MJ, Castillo-Carranza DL, Lasagna-Reeves CA, Gerson JE, Paulucci-Holthauzen AA, et al. Pathological interface between oligomeric alpha-synuclein and tau in synucleinopathies. *Biol Psychiatry* (2015) 78:672–83. doi: 10.1016/j.biopsych.2014.12.019
14. Parnetti L, Castrioto A, Chiasserini D, Persichetti E, Tambasco N, El-Agnaf O, et al. Cerebrospinal fluid biomarkers in Parkinson disease. *Nat Rev Neurol.* (2013) 9:131–40. doi: 10.1038/nrneurol.2013.10
15. Hong Z, Shi M, Chung KA, Quinn JF, Peskind ER, Galasko D, et al. DJ-1 and alpha-synuclein in human cerebrospinal fluid as biomarkers of Parkinson's disease. *Brain* (2010) 133(Pt 3):713–26. doi: 10.1093/brain/awq008
16. Montine TJ. CSF Aβ(42) and tau in Parkinson's disease with cognitive impairment. *Mov Disord.* (2010) 25:2682–5. doi: 10.1002/mds.23287
17. Mollenhauer B, Locascio JJ, Schulz-Schaeffer W, Sixel-Doring F, Trenkwalder C, Schlossmacher MG. alpha-Synuclein and tau concentrations in cerebrospinal fluid of patients presenting with parkinsonism: a cohort study. *Lancet Neurol.* (2011) 10:230–40. doi: 10.1016/S1474-4422(11)70014-X
18. Hall S, Ohrfelt A, Constantinescu R, Andreasson U, Surova Y, Bostrom F, et al. Accuracy of a panel of 5 cerebrospinal fluid biomarkers in the differential diagnosis of patients with dementia and/or parkinsonian disorders. *Arch Neurol.* (2012) 69:1445–52. doi: 10.1001/archneurol.2012.1654
19. Kang JH, Irwin DJ, Chen-Plotkin AS, Siderowf A, Caspell C, Coffey CS, et al. Association of cerebrospinal fluid beta-amyloid 1-42, T-tau, P-tau181, and alpha-synuclein levels with clinical features of drug-naive patients with early Parkinson disease. *JAMA Neurol* (2013) 70:1277–1287. doi: 10.1001/jamaneurol.2013.3861
20. Kang JH, Mollenhauer B, Coffey CS, Toledo JB, Weintraub D, Galasko DR, et al. CSF biomarkers associated with disease heterogeneity in early Parkinson's disease: the Parkinson's Progression Markers Initiative study. *Acta Neuropathol.* (2016) 131:935–49. doi: 10.1007/s00401-016-1552-2
21. Hall S, Surova Y, Ohrfelt A, Blennow K, Zetterberg H, Hansson O. Longitudinal Measurements of Cerebrospinal Fluid Biomarkers in Parkinson's Disease. *Mov Disord.* (2016) 31:898–905. doi: 10.1002/mds.26578
22. Irwin DJ, Lee V. MY, Trojanowski JQ. Parkinson's disease dementia: convergence of α-synuclein, tau and amyloid-β pathologies. *Nat Rev Neurosci.* (2013) 14:626–36. doi: 10.1038/nrn3549
23. Kang J. H. Cerebrospinal Fluid Amyloid beta1-42, Tau, and alpha-synuclein predict the heterogeneous progression of cognitive dysfunction in Parkinson's Disease. *J Mov Disord.* (2016) 9:89–96. doi: 10.14802/jmd.16017
24. Majbour NK, Vaikath NN, Eusebi P, Chiasserini D, Ardah M, Varghese S, et al. Longitudinal changes in CSF alpha-synuclein species reflect Parkinson's disease progression. *Mov Disord.* (2016) 31:1535–42. doi: 10.1002/mds.26754
25. Stewart T, Liu C, Ginghina C, Cain KC, Auinger P, Cholerton B, et al. Cerebrospinal fluid alpha-synuclein predicts cognitive decline in Parkinson disease progression in the DATATOP cohort. *Am J Pathol.* (2014) 184:966–75. doi: 10.1016/j.ajpath.2013.12.007
26. Forland MG, Ohrfelt A, Dalen I, Tysnes OB, Blennow K, Zetterberg H, et al. Evolution of cerebrospinal fluid total alpha-synuclein in Parkinson's disease. *Parkinsonism Relat Disord.* (2018) 49:4–8. doi: 10.1016/j.parkreldis.2018.01.018
27. Buongiorno M, Antonelli F, Compta Y, Fernandez Y, Pavia J, Lomena F, et al. Cross-Sectional and Longitudinal Cognitive Correlates of FDDNP PET and CSF Amyloid-beta and Tau in Parkinson's Disease1. *J Alzheimers Dis.* (2017) 55:1261–72. doi: 10.3233/JAD-160698
28. Parkinson Progression Marker Initiative. The Parkinson Progression Marker Initiative (PPMI) *Prog Neurobiol.* (2011) 95:629–35. doi: 10.1016/j.pneurobio.2011.09.005
29. Parnetti L, Tiraboschi P, Lanari A, Peducci M, Padiglioni C, D'Amore C, et al. Cerebrospinal fluid biomarkers in Parkinson's disease with

dementia and dementia with Lewy bodies. *Biol Psychiatry* (2008) 64:850–5. doi: 10.1016/j.biopsych.2008.02.016

30. Alves G, Bronnick K, Aarsland D, Blennow K, Zetterberg H, Ballard C, et al. CSF amyloid-beta and tau proteins, and cognitive performance, in early and untreated Parkinson's disease: the Norwegian ParkWest study. *J Neurol Neurosurg Psychiatry* (2010) 81:1080–6. doi: 10.1136/jnnp.2009.199950
31. Parnetti L, Chiasserini D, Bellomo G, Giannandrea D, De Carlo C, Qureshi MM, et al. Cerebrospinal fluid Tau/alpha-synuclein ratio in Parkinson's disease and degenerative dementias. *Mov Disord.* (2011) 26:1428–35. doi: 10.1002/mds.23670
32. Emmanouilidou E, Melachroinou K, Roumeliotis T, Garbis SD, Ntzouni M, Margaritis LH, et al. Cell-produced alpha-synuclein is secreted in a calcium-dependent manner by exosomes and impacts neuronal survival. *J Neurosci.* (2010) 30:6838–51. doi: 10.1523/JNEUROSCI.5699-09.2010
33. Danzer KM, Kranich LR, Ruf WP, Cagsal-Getkin O, Winslow AR, Zhu L, et al. Exosomal cell-to-cell transmission of alpha synuclein oligomers. *Mol Neurodegener* (2012) 7:42. doi: 10.1186/1750-1326-7-42
34. Mollenhauer B, Cullen V, Kahn I, Krastins B, Outeiro TF, Pepivani I, et al. Direct quantification of CSF alpha-synuclein by ELISA and first cross-sectional study in patients with neurodegeneration. *Exp Neurol.* (2008) 213:315–25. doi: 10.1016/j.expneurol.2008.06.004
35. Mollenhauer B, Parnetti L, Rektorova I, Kramberger M, Pikkarainen M J., Schulz-Schaeffer W, et al. Biological confounders for the values of cerebrospinal fluid proteins in Parkinson's disease and related disorders. *J Neurochem.* (2015) 139(Suppl. 1):290–317. doi: 10.1111/jnc.13390
36. Hansson O, Zetterberg H, Buchhave P, Londos E, Blennow K, Minthon L. Association between CSF biomarkers and incipient Alzheimer's disease in patients with mild cognitive impairment: a follow-up study. *Lancet Neurol.* (2006) 5:228–34. doi: 10.1016/S1474-4422(06)70355-6
37. Toledo JB, Korff A, Shaw LM, Trojanowski JQ, Zhang J. CSF alpha-synuclein improves diagnostic and prognostic performance of CSF tau and Abeta in Alzheimer's disease. *Acta Neuropathol.* (2013) 126:683–97. doi: 10.1007/s00401-013-1148-z
38. Sonnen JA, Montine KS, Quinn JF, Kaye JA, Breitner JC, Montine TJ. Biomarkers for cognitive impairment and dementia in elderly people. *Lancet Neurol.* (2008) 7:704–14. doi: 10.1016/S1474-4422(08)70162-5
39. Parnetti L, Farotti L, Eusebi P, Chiasserini D, De Carlo C, Giannandrea D, et al. Differential role of CSF alpha-synuclein species, tau, and Aβ42 in Parkinson's Disease. Front Aging Neurosci (2014) 6:53. doi: 10.3389/fnagi.2014.00053
40. Stancu IC, Vasconcelos B, Terwel D, Dewachter I. Models of β-amyloid induced Tau-pathology: the long and "folded" road to understand the mechanism. *Mol Neurodegener.* (2014) 9:51. doi: 10.1186/1750-1326-9-51
41. Atsmon-Raz Y, Miller Y. Non-Amyloid-beta Component of Human alpha-Synuclein Oligomers Induces Formation of New AbetaOligomers: insight into the mechanisms that Link Parkinson's and Alzheimer's Diseases. *ACS Chem Neurosci.* (2016) 7:46–55. doi: 10.1021/acschemneuro.5b00204
42. Ferini-Strambi L, Marelli S, Galbiati A, Rinaldi F, Giora E. REM Sleep Behavior Disorder (RBD) as a marker of neurodegenerative disorders. *Arch Ital Biol.* (2014) 152:129–46. doi: 10.12871/000298292014238
43. Postuma RB, Gagnon JF, Rompre S, Montplaisir JY. Severity of REM atonia loss in idiopathic REM sleep behavior disorder predicts Parkinson disease. *Neurology* (2010) 74:239–44. doi: 10.1212/WNL.0b013e3181ca0166
44. Prashanth R, Dutta Roy S, Mandal PK, Ghosh S. High-Accuracy Detection of Early Parkinson's disease through multimodal features and machine learning. *Int J Med Inform.* (2016) 90:13–21. doi: 10.1016/j.ijmedinf.2016.03.001
45. Howell MJ, Schenck CH. Rapid eye movement sleep behavior disorder and neurodegenerative disease. *JAMA Neurol.* (2015) 72:707–12. doi: 10.1001/jamaneurol.2014.4563
46. Goldman JG, Andrews H, Amara A, Naito A, Alcalay RN, Shaw LM, et al. Cerebrospinal fluid, plasma, and saliva in the BioFIND study: relationships among biomarkers and Parkinson's disease features. *Mov Disord.* (2018) 33:282–8. doi: 10.1002/mds.27232
47. Zhang WJ, Shang XL, Peng J, Zhou MH, Sun WJ. Expression of prion protein in the cerebrospinal fluid of patients with Parkinson's disease complicated with rapid eye movement sleep behavior disorder. *Genet Mol Res.* (2017) 16. doi: 10.4238/gmr16019022
48. Mollenhauer B, Zimmermann J, Sixel-Doring F, Focke NK, Wicke T, Ebentheuer J, et al. Monitoring of 30 marker candidates in early Parkinson disease as progression markers. *Neurology* (2016) 87:168–77. doi: 10.1212/WNL.0000000000002651
49. Leaver K, Poston KL. Do CSF Biomarkers Predict Progression to Cognitive Impairment in Parkinson's disease patients? A systematic review. *Neuropsychol Rev.* (2015) 25:411–23. doi: 10.1007/s11065-015-9307-8
50. Brier MR, Gordon B, Friedrichsen K, McCarthy J, Stern A, Christensen J, et al. Tau and Abeta imaging, CSF measures, and cognition in Alzheimer's disease. *Sci Transl Med.* (2016) 8:338ra366. doi: 10.1126/scitranslmed.aaf2362
51. Rodrigues FB, Byrne L, McColgan P, Robertson N, Tabrizi SJ, Leavitt BR, et al. Cerebrospinal fluid total tau concentration predicts clinical phenotype in Huntington's disease. *J Neurochem.* (2016) 139:22–5. doi: 10.1111/jnc.13719

Permissions

All chapters in this book were first published by Frontiers; hereby published with permission under the Creative Commons Attribution License or equivalent. Every chapter published in this book has been scrutinized by our experts. Their significance has been extensively debated. The topics covered herein carry significant findings which will fuel the growth of the discipline. They may even be implemented as practical applications or may be referred to as a beginning point for another development.

The contributors of this book come from diverse backgrounds, making this book a truly international effort. This book will bring forth new frontiers with its revolutionizing research information and detailed analysis of the nascent developments around the world.

We would like to thank all the contributing authors for lending their expertise to make the book truly unique. They have played a crucial role in the development of this book. Without their invaluable contributions this book wouldn't have been possible. They have made vital efforts to compile up to date information on the varied aspects of this subject to make this book a valuable addition to the collection of many professionals and students.

This book was conceptualized with the vision of imparting up-to-date information and advanced data in this field. To ensure the same, a matchless editorial board was set up. Every individual on the board went through rigorous rounds of assessment to prove their worth. After which they invested a large part of their time researching and compiling the most relevant data for our readers.

The editorial board has been involved in producing this book since its inception. They have spent rigorous hours researching and exploring the diverse topics which have resulted in the successful publishing of this book. They have passed on their knowledge of decades through this book. To expedite this challenging task, the publisher supported the team at every step. A small team of assistant editors was also appointed to further simplify the editing procedure and attain best results for the readers.

Apart from the editorial board, the designing team has also invested a significant amount of their time in understanding the subject and creating the most relevant covers. They scrutinized every image to scout for the most suitable representation of the subject and create an appropriate cover for the book.

The publishing team has been an ardent support to the editorial, designing and production team. Their endless efforts to recruit the best for this project, has resulted in the accomplishment of this book. They are a veteran in the field of academics and their pool of knowledge is as vast as their experience in printing. Their expertise and guidance has proved useful at every step. Their uncompromising quality standards have made this book an exceptional effort. Their encouragement from time to time has been an inspiration for everyone.

The publisher and the editorial board hope that this book will prove to be a valuable piece of knowledge for researchers, students, practitioners and scholars across the globe.

List of Contributors

Md. Mamun Al-Amin, Md. Faiyad Rahman Choudhury, Al Saad Chowdhury, Tahsinur Rahman Chowdhury, Preeti Jain and Hasan Mahmud Reza
Department of Pharmaceutical Sciences, North South University, Dhaka, Bangladesh

Mohsin Kazi, Musaed Alkholief and Sultan M. Alshehri
Department of Pharmaceutics, College of Pharmacy, King Saud University, Riyadh, Saudi Arabia

Hans-Peter Müller and Jan Kassubek
Department of Neurology, University of Ulm, Ulm, Germany

Vincent Grollemund
Laboratoire d'Informatique de Paris 6, Sorbonne University, Paris, France
FRS Consulting, Paris, France

P. Nigel Leigh
Hurstwood Park Neurological Centre, Haywards Heath, West Sussex, United Kingdom

Giorgia Querin
Laboratoire d'Imagerie Biomédicale, INSERM, CNRS, Sorbonne Université, Paris, France
APHP, Département de Neurologie, Hôpital Pitié-Salpêtrière, Centre Référent SLA, Paris, France

Pierre-François Pradat
Laboratoire d'Imagerie Biomédicale, INSERM, CNRS, Sorbonne Université, Paris, France
APHP, Département de Neurologie, Hôpital Pitié-Salpêtrière, Centre Référent SLA, Paris, France
Northern Ireland Center for Stratified Medecine, Biomedical Sciences Research Institute Ulster University, C-TRIC, Altnagelvin Hospital, Londonderry, United Kingdom

François Delbot
Laboratoire d'Informatique de Paris 6, Sorbonne University, Paris, France
Département de Mathématiques et Informatique, Paris Nanterre University, Nanterre, France

Jean-François Pradat-Peyre
Laboratoire d'Informatique de Paris 6, Sorbonne University, Paris, France
Département de Mathématiques et Informatique, Paris Nanterre University, Nanterre, France
Modal'X, Paris Nanterre University, Nanterre, France

Peter Bede
Laboratoire d'Imagerie Biomédicale, INSERM, CNRS, Sorbonne Université, Paris, France
APHP, Département de Neurologie, Hôpital Pitié-Salpêtrière, Centre Référent SLA, Paris, France
Computational Neuroimaging Group, Trinity College, Dublin, Ireland

Mara Cercignani
Clinical Imaging Sciences Centre, Brighton and Sussex Medical School, Falmer, United Kingdom

Andrew W. Barritt
Clinical Imaging Sciences Centre, Brighton and Sussex Medical School, Falmer, United Kingdom
Hurstwood Park Neurological Centre, Haywards Heath, West Sussex, United Kingdom

Matt C. Gabel
Department of Neuroscience, Trafford Centre for Biomedical Research, Brighton and Sussex Medical School, Falmer, United Kingdom
Department of Neuroscience, Trafford Centre for Biomedical Research, Brighton and Sussex Medical School, Falmer, United Kingdom

Stacey Li Hi Shing, Rangariroyashe H. Chipika, Eoin Finegan, Deirdre Murray, Orla Hardiman and Peter Bede
Computational Neuroimaging Group, Academic Unit of Neurology, Biomedical Sciences Institute, Trinity College Dublin, Dublin, Ireland

Mohamed Mounir El Mendili
Department of Neurology, Icahn School of Medicine at Mount Sinai, New York, NY, United States
Biomedical Imaging Laboratory (LIB), Sorbonne University, CNRS, INSERM, Paris, France

Giorgia Querin and Pierre-François Pradat
Biomedical Imaging Laboratory (LIB), Sorbonne University, CNRS, INSERM, Paris, France
Department of Neurology, Pitié-Salpêtrière University Hospital (APHP), Paris, France

Peter Bede
Biomedical Imaging Laboratory (LIB), Sorbonne University, CNRS, INSERM, Paris, France
Department of Neurology, Pitié-Salpêtrière University Hospital (APHP), Paris, France
Computational Neuroimaging Group, Trinity College Dublin, Dublin

Gaétan Le Chat
FRS Consulting, Paris, France

Thanuja Dharmadasa
Brain and Mind Centre, University of Sydney, Sydney, NSW, Australia

William Huynh
Brain and Mind Centre, University of Sydney, Sydney, NSW, Australia
Prince of Wales Clinical School, University of New South Wales, Sydney, NSW, Australia

Steve Vucic
Western Clinical School, University of Sydney, Sydney, NSW, Australia

Matthew C. Kiernan
Brain and Mind Centre, University of Sydney, Sydney, NSW, Australia
Institute of Clinical Neurosciences, Royal Prince Alfred Hospital, Sydney, NSW, Australia

Serena Stanga, Bernadette Tasiaux, Jean-Noël Octave and Pascal Kienlen-Campard
Alzheimer Research Group, Institute of Neuroscience, Université Catholique de Louvain, Brussels, Belgium

Liliana Brambilla and Daniela Rossi
Laboratory for Research on Neurodegenerative Disorders, Istituti Clinici Scientifici Maugeri SpA SB - IRCCS, Pavia, Italy

Vincent van Pesch
Unité de Neurochimie, Institute of Neuroscience, Université Catholique de Louvain, Brussels, Belgium
Neurology Department, Cliniques Universitaires Saint-Luc, Brussels, Belgium

Anh H. Dang
Unité de Neurochimie, Institute of Neuroscience, Université Catholique de Louvain, Brussels, Belgium

Adrian Ivanoiu
Neurology Department, Cliniques Universitaires Saint-Luc, Brussels, Belgium

Koen Poesen
Department of Neurosciences, Laboratory for Molecular Neurobiomarker Research, KU Leuven, Leuven, Belgium
Laboratory Medicine, University Hospitals Leuven, Leuven, Belgium

Efstratios Karavasilis and Nikolaos Kelekis
Second Department of Radiology, University General Hospital Attikon, National and Kapodistrian University of Athens, Athens, Greece

Philip Van Damme
Laboratory of Neurobiology, Department of Neurosciences, KU Leuven and Center for Brain & Disease Research VIB Leuven, Leuven, Belgium
Department of Neurology, Neuromuscular Reference Centre, University Hospitals Leuven, Leuven, Belgium

Yong Chen, Kailin Xia and Lu Chen
Department of Neurology, Peking University Third Hospital, Beijing, China

Dongsheng Fan
Department of Neurology, Peking University Third Hospital, Beijing, China
Key Laboratory for Neuroscience, Ministry of Education/National Health Commission, Peking University, Beijing, China

Foteini Christidi, Michail Rentzos and Ioannis Evdokimidis
First Department of Neurology, Aeginition Hospital, National and Kapodistrian University of Athens, Athens, Greece

Peter Bede
Computational Neuroimaging Group, Academic Unit of Neurology, Trinity College Dublin, Dublin, Ireland

Vanessa X. Tan and Gilles J. Guillemin
Macquarie University Centre for MND Research, Department of Biological Sciences, Faculty of Medicine and Health Sciences, Macquarie University, Sydney, NSW, Australia

Silvia Basaia, Edoardo G. Spinelli and Federica Agosta
Neuroimaging Research Unit, Institute of Experimental Neurology, Division of Neuroscience, Vita-Salute San Raffaele University, Milan, Italy

Massimo Filippi
Neuroimaging Research Unit, Institute of Experimental Neurology, Division of Neuroscience, Vita-Salute San Raffaele University, Milan, Italy
Department of Neurology, Institute of Experimental Neurology, Division of Neuroscience, San Raffaele Scientific Institute, Vita-Salute San Raffaele University, Milan, Italy

Siobhan E. Kirk and Timothy J. Tracey
The Australian Institute for Bioengineering and Nanotechnology, The University of Queensland, Brisbane, QLD, Australia

Dong Woo Kang and Chang Uk Lee
Department of Psychiatry, Seoul St. Mary's Hospital, College of Medicine, The Catholic University of Korea, Seoul, South Korea

Frederik J. Steyn
The Australian Institute for Bioengineering and Nanotechnology, The University of Queensland, Brisbane, QLD, Australia
Centre for Clinical Research, The University of Queensland, Brisbane, QLD, Australia

Shyuan T. Ngo
The Australian Institute for Bioengineering and Nanotechnology, The University of Queensland, Brisbane, QLD, Australia
Centre for Clinical Research, The University of Queensland, Brisbane, QLD, Australia
Queensland Brain Institute, The University of Queensland Brisbane, QLD, Australia

Se Hee Yun
Seocho Center for Dementia, Seoul, South Korea

Chang Tae Hahn
Department of Psychiatry, Daejeon St. Mary's Hospital, College of Medicine, The Catholic University of Korea, Seoul, South Korea

Hyun Kook Lim
Department of Psychiatry, Yeouido St. Mary's Hospital, College of Medicine, The Catholic University of Korea

Eoin Finegan, Rangariroyashe H. Chipika, Stacey Li Hi Shing, Orla Hardiman and Peter Bede
Computational Neuroimaging Group, Biomedical Sciences Institute, Trinity College Dublin, Dublin, Ireland

Jose-Luis González De Aguilar
Université de Strasbourg, UMR_S1118, Strasbourg, France,
INSERM, U1118, Mécanismes Centraux et Périphériques de la Neurodégénerescence, Strasbourg, France

Mary Kay Floeter
National Institute of Neurological Disorders and Stroke, National Institutes of Health, Bethesda, MD, United States

Tania F. Gendron
Department of Neuroscience, Mayo Clinic, Jacksonville, FL, United States

Pei-Chen Hsieh, Han-Tao Li, Chun-Wei Chang, Yih-Ru Wu and Hung-Chou Kuo
Department of Neurology, Linkou Chang Gung Memorial Hospital, College of Medicine, Chang Gung University, Taipei, Taiwan

Carolina Barnett
Division of Neurology, Department of Medicine, University of Toronto and University Health Network, Toronto, ON, Canada

Zhi-Li Wang, Mingsheng Liu, Kang Zhang, Shuangwu Liu and Qingyun Ding
Department of Neurology, Peking Union Medical College Hospital, Chinese Academy of Medical Sciences, Beijing, China

Liying Cui
Department of Neurology, Peking Union Medical College Hospital, Chinese Academy of Medical Sciences, Beijing, China
Neurosciences Center, Chinese Academy of Medical Sciences, Beijing, China

Yana Yunusova
Department of Speech Language Pathology, University of Toronto, Toronto, ON, Canada
Hurvitz Brain Sciences Research Program, Sunnybrook Research Institute, Toronto, ON, Canada
Volcal Tract Visualization Lab, Toronto Rehabilitation Institute, University Health Network, Toronto, ON, Canada

Emily K. Plowman
Swallowing Systems Core, Department of Speech, Language, and Hearing Sciences, University of Florida, Gainesville, FL, United States

Jordan R. Green
Department of Communication Sciences and Disorders, MGH Institute of Health Professions, Boston, MA, United States
Speech and Hearing Biosciences and Technology Program, Harvard University, Cambridge, MA, United States
Institute of Health Policy, Management and Evaluation, Dalla Lana School of Public Health, University of Toronto, Toronto, ON, Canada

Peter Bede
Computational Neuroimaging Group, Academic Unit of Neurology, Trinity College Dublin, Dublin, Ireland

Sanjay Kalra
Division of Neurology, Department of Medicine, Neuroscience and Mental Health Institute, University of Alberta, Edmonton, AB, Canada

Mahsa Dolatshahi, Shayan Pourmirbabaei, Aida Kamalian, Amir Ashraf-Ganjouei and Mohammad H. Aarabi
Faculty of Medicine, Tehran University of Medical Sciences, Tehran, Iran

Mehdi Yaseri
Department of Epidemiology and Biostatistics, School of Public Health, Tehran University of Medical Sciences, Tehran, Iran

Index

Printed in the USA
CPSIA information can be obtained
at www.ICGtesting.com
LVHW080055211023
761596LV00010BA/2068

9 781639 897896